Foundations of
ANIMAL DEVELOPMENT

Foundations of
ANIMAL DEVELOPMENT

ARTHUR F. HOPPER and
NATHAN H. HART
Rutgers University

New York Oxford
OXFORD UNIVERSITY PRESS 1980

Library of Congress Cataloging in Publication Data

Hopper, Arthur F   1917–
    Foundations of animal development.

    Bibliography: p.
    Includes index.
    1. Developmental biology.   I. Hart, Nathan H.,
1936–   joint author.   II. Title.
OL971.H79   591.3   78-26678
ISBN 0-19-502569-5

Preface

The teacher of an introductory course in animal embryology or animal development is faced with the difficult task of determining the content of his course and the methodology of its presentation. By its very nature, the subject matter is difficult to define and delineate. The essence of development is change over time and this is reflected at all levels of structural organization from the molecular to the organismal. In selecting material for such a course, one is also influenced by the students' varied interests and backgrounds. Some students may be terminating their biological training at the level of the college or university, while others may intend to pursue advanced professional training in the disciplines of biology, medicine, dentistry, and so on. Such considerations have influenced our approach to and selection of material for the writing of this textbook. From the very beginning, we realized that it would be impossible to design a format and provide coverage which would satisfy the needs of all teachers of this subject area.

We have endeavored to set forth in direct and readable form an account of the ontogenetic development of organisms through an integration of descriptive, experimental, and biochemical approaches. The focus is the whole embryo and the sequence of events by which the form and structure of its body and constituent organ systems emerge from the superficially simple-appearing egg. Concurrently, the book attempts to set the subject of development in a modern context by recognizing and formulating major questions associated with these events and by analyzing, where appropriate, the underlying mechanisms. There is an emphasis on the basic, morphological aspects of development. Central to our thinking is the belief that insights into the complexities of the developmental process are diminished unless the student is thoroughly familiar with this type of information. Students working with this book will be prepared to study in more detail a specialized area of development which might be assigned by the teacher or to meet the challenge afforded by an advanced course in embryology or developmental biology.

The book may be divided into two parts. The first part gives consideration to the onset of development (gametogenesis, fertilization, and cleavage), the rearrangements of embryonic cells and the organization of the early embryo, tissue interactions and the basis of cellular differentiation, and principles of morphogenesis. Concepts and principles are introduced which provide a background against which the second part of the book, the development of various organ systems, can be examined in detail. Our comprehensive survey of the development of the organ systems includes an analysis of the mechanisms responsible for their form and structure. Emphasis is placed on the development of the mammal, a treatment which reflects an increasing interest in this group by investigators as a source for the study of developmental processes.

The authors are grateful to the many people who have assisted in the preparation of this book. We express particular thanks to friends and colleagues who generously provided photographs and illustrations, and to the publishers who have permitted reproduction of previously published illustrations. The names of these colleagues appear in the legends of the textbook figures. A special word of thanks to Ms. Diane Abeloff, our illustrator, who patiently listened to us and then carefully designed and drew what was requested. We are indebted to Mrs. Elaine Derry who typed the book manuscript and in the process made some helpful suggestions.

Finally, we express our gratitude to the staff at Oxford University Press, especially to Mr. Robert Tilley, whose encouragement did much to bring this book to completion.

NATHAN H. HART
ARTHUR F. HOPPER

New Brunswick, N.J.
June 1979

Contents

Foundations of
ANIMAL DEVELOPMENT

1

Introduction

The existing individuals of any species have a finite lifespan. Thus, if a species is to persist, each generation of individuals must possess some mechanism whereby it can produce the next generation. The process whereby individuals of a species are perpetuated is called reproduction. In vertebrates the process is concerned with the production of specialized reproductive (germ) cells in the male and the female whose union results in the formation of a fertilized egg (*zygote*), which will develop into a new individual.

Embryology is the field of biology that involves the description and analysis of the development of the individual. Insofar as descriptive embryology is, historically, an anatomical science, the term developmental anatomy may be applied to this aspect of embryology. However, the analysis of the factors underlying and controlling the complex changes that occur as a single-celled fertilized egg develops into a multicellular adult is the major concern of most modern embryologists who apply to their investigations the techniques of such disciplines as physiology, biochemistry, radioisotope analysis, radiation biology, molecular biology, and genetics.

EMBRYOLOGY, DEVELOPMENT, AND ONTOGENY

Generally speaking, an embryo is regarded as something in a developmental or rudimentary condition. In biology, we can assign a more specific definition to the embryonic state: It is one that encompasses the development of the individual up to the time of hatching or, in mammalian species, up to the time of birth. In mammalian embryology, the prenatal period may be divided into two stages: (1) the period of the embryo, covering development up until the individual attains the form—but, of course, not the size—of the adult, and (2) the period of the fetus, covering the remainder of the prenatal period until birth.

Dramatic as the events of birth and hatching are, we must not consider them as representing the termination of the development of an individual. To be sure, the change from an aquatic to a gaseous environment does indeed represent, in many species, a dramatic change to which an individual must adjust. But since the systems that support an individual in its aquatic envirnoment are exactly those that continue, with only minor adjustments, to support it in its gaseous environment, birth and hatching do not represent sharp changes in the continuing development of an organism. They represent only a single point in a process of continuing, progressive change.

The term *development,* then, is not synonymous with embryology but includes the entire lifespan of the individual from fertilization to death. Development is simply defined as progressive change. It includes both prenatal and postnatal stages leading to structural and functional maturity. In turn, these stages are followed, after a certain length of time, by the changes associated with senescence, which lead ultimately to death. Development proceeds in an orderly sequence, and each change leaves the organism in a state different from its previous one and, generally, unable to return to it. Unfortunately, the term development often carries with it the connotation that the progressive change is for the better or towards a higher plane. If we include this meaning in the term, there is then a point in a life history at which development stops. Or rather, there are many points, since the time at which each organ system reaches its maximum development varies considerably. However, we should consider development as taking the entire lifespan of the individual into account and as synonymous, in this sense, with the term *ontogeny.*

Ontogeny and Phylogeny

Ontogeny, the development of the individual, is only one very small phase of a much larger developmental sequence, *phylogeny*—the historical development of the species; that is, the evolution of the species. Early in the 19th century a German scientist, Johann F. Meckel, proposed that there was a relationship between the embryos of higher forms and the adults of lower forms, the former progressing through stages in which they bore a marked resemblance to the latter. After Charles Darwin's theory on evolution appeared in the mid 1800s Meckel's views were reconsidered and rephrased in evolutionary terms by another German scientist, Ernest H. Haeckel, who expressed in the succinct phrase "ontogeny recapitulates phylogeny" what has come to be known as the *recapitulation theory.* This implied that the embryos of each species progress through stages in which they resemble the structure of adults belonging to their evolutionary line. Although this theory is a fascinating one—one that a superficial consideration of the embryonic development of the higher animal forms appears to support—it goes beyond the facts. It is not correct to consider that the human embryo is at one stage of its development comparable to a fish because at that time it has developed the fishlike characteristics of five branchial (gill) arches, an undivided heart, and a head kidney.

It is closer to fact to note that certain organs in the embryos of higher forms may in some respects resemble the same organs in the embryos of lower forms, as was indeed proposed by the well-known German embryologist, Karl E. von Baer, in his 1839 monograph on embryology. However, it is still not correct to consider that any embryonic stage of a higher species is comparable to any embryonic stage of a lower one. The embryos of all species are specific unto themselves, and a human embryo is always a human embryo. Despite the fact that it at one time develops branchial arches, a human embryo is never the counterpart of a fish, or even a fish embryo.

The development of a number of organs illustrates another relationship between ontogeny and phylogeny. Structures that appear in the embryo as phylogenetic holdovers often function in the embryo before they are replaced by evolutionarily more recent acquisitions. Some structures that function in the embryo and are then superseded by later developing structures may degenerate and disappear, or they may be retained as nonfunctional vestigial structures. However, many structures, after giving up their original function may be retained and diverted to an entirely different function. This is illustrated by the conversion of the excretory (mesonephric) duct of the embryonic kidney to a major part of the genital duct (vas deferens) of the adult male. Another example is the conversion of the branchial arches and pouches into a variety of structures in the adult mammal, none of which have anything to do with the respiratory function of these structures in the fish.

Although many evolutionarily older parts are lost along the way, it appears that the higher forms are basically conservative and reluctant to abandon completely their phylogenetic inheritance; for, whenever possible, they convert older structures into functional parts of a newer system.

PREFORMATION AND EPIGENESIS

The earliest studies of embryology, which go back to Aristotle's observations on sharks and chicks, were generally concerned with the description of the development of different species. Before the advent of the microscope in the 18th century and the concept of the cell theory in the 19th, any real knowledge of the principles of embryology, especially of the earliest stages, was limited. William Harvey, who is most well-known for his writings on the circulation of the blood, probably made a more original contribution to science by stating in 1651 that all animals develop from eggs in a manner in which complexity of form gradually appears where uniformity previously existed. Over a hundred years later, Harvey's observations were further enlarged on by Kaspar F. Wolff who described the embryo as first consisting of a formless array of "globules" (cells) that gradually are arranged into organ rudiments and then into organs, more and more complex structures appearing in a stepwise fashion as development proceeds. This concept of development is called *epigenesis*.

In opposition to the epigenetic theory, there arose, also in the middle of the 18th century, the *preformation* theory of embryonic development. This theory stated that development consists merely of a growth or unfolding of structures which already exist preformed, but in a miniature state, in the germ cells. The theory emerged with the development of the microscope and its use in the examination of eggs and sperm. Investigators with somewhat fertile imaginations claimed to see fully formed tiny adults in eggs and sperm. Some of the leading microscopists of the time became involved in a controversy over whether the preformed adult resides in the egg (they were called ovists) or in the sperm (spermists). Further analysis and more careful observation saw the end of the preformation theory (at least in the form in which it was proposed in the 18th century) and development was considered to be epigenetic in nature. The fertilized egg is a simple "undifferentiated" cell from which, through an orderly series of developmental transformations, are produced differentiated structures that make up the organs and organ systems of the adult. The bold statement that epigenesis means the development of the complex from the simple may present the erroneous impression that the egg is a simple, uncomplicated cell. As we shall see, it is in reality a highly complex cell—made so by the tremendous synthetic activity that takes place during oogenesis. It contains a multitude of enzymes and other substances necessary both for normal cellular metabolism and for the early differentiation of the embryo.

STAGES OF DEVELOPMENT

Fertilization

Embryonic development starts with the union of the haploid egg and sperm and this process of *fertilization* produces the diploid *zygote*. This union not only restores the diploid number characteristic of the species but also provides the stimulus for the beginning of development. Prior to the fusion of the gametes, the cells of the germ line undergo a maturation process, *gametogenesis,* which is marked by a type of division called *meiosis* in which the diploid number is halved. In both *spermatogenesis,* the development of sperm, and *oogenesis,* the development of eggs, many significant events take place. These include the storage of nutrient and informational materials, the formation of accessory membranes in the egg, the condensation of the nuclear material, and the formation of locomotor structures in the sperm.

Cleavage

Fertilization is followed by a period of rapid cell multiplication, a period known as *cleavage,* in which the single-celled zygote is changed into a multicellular structure. The cleavage cells are known as *blastomeres.* During the cleavage stage, cell division is so rapid that the cells do not increase in size between divisions, and thus the embryo remains about the same size and the individual blastomeres become progressively smaller. Cell division, of course, does not stop at the end of the cleavage period but continues throughout development. However, after the cleavage stage, cell division no longer appears as the dominant feature of development. Cleavage patterns vary in different species, a large part of the variation being dependent upon the amount and distribution of the inert yolk that may be present in the ovum.

Blastulation

Cleavage leads to the formation of the *blastula,* which usually consists of a group of cells surrounding a cavity, the *blastocoele.* In the mammal, the embryo at this time is known as the *blastocyst.* The cells of the blastula may be arranged either in a single layer or in a number of layers.

Gastrulation

Gastrulation is a period of cellular movements in which the cells of the blastula are rearranged, some moving into the inside of the embryo and some remaining on the outside. During gastrulation the blastocoele is obliterated and a new cavity, the *gastrocoele,* develops. In most species the gastrocoele may also be called the *archenteron,* marking it as the forerunner of the gut tube. The gastrula is a layered structure, not in the sense that there is more than a single tier of cells but in the sense that the movements of gastrulation give rise to sheets of cells that are known as the *primary germ layers*. These consist of an outer, a middle, and an inner layer, respectively, *ectoderm, mesoderm,* and *endoderm.*

Neurulation and the Establishment of the Organ Rudiments

Gastrulation is quickly followed by the formation of the neural plate and the neural tube and by the elaboration of other axiate structures such as the somites and the alimentary tract. The paired somites develop lateral to the neural tube from the most medial region of the mesoderm. They will form parts of the skeletal, muscular, and integumentary systems. Lateral to the somites, the mesoderm splits into two layers, one of which becomes associated with the overlying ectoderm and the other with the underlying endoderm. The cavity formed between these two layers of mesoderm is the *coelom.* Thus, immediately after gastrulation we begin to see morphological changes in which the primary germ layers of the gastrula develop into structures that represent the earliest stages in the formation of specific organs. These structures are then called *primary organ rudiments.*

Organogenesis

The development of the primary organ rudiments is the first stage in *organogenesis* (organ formation). The formation of the neural tube and the alimentary tract occurs during and shortly after gastrulation. Other organ rudiments develop later. Each rudiment consists of a group of cells with special properties. They are segregated from other cells and groups of cells in the embryo and are destined to develop into specific organs. An organ rudiment is often called an *anlage.* Organogenesis is an extensive period in development during which a number of rather complicated mechanisms interact to form the organ rudiments and in turn guide their differentiation into the adult state, where each organ then becomes capable of performing its particular physiological function. Some of the processes involved are cell movements, changes in cell size and shape, cell death, epithelial-mesenchymal interaction, histogenesis, and growth. In addition to describing the development of the individual organ systems in the latter part of this text, we will discuss the general principles of organogenesis more fully in Chapter 13.

DESCRIPTIVE AND EXPERIMENTAL EMBRYOLOGY

As mentioned previously, the earliest studies of embryology were primarily descriptive. It was not until the late 1800s and early 1900s that experimental manipulation of the embryo was introduced as a method of analysis of the underlying factors controlling the events of development. Some of these studies that form the basic framework of modern experimental embryology included studies in Germany by Wilhelm Roux and Hans Driesch on the separation and subsequent development of the early blastomeres of the frog and sea urchin embryos. In the United States, E. B. Wilson and E. G. Conklin carefully traced the precise contributions of the early blastomeres of invertebrate embryos to the future structure of the animal. The famous German embryologist, Hans Spemann, and his colleagues perfected grafting techniques in amphibian embryos and thereby pointed out the importance of interaction between groups of cells. Although advances in genetics, biochemistry, microscopy, and molecular biology have skyrocketed our knowledge of the basic mechanisms of development, many of the questions raised in the studies of these eminent experimental embryologists remain as problems still under active investigation today.

Experimental Analysis of Early Development

The union of the egg and the sperm may seem on the surface a rather simply, although an obviously important, event. However, the process of fertilization presents a number of interesting problems that include, in addition to the mechanism of the development of the gametes, the role of chemical substances in egg–sperm interaction, the mechanism of sperm penetration, the prevention of polyspermy, and the immediate reaction of the egg to sperm penetration.

During cleavage we are concerned with understanding the mechanism of cell division and the control of its pattern and rate. The interaction between the nucleus and the cytoplasm is also of particular interest in this period of development.

Gastrulation is a time when the investigation of cell movements is of importance. The formation of the germ layers introduces the problem of the mechanism of cell segregation. In addition, germ layer formation is one of the first indications of differentiation in the embryo. The three germ layers are clearly distinguished from one another not only by their respective locations, but also by the specific tissues and organs each layer forms.

The Germ Layer Concept

The germ layer concept states that each of the three germ layers is marked to develop into its own specific tissues and organs. Epidermis and neural structures will be formed from ectoderm; the alimentary tract and its accessory organs from endoderm; and muscle, connective tissue, and the urogenital system from mesoderm. Because of the simplicity of this concept and because of its inclusion in all textbooks of embryology, and its reinforcement in the laboratory by the use of colored pencils to denote the germ layer origin of the tissues and the organs, the histological performance of the germ layers is one of the facts longest remembered by most embryology students. However, this emphasis may serve to give a false idea of realism to the germ layers and to imply a specificity not supported by the facts.

The germ layer concept played an important role in comparative embryology when it was shown that the germ layers were similar throughout the entire animal kingdom—although only ectoderm and endoderm appear in some invertebrates—and that their formation and fates were essentially the same in all animal species. During the debate on the theory of evolution in the 1800s, this similarity of origin and fate was used as one of the strongest confirmations of the principles of evolution. However, these earlier concepts assigned to the germ layers an absolute specificity and a reality that does not exist as well as a controlling force that is not warranted. E. B. Wilson noted that the typical relationships between the germ layers and the structures that are derived from them can be experimentally changed and he stated that if this is the case, these relationships can not be causally connected and the germ layers themselves do not have any intrinsic morphological value. Experiments conducted to change the fate of the germ layers will be described in a later chapter where it will be seen that the cells of any germ layer may be induced to overstep the classical boundaries of their own particular layer and to exhibit a variety of potentialities for the formation of tissues and organs of other germ layers. Thus, the germ layers are not regions of fixed specificities; nor are they causally related to the development of particular tissues or organs.

The value of the germ layer concept lies in the fact that germ layer formation is the first overt indication of the beginnings of differentiation. The establishment of the germ layers may be looked upon as the embryo's method of sorting out and locating its constituent parts in such a manner that, under normal circumstances, cells in a particular layer will form particular structures. Each germ layer is a region to which the building blocks for later organ formation are consigned. As labels and markers to indicate future differentiation, they aid in our understanding of the events of development. However, the germ layer concept tells us nothing about the underlying factors responsible for these differentiations.

Induction and Tissue Interactions

The early development of the nervous system has been the subject of investigation for many years. One major consideration is the influence of one part of the embryo on another resulting in the differentiation of specific organs, a phenomenon known as *induction*. The inductive influence of the middle mesoderm on the overlying ectoderm was considered such an important factor in the development of the axiate pattern of the embryo that Spemann termed the tissue responsible for induction, the *organizer*. The nature of the organizing substance and the mechanism of inductive processes are still the subject of considerable investigation.

DIFFERENTIATION AND DETERMINATION

Differentiation

Development has been defined as progressive change taking place over the lifetime of the individual. Nowhere in the lifespan is progressive change more evident than in the embryonic stages of development, and it is therefore understandable why embryologists are concerned with the causal processes underlying these changes. The progressive changes in the embryo by which its cells acquire their distinctive structures and functions is called *differentiation*. In differentiation, the cells become phenotypically different from other cells and from their precursors.

Although the formation of the germ layers is the first easily recognizable evidence of differentiation, some differentiation does occur before this time. The pregastrular cellular specialization associated with the acquisition of locomotor capability represents an early differentiation of the blastula cells of the teleost. An ultrastructural change that results in the appearance of intercellular junctions between trophoblast (membrane) cells of the mammalian blastocyst is another example of early differentiation.

One aspect of differentiation results in the development of groups of similar cells that have acquired the ability to perform a certain specific function. Such groups of cells are known as tissues and their differentiation is called *histogenesis*. For example, the cells lying along the middorsal axis of the amphibian gastrula differentiate into neural tissue whose function is to transmit nerve impulses. Histogenesis of the somites gives rise to connective tissue (dermis and bone) and to muscular tissue.

The part of development that deals with the assembling and molding of embryonic tissues into complex, highly structurated and fully functional organs we have termed organogenesis. *Growth* and *morphogenesis* are integral parts of organ formation. Growth is simply the increase in the size of an organism or its parts as the result of the synthesis of protoplasm or substances such as bone, cartilage matrix, or connective tissue fibers that form a part of the extracellular material of tissues or organs.

Gene Control of Differentiation
The structural and functional characteristics of a cell depend upon the nature of its proteins. The nature of its proteins in turn depends upon the expression of the genetic information contained in the cell's genome. Differentiation, then, is the function of gene activity, the sequence of each protein reflecting the linear sequence of the nucleotide-containing coding units of a gene. This, of course, immediately raises the problem of how cells, each one of which is known to have exactly the same genome, can synthesize different proteins in different tissues of the body. The only logical answer is that the entire genome is not active continually in every cell and only a small part of the DNA is transcribing in any given cell, the activity differing in different cells. In other words, differentiation is the expression of variable gene activity.

This brings us only a step closer to the solution of the mechanism of differentiation since we are still left with the question of why different parts of the genome are turned on or off in different cells. The answer to the question most probably lies in regional differences in the environment, both extracellular and intracellular. It is usually proposed that a cyclic interaction between the environment and the genome occurs so that the environment specifies which part of the genome will function and the genome in turn modifies the environment. Nucleocytoplasmic interaction will be the subject of Chapter 11. Basically, the interplay between nucleus and cytoplasm is considered to be the force that moves the cell along a specific pathway of differentiation and is thus responsible for development.

Determination

Another concept which often appears in embryology is that of *determination*. At one time in its development every egg is probably totipotent and indeed in many eggs individual blastomeres of the 2-,

4- or even 8-cell stage are capable of forming an entire—although smaller—individual. As development proceeds, the potency of the cells becomes progressively restricted and the lines of development open to them become fewer. That is, they gradually become "determined" to develop in a certain direction. Determination thus involves a series of events that results in a change from an indefinite to a definite condition. An area of the embryo first becomes determined toward some particular formation and then within this area continuing determination defines the fates of smaller groups of cells until eventually each cell becomes determined to differentiate in a single specific direction. Although determination can be simply visualized as progressive restriction of potencies and although in this sense determination is a single underlying principle in the development of every organ and its parts, the causative agents behind the events of determination are multiple. That is, the mechanism of the determination of a region of the frog egg to become a limb is entirely different from that which determines what part of this limb bud will become muscle, which is in turn certainly different from the determination that a muscle cell will synthesize actin and myosin.

TOPOGRAPHIC TERMINOLOGY

In anatomy it is important that we use well-defined terms by which we may relate parts of the body to other parts. Such terms as "under," "over," "up," "down," and so on vary according to the position of the body and are generally not used in descriptive anatomy.

The terms *ventral, dorsal, cranial,* and *caudal* are in common usage and should require no definition. However, there are some terms used in human anatomy that may be confusing. For the purpose of description in human anatomy, the body is assumed to be in what is known as the anatomical position: erect, with the hands at the sides and the palms directed forward. In this position, the normal direction in which a person would move is called *anterior,* the opposite direction being *posterior.* Thus, anterior is synonymous with ventral and posterior with dorsal. Two other terms are also used, *superior* or toward the head, synonymous with cranial, and *inferior* or toward the feet, synonymous with caudal. *Rostral* is a term that means toward the cranial end of the nervous system.

2

The Reproductive System
and the Germ Cells

"Ex ova omnia" is a statement made by the physiologist William Harvey in the 17th century. The *ovum* from which everything arises is the mature female *germ cell*. It usually develops into a new individual only after uniting with a male germ cell, the *spermatozoon*. Germ cells are highly specialized cells that are generally considered to be formed from stem cells called *primordial germ cells,* set aside from the body (somatic) cells early in development. There is convincing evidence in a number of species that the primordial germ cells are unique in their possession of a specific cytoplasmic component known as the *germ (germinal) plasm.* The germ plasm undergoes a precocious segregation into only a few cells of the early embryo which then become the primordial germ cells, the stem cells for the germ line in each new individual.

The germ plasm presents a number of scientific problems such as its chemical nature, the method of its segregation into the primordial germ cells, and the mechanism of its action. These will be discussed in the chapter on the development of the reproductive system. In addition, it presents a philosophical problem. If we consider that the germ plasm is the factor that determines the germ line in each new individual and then becomes a part of every germ cell formed by the individual, we are faced with the question of its immortality. Since each individual, in turn, is the product of germ cells from his previous generation, this specialized material, the germ plasm, is the substance that links each individual to both his previous and his future generations. We may then conclude that it is self-perpetuating and lives on indefinitely and in each generation is retained in a temporary body before it passed on to the next generation.

The formation of mature male and female gametes from their respective stem cells is known as *gametogenesis. Spermatogenesis* refers to the production of spermatozoa and *oogenesis* refers to the production of *ova.* Although gametogenesis is not, strictly speaking, a part of the study of embryology, a knowledge of its processes is fundamental. This, in turn, leads us to a brief consideration of the anatomy of the male and female reproductive systems where these processes take place.

15

THE MALE REPRODUCTIVE SYSTEM

The male reproductive system (Fig. 2–1 A,B) consists of the primary sex organs, the *testes,* and a set of accessory organs which includes the tubes and tubules through which the sperm pass to the outside, various glands that empty their secretions into these passageways, and a copulatory organ, the *penis,* by means of which sperm are deposited in the female reproductive tract. Not part of the reproductive system, but certainly associated with reproduction, are the body modifications characteristic of the different sexes, the *secondary sexual characteristics.* These include in the male such features as the higher coloration in fishes and birds, the cock's comb in the chicken, the thumb pad in the frog and the enlarged larynx, the beard and the pattern of the pubic and cranial hair in man.

The Testes

Although the testes develop in the abdominal cavity, they are, in the adults of most mammals, suspended in a sac, the *scrotum,* outside of the abdominal cavity. They perform a dual function: (1) the production of sperm, and (2) the synthesis and secretion of male sex hormones, called *androgens.* Testosterone is the principal testicular hormone. Spermatogenesis takes place within a set of tortuous tubes, the *seminiferous tubules,* which are lined with *germinal epithelium.* Located between the seminiferous tubules are cells known as *interstitial* or *Leydig cells* that produce the testosterone. Testosterone is responsible for the maintenance of the accessory sexual structures and the continued expression of the secondary sexual characteristics.

The Reproductive Tract

The path by which the sperm reach the outside may be traced by reference to Figure 2–1 A,B. Ducts, nerves, and blood vessels enter and leave the testis at its posterocephalic margin, a region known as the *mediastinum.* Radiating out from the mediastinum are connective tissue septa that divide the testis into over 200 lobules each containing a number of highly convoluted seminiferous tubules. As the seminiferous tubules approach the mediastinum, those in each lobule unite to form straight tubules, *tubuli recti.* The tubuli recti enter the mediastinum and form a branched network, the *rete testis.* From the rete, a number of ducts, the *vasa efferentia,* carry the sperm into a single common duct, the *epididymis.* The convoluted epididymis, over 15 feet long in man, lies along the posterior aspect of the testis. The epididymis, in turn, connects with the *vas deferens*

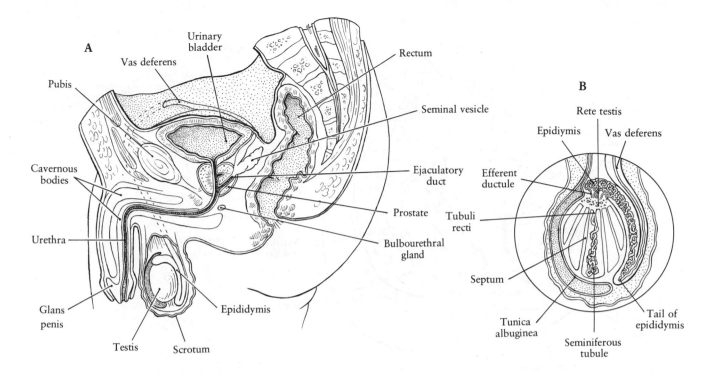

Pubis

Vas deferens

Urinary bladder

Rectum

Seminal vesicle

Cavernous bodies

Ejaculatory duct

Prostate

Urethra

Bulbourethral gland

Glans penis

Epididymis

Testis   Scrotum

B

Rete testis

Epidiymis   Vas deferens

Efferent ductule

Tubuli recti

Septum

Tunica albuginea

Seminiferous tubule

Tail of epididymis

which passes craniad out of the scrotal sac through the inguinal canal into the abdominal cavity. Here it opens into the *urethra* as the *ejaculatory duct* just after it is joined by the duct of the *seminal vesicle*. This portion of the urethra is surrounded by the *prostate gland*, which also empties its secretions into the urethra. Secretions from the seminal vesicles and the prostate form a large part of the ejaculate. From the point of entrance of the vas deferens into the urethra, the urethra in the male is a common pathway for both the urinary and the reproductive systems.

2–1   A, sagittal section of the pelvic region of the male; B, sagittal section of the testis and scrotal sac.

THE FEMALE REPRODUCTIVE SYSTEM

The female reproductive system consists of the gonads, the *ovaries*, and the accessory sex organs, the *uterine tubes, uterus,* and *vagina.* The external genitalia consist of the *labia minora,* the *labia majora,* and the *clitoris* (Fig. 2–2).

The Ovaries

The ovaries are paired organs lying within the pelvic cavity on either side of the uterus, attached to the posterior surface of the

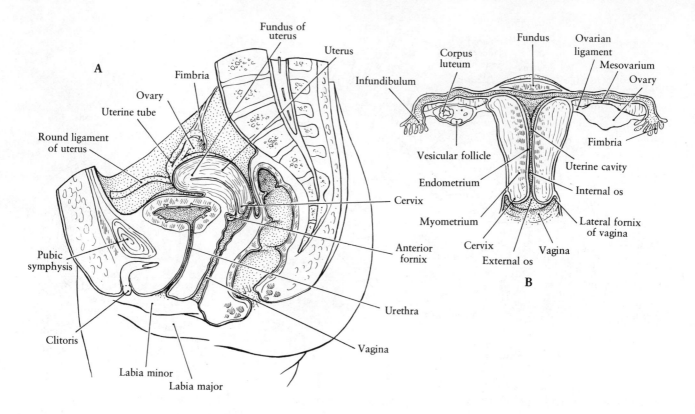

A

Fundus of
uterus

Uterus

Fimbria

Ovary

Uterine tube

Round ligament
of uterus

Pubic
symphysis

Clitoris

Labia minor

Labia major

Cervix

Anterior
fornix

Urethra

Vagina

B

Corpus
luteum

Fundus

Ovarian
ligament

Infundibulum

Mesovarium

Ovary

Vesicular follicle

Fimbria

Endometrium

Uterine cavity

Myometrium

Internal os

Cervix

Vagina

Lateral fornix
of vagina

External os

broad ligaments by a mesentery known as the *mesovarium*. The broad ligaments are folds of peritoneum that extend from the sides of the uterus to the sides of the pelvic walls. Each ovary is also attached to the uterus by an *ovarian ligament.*

Beneath the outer peritoneal covering of the ovary, the serosa, is a single layer of cuboidal or low columnar germinal epithelium. Below the germinal epithelium, subdivided by a network of connective tissue, are nests of undeveloped *primary follicles, developing follicles,* and *corpora lutea.* The sequence of development of the ovarian follicles and the formation of the corpora lutea after ovulation will be described in a later chapter.

During the embryonic development of the ovary, cells from the germinal epithelium move into the ovarian cortex to form the primary follicles. It has been estimated that there may be as many as 400,000 primary follicles in the human ovary at the time of birth. While there is a possibility that some germ cells may be formed from the germinal epithelium postnatally, it is more probable that all of the follicles which develop to maturity after puberty are those that are already present in the ovaries at the time of birth. Since in humans only a single ovum is normally released from the ovaries each month during the reproductive lifetime of the individual, it is

2–2 A, sagittal section through the pelvic region of the female; B, posterior view of the ovaries, uterine tubes, and uterus.

apparent that a tremendous number of ova never mature but instead undergo atresia.

The Reproductive Tract

The open, fimbriated ends of the *uterine tubes* (*oviducts*) encircle one pole of each ovary. Each uterine tube follows a C-shaped course back toward its opening into the uterus. The uterus is a thick-walled muscular organ situated between the bladder anteriorly and the rectum posteriorly. This pear-shaped organ can be divided into, in order from its cranial to its caudal end, the *fundus,* the *corpus,* the *isthmus,* and the *cervix.* The rather small uterine cavity opens through the cervix into the vagina. The cervix of the uterus projects downwards into the vagina so that a recess, the *fornix,* is formed between the two. Since the cranial end of the uterus is tipped anteriorly, the posterior fornix is deeper and the posterior wall of the vagina is longer than the anterior. The slit-shaped cavity of the vagina opens into the *vestibule* between the labia minora. The urethra opens into the vestibule anterior to the opening of the vagina.

Sperm are deposited in the vagina and pass through the reproductive tract of the female to the upper part of the uterine tubes where, if an egg is present, fertilization takes place. The fertilized egg then passes back down through the uterine tube and into the uterus where it implants and develops.

CELL DIVISION IN SOMATIC CELLS AND GERM CELLS

Mitosis

All of the body or somatic cells are normally diploid. That is, they have two full sets of homologous chromosomes, having received one set from each parent. Each cell contains the same number of chromosomes, a number characteristic of the species (46 in man). Cell reproduction is accomplished by mitotic divisions in which each daughter cell receives a chromosome complement that is exactly the same as that of the parent cell.

Cell division has been studied in innumerable plant and animal cells and is known to consist of a fairly complicated process divided into different phases progressing from *prophase* through *metaphase* and *anaphase* to *telophase* (Fig. 2–3). In prophase, the chromosomes become increasingly coiled and condensed and at the end of prophase, individual chromosomes may be seen with the aid of the

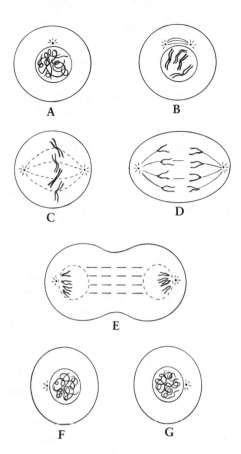

2–3 Mitotic division in a cell with two pairs of chromosomes. For description see text.

light microscope. Each chromosome is seen to be double, made up of two *chromatids*. During prophase, the nuclear membrane begins to break down and the nucleolus disappears. In metaphase, a *spindle* develops whose fibers radiate from *centrioles* located at opposite poles of the cell. The chromosomes become aligned in a plane passing through the middle of the cell, the metaphase plate. Spindle fibers attach to the *centromere* (*kinetochore*) of each chromosome. At anaphase, the centromeres divide and the sister chromatids move toward opposite poles with the centromeres leading the way. Each of the chromatids may now be called a daughter chromosome. Movement to the opposite poles is completed at telophase when the nuclear membrane develops, the nucleolus reappears, the chromosomes uncoil, and the spindle disappears. Cell division, *cytokinesis*, divides the telophase cell into two daughter cells, each with identical genetic material.

The actual process of mitosis usually occupies only a small part of what is known as the *cell cycle*. The major part of the cell cycle is spent in what has been termed the *interphase*, that is, the period between mitotic divisions, a period when the individual chromosomes are not visible. However, interphase is not a period of inactivity—as the term resting phase, which was once its synonym, implied—but one of considerable metabolic and synthetic activity.

The technique of autoradiography has been an extremely useful tool in the analysis of the cell cycle and in particular in demonstrating that one phase of the cycle shortly before mitosis is the time when the cell synthesizes DNA. This phase is the S-phase, and during this period—and this period only—is a radioactive precursor of DNA, tritiated thymidine, taken up by the cell. A G_1-phase before and a G_2-phase after the S-phase complete the cycle (Fig. 2–4). Synthesis of DNA indicates that chromosome replication is occurring; thus shortly before mitotic division—during the G_2 phase—each nucleus contains an amount of DNA which is double that of the presynthetic cell. This material is then halved at mitosis and the diploid value restored in each daughter cell (Fig. 2–5).

Meiosis

Although the *spermatogonia* and *oogonia* are diploid cells and divide mitotically to reproduce themselves, the mature germ cells that are derived from them contain only half the number of chromosomes characteristic of the somatic and stem cells of the species. They are haploid. At fertilization, the union of the 1N or haploid cells restores the diploid number. If the germ cells were not haploid,

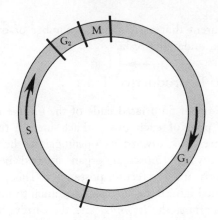

2–4 Diagram of the cell cycle. S, synthetic phase; M, mitosis; G_1 and G_2, presynthetic and postsynthetic phases, respectively.

2–5 Diagram illustrating the amount of DNA present in the cell nucleus during the different stages of the cell cycle in mitosis (A) and meiosis (B).

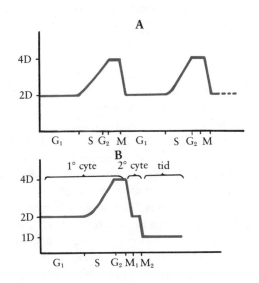

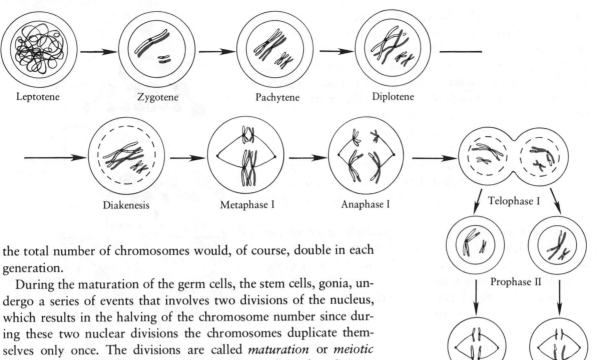

Leptotene   Zygotene   Pachytene   Diplotene

Diakenesis   Metaphase I   Anaphase I

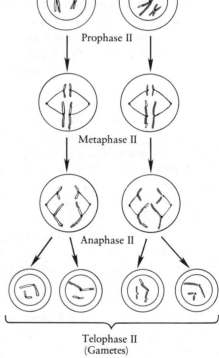

Telophase I

Prophase II

Metaphase II

Anaphase II

Telophase II
(Gametes)

the total number of chromosomes would, of course, double in each generation.

During the maturation of the germ cells, the stem cells, gonia, undergo a series of events that involves two divisions of the nucleus, which results in the halving of the chromosome number since during these two nuclear divisions the chromosomes duplicate themselves only once. The divisions are called *maturation* or *meiotic* divisions, although it is only in the prophase of the first division that the chromosomes behave differently than they do in ordinary mitosis.

Meiosis I. Meiosis I is characterized by a long and complicated prophase that is divided into a number of stages (Fig. 2–6). The first stage is *leptotene* when the chromosomes condense into long, threadlike, loosely coiled structures. Although the leptotene chromosomes are not visibly double, DNA synthesis studies show that each chromosome has already duplicated itself in the preceding S-phase.

The next stage is *zygotene,* when homologous segments of maternal and paternal chromosomes—and thus the chromosomes themselves—pair. Pairing of homologous chromosomes is known as *synapsis,* and it results in a nucleus that appears to have only the haploid number of chromosomes although neither the number of chromosomes nor the amount of DNA has changed.

In the next stage, *pachytene,* the shortening and thickening of the chromosomes, which was begun in zygotene, continues. Each synaptic pair is called a *bivalent.* It is now possible to determine that each bivalent consists of four chromatids, forming what is known as a *tetrad.*

In the next stage, *diplotene,* the individual chromatids are more apparent. In synapsis in leptotene, homologous chromosomes

2–6   Meiotic divisions in a germ cell with two pairs of chromosomes. (For description see text.)

paired over their entire lengths. Now, in diplotene, sister chromatids are still closely paired but maternal and paternal chromatids have begun to repel each other and to separate. However, they still remain attached at certain points known as *chiasmata*. Each chiasma represents a region where there has been an exchange, a crossing over, between chromatids of maternal and paternal origin. One or more chiasmata may appear in each bivalent.

The next stage is *diakenesis* and the chromosomes are maximally shortened and thickened. The chiasmata become terminalized, that is, they move toward the ends of the bivalents. Diakenesis is the last stage in prophase I and is accompanied by the disappearance of the nucleolus and the nuclear membrane and the formation of the spindle apparatus.

The bivalents take up position on the equatorial plate of the spindle during metaphase and spindle fibers from opposite poles attach to each homologous chromosome at its kinetochore. During anaphase, homologous chromosomes move toward the opposite poles. Anaphase I ends with a haploid set of chromosomes at each pole. However, each is a double structure, consisting of two chromatids, known as a *dyad*.

Telophase I is short and usually abortive, and the cell moves rapidly into the next division. When a short interphase does occur, it is only a transition stage and no DNA synthesis or chromosome duplication takes place. Thus, following the first maturation division, each daughter cell contains a haploid number of chromosomes. However, each chromosome is double—due to DNA synthesis in the previous S-phase—and the amount of DNA present is characteristic of a diploid cell (Fig. 2–5 B). Each duplicated chromosome is of either maternal or paternal origin, except where crossing over has produced interchanges.

Meiosis II. Although the second maturation division is preceded by an abortive interphase in which there is no S-phase, the nuclear division is exactly the same as that which occurs during normal mitosis. If an interphase stage is lacking, no prophase occurs; and the dyads align along the equatorial plate of the spindle and separate into two units, each of which is consigned to a daughter cell. Each daughter cell now contains the haploid number of chromosomes and also an amount of DNA characteristic of a haploid nucleus (Fig. 2–5 B). The above brief description of maturation divisions may be applied to the formation of the germ cells in each of the sexes.

A diagrammatic representation of the separation of the germ line cells from the somatic line cells and the proliferation and meiotic divisions of the male and female germ cells is shown in Figure 2–7. Each spermatogonium forms four mature sperm while, as will be

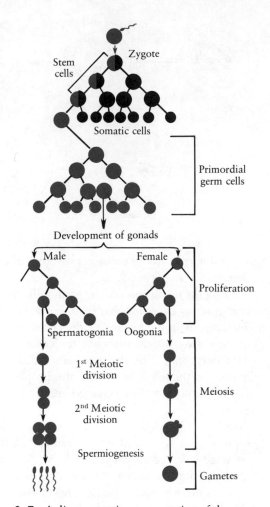

2–7 A diagrammatic representation of the separation, following fertilization, of the germ line cells from the somatic line cells and the proliferation and meiotic divisions of the male and female germ cells.

described in the next chapter, each oogonium forms only a single mature ovum.

REFERENCES

Smith, L. D. 1975. Germinal plasm and primordial germ cells. 33rd Symposium, The Society for Developmental Biology. Eds., C. L. Markert and J. Papaconstantinou. New York: Academic Press.

3

Spermatogenesis

In the previous chapter we noted that the seminiferous tubules of the testes were lined with germinal epithelium. The cells of the germinal epithelium are made up of male germ cells in all stages of transition from spermatogonia to mature sperm. A cross section of a testis will show as its main feature seminiferous tubules cut in many different planes. For a study of spermatogenesis, tubules cut in cross section should be selected. Three such tubules from a human testis are represented in Figure 3–1.

SPERMATID DEVELOPMENT

The most immature cells, the spermatogonia, are found forming a few layers closest to the basement membrane of the tubule. These are the cells that divide mitotically to produce more spermatogonia. Successive steps in the formation of spermatozoa will be seen progressing from the periphery of the tubule to its lumen. The first step, the formation of *primary spermatocytes,* does not involve cell divisions but results from the growth of certain spermatogonia to about double the size of the original cells. Each primary spermatocyte now goes through the two maturation or meiotic divisions, first forming two secondary spermatocytes and from these four *spermatids,* each with the haploid number of chromosomes. Since the secondary spermatocytes divide rapidly without going through an interphase, they are often difficult to locate in sections of the seminiferous tubules.

SPERMATID MATURATION

After the formation of the four spermatids from each of the original spermatogonia, spermatogenesis is still not complete. The task of the mature spermatozoon is to carry to and introduce into the egg the genetic material of the male parent. Spermatids are not adapted to carry out this function and must undergo extensive morphological and biochemical modification before they are capable of doing so. This process is called *spermatid maturation* or *spermiogenesis.* It does not involve any cell division but is concerned with getting

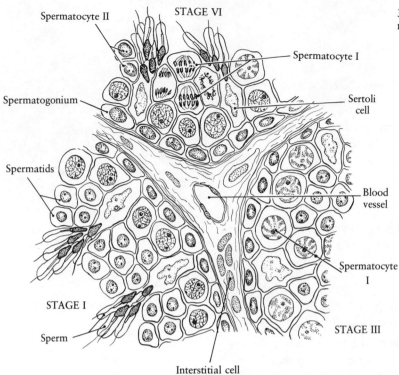

Spermatocyte II   STAGE VI

Spermatocyte I

Spermatogonium

Sertoli cell

Spermatids

Blood vessel

STAGE I

Spermatocyte I

Sperm

STAGE III

Interstitial cell

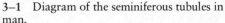

3–1 Diagram of the seminiferous tubules in man.

rid of those structures not necessary for the task at hand and modifying those structures that are retained to form a highly specialized cell geared for motility and penetration. Spermatozoa are spermatids "stripped for action." The remodeling of the spermatid will be followed by considering in turn the parts of the mature sperm (Fig. 3–2) and the processes by which they are formed. A diagram of a mature sperm, which includes the cellular components of the spermatid that contribute to its formation, is shown in Figure 3–3.

The Head

The nucleus of the spermatid becomes the major part of the *head* of the sperm, forming a small compact mass of chromatin in a shape characteristic of the species. The human sperm is oval when viewed on its flat surface and lanceolate when viewed on its edge. The amount of nuclear material appears to be smaller in the sperm than in the spermatid, but this is due to a condensation of the chromatin rather than any reduction in amount. In sections prepared for electron microscopy, the condensed chromatin in the mammalian sperm appears homogeneous or coarsely granular, although freeze-

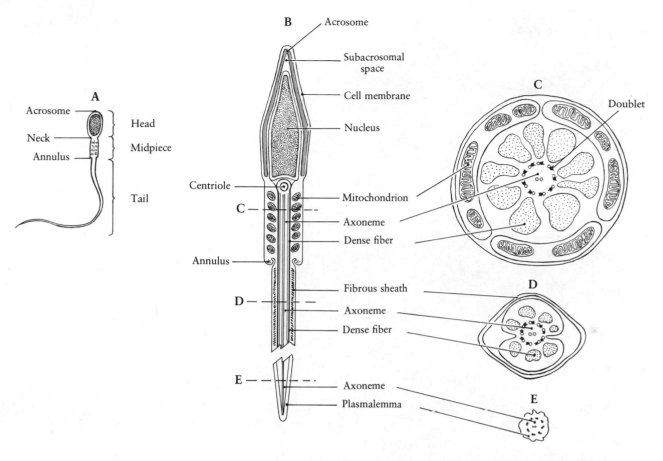

A
Acrosome
Neck
Annulus
Head
Midpiece
Tail

B
Acrosome
Subacrosomal space
Cell membrane
Nucleus
Centriole
Mitochondrion
Axoneme
Dense fiber
Annulus
Fibrous sheath
Axoneme
Dense fiber
Axoneme
Plasmalemma

C
Doublet

D

E

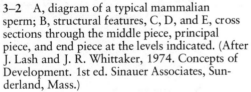

3–2 A, diagram of a typical mammalian sperm; B, structural features, C, D, and E, cross sections through the middle piece, principal piece, and end piece at the levels indicated. (After J. Lash and J. R. Whittaker, 1974. Concepts of Development. 1st ed. Sinauer Associates, Sunderland, Mass.)

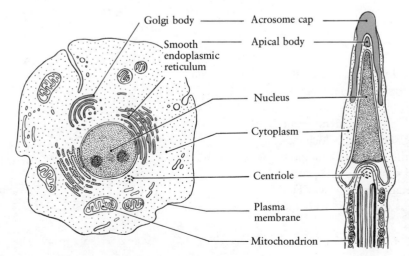

Golgi body
Smooth endoplasmic reticulum
Nucleus
Cytoplasm
Centriole
Plasma membrane
Mitochondrion
Acrosome cap
Apical body

3–3 A generalized diagram of the role of the cellular elements of the spermatid in the formation of the structures of the mature sperm. (After R. Hadek, 1969. Mammalian Fertilization. Academic Press, New York.)

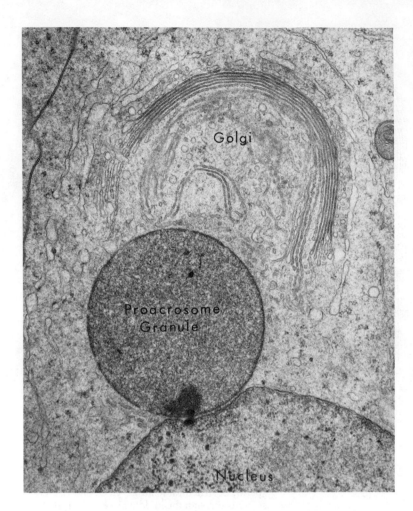

3–4 Formation of the acrosome in an insect, showing the relation to the Golgi apparatus. (From D. M. Phillips, 1974. Spermiogenesis. Academic Press, New York.)

etching studies reveal a structural order in the form of lamellae parallel to the flattened surfaces.

The Acrosome

The *acrosome* appears as a membrane-bounded vesicle covering the anterior end of the head. It is of almost universal occurrence in all sperm so far examined with the exception of some fishes and some insects. It shows a wide variety of shapes and sizes in different species. The acrosome develops in the Golgi complex, which becomes oriented close to the anterior end of the head early in spermatid maturation. Frequently the acrosome first appears as a proacrosomal vesicle between the Golgi complex and the nucleus (Fig. 3–4). It is not surprising that the acrosome is associated with the

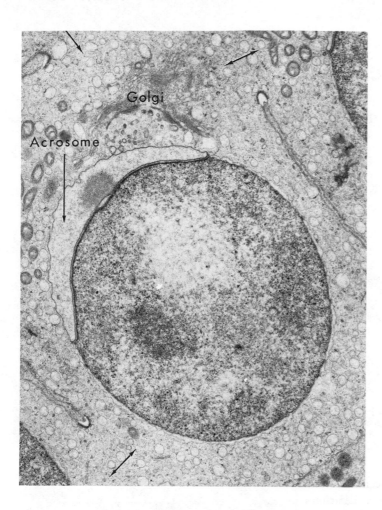

3–5   An early stage in the formation of the acrosome in the rabbit. (From D. M. Phillips, 1974. Spermiogenesis Academic Press, New York.)

Golgi complex since the acrosome is a specialized secretion granule containing lytic enzymes and the Golgi apparatus is known to be involved in the formation of secretion granules. The action of these acrosomal lytic enzymes will be described in the section on fertilization. As the original acrosome vesicle enlarges, it spreads over the anterior surface of the nucleus (Fig. 3–5) and eventually covers somewhat more than the anterior half. An acrosomal granule forms a small distinct element in the human sperm, and the acrosomal vesicle forms what is often referred to as the *anterior head cap,* although the term *acrosomal cap* better reflects its origin.

Neck and Flagellum

The *neck* is the small region just posterior to the head and connects it to the *middle piece.* The important developmental processes oc-

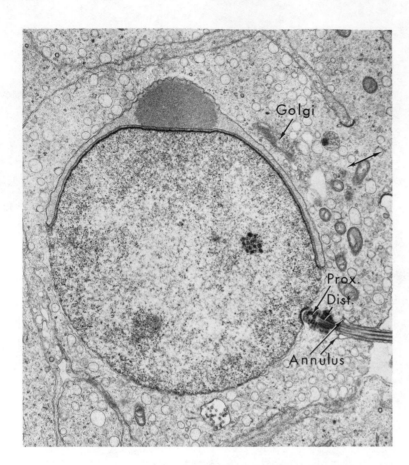

3–6 Centrioles and annulus of the maturing rabbit spermatid at a stage later than that shown in Figure 3–5. (From D. M. Phillips, 1974. Spermiogenesis. Academic Press, New York.)

curring in the neck region are concerned with the centrioles and the formation of the *flagellum*. The spermatid has two centrioles located just below the plasma membrane, a *proximal centriole* closest to the nucleus, and a *distal centriole*. The flagellum develops in association with the distal centriole. The centrioles move from their original peripheral position toward the nucleus and the proximal centriole assumes a position indenting the posterior pole of the nucleus (Fig. 3–6). Early in spermiogenesis the plasma membrane becomes associated with an electron dense material lying just distad of the centriole pair. It is called the *chromatid body*. This structure, of as yet unknown origin, will form the *annulus*. As the centrioles migrate toward the nucleus, the plasma membrane retains its connection with the developing annulus and forms an involution around the flagellum (Fig. 3–7). The annulus later moves distally and marks the end of the middle piece. It is sometimes called the *ring centriole*. This is a rather unfortunate term since the annulus, although closely associated with the centrioles, does not develop from them; and electron microscopy studies show that it does not have the structure characteristic of a centriole.

The flagellum develops a central axial structure, the *axoneme*, which consists of two central single tubules surrounded by nine pairs of tubules or doublets. This structure is characteristic of the axial filaments of flagellae and cilia developed as locomotor organs in a variety of animals. Surrounding the axoneme in the mammalian sperm are nine outer *dense fibers,* each associated with one of the nine doublets. A fibrous sheath forms the outer covering (Fig. 3–2).

The Middle Piece

The *middle piece* consists of the flagellum surrounded by a mitochondrial element. The mitochondrial sheath is in the form of a helical structure located outside of the dense fibers. The middle piece extends from the neck to the annulus (Fig. 3–2).

The Principal Piece and the End Piece

The *principal piece* and the *end piece* run from the annulus to the tip of the flagellum. The axoneme is present as the core in both of these regions. In the principal piece the nine-plus-two tubular structure is surrounded by seven dense fibers instead of nine as in the middle piece. The fibrous shcath that surrounds the dense fibers shows two longitudinally running columns on opposite sides of the flagellum, each making contact with a doublet (Fig. 3–2). The dense fibers of these doublets are the two that are missing from the original nine found in the middle piece. Progressing toward its tip, the flagellum gradually tapers as the dense fibers and the fibrous sheath become thinner and eventually disappear. Approximately the last five microns of the tail, the end piece, consist of the axoneme covered by only a thin layer of cytoplasm and its plasmolemma.

THE MATURE SPERM

The mature sperm is thus a specialized cell that is efficiently packaged to carry the paternal DNA condensed in its head to the vicinity of the ovary. As a locomotor organ, it uses the flagellum, with special contractile elements, the dense fibers, to which energy is supplied by the mitochondria of the middle piece. Once contact with the ovum is made, the acrosome functions to penetrate the egg membranes and the male nucleus moves into the cytoplasm of the

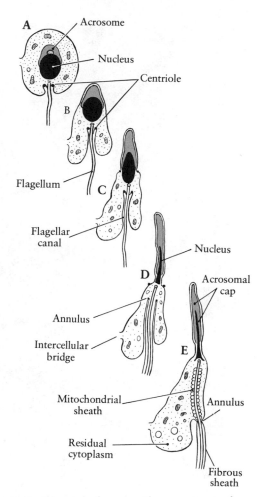

3–7 Diagram of spermatid maturation in the guinea pig. (After D. W. Fawcett, W. A. Anderson and D. M. Phillips, 1971. Dev. Biol. 26:220.)

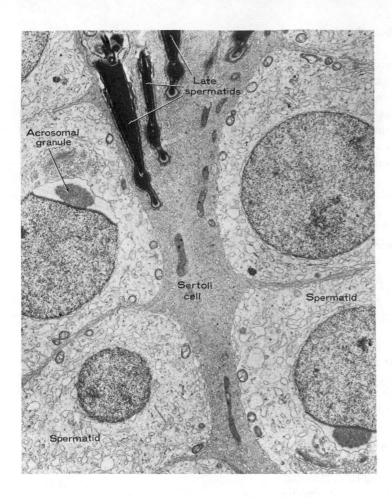

Acrosomal granule

Late spermatids

Sertoli cell

Spermatid

Spermatid

3–8 Relationship of a Sertoli cell to maturing spermatids. Sertoli-cell processes passing between younger spermatids. Advanced spermatids found in recesses at the luminal end of a Sertoli cell. (Courtesy of D. W. Fawcett.)

egg. As part of the package, the sperm centriole moves into the cytoplasm and there it functions in forming the achromatic spindle apparatus of the first division of the zygote nucleus.

SERTOLI CELLS

In addition to its germinal elements, the seminiferous tubules also contain a population of sessile cells, the *Sertoli cells*. They are individual columnar cells with processes extending laterally and toward the lumen of the seminiferous tubule. These processes pass between, and sometimes completely around, the germinal elements with which they are associated—the spermatozoa at the basal level and the clusters of spermatids undergoing maturation at the lumenal level (Fig. 3–8).

Sertoli cells are often considered to function in the sustenance of the germinal elements and the regulation of the spermatogenic cycle, although no unequivocal evidence for these functions has been reported. Evidence has been presented in support of a number of other possible functions. The seminiferous tubules have the capacity to synthesize androgens, although not in amounts large enough to contribute significantly to circulating steroids. It is possible that androgen produced by the Sertoli cells may instead act locally in the support of germ cell maturation. In addition, electron microscope (EM) studies of the later stages of spermatid maturation suggest that the Sertoli cells may control the release of the sperm into the lumen of the seminiferous tubule. The sperm flagellum is immobile at this time, and sperm release may be effected by movement of the Sertoli cell cytoplasm (Fig. 3–9). Other suggested functions are the maintenance of the blood-testis barrier and the elaboration of the fluid necessary for the transport of sperm along the tubules.

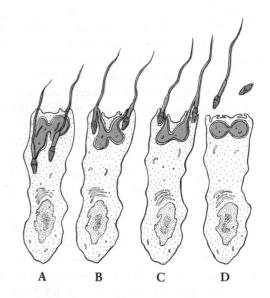

3–9 Stages in the release of sperm by a Sertoli cell. A, spermatid deep within the cytoplasm of a Sertoli cell. Spermatid cytoplasm between the spermatid head and the lumen of the seminiferous tubule; B, beginning of sperm extrusion, with cytoplasmic remnant retained in a Sertoli cell; C, extrusion continued, with sperm connected to the cytoplasmic remnant by a narrow neck; D, sperm free, with cytoplasmic remnant remaining in a Sertoli cell. (From D. W. Fawcett, 1975. Handbook of Physiology, Section 7, Endocrinolgy Vol. 5. D. W. Hamilton and R. O. Greep, eds. The American Physiological Society, Bethesda.)

CYCLE OF THE SEMINIFEROUS TUBULE

Examination of cross sections of the rodent testis early showed that associations of cells with fixed compositions occurred regularly. That is, the cell types (stages in spermatogenesis and spermatid maturation) did not occur in a haphazard fashion but various stages of spermatid maturation were always associated with certain types of spermatogonia and spermatocytes. This suggested that each of these associations or stages followed each other in an orderly progression giving rise to what was termed the cycle of the seminiferous tubule. Although the histological appearance of the human seminiferous tubule was at first thought not to fit into this pattern and to show a haphazard arrangement of germinal elements, it was subsequently shown that there are, in fact, six types of cell associations in man and thus six stages in the cycle of the seminiferous tubule. These stages continually succeed each other in an orderly sequence. The fact that in man these stages may sometimes show irregularities made the original definition of the human cycle difficult.

MALE INFERTILITY

In about 25 percent of the couples who are unable to conceive, infertility is attributable to defective production of spermatozoa. Thus, it is important to establish criteria for the evaluation of the ejaculate. Such criteria usually consider semen volume as well as sperm density, motility, and morphology. While no rigid line of demarcation between fertile and infertile males may be drawn at any specific level for any of the above criteria, a number of guidelines are considered indicative in semen analysis. Although three milliliters is given as the mean semen volume, there does not seem to be too much relation between volume and ease of conception; consequently, semen volume is probably the least reliable criterion of fertility. Sperm density is important, but there is no established level below which a male should be considered infertile. For some time, 60 million sperm per milliliter was considered to be borderline, but some men with counts less than 20 million per milliliter have proven to be fertile and, in one study of 2000 men with counts between 20 and 40 million, 47 percent proved to be fertile.

Sperm motility is important. However, its importance is not in moving the sperm through the female reproductive tract following insemination. Sperm move far too slowly to traverse this distance in the allotted time on their own power and rely on muscular contractions and the beat of the cilia of the reproductive passages. The sperm's own locomotor efforts may be important in traversing the narrow uterotubal junction. Once in the region of the egg, motility does become important and at least 40 percent motile sperm is considered a minimum standard to permit fertilization. The quality of the progression must also be considered; active progression rather than random circling is the desired type of movement.

Not all sperm are normal morphologically, and a variety of abnormal sperm are seen on examination of any semen sample (Fig. 3–10). If the percentage of abnormal forms exceeds 20 percent, impaired fertility may be expected.

In evaluating male fertility it is thus not possible to set absolute standards. The only absolute standard for sterility, since it takes but a single sperm to fertilize an egg, would be a semen sample with no motile sperm. However, certain minimum standards in semen volume, sperm concentration, mobility, and morphology may be considered in classifying individuals as potentially fertile or subfertile.

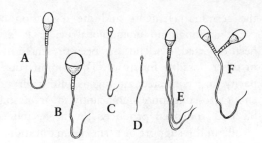

3–10   Some types of abnormal sperm.

REFERENCES

Clermont, Y. 1963. The cycle of the seminiferous epithelium in man. Am. J. Anat. 112:35–52.

Fawcett, D. W. 1972. Observations on cell differentiation and organelle continuity in spermatogenesis. In: International Symposium on the Genetics of the Spermatozoan. Eds., R. A. Beatty and S. Gluecksonn-Waelsh. Edinburgh, New York: Department of Genetics University of Edinburgh.

Fawcett, D. W. 1975. Ultrastructure and function of the Sertoli cell. In: Handbook of Physiology-Endocrinology, V, Section 7, pp. 21–25. Eds., D. W. Hamilton and R. O. Greep. Baltimore: Williams and Wilkins.

Koehler, J. K. 1970. A freeze-etching study of rabbit spermatozoa with particular reference to head structures. J. Ultrastruct. Res. 33:598–610.

4

Oogenesis

A single cell, the oocyte, represents the connecting link between the ongoing generation and the next generation. As such, it is a highly specialized cell that is capable of expressing and maintaining the characteristics of the species. *Oogenesis* constitutes a continuum of events and processes involved in the origin, growth, and differentiation of the oocyte or egg cell from stem cells in the ovary. The transformations from stem cell to mature ovum are complex, embracing cellular, molecular, and physiological phenomena.

The egg cell in all animals is nonmotile and quite large by comparison to the somatic cells of the body. The importance of a careful examination of the growth and differentiation of the oocyte was clearly articulated by E. B. Wilson, an eminent cytologist, in 1896 when he stated that embryogenesis begins in oogenesis. Ample evidence currently available suggests that the development of the early embryo is in great measure controlled by the egg cell. In other words, the information controlling the early development of the embryo is somehow programmed into the oocyte during oogenesis. How and in what form this developmental information is stored in the egg cell is an area of active investigation.

In addition to storing developmental information, the ovum also carries the nutrients (i.e., yolk) to provide building materials and energy for the support of the early embryo. The synthesis and packaging of these materials is a major process in oogenesis.

An equally important aspect of oogenesis is the extent to which the programming of developmental information and the packaging of yolk materials are regulated by factors outside of the oocyte. We know that the growth and differentiation of the oocyte are under endocrine control (Chapter 5). However, the nature of the mechanisms by which hormones act upon the oocyte remains to be fully determined.

In the pages that follow, we summarize how oogenesis changes the egg cell into a cell specialized to undergo meiosis, to participate in fusion with the male gamete, and to store information and materials that are essential to development following fertilization.

ORGANIZATION OF THE OVUM

Descriptions of oogenesis often seem confusing because of the variety of terms used to refer to the "egg cell." During its growth and differentiation within the ovary, the egg cell is an *oocyte.* In order to emphasize homological relationships with the male sex cell, it is more appropriately termed the *primary oocyte.* At the end of the period of growth, differentiation, and maturation, the oocyte can be termed the *ovum* or *mature egg cell.*

As in the development of the male gamete, oocytes arise from stem cells in the ovary called *oogonia.* Oogonia are often difficult to identify in ordinary histological sections of the ovary because of their proximity to the germinal epithelium of this organ. In most chordates, the population of oogonial cells increases in number by ordinary mitotic divisions. However, in the human female, the ovary at birth has few if any oogonial cells. Most of these cells have been converted into a finite stock of primary oocytes. Without considering details, it can be said that as soon as the oogonia reach a size of 10 to 20 micrometers in the mammal, depending upon the species, the differentiation of the primary oocyte has begun. The transformation of the stem cell into the primary oocyte is accompanied by an enlargement of the nucleus and rearrangement of the chromatin material.

The period of growth and differentiation of the primary oocyte is macroscopically expressed in most vertebrates as a dramtic increase in size, a change that may take place over a time interval of several days or several years. During this time, the primary oocyte becomes surrounded or enclosed by an epithelium of *follicle cells,* the latter being special cells presumably originating from the germinal epithelium of the ovary. For example, in the newborn human, the several hundred thousand oocytes are each surrounded by a single layer of follicle cells. These *unilaminar follicles* characterize the female ovary during the postembryonic period of sexual immaturity (Fig. 4–1).

With the onset of sexual maturity in the mammal, some of these unilaminar follicles begin to increase in size (Fig. 4–2). The simple columnar-shaped cells of the primary follicles multiply, first forming a double (*secondary follicle*) and finally a stratified cuboidal epithelium around the oocyte. At about the time that the growth of the primary oocyte ceases (140 μm in diameter in the human female), small, fluid-filled irregular spaces appear between the follicle cells. These gradually coalesce to form a single, large cavity, the *follicular antrum,* filled with a fluid known as the *liquor folliculi* (Fig. 4–3). Autoradiographic studies have shown that the elaboration of the liquor folliculi is due to the secretory activity of the

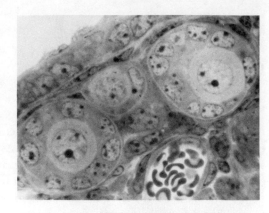

4–1   Quiescent oocyte in a primary follicle in the cortex of a mature mouse ovary. (From L. Zamboni, 1970. Biol. Reprod. Suppl. 2, 44.)

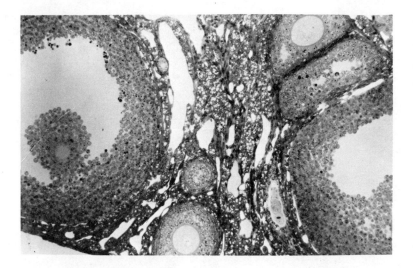

4–2 A section through the mouse ovary to show follicles in various stages of maturation. A young Graafian follicle with the forming cumulus oophorus can be seen to the left. (From L. Zamboni, 1972. Oogenesis. J. Biggers and A. Schuetz, eds. University Park Press, Baltimore.)

follicle cells. The continued increase in the volume of the liquor folliculi separates the primary oocyte, ensheathed by several layers of follicle cells, from the remaining follicle cells. The primary oocyte with its halo of follicle cells, termed the *cumulus oophorus,* now occupies an eccentric position in the antral cavity (Fig. 4–3). The large (20–25 mm in diameter) and vesicular follicle is now termed the *Graafian follicle.* Figure 4–4 summarizes in diagrammatic form the various changes in the primary oocyte and its associated follicle cells which lead to the formation of the Graafian follicle.

Note that the antral cavity of the Graafian follicle is invested by follicle cells arranged as a stratified cuboidal epithelium. These constitute the structural layer known as the *stratum granulosum.* Outside of the stratum granulosum, the connective tissue of the ovary typically condenses around the growing follicle as the *theca folliculi.* As the antral cavity enlarges with fluid accumulation, the Graafian follicle pushes closer to the surface of the ovary. Rupture of the wall of the Graafian follicle results in the release of the oocyte with its surrounding 12 to 15 layers of follicle cells. The stratum granulosum and the theca folliculi then rearrange themselves to form the *corpus luteum.*

Close examination of the primary oocyte in the Graafian follicle shows that, in addition to follicle cells, it is surrounded by a transparent, noncellular envelope, the *zona pellucida* (Fig. 4–5). This envelope is approximately 15 micrometers in thickness and very rich in acid mucopolysaccharides. A narrow fluid-filled space, the *perivitelline space,* can be identified between the zona pellucida and the plasmalemma of the oocyte (oolemma).

Our understanding of the structural changes in the oocyte, as well as the interrelationships between the oocyte and the surround-

4–3 Formation of the antral cavity in a mouse follicle. (From L. Zamboni, 1970. Biol. Reprod. Suppl. 2, 44.)

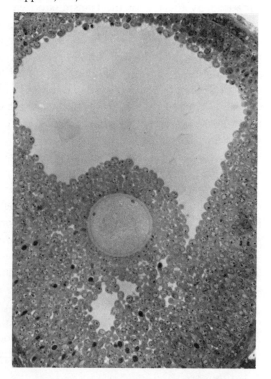

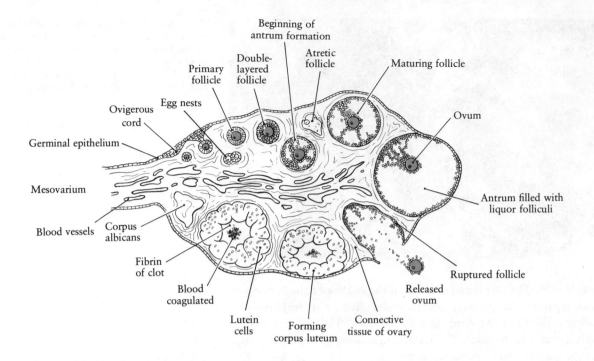

ing environment of follicle cells, during oogenesis has been greatly enhanced by the use of the transmission electron microscope and various labeling techniques. Typically, the young oocyte of the primary follicle is rather simple in appearance and structural organization (Fig. 4–6). The cytoplasm tends to be rather transparent and granular. The granules are undoubtedly particles of ribonucleoprotein. In the mammalian oocyte, the nucleus is large and spheroidal in shape. Most of the organelles of the cell are clustered in a limited region around the nucleus. Electron microscopic studies have shown that the perinuclear organelles consist mostly of *endoplasmic reticulum,* closely packed *mitochondria, lysosomes,* and a prominent *Golgi complex.* A particularly interesting organelle, the *annulate lamellae,* has been observed in the young human oocyte (Fig. 4–7). Annulate lamellae are stacks of parallel, paired membranes interrupted at regularly spaced intervals by pores or annuli. Similar structures have been found in the sea urchin oocyte in association with ribosomelike particles. Presumably, these annulate lamellae arise by blebbing activity of the nuclear membrane. The functional significance of these structures during oogenesis is not known.

The number and distribution of many of these cytoplasmic organelles undergo a marked change with continued growth and maturation of the primary oocyte. The mitochondria increase in number and become more uniformly distributed throughout the cy-

4–4 Schematic diagram of the mammalian ovary showing the sequence of events in the origin, growth, and eventual rupture of the Graafian follicle. Start at the mesovarium and follow in a clockwise direction. Note also the formation and regression of the corpus luteum.

4–5 Human oocyte in antral follicle. Note the zona pellucida and the surrounding cumulus cells. Organelles are distributed throughout the oocyte cytoplasm. (From L. Zamboni, 1972. Oogenesis. J. Biggers and A. Schuetz, eds. University Park Press, Baltimore.)

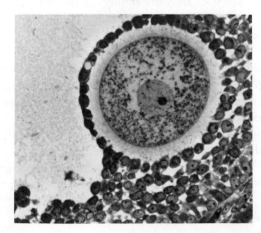

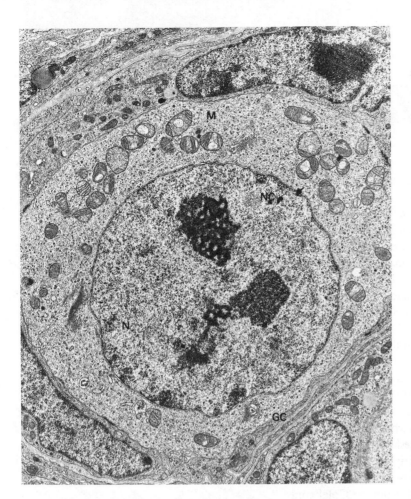

4–6 Electron micrograph of a young oocyte of the mouse ovary showing the distribution of Golgi material (GC), mitochondria (M), and endoplasmic reticulum. N, nucleus; NC, nucleolus. (Courtesy of E. Anderson.)

4–7 Annulate lamellae in the cytoplasm of the human oocyte. (From L. Zamboni, 1972. Oogenesis. J. Biggers and A. Schuetz, eds. University Park Press, Baltimore.)

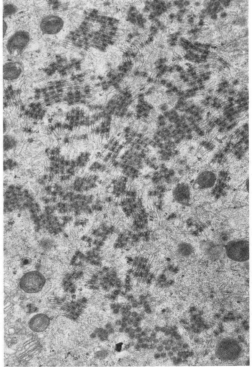

toplasm. The elements of the endoplasmic reticulum become pronounced. Their association with numerous ribosomes is functionally associated with the dramatic increase in protein synthesis, which is known to take place during the growth stage of the primary oocyte.

One of the most dynamic transformations in the cytoplasm of the maturing oocyte involves the Golgi complex. The Golgi complex has been implicated in a variety of animals in the formation of a population of vesicles known as the *cortical granules* (or *cortical alveoli*). These spheroidal-shaped bodies have been identified in the peripheral cytoplasm of the mature egg in frogs, echinoderms, teleost fishes, bivalve molluscs, and several mammalian species (including the rabbit, hamster, and man [Fig. 4–8]). They are apparently absent in the ova of urodeles, insects, birds, and several mammals (e.g., the rat and the guinea pig).

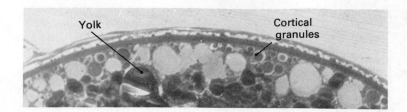

Yolk

Cortical granules

4–8 A section through the mature egg of the zebra fish (teleost) showing the cortical granules.

Cortical granules are membrane-bound spheres that range in size from about 0.5 micrometers (sea urchin) to 20 micrometers (zebrafish) (Fig. 4–8). Positive staining reactions with periodic acid Schiff reagent (PAS) and Alcian blue indicate that their contents are rich in acid mucopolysaccharide. Several hydrolytic enzymes, including acid phosphatase and beta glucanase, have also been identified as constituents of the cortical granules in sea urchins. From studies with fish, amphibian, and echinoderm oocytes, it can be concluded that the proteinaceous component of the granule is probably manufactured in the endoplasmic reticulum and the polysaccharide component(s) in the Golgi complex.

The modification of the Golgi complex into the cortical granules appears to occur throughout the cytoplasm of the oocyte. In forms like the rabbit and man, the Golgi complex is observed to divide into aggregates of vesicular and tubular elements (Fig. 4–9 A). These become filled with an electron-dense material. The mature cortical granule, approximately 300 to 500 millimicrons in diameter, is produced through the coalescence of these vesicles with their contents. These then migrate to the extreme periphery of the oocyte where they are organized into several layers beneath the oolemma (Fig. 4–9 B). The fusion of vesicles pinched off from the Golgi complex also appears to be the method of cortical granule formation in other invertebrate and vertebrate organisms.

Ultrathin sections of sea urchin oocytes have revealed that the organization of the cortical granule is very complex. The mature granule is limited peripherally by a unit membrane approximately 50 Å in thickness. The unit membrane is close to but distinctly separate from the adjacent oolemma. The contents of the cortical granule consist of a large, centrally located electron-dense mass (250–500 Å) and several lighter hemispheric-shaped globules (200–300 mμ in diameter) (Fig. 4–10). Studies with other sea urchins, such as *Arbacia* and *Strongylocentrotus*, indicate that there is considerable variation in the appearance, shape, and arrangement of the components of the cortical granules. By contrast, the cortical granules in fishes and amphibians are quite homogeneous in appearance (Fig. 4–11).

The cortical granules of the mature ovum are associated with and

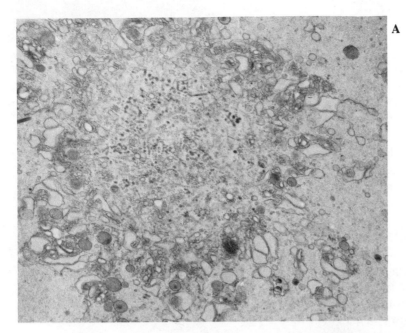

A

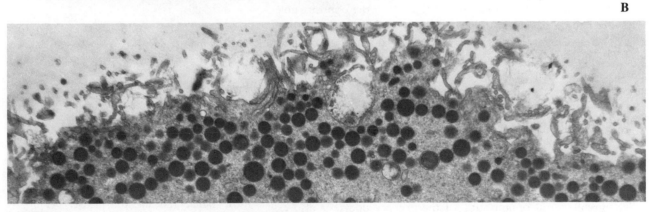

B

4-9 A, cortical granule formation in the Golgi complex of a human oocyte; B, cortical granules located in the cortex of the human oocyte. (From L. Zamboni, 1972. Oogenesis. J. Biggers and A. Schuetz, eds. University Park Press, Baltimore.)

part of a peripheral layer of cytoplasm whose physical properties are quite different from the rest of the cytoplasm of the cell. If sea urchin ova, for example, are subjected to moderate centrifugation, the inclusions in the interior of these cells, such as mitochondria, ribosomes, and yolk particles, are movable and easily displaced. By contrast, the cortical granules and the cytoplasm in which they are embedded remain intact and undisturbed. Although there are some differences of opinion, it is generally recognized that these experimental results offer proof for the existence of a peripheral zone of cytoplasm, termed the *cortical cytoplasm*. It forms a layer several micrometers in thickness and is viewed as being more viscous than the rest of the ooplasm. Recent evidence tends to suggest that the cortical cytoplasm possesses a cytoskeletal network of actinlike microfilaments that probably function to protect the egg cell against mechanical deformation. The cortex of the egg cell also appears to be a site for the storage of information that is important to the development of the future embryo. Unraveling the nature of the cortical information and determining its influence upon the processes of embryogenesis has been a very difficult task. We will examine the significance of this specialized area of the ovum in later chapters.

The advanced primary oocyte emerges as a highly differentiated cell with a variety of organelles and inclusions, such as mitochondria, ribosomes, membrane complexes (endoplasmic reticulum, the Golgi complex), pigment granules, and yolk particles (see section that follows on vitellogenesis), embedded in a liquidlike cytoplasm. Many of these cellular constituents become localized in specific areas of the oocyte during its growth and maturation, giving a distinct *polarity* to the cell. For example, there is in most animals an enormous increase in the number of ribosomes during the growth phase of the oocyte. However, instead of being arranged at random in the ooplasm, they are distributed along a gradient in decreasing numbers from one pole of the cell to the opposite pole. The distribution of mitochondria follows a similar pattern. Also, in the oocytes of many vertebrates, particularly those with moderate to large amounts of yolk (frogs, fishes, birds), the yolk inclusions or particles are smaller and more loosely packed at one end of the cell; they progressively become larger and more tightly packed toward the opposite end of the cell. This stratification permits us to refer to the region of the oocyte containing the nucleus and few yolk inclusions—but rich with ribosomes and mitochondria—as the *animal pole*. The opposite or yolk-filled region of the oocyte is termed the *vegetal pole*. The imaginary line passing from the animal pole to the vegetal pole is the *animal-vegetal axis*.

The architectural organization of the primary oocyte is also expressed in many animal species in regional differences in the appearance of the ooplasm. In the ova of many amphibians, dark brown or black pigment granules are located in the cortical cytoplasm of the animal hemisphere (Figs. 4–11; 4–12 A). This is in sharp contrast to the vegetal hemisphere, which appears colorless or white because of the densely packed mass of yolk and few pigment granules. Although the transition from dark to light is macroscopically distinct, there is an intermediate or *marginal zone* where the pigment granules are intermediate in intensity. The mature egg of the tunicate or ascidian, *Styela*, possesses yellow pigment granules uniformaly distributed throughout the cortical cytoplasm (Fig. 4–12 B). In several species of mollusc (*Dentalium, Ilyanassa*), the fully grown oocyte shows three distinct cytoplasmic areas (Fig.

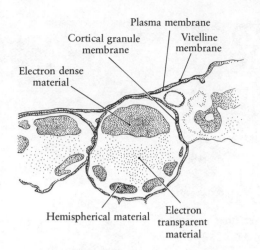

4–10 Reconstruction from electron micrographs of a section through the cortical granule of the egg of the sea urchin, *Clypeaster*. (After Y. Endo, 1961. Exp. Cell Res. 25, 383.)

4–11 A cortical granule (CG) in the mature oocyte of the frog. Note also the distribution of pigment granules (PG) and yolk platelets (YP). (From N. Kemp and N. Istock, 1967. J. Cell Biol. 34, 111.)

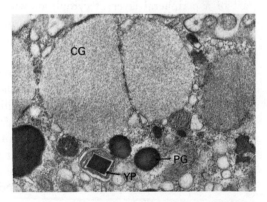

4–12 C). These are: a yolk-free, clear, unpigmented zone of transparent cytoplasm at the vegetal pole (*vegetal polar plasm*); a narrow, pigment-free zone of cytoplasm at the animal pole (*animal polar plasm*); and an intervening zone of cytoplasm filled with yolk particles and pigment granules. Similar animal and vegetal polar plasms are observed in the ovum of the snail (*Limnaea*). These cytoplasmic regions apparently differentiate just as the ovum leaves the ovary. Additionally, six lenticular-shaped patches of cytoplasm, known as *subcortical accumulations,* have been described by Raven as occurring at the equator of the snail oocyte (Fig. 4–13). Their significance is very much in doubt. However, the positions of the subcortical accumulations directly reflect the locations of six follicle cells that surround the oocyte during its development, thus suggesting that the organization of the ooplasm is, in part, brought about or dictated by cells accessory to the primary oocyte.

Since pigment granules are perhaps the most visible expression of oocyte differentiation, it is logical to ask if they play a key role in the future development of the embryo. It is unlikely that pigment granules are very important to the growth and differentiation of the embryo. However, we can consider that the uneven distribution of pigment granules may very well reflect a more subtle organization of the ooplasm into qualitatively different regions that subsequently are vital to the specific differentiations of the embryo.

In most animal species the oocyte develops in close association with a population of accessory or follicle cells. These accessory cells have been shown to be essential to the complete structural and physiological maturation of the oocyte. They participate in such activities of the ovary as transportation of yolk materials into the oocyte, stimulation of nuclear maturation (i.e., reduction divisions), and formation of investing layers of membranes around the oocyte.

The close functional relationship between the primary oocyte and its surrounding cellular environment is indicated by several structural specializations of the oolemma. One of the earliest structural changes to occur in the maturing oocyte of many invertebrates and vertebrates is the appearance of numerous fingerlike projections of the oolemma. These *microvilli,* which increase substantially the surface area of the oocyte, develop rapidly and uniformly over the whole surface of the oocyte. They interdigitate with similar cytoplasmic extensions of the investing follicle cells (Fig. 4–14). With the light microscope, this zone of projecting and overlapping microvilli gives a distinct striated appearance to the region of the primary follicle beyond the oolemma. This region of the primary follicle is termed the *zona radiata* in the mammals.

Electron microscopic studies provide strong evidence that the microvilli function in the exchange and transport of substances be-

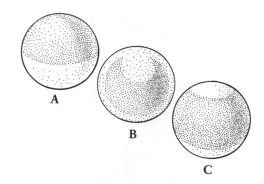

4–12 Superficial views of the mature oocyte of the frog (A), tunicate (B), and mollusc (C) to show regional differences in the cytoplasm.

4–13 A view from the vegetal pole showing positions of the subcortical accumulations (SCA) as proposed by Raven in the egg of the snail. (After C. Raven, 1970. Int. Rev. Cytol. 28, 1.)

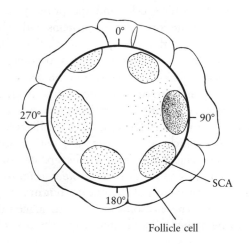

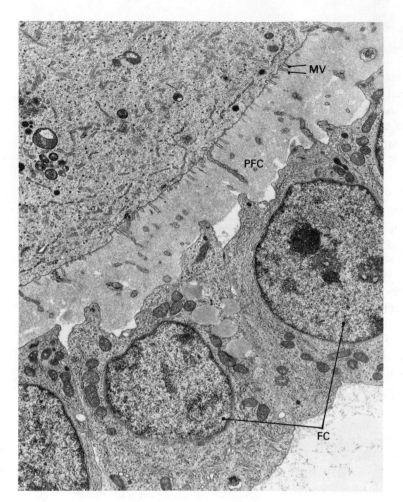

4–14 An electron micrograph showing microvilli (MV) extending from the surface of the mouse oocyte and interdigitating with projections (PFC) from the investing follicle cells (FC). (Courtesy of E. Anderson.)

4–15 Electron micrograph of a longitudinal section through a projection of an ovarian follicle cell (hen) termed the lining body. The lining body indents but does not penetrate the cell membrane of the oocyte. (From R. Bellairs, 1971. Developmental Processes of Higher Vertebrates. University of Miami Press, Coral Gables.)

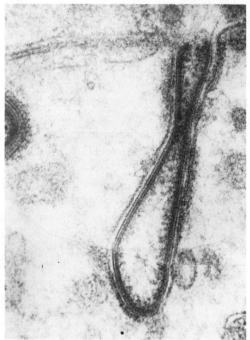

tween the follicle cells and the primary oocyte. Oocytes actively engaged in the formation of proteins and yolk often show small inpocketings at the bases of these microvilli. Subsequently, after sequestering fluids, these pockets become pinched off and form membrane-bound vesicles within the ooplasm. This process of "cell drinking" is referred to as *micropinocytosis*. By the time the oocyte has reached its full size, micropinocytosis is greatly diminished or no longer visible. Hence, the microvilli of both the oocyte and the adjacent follicle cells are generally withdrawn.

In the chick, the follicle cells are drawn out into club-shaped projections known as *lining bodies* (Fig. 4–15). These push deep into the cytoplasm of the oocyte, but never apparently penetrate its oolemma. There is some evidence to suggest that these lining bodies may be nipped off and engulfed by the oocyte. Their fate within the oocyte remains a mystery. Similar specializations of follicle cells have been observed in the primary oocytes of some turtles.

In addition to follicle cells, some insects, molluscs, and annelids rely on a special system of accessory cells, known as *nurse cells*, for the transfer of mateials (such as yolk) into the oocyte. Nurse cells immediately surround the oocyte and are joined to it by a network of *intercellular bridges*. Since there is direct cytoplasmic continuity between oocyte and nurse cell, no microvilli are required.

VITELLOGENESIS

Growth and increase in size of the primary oocyte are conspicuous features of oogenesis. Although an increase in volume of cytoplasm contributes to the growth of the oocyte, much of the change is due to the deposition and stockpiling of foodstuffs. The growth phase of the primary oocyte may span a considerable period of time. In some frogs, for example, the development of the mature ovum occurs over an interval of approximately three years. During this time the oocyte increases from a cell size of about 50 micrometers to one of about 1500 micrometers in diameter. This corresponds to an increased volume of approximately 27,000-fold. However, most of the change in size occurs during the third year when deposition of yolk within the cell is particularly intense. By contrast, the size of the hen's egg changes very rapidly during the 14-day period immediately preceding ovulation. The volume of the oocyte increases some 200-fold, with most of the yolk being laid down within the six-day period before the egg leaves the ovary (Fig. 4–16).

The phase of oogenesis during which nutritive material or *yolk* is deposited and accumulated within the primary oocyte is termed *vitellogenesis*. For all animals studied, this vital step or process begins after the oocyte enters the first prophase stage of nuclear maturation or meiosis.

The term yolk or *deutoplasm* as used in the literature appears to have several meanings. Yolk is often used to refer to the reserve foodstuffs in mature ova, including fat droplets and glycogen granules. In the strict sense of its definition, however, yolk refers to reserve materials present in special cytoplasmic inclusions laid down during oogenesis and present in the developing embryo. The chief constituents of these yolk inclusions or bodies are phospholipids, proteins, and carbohydrates. Depending upon the animal, the structural organization and composition of yolk will vary. In forms like cephalochordates and echinoderms, most of the yolk is proteinaceous (*proteoid yolk*) and distributed throughout the ovum as fine *granules*. By contrast, less than 50 percent of the dry weight of

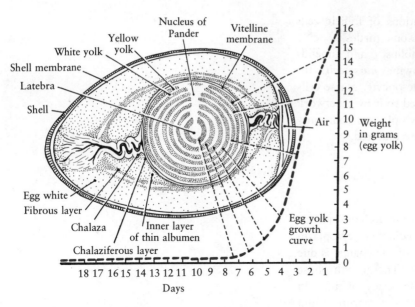

Nucleus of Pander

Yellow yolk

Vitelline membrane

White yolk

Shell membrane

Latebra

Shell

Air

Egg white

Fibrous layer

Chalaza

Inner layer of thin albumen

Chalaziferous layer

Egg yolk growth curve

Weight in grams (egg yolk)

16
15
14
13
12
11
10
9
8
7
6
5
4
3
2
1
0

18 17 16 15 14 13 12 11 10 9 8 7 6 5 4 3 2 1

Days

4–16 Diagram showing the structural organization of the hen's egg at the time of laying. The graph indicates the rate of growth of the egg, measured by weight of yolk in grams, during the 18 days preceding oviposition (laying). (After E. Witschi, 1956. Development of Vertebrates. W. B. Saunders Company, Philadelphia.)

the mature egg cell is yolk protein in the amphibian. Lipids constitute about 25 percent of the dry weight of the amphibian ovum and are distributed in the cytoplasm in the form of inclusions known as *lipochondria*. Most of the protein yolk in the amphibian oocyte is found in the form of large, flattened crystalline bodies termed *yolk platelets*. Similar inclusions with a crystalline structure are identifiable in the oocytes of cyclostomes, elasmobranchs, and bony fishes. Avian yolk is a combination of water (48.7%), proteins (16.6%), phospholipids (32.6%), and carbohydrates (1.0%). Vitamins A_1, B_1, B_2, and D are also present. Most of the yolk is in liquid form. Approximately 25 percent of the yolk is organized as *yolk globules* or *yolk spheres*.

It is not surprising that differences in the amount and distribution of yolk within the mature ovum exist among members of the animal kingdom. The egg of the bird has a large and generous supply of yolk, sufficient to provide for rapid and complete development. The chick is, in fact, a small adult upon emergence from the shell and fully capable of taking care of its own needs. Ova with large amounts of yolk are termed *polylecithal* or *megalecithal* and can be found in teleost fishes, elasmobranch fishes, reptiles, and birds. Generally, the active cytoplasm in a polylecithal egg is restricted to a thin layer on the surface of the yolk and thickened disc (with the nucleus) at the animal pole. By contrast, the yolk in the ovum of a frog or salamander is moderate in amount (*mesolecithal*), sufficient to carry the developing embryo only to the larval or tadpole stage. The tadpole is then able to secure enough food for its growth and development into a small frog. The yolk in polyle-cithal and mesolecithal ova tends to be localized at the vegetal pole, a condition referred to as being *telolecithal*. The amount of the yolk in the ova of echinoderms, lower chordates (cephalochordates, urochordates), and mammals is small (*oligolecithal* or *microlecithal*) and rather evenly distributed throughout the ooplasm (*isolecithal* or *homolecithal*). Arthropods, especially insects, have an unusual distribution of yolk in their ova. The yolk lies in the interior of the cell, surrounding a mass of cytoplasm containing the nucleus. Such an egg is termed *centrolecithal*.

Within recent years, studies by a number of investigators have greatly increased what we know concerning the sources of the constituents of the yolk inclusions and the mechanisms by which yolk is packaged within the primary oocyte. We now know more, for example, about the sites of synthesis for the precursors of protein and carbohydrate yolk as well as the organelles charged with fashioning the yolk into a cytoplasmic inclusion. In general, yolk production results from precursors synthesized either within (*autosynthetic*) or outside (*heterosynthetic*) of the primary oocyte. A variety of organelles including the endoplasmic reticulum, the Golgi complex, and the mitochondria have been identified as possible sites for the assembly of yolk within the oocyte.

Techniques employing the electron microscope and radioactively labeled amino acids have provided clear evidence that the precursors of protein yolk in both invertebrates and vertebrates are commonly manufactured outside of the primary oocyte and subsequently sequestered within it. If the ovaries of insects are exposed to a tritiated amino acid, such as ^{3}H-leucine, radioactivity is initially detected in the accessory cells surrounding the oocyte. Shortly thereafter, the radioactive label is present throughout the cytoplasm of the oocyte. Similar labeling methods have been used to trace the source of yolk in amphibians and birds. Here, the yolk precursors, in the form of a lipophosphoprotein, are synthesized in the liver and transported in the plasma of the bloodstream to the follicular epithelium around the oocytes. The lipophosphoprotein passes through the follicle cells and is incorporated into the oocyte by micropinocytosis. One within the ooplasm, the *yolk vesicles* produced by this process may coalesce to form the large yolk inclusions of the mature ovum. Based upon observations in the cockroach, Anderson proposes that exogenous proteins and polysaccharides may initially be adsorbed onto specialized areas of the oolemma containing a sticky, matted substance or *bristle coat* (Fig. 4–17). These areas then become invaginated and pinched off to form *coated vesicles* or precursors to the yolk bodies.

Yolk bodies are fashioned in quite different ways in other ani-

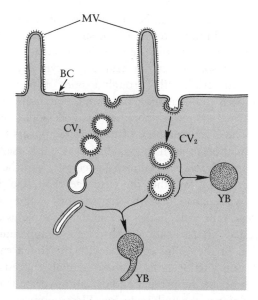

4–17 A diagrammatic section through the oolemma of the cockroach oocyte to show the formation of yolk bodies. The surface of the oolemma is thrown into a number of microvilli (MV). Areas between the microvilli show a sticky, matted substance termed bristle coat (BC). Micropinocytic or coated vesicles form, some of which are small (CV_1) and some which are large (CV_2). The large vesicles fuse to form dense-cored yolk bodies (YB). The small coated vesicles fuse to form tubular structures; some of these fuse with larger coated vesicles to form yolk bodies (YB). Exogenous proteins and polysaccharides are probably adsorbed onto the bristle coat and then taken into the ooplasm by micropinocytosis. (From E. Anderson, 1969. J. Microsc. 8, 721.)

mals. The yolk bodies in the ova of the crayfish and lobster are formed in the cisternae of the smooth endoplasmic reticulum. Granules of protein yolk are initially visible in the cisternae of the rough endoplasmic reticulum near the oocyte nucleus. After being transported peripherally through a series of interconnecting tubes to the smooth endoplasmic reticulum, the granules aggregate and are then pinched off into the ooplasm as yolk bodies (Fig. 4–18).

The Golgi complex of the oocyte appears to be a center of yolk formation in such diverse forms as the horseshoe crab, the hydrozoan jellyfish, the killifish (a teleost), and the African-clawed frog (*Xenopus*). Whether the cisternae of the Golgi complex synthesize as well as assemble the constituents of the yolk bodies is still unclear. The yolk bodies are initially visible as a collection of small vesicles in association with the Golgi apparatus. The close association of the Golgi complex with the rough endoplasmic reticulum during vitellogenesis in these animals suggests that the latter may synthesize the protein and/or carbohydrate that is packaged by the Golgi into the yolk inclusion. Electron micrographs of amphineuran (*Mollusca*) oocytes actively engaged in vitellogenesis show that vesicles evaginated from the endoplasmic reticulum appear to be transferred to the Golgi complex.

There is little doubt that several methods may be used by the oocyte in producing yolk bodies. The formation of protein yolk in a dual fashion is amply illustrated in both amphibians and fishes. In addition to the fusion of micropinocytotic vesicles, the yolk bodies are formed as large crystalline inclusions inside of modified mitochondria (Fig. 4–19). Because the oocyte mitochondria in *Rana* appear to contain all the components required for protein synthesis, it is probable that the yolk proteins in this frog are synthesized as well as packaged in the mitochondria. By contrast, the yolk platelet proteins of *Xenopus* appear to be manufactured outside of the mitochondria with subsequent transfer to these organelles by micropinocytosis.

Following release from the mitochondria, the yolk platelets of the frog ovum are seen as large, membrane-bound, ovoid crystalline structures that are flattened in one plane. Each platelet consists of a proteinaceous core surrounded by a superficial granular coat of polysaccharide. Analysis of the platelet shows the presence of two prominent yolk proteins, *phosvitin* (molecular weight of 35,000) and *lipovitellin* (molecular weight of 40,000). Two molecules of phosvitin are joined to each molecule of lipovitellin to form the organizational unit of the yolk crystal. Phosvitin and lipovitellin are also prominent components of yolk protein in the bird egg.

The mature egg of the mammal is often described as having no yolk. Within the framework of our loose definition of this term,

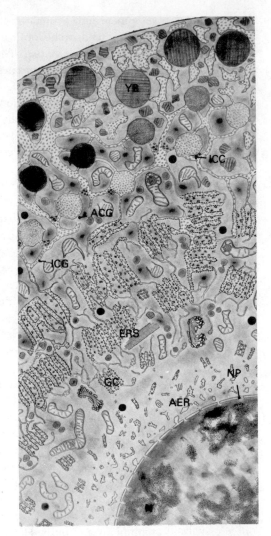

4–18 Differentiation and growth of the crayfish oocyte showing the role of the endoplasmic reticulum in the formation of proteinaceous yolk. The structures shown are nucleus (N), nuclear pores (NP), Golgi complex (GC), agranular endoplasmic reticulum (AER), differentiated stacks of rough-surfaced endoplasmic reticulum (ERS), intercommunicating smooth-surfaced cisternae (ICC), intracisternal granules (ICG), aggregates of intracisternal granules (ACG), immature yolk bodies (IYB), and mature yolk bodies (YB). (From H. Beams and R. Kessel, 1963. J. Cell Biol. 18, 621.)

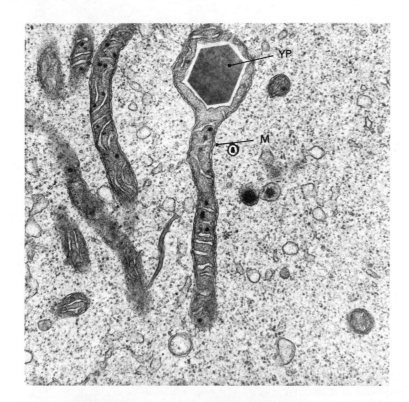

4–19 Two views of the yolk platelet (YP) in varying degrees of growth inside the mitochondrion (M) of a frog. (From R. Kessel, 1971. Z. Zellforsch. Mikrosk. Anat. 112, 313.)

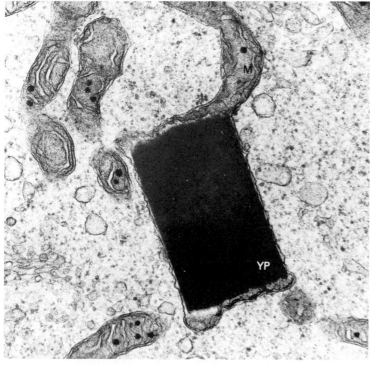

yolk is definitely present in mammalian eggs in the form of lipid droplets and glycogen granules. Whether distinct inclusions of a protein-lipid nature are part of the organization of the egg is still an open question. In the mouse, rat, and hamster, multiple stacks of fibrous material appear in the cytoplasm of young oocytes. These continue to accumulate within the ooplasm until the oocyte is mature. Interestingly, these fibrous stacks disappear during the preimplantation period of the embryo. Perhaps this fibrous material is being used as an energy source by the embryo during the interval between fertilization and implantation. Large yolklike vesicles filled with flocculent material have also been identified in the ova of rabbit, ferret, and sheep.

THE OOCYTE NUCLEUS

Most of our discussion to this point has been directed at activities that occur at the surface and in the cytoplasmic compartment of the primary oocyte. Simultaneously, however, complex synthetic activities, which are important to the storage of information to be used by the developing embryo, take place in the nucleus.

The nucleus of the primary oocyte, particularly during vitellogenesis, is characterized by its relatively large size and swollen appearance. In this condition, it is often referred to as the *germinal vesicle*. The main components of the germinal vesicle are the *nuclear envelope,* the *chromosomes,* the *nucleoli,* and the *nuclear sap* or *nucleoplasm.*

The large size of the nucleus of the growing oocyte has been of decided advantage in studies designed to probe the structure and function of this organelle during oogenesis. With the amphibian oocyte, it is a rather simple procedure to manually isolate the nucleus using a pair of fine forceps. Ultrathin sections of the isolated nucleus show that the nucleoplasm is granulofibrillar and limited by a bilaminar envelope that is perforated with regular arranged *nuclear pores or annuli.* Close analysis tends to indicate that these pores are not simple openings in the nuclear membrane. Rather, each pore appears to be closed by a granularlike material. Commonly, aggregates of dense fibrous material can be seen projecting through these pores, suggesting that these annuli act to control the passage of material from nucleus to cytoplasm. Experiments in which ions and low molecular weight proteins have been injected into amphibian oocytes give clear evidence that the nuclear envelope is very selective in its permeability.

Suspended in the nucleoplasm of the germinal vesicle are chromosomes and nucleoli. Both of these structures actively engage in the synthesis of ribonucleic acid (RNA) during the growth and differentiation of the oocyte. As in the case of the primary spermatocyte, distinct and characteristic changes in the configuration of the chromosomes become visible in the primary oocyte. In extremely young oocytes, for example in the ovaries of newborn mice or tiny *Xenopus* toads prior to metamorphosis, the chromosomes are observed to be in leptotene or early zygotene state of meiosis. By four days of age in mice, the chromosomes are in the diplotene stage of meiosis. They will remain in such a configuration until the time of ovulation.

Shortly after the onset of vitellogenesis, the arrested chromosomes attain a high degree of extension and assume what is commonly known as the lampbrush configuration (Fig. 4–20). Thin threads or loops characteristically branch out at right angles to the long axis of each chromosome, thus suggesting the appearance of lampbrushes used for cleaning petroleum lamps before the invention of the electric light. Such lampbrush chromosomes have been observed in the nuclei of oocytes in a wide variety of both vertebrates and invertebrates, including man (Table 4–1).

The structure of the typical lampbrush chromosome as proposed by Gall and Callan is shown in Figure 4–20. The main axis of each chromosome consists of two homologous chromatids, which are closely paired. The chromatid is considered to be a single, long fiber of double-stranded deoxyribonucleic acid (DNA). The paired loops represent uncoiled segments of the DNA fiber on adjacent regions of the sister chromatids. In the salamander (*Triturus*), there are some 20,000 loops in the whole set of chromosomes with the average loop being about 50 micrometers in length. Thus, there are about 5000 loops per haploid set of chromosomes. It has been estimated that *Plethodon,* also a salamander, may have as many as 10,000 loops per chromosomal set.

The configuration of the lampbrush chromosome is suggestive of intensive and widespread gene activity in the nucleus. When lampbrush chromosomes are manually isolated and exposed in a culture medium to a radioactive precursor of RNA (^{3}H-uridine), the results of autoradiography indicate that most of the label is detected along the length of the lateral loops. Newly synthesized proteins can also

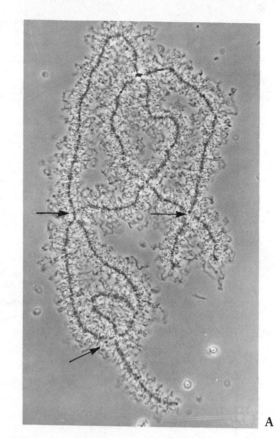

A

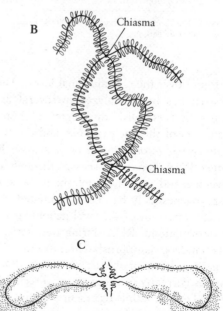

B

Chiasma

Chiasma

C

4–20   A, a phase contrast photomicrograph of an isolated lampbrush chromosome from the oocyte nucleus of the salamander, *Triturus viridescens*—note the multiple, paired loops extending from the axes of the homologous chromatids, which are held in a tetrad configuration by chiasmata (arrows); B, a diagrammatic sketch of a pair of lampbrush chromosomes joined by two chiasmata; C, an interpretation of chromosome structure as two continuous chromatids. (Micrograph Courtesy of J. Gall.)

Table 4–1 Occurrence of lampbrush chromosomes in animal oocytes and the duration of the lampbrush stage

Species and affiliation of animals in which lampbrush chromosomes have been reported	Estimated duration of lampbrush stage (where available)
Deuterostome	
Chaetognath	
Arrow worm	
Echinoderm	
Sea urchin	
Chordate	
Cyclostome	Several months in lamprey
Shark	
Teleost	
Amphibian	
Urodele	About seven months in *Triturus*
Anuran	Four to eight months in *Xenopus*, 30–40 days in *Engystomops*
Reptile	Some months in lizards
Bird	Three weeks in chick
Mammal	Perhaps years in man
Protostome	
Mollusk	
Gastropod	
Cephalopod	
Insect	
Orthopteran	Three months in cricket

From E. Davidson and B. Hough, 1972. In: Oogenesis. Eds. J. Biggers and A. Schuetz. Baltimore, University Park Press.

be found over the chromosomal loops. The nature of the RNA synthesized has been analyzed in several animal species using techniques that establish the degree of homology between the base sequences of the nuclear DNA and the RNA. Some of the RNA is quite clearly *informational* or *messenger* RNA (mRNA). This messenger RNA apparently passes through the annuli of the nuclear envelope and into the ooplasm to be stored for use during early embryogenesis. It has been estimated that in *Xenopus* approximately 3 percent of the total genome is involved in the production of informational RNA during oogenesis. Based upon studies with salamanders, lampbrush chromosome RNA transcripts are very large, consisting of at least 5×10^4 to 10×10^4 nucleotides in length. Studies currently in progress are directed at determining how much of the DNA length is represented in the lampbrush messenger molecules, rates of RNA synthesis, and the base sequence complexity of the total loop transcripts. Conceivably, then, we might be able to establish the number of genes involved in the informational programming of the oocyte.

A second major site of RNA synthesis in the primary oocyte is the nucleoli. Nucleoli are extrachromosomal bodies set aside within the nucleus for the specific production of ribosomal RNA (rRNA). The oocytes of different animal species show variable numbers of nucleoli. In most invertebrates, the nucleolus is a large, single, spheroidal-shaped organelle. By contrast, the oocytes of vertebrates commonly have hundreds of nucleoli of various sizes distributed just inside the nuclear envelope. There are about 600 nucleoli in the germinal vesicle of *Triturus* and about twice this number in *Xenopus*.

Ultrathin sections of a typical nucleolus show a bipartite structure with a granular cortex surrounding a central fibrillar core (Fig. 4–21A). In *Triturus*, the core has been isolated from the granular cortex, dispersed, and examined under the electron microscope. The core consists of thin circular axial fibers along which, at regularly spaced intervals, are groups of 80 to 100 short-to-long fibrils (Fig. 4–21B). If treated with selected digestive enzymes, deoxyribonuclease (DNAase) is observed to dissolve the main core axis. These results allow us to conclude that each core fiber is composed of DNA, the fibrils are RNA, and both nucleic acids are coated with protein. Elegant studies by Gall, MacGregor, and Miller permit the view that the fibrils are growing chains of rRNA being transcribed from segments of DNA. Indeed, each segment of DNA is a single gene coding for rRNA. Hence, as many as 80 to 100 precursor rRNA molecules are being synthesized simultaneously on each rRNA gene.

Since vertebrate oocyte nuclei contain many nuceloli, there must be many copies of genes coding for nucleolar rRNA. The replication of rRNA genes that takes place during oogenesis is known as *gene amplification*. Amplification is generally thought to occur at the pachytene stage of early oocyte development. It has been demonstrated in amphibian oocytes that the extra genes originate from specific, condensed regions (caps or nucleolar-organizing regions) of the chromosomes. The importance of ribosomal gene amplification is shown in the fact that it would take, in the absence of the extra ribosomal genes, some 500 years for the frog to synthesize the rRNA that normally is made during a three-year period.

In all growing oocytes, the overwhelming majority of the newly synthesized stable RNAs are of the ribosomal type. The large amount of rRNA has posed severe problems in characterization of other RNA species in total RNA extracts. At the end of oogenesis, there is a sharp decrease in RNA synthesis. The number of nucleoli

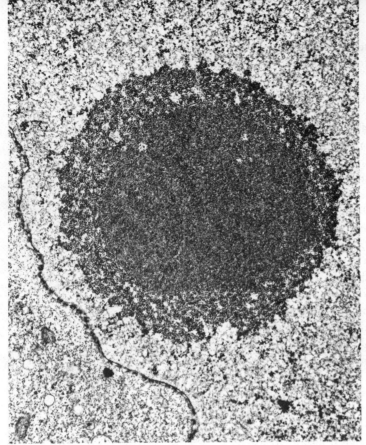

A

4–21   A, an ultrathin section of an extra-chromosomal nucleolus from the oocyte of a salamander to show a compact fibrous core surrounded by a granular cortex (From O. L. Miller and B. Beatty, 1969. J. Cell Physiol. 74 Suppl. 1, 225); B, a portion of the dispersed core of the extrachromosomal nucleolus showing the active (RNA-producing fibrils) and nonactive segments of the DNA. (From O. L. Miller and B. Beatty, 1972. Oogenesis. J. Biggers and A. Schuetz, eds. University Park Press, Baltimore.)

B

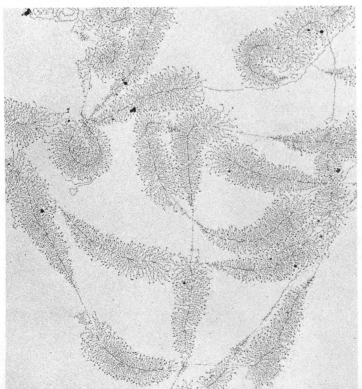

becomes reduced and the lampbrush chromosomes undergo condensation.

OOCYTE MATURATION

When the primary oocyte has reached the end of its growth period, it is ready to undergo the reduction divisions. The resumption of the meiotic process is marked by the breakdown of the germinal vesicle and the migration of the synaptic chromosomal pairs to a position beneath the oolemma. Here, an achromatic figure is formed with the spindle fibers oriented perpendicularly to the surface of the oocyte. The primary oocyte is then divided unequally into a large *secondary oocyte* and a small *polar body (polocyte)*. The second reduction proceeds in a similar fashion, resulting in the production of a mature egg cell (ovum or ootid) with a haploid set of chromosomes. The first polar body may divide to form two polocytes. Theoretically, at least, each primary oocyte produces a mature egg cell and three abortive polar bodies during meiosis (Fig. 4–22).

With the exception of some invertebrates, including the echinoderms, completion of the reduction divisions is dependent upon the entrance of sperm into the egg cell at the time of fertilization. In *Ascaris* (nematode) and *Nereis* (marine annelid), both reduction divisions occur after the sperm cell has been incorporated into the egg cell. In *Styela* the spindle apparatus for the first reduction division is formed as the ovum is discharged into the sea water. Continuation of meiosis is then dependent upon penetration by the male gamete. In *Amphioxus* and most vertebrates, the meiotic process is initiated in the ovary but then arrested in metaphase of the second reduction division. It is still unclear as to why the reduction divisions of the oocyte progress to different stages in different animal species.

The progression of events from breakdown of the membrane of the germinal vesicle through the reduction divisions is known as the period of *oocyte maturation* (nuclear and cytoplasmic). The significance of the breakdown of the germinal vesicle is severalfold. First, the chromosomes are released from the nucleoplasm, thereby permitting their migration to a position beneath the oolemma in anticipation of the physical division of the ovum. Second, the contents of the germinal vesicle appear to be significant to a series of important developmental steps following fertilization, including conditioning of the cytoplasm of the ovum in preparation for cleavage and the early differentiation of specific parts of the embryo. Whether the germinal vesicle material is also necessary to condition the cy-

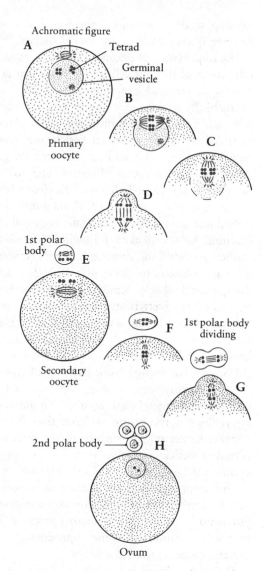

4–22 Reduction divisions in an oocyte. A, an oocyte before the onset of the meiotic divisions showing two tetrads in the germinal vesicle (nucleus) and the achromatic figure; B, C, D, first meiotic divisions; E, the formation of first polar body with achromatic figure in preparation for second meiotic division; F, G, second meiotic division including division of the first polar body; H, meiosis completed.

toplasm so that the ovum can be activated at fertilization remains an open question for many animal species.

The importance of germinal vesicle breakdown for continued development of the egg cell was pointed out at the beginning of this century in classical experiments by Delage on oocytes of *Asterias* (starfish). By shaking ripe ova in a vial, Delage discovered that each cell could be fragmented into two spherical halves. If fragmentation occurred when the germinal vesicle was still intact, it was determined that the nucleated half (i.e., with the germinal vesicle) would cleave after the addition of sperm. The nonnucleated (i.e., without the germinal vesicle) half failed to cleave following exposure to a sperm suspension. However, if fragmentation of mature ova occurred just after dissolution of the germinal vesicle membrane, both resulting halves cleaved following the addition of sperm. These studies provided the first experimental evidence that the ability of the egg cytoplasm to cleave was dependent upon the nucleoplasm of the germinal vesicle. Similar results have been obtained using the eggs of other invertebrates, such as *Nereis* and *Arbacia*.

Several intensive investigations have focused on the mechanisms initiating germinal vesicle breakdown. Kanatani and his colleagues have isolated and purified a *meiosis-inducing factor* or substance (MIS; ovarian factor) from extracts of ripe starfish ovaries. Identified as l-methyladenine, this simple purine base induces dissolution of the nuclear membrane within 30 minutes of treatment. Interestingly, there is increasing evidence that the meiosis-inducing factor appears to act on the surface of the oocyte rather than upon the germinal vesicle directly. It has been suggested, therefore, that events leading to germinal vesicle breakdown are mediated by some substance produced at the surface of the oocyte following stimulation by l-methyladenine. In the intact starfish, a gonadotrophiclike polypeptide (radial nerve factor) released from the radial nerve probably stimulates the production and/or release of 1-methyladenine from the ovary.

Techniques involving removal of the nucleus (*enucleation*) have permitted further examination of the role of the germinal vesicle in oocyte maturation as induced by l-methyladenine. Isolated ova, from which the germinal vesicles were removed, have been treated with l-methyladenine and then exposed to a sperm suspension. Most of the ova become fertilized, based upon elevation of a fertilization membrane. However, none of the fertilized eggs undergo cleavage. Hence, in the starfish, maturation of the cytoplasm for activation (or fertilization) is not dependent upon breakdown of the germinal vesicle.

Studies utilizing the ova of frogs and fishes indicate that the germinal vesicle can be induced to break down by exposure to pituitary extracts. However, the pituitary gonadotrophins do not appear to act directly upon the egg cell to initiate this change. For example, if one removes by dissection the follicle cells surrounding the mature ovum of the frog (*Rana*) and then treats the latter with pituitary hormones, the germinal vesicle of the egg cell remains intact. By contrast, this same "naked" ovum when treated with steroid hormones such as progesterone is induced to undergo meiosis. Results from several investigations, mainly from the laboratories of Smith and Ecker, have shown that pituitary-induced maturation is sensitive to actinomycin D (an inhibitor that blocks the formation of mRNA), but that progesterone-induced maturation is not.

One can conclude that the follicle cells surrounding the frog ovum are stimulated by pituitary hormones to produce mRNA. This mRNA conceivably then directs the synthesis of a progesteronelike substance that is released from the follicle cells. Similar to the system in the echinoderm, the meiosis-inducing factor or progesteronelike substance acts on or just inside the surface of the ovum. Many new kinds of proteins appear in the cytoplasm after stimulation of the egg cell by progesterone. It is suggested that one of these stimulates the breakdown of the germinal vesicle, thereby permitting the mixing of the nucleoplasm with the egg cytoplasm. Cleavage will not occur in the amphibian egg unless this mixing of nucleoplasm and ooplasm is allowed to take place.

OVULATION

The release or discharge of the mature egg through the surface of the ovary is the event known as *ovulation*. In the mammal, as the Graafian follicle swells, it pushes against the surface of the ovary and causes the latter to bulge locally (Fig. 4–23). At this site the wall of the ovary gradually becomes thinner, attenuated, and avascular. Rupture of the ovarian surface and the wall of the Graafian follicle releases the ovum, surrounded by its investment of follicle cells, with the antral fluid into the peritoneal cavity. Although the egg cell is technically liberated into the peritoneal cavity, the favorable positioning in the mammal of the infundibulum of the oviduct virtually assures its reception of the ovulated egg.

The mechanism that stimulates the rupture of the ovarian follicle is still imperfectly understood. Although a sudden elevation in the pressure of the antral fluid was an early hypothesis, it is now not deemed critical to the ovulatory step. There is some evidence to suggest that lytic enzymes, produced under the influence of pituitary hormones, may act to weaken the follicle wall. More recently, stud-

A

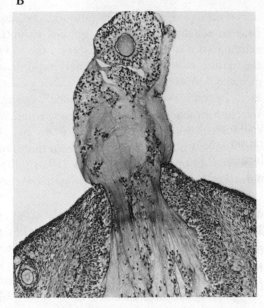

B

4–23 A, photographs showing the sequence of ovulation in the rabbit. The arrow in (1) points to the stigma or site where follicle will rupture along the wall of the ovary. The stigma represents an attenuation of the stratum granulosum and the theca. The arrows in (3) show the expulsion of thin follicular fluid. The egg is finally shed with a surrounding halo of follicle cells (6); B, a micrograph of the cumulus oophorus with follicular fluid being discharged from the ovary in the rabbit. (Courtesy of R. Blandau.)

ies with the electron microscope have shown myofilaments, similar to those in striated muscle, to be present in cells of the connective tissue of the ovary and in the cells of the theca of several mammalian species. These contractile cells may play a functional role in ovulation, but just how and to what extent they are necessary is not clear.

ACCESSORY ENVELOPES

As in the case of the mammalian egg cell, the primary oocyte of most animals becomes surrounded by a series of envelopes during oogenesis. Despite the fact that the subject of egg membranes is an old one, information on their formation is confusing and often contradictory. Hence, there is no general agreement on their nomenclature. We will use the scheme proposed by Ludwig (1874) to classify egg envelopes.

A membrane produced by the oocyte itself is a *primary envelope*. Examples include the *vitelline membrane* of the mature ovum of echinoderms and cephalochordates. In the sea urchin, the vitelline membrane is about 30 Å in thickness and tightly bound to the oolemma. A membrane produced as a result of the secretory actively of follicle cells is termed a *secondary envelope*. Lying between the primary oocyte and the follicular cells, these include the vitelline membrane of insects, molluscs, amphibians, reptiles, and birds; the *chorion* of urochordates and fishes; the *zona pellucida* of mammals; and the *jelly coat* of sea urchins. All of these are noncellular in construction. *Tertiary membranes* are investments added to the ovum after it has been discharged into the oviduct. These include the jelly coats surrounding the frog egg; the leatherylike capsule of the shark egg; and the albumen, shell membranes, and calcareous shell of the chick egg.

Without question the most complicated membranes are found in bird eggs. The innermost membrane is the vitelline membrane. Although initially granular in appearance, a complex system of fibers is deposited in this envelope just before ovulation. Once ovulation has taken place, other membranes are added by the secretory activity of cells of the genital tract (Fig. 4–24). Following the addition to the vitelline membrane of a complex fibrous layer of material, the egg white or albumen is added. Further down the oviduct, two fibrous shell membranes are added to surround the albumen. A calcareous shell is laid down directly onto the outer shell membrane following entrance of the ovum into the uterus. The calcareous membrane is composed chiefly of calcium, the source of which appears to be the long bones of the laying hen. The relationships between these five accessory membranes are summarized in Figure 4–16.

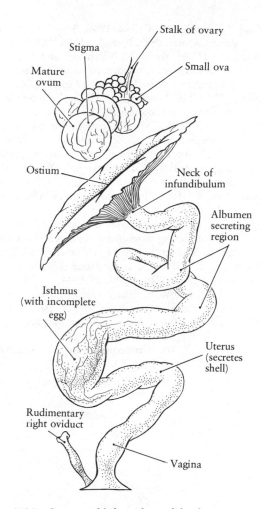

4–24 Ovary and left oviduct of the domestic fowl.

REFERENCES

Anderson, E. and H. Beams. 1960. Cytological observations on the fine structure of the guinea pig ovary with special reference to the oogonium, primary oocyte, and associated follicle cells. J. Ultrastruct. Res. 3:432–446.

Balinsky, B. I. 1975. An Introduction to Embryology. Philadelphia: W. B. Saunders.

Biggers, J. D. and A. W. Schuetz (eds.). 1972. Oogenesis. Baltimore: University Park Press.

Delage, Y. 1901. Etudes experimentales chez les Echinodermes. Arch. Zool. Exp. Gen Ser 9:285–326.

Endo, Y. 1961. Changes in the cortical layer of sea urchin eggs at fertilization as studied with the electron microscope. I. *Clypeaster japonicus*. Exp. Cell Res. 25:383–397.

Gall, J. G. and H. G. Callan. 1962. ³H-Uridine incorporation in lampbrush chromosomes. Proc. Nat. Acad. Sci. U.S.A. 48:562–570.

Kanatani, H., H. Shirai, K. Nahanishi, and T. Kurokawa. 1969. Isolation and identification of meiosis inducing substance in starfish, *Asterias amurensis*. Nature (London). 221:273–274.

Kemp, N. and N. Istock. 1967. Cortical changes in growing oocytes and in fertilized or pricked eggs of *Rana pipiens*. J. Cell Biol. 34:111–121.

Kessel, R. G. 1971. Cytodifferentiation in the *Rana pipiens* oocyte. II. Intramitochondrial yolk. Z. Zellforsch. Mikrosk. Anat. 112:313–331.

Longo, F. J. and E. Anderson. 1974. Gametogenesis. In: Concepts of Development. Eds., J. Lash and J. R. Whittaker. Stamford, Conn.: Sinauer Associates.

Massover, W. 1971. Intramitochondrial yolk crystals of frog oocytes. J. Cell Biol. 48:266–279.

Miller, O. L., B. Beatty, and B. Hamkalo. 1972. Nuclear structure and function during amphibian oogenesis. In: Oogenesis. Eds., J. Biggers and A. Schuetz. Baltimore: University Park Press.

Raven, C. P. 1970. The cortical and subcortex of cytoplasm of the *Lymnaea* egg. Int. Rev. Cytol. 28:1–44.

Smith, L. D. and R. E. Ecker. 1969. Role of the oocyte nucleus in physiological maturation in *Rana pipiens*. Dev. Biol. 19:281–309.

Wilson, E. B. 1896. On cleavage and mosaic-work. Wilhelm Roux' Arch. Entwicklungsmech. Org. 3:19–26.

Zamboni, L. 1970. Ultrastructure of mammalian oocytes and ova. Biol. Reprod. Suppl. 2:44–63.

5

The Physiology of Reproduction

The primary function of the gonads is the production of eggs and sperm. However, both the ovary and the testis also synthesize and secrete hormones whose function is to maintain the reproductive system in a state best suited to promote the development, delivery, and union of the germ cells that the gonads produce.

The sex hormones are given the general names of *androgens,* male producing, and *estrogens,* female producing. Regardless of the sex, both types of hormones are produced in all individuals, although the male produces a preponderance of androgens and the female a preponderance of estrogens.

FEMALE REPRODUCTIVE ACTIVITY

Reproductive activity in the female shows a cyclic pattern of rather complex, interrelated behavior of the ovary, the pituitary gland, the hypothalamus, and the reproductive tract. The ovary and the reproductive tract show periods of activity and inactivity that are marked by and under the control of the cyclic activity of the hypothalamus and the pituitary.

The Estrous Cycle

In nonprimate mammals, the hormonal interplay results in the female periodically reaching a state in which she is receptive to the male. When in this condition, she is said to be in heat or in *estrus* and the cycles are thus termed *estrous cycles.* Estrous cycles in different species vary in length, but essentially they all show the following phases:

1. *Diestrus*—a period of quiescence, which in some species may be prolonged into an extended seasonal period of sexual inactivity termed *anestrus.* During the diestrus, the ovarian follicles are small, the reproductive tract is shrunken and anemic, and the glands of the uterine lining, the endometrium, are collapsed.

2. *Proestrus*—a period of reawakening of reproductive activity just prior to estrus. The ovarian follicles are maturing, the uterine lining is growing rapidly, and its vascularity is increasing.

3. *Estrus*—the period of receptivity and the time when ovulation

occurs. Ovulation is usually spontaneous but in a few species occurs only when induced by copulation. This stage is the continuation and culmination of proestrus; all the manifestations of proestrus reach their peaks in estrus.

4. *Metestrus*—the period following estrus and ovulation when the follicles develop into corpora lutea. If fertilization does not take place, the corpora lutea regress and the reproductive tract returns to its state of quiescence, losing its vascularity and motility.

Thus, the estrous cycle pivots about a periodic attainment of sexual receptivity at which time ovulation takes place. Ovulation is the result of the maturation of the Graafian follicle and the events leading up to ovulation are concerned with follicular growth. This period (proestrus and the beginning of estrus up to the time of ovulation) may be called the *follicular phase* of the cycle. Following ovulation, the corpus luteum becomes the dominant feature of the ovary and, until it regresses, marks the *luteal* phase of the cycle.

In the rat and the mouse, two favorite laboratory animals, estrous cycles are continuous throughout the year. Each cycle lasts four to six days, the estrous phase lasting about 12 hours at which time ovulation occurs spontaneously. These animals are thus continuous breeders. This is the exception to what we see in the natural environment where reproductive activity is generally restricted to a particular season. Seasonal breeders generally reflect a response to the environment in that sexual activity takes place at a time when environmental conditions are most likely to be kindest to the pregnant mother and the newborn offspring. Most mammals in temperate climates bear their young in the spring or summer when conditions for the survival of the young are optimal. Seasonal breeders may be *monestrous*—one cycle per year—or *polyestrous*—a number of consecutive cycles during the breeding season or more than one breeding season per year.

Hormonal Control of the Estrous Cycle
Cyclic activity in the female is controlled by trophic hormones (*gonadotrophins*) secreted by the anterior lobe of the pituitary gland. Following hypophysectomy, all cyclic activity stops but may be restored by injections of the appropriate pituitary extracts. The pituitary gonadotrophins influencing ovarian activity are *follicle-stimulating hormone* (FSH), *luteinizing hormone* (LH) and *luteotrophic* hormone (LTH). The ovary itself secretes *estrogens* and *progesterone* in response to the stimuli of the trophic hormones of the pituitary. These ovarian hormones control the cyclic changes in the reproductive tract that periodically prepare it for the anticipated reception of the fertilized egg.

The blood levels of the ovarian hormones in turn influence the release of the pituitary gonadotrophins. The feedback from the ovary to the pituitary may be positive—resulting in an increase in the release of the trophic hormone—or negative—resulting in a decrease. Although a small part of this ovarian feedback may be ascribed to a direct effect on the pituitary gland itself, the major pathway is through the brain, specifically the *hypothalamus,* a subdivision of the diencephalon. The concept of neural control over gonadotrophin release dates back to the 1940s when it was proposed that specific substances secreted by neurons in the hypothalamus were carried to the pituitary gland by way of a *hypothalamic–hypophyseal portal system.*

The hypothalamus is the region of the diencephalon lying closest to the pituitary gland. In fact, a part of the pituitary gland—its posterior lobe—is formed by a ventral evagination of the hypothalamus, to which it remains attached by a stalk. However, it is the anterior lobe of the pituitary, formed by an evagination of the roof of the oral cavity, which secretes the gonadotrophins. The hypothalamic control over gonadotrophin output is mediated through what are termed neural releasing factors. A specific *LH-releasing factor* (LH-RF) was reported in 1960 and shortly thereafter a *FSH-releasing factor* (FSH-RF) was demonstrated. Although there is considerable evidence in favor of separate LH- and FSH-releasing factors, some investigators propose that only a single combined factor exists.

There are two types of hypothalamic mechanisms controlling the cyclic release of the pituitary gonadotrophins. The first, a tonic control mechanism, stimulates a continuous release of gonadotrophins in quantities sufficient to maintain follicular growth and estrogen secretion. Luteinizing hormone–releasing factor and FSH-RF needed for the tonic control are produced in an area called the *hypophysiotrophic area* (HTA) of the hypothalamus. The HTA is in the median basal region of the hypothalamus and includes the *arcuate* and *ventromedial nuclei* (Fig. 5–1). This region contains neurons that secrete LH-RF and FSH-RF. The releasing factors are transported along the axons and released at the axon terminals from where they pass in the portal circulation to the anterior lobe of the pituitary gland. In addition to the tonic mechanism, a cyclic mechanism also exists. It functions periodically to secrete sufficient additional FSH-RF and LH-RF to induce surges of LH and FSH secretion by the pituitary. These surges occur during estrus, at the time when the follicle is mature, and are the stimulus for ovulation. A different, more rostral region, including the *preoptic* and the *anterior hypothalamic areas* (Fig. 5–1) contains these secretory neurons. Their axons impinge on the neurons of the HTA.

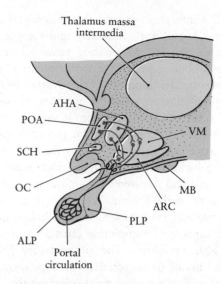

5–1 Diagram of hypothalamic areas secreting tonic and cyclic-releasing factors controlling pituitary gonadotropins. AHA, anterior hypothalamic area; ALP, anterior lobe of pituitary; ARC, arcuate nucleus; MB, mammillary body; OC, optic chiasma; PLP, posterior lobe of pituitary; POA, preoptic area; SCH, superchiasmatic nucleus; VM, ventromedian nucleus.

The interplay between the pituitary, the ovary, and the hypothalamus is still not completely understood; in addition, there are, of course, species differences. However, a generalized pattern, although one certainly not applicable to all species, may be described. The early development of the ovarian follicle proceeds without any trophic influence from the pituitary. However, development beyond the stage at which the ovum is surrounded by four layers of granulosa cells is dependent upon gonadotrophins. In the absence of a negative estrogen feedback to the hypothalamus at the time when the follicle is first developing, increasing amounts of FSH are synthesized and released by the pituitary, stimulating the further development of the follicle. When the theca interna forms, its cells synthesize and release estrogens. Follicle-stimulating hormone alone is not capable of stimulating estrogen secretion. Luteinizing hormone is also necessary. The preovulatory follicle also secretes small amounts of progesterone. The dependence of follicular growth on FSH and of estrogen production on the added stimulus of LH has led to the concept that FSH is primarily a morphogenic hormone and LH is primarily a steroidogenic hormone. The secretion of increasing amounts of estrogen by the maturing follicle exerts a positive feedback effect and results in a surge of gonadotrophin release—both FSH and LH. The LH surge is higher than the FSH, and the two may not be completely coordinated (Fig. 5–2). The LH surge, in spontaneous ovulators, induces ovulation. In the rat, the surge occurs in the afternoon of proestrus and is followed by ovulation about 10 hours later. Luteinizing hormone is secreted in amounts considerably higher than needed, as ovulation can be induced by LH levels much lower than those that normally occur. If LH is blocked, FSH alone can induce ovulation, although under these conditions, the corpus luteum does not develop. Following their preovulatory peaks, both FSH and LH fall to levels comparable to those present before the surge.

During the follicular phase of the cycle, estrogens stimulate uterine growth while during the luteal phase, progesterone stimulates the estrogen-primed uterus to differentiate into an organ optimally prepared to receive and nourish the fertilized egg. Estrogens are primarily growth hormones and progesterone is primarily a differentiation hormone.

The control of the development of the corpus luteum and the secretion of progesterone presents an excellent example of the great diversity in the mechanisms controlling the reproductive cycles in different species. The corpus luteum of the pig is completely autonomous and functions without any trophic stimulus. The guinea pig needs hypophyseal support for only the first three or four days

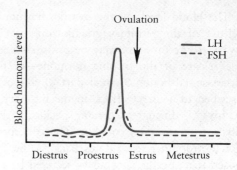

5–2 Schematic diagram of serum concentrations of LH and FSH during the estrous cycle of the rat.

and after this is autonomous. The sheep and the human female require the continual trophic stimulus of LH, while rats and mice require not only LH but also the LTH, *prolactin*.

The length of the luteal phase also shows considerable species variation. In the rat, mouse, and hamster, this phase of the cycle is short, and the corpus luteum regresses after only a brief and insignificant existence. On the other hand, in most domestic animals, such as the sheep, the cow, and the horse, the luteal phase is the longest part of the cycle.

The mechanisms controlling the regression of the corpus luteum are not completely known but may involve a decline in LTH, the appearance of a luteolytic factor, or a combination of both. Considerable species difference again exists, as has been demonstrated by numerous experiments on the effects of hypophysectomy and/or hormone administration on the maintenance of the corpus luteum. An important part of the evidence dates back to Leo Loeb who, in 1923, showed that hysterectomy prolonged the lifespan of the corpus luteum in the ewe. Studies from other laboratories have supported Loeb's observations and shown that in a number of species, including cows, sheep, pigs, and guinea pigs, that the uterus exerts a lytic effect on the corpus luteum. Hysterectomy removes the lytic principle and thereby prolongs the life of the corpus luteum. If only one horn of the uterus is removed, the corpus luteum on the operated side will persist while that on the unoperated side will regress at the normal time. The action is thus a local one. There is some indication that the lytic effect is produced only after the uterus has been exposed to progesterone for a certain length of time. If sheep are given continuous injections of progesterone before they are induced to ovulate, the corpus luteum regresses almost as soon as it is formed. Thus, there appears to be in some species a local utero-ovarian interaction whereby progesterone secreted by the mature corpus luteum induces the synthesis of a lytic agent in the uterine endometrium which, in turn, then "murders" the corpus luteum. The uterus is then implicated as playing an important role in controlling the periodicity of the estrous cycle. However, the evidence is still circumstantial, and it has not been demonstrated unequivocally by extraction, purification, and injection that a specific luteolytic substance exists. Perhaps the best demonstration is seen in the fact that uterine flushings from sows in days 14 to 18 of a 20-day estrous cycle will destroy luteal cells grown in vitro, while flushing at other stages of the cycle will not. Prostaglandin F_{2a} has been proposed as a possible agent, but it requires large amounts of this compound to produce corpus luteum regression experimentally.

The Menstrual Cycle

Cyclic phenomena associated with the reproductive activity of the female also occur in primates. The cycles are called *menstrual* cycles. Their overt manifestation is a periodic *menstruation,* every three to five weeks, associated with a physiological breakdown of the uterine lining (the endometrium) resulting in a blood-stained vaginal discharge, the *menses.*

Menstrual cycles are quite comparable to estrous cycles and are controlled by the same interplay of ovarian, pituitary, and hypothalamic hormones as are the estrous cycles. The menstrual cycle has a preovulatory follicular phase that ends in spontaneous ovulation and is followed by a postovulatory luteal phase, as does the estrous cycle. The major differences between the two are menstruation and the absence of any periodicity of sexual activity in the primates. In the nonprimate mammals, a period of sexual receptivity at which time ovulation occurs, provides a mechanism by which mating takes place only at the time of the cycle most likely to result in fertilization. A considerably higher percentage of fertile mating is then expected, much higher than in the primates, whose time of ovulation bears no relation to mating.

The menstrual cycle is considered to begin on the first day of menstruation. This may be, however, somewhat of an unfortunate choice since, as we shall see, menstruation actually represents the terminal stage of the cycle. The follicular stage of the cycle starts immediately after menstruation. During this stage, the follicles mature under the influence of FSH and small amounts of LH (Fig. 5–3). The follicle secretes large amounts of estrogens and little, if any, progesterone (Fig. 5–3). The estrogens stimulate the rapid growth of the uterine endometrium. New uterine glands are formed which, however, during the follicular phase, do not branch and contain only small amounts of glycogen. Ovulation occurs spontaneously approximately in the middle of the cycle. About 24 hours before ovulation, LH titers start to increase and reach a sharp preovulatory peak in midcycle apparently owing to the influence of increasing amounts of estrogen secreted by the vesicular follicle. The surge in LH secretion lasts for one to three days and is associated with a corresponding increase in FSH secretion. The FSH surge, however, is neither so pronounced nor consistent as the LH surge. Following their midcycle peaks, the levels of both LH and FSH fall to levels lower than those seen during the preovulatory stage.

Following ovulation, the corpus luteum develops and, under the stimulation of LH, secretes increasing amounts of progesterone (Fig. 5–3). In the luteal phase, the reproductive tract, already

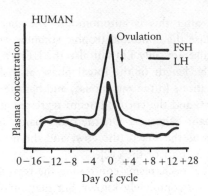

5–3 FSH and LH levels during the menstrual cycle determined by radioimmunoassay of plasma and urinary extracts. (From V. C. Stephans, 1969. J. Clin. Endocrin. 29, 904.)

primed by estrogen, differentiates further under the additional stimulation of progesterone. Development at this time involves cellular changes associated with secretion of the uterine glands rather than with growth. The glands become serrated and branched, the nuclei of their cells assume a basal position characteristic of secretory epithelia, and glycogen is secreted into the lumen of the glands. Secretory activity reaches its maximum about the middle of the luteal phase, at about the time implantation will take place if fertilization occurs during that cycle. If fertilization does not occur, functional degeneration of the corpus luteum begins about 8 to 10 days after ovulation. In the human, hysterectomy has no influence on the lifespan of the corpus luteum, and evidence is against a uterine luteolytic agent causing regression of the corpus luteum. One may then propose the concept of an inherent lifespan of the corpus luteum (certainly an easy way out) or search for other regulatory mechanisms. One suggestion is that regression may be the result of an intraovarian action of steroid hormones, possibly estrogens.

Following the regression of the corpus luteum, the uterine endometrium reacts to the subsequent low levels of progesterone and estrogen by undergoing degenerative changes. The uterine glands involute. Constriction of the muscular walls of certain arteries produces local areas of restricted blood supply (*ischemia*), which leads to necrosis. This breakdown of the endometrial lining results in an extravasation of blood and cellular debris into the uterine lumen and the appearance of a vaginal discharge marking the end of the old cycle—or the beginning of the new. Since the cyclic build up of the uterus is solely in preparation for the reception of the fertilized egg, menstruation has been aptly characterized as the reaction of a disappointed uterus.

Ovulation

There is no external manifestation of ovulation in humans and, it is difficult therefore to pinpoint the time of its occurrence. This is unfortunate, because in any attempt to increase (or decrease) the chance of pregnancy, it is important to be able to predict the time of ovulation with some degree of accuracy. The fertilizable life of the human ovum is no more—and probably less than—48 hours, and that of the sperm is only slightly longer.

One of the earliest methods of attempting to determine the time of ovulation was by daily measurement of early morning body temperature. Temperature changes are, of course, subject to wide variation depending upon a number of circumstances but, in general, it has been shown—following the examination of many temperature graphs—that the temperature is lower during the preovulatory period than following ovulation (Fig. 5–4). In some cases there may even be a small drop in temperature just preceding ovulation. The entire range of the temperature change is not more than 1 to 1.5 degrees and the efficiency of predicting the time of ovulation by this method is not without its pitfalls.

The cyclic secretion of estrogens and progesterone results in characteristic changes of the reproductive tract. In the nonprimate mammal, examination of smears obtained by inserting a cotton swab into the vagina (the *vaginal smear technique*) allows these changes to be used very easily to determine what stage of the estrous cycle the animal is in. However, vaginal cytology in humans has been of little predictive value in determining the time of ovulation, although changes have been shown to occur. Considerable training and experience may enable an examiner to distinguish in general between the estrogenic and progestational phases of the cycle, but this method is of limited value in predicting the time of ovulation.

Another method used to determine changes in hormone levels indirectly has been by noting their effects on the vascularity of the rat ovary. Some investigators have claimed considerable success with this method.

Recently, advances have been made in the methods available for the direct determination of hormone levels in the blood, such as radioimmunoassay. The use of these methods has given a clear-cut picture of changes in hormone levels during the menstrual cycle. For example, the time of the preovulatory surge in LH presents an excellent indication of the midcycle occurrence of ovulation.

Pregnancy is an obvious positive evidence of ovulation and in the case of isolated coitus or artificial insemination may be used to indicate the approximate time of ovulation. Most studies report that insemination results in pregnancy when it takes place around midcycle. Direct observations of the ovary by *culdoscopy* also have confirmed the fact that ovulation occurs near midcycle. It is probable that in the large majority of cases ovulation normally takes place within a rather short period covering from three days before to two days after midcycle. However, deviation from this mean is often considerable and, indeed, ovulation may occur on any day of the cycle. In addition, the length of the menstrual cycles in many women is not regular—particularly in younger women and those approaching menopause—and thus the midcycle time may vary from one cycle to the next. Of course, the precise midcycle time for any given cycle cannot be determined until after the cycle is completed.

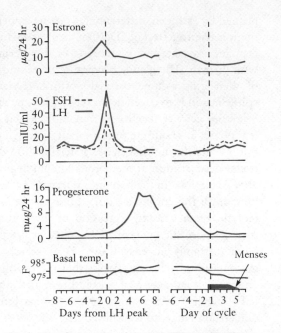

5–4 Basal temperature, serum FSH and LH, and urinary estrone and progesterone concentrations related to LH midcycle peak and days from menstruation. (After U. Goebelsmann, A. R. Midgley, Jr., and R. B. Jaffe, 1969. J. Clin. Endocrin. 29, 1222.)

HORMONES OF PREGNANCY

Human Chorionic Gonadotrophin (HCG)

In the normal menstrual cycle in the absence of pregnancy, the corpus luteum functions in steroidogenesis for only a limited period of less than 10 days before it undergoes regression. However, if fertilization occurs, the corpus luteum does not regress but continues to function throughout pregnancy. The factor responsible for the maintenance of the corpus luteum is introduced by the developing embryo, which begins to implant in the uterine wall about one week after fertilization—about in the middle of the luteal phase of the cycle. Implantation takes place when the embryo is in the blastocyst stage. It consists of a thin-walled vesicle (the trophoblast) enclosing a fluid-filled cavity (the blastocyst cavity) and a small mass of cells at one pole, which will ultimately form the embryo proper. The trophoblast proliferates rapidly after implantation and actively invades the maternal uterine tissues, forming the fetal part of the placenta. The trophoblast—which forms the embryonic membrane called the chorion—secretes a hormone that in the human is called *human chorionic gonadotrophin* (HCG). It is the luteotrophic action of this hormone that maintains the corpus luteum. Human chorionic gonadotrophin is detectable in the maternal blood during the second week of pregnancy, reaches a peak during the 7th and 12th weeks, and then drops sharply to levels about one-fifth to one-tenth of peak values until term (Fig. 5–5).

Human chorionic gonadotrophin resembles LH in many of its actions but also has some of the properties of LTH, one of which is to stimulate the continued secretion of progesterone by the corpus luteum of pregnancy. The precise physiological role of HCG has not yet been determined, although a number of possible functions have been suggested. These include the stimulation of placental steroid synthesis and the stimulation of the growth of the fetal adrenal gland. In addition, HCG may play a role in sex differentiation and in altering the immunological reactivity of the maternal tissues by local immunosuppressive action on the maternal leucocytes in the region of the invading trophoblast.

Pregnancy Tests
Whatever the physiological function of HCG may be, there is no doubt of its value to the obstretician who uses its presence as a basis for pregnancy tests. It might well be stated that HCG is an invention of the obstretician in order to have available a highly reliable method for the early determination of the fact of pregnancy.

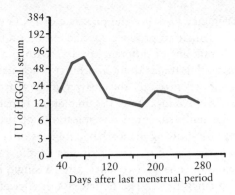

5–5 Ranges in values of urinary excretion of HCG during pregnancy. (From S. Brody and G. Carlstrom, 1965. J. Clin. Endocrin. 25, 792.)

Pregnancy tests use the presence of HCG in the urine of the pregnant female to produce specific effects on the reproductive systems of a number of different species. With our characteristic penchant for getting things done in a hurry, each new pregnancy test that is developed gives us the answer in a shorter period of time. The *Ascheim-Zondek* tests use immature female mice that respond to twice daily subcutaneous injections of pregnancy urine for three days by showing hemorrhagic follicles or corpora lutea when examined on day five. The endpoint of the rabbit (*Friedman*) test is ovulation one to two days after a single intravenous injection of pregnancy urine. The female South African clawed toad responds by ovulating in 12 hours, while the male frog will show sperm in the cloaca in 6 hours if the test is positive.

The more recently developed serological tests are by far the most rapid; the results are available in 10 to 15 minutes. Serological tests involve the capacity of the HCG in pregnancy urine, when mixed with a solution containing HCG antibody, to block this antibody. When the solution containing the blocked antibody is mixed with another solution containing HCG antigen, no precipitate forms. In view of the fact that the pregnant female can now determine in a quarter of an hour that she has eight and a half months before the final outcome, we have here an excellent example of the old saying "hurry up and wait."

Human Chorionic Somatomammotrophin (HCS)

This hormone, detected in the human placenta in the early 1960s, has been shown to have both a somatotrophic and lactogenic effect. It has been variously called human placental lactogen (HPL), chorionic growth hormone-prolactin (CGP), and human chorionic somatomammotrophin (HCS). It is detectable at the sixth week of pregnancy and, unlike HCG, does not peak and then fall, but increases progressively to reach a maximum at about 35 weeks. The increase in HCS parallels the increase in placental mass and the ratio of HSC to placental weight remains constant throughout pregnancy. Its physiological role is not known. It has been suggested that it might function in diverting glucose from maternal to fetal tissues, where the energy requirements are met almost exclusively by the metabolism of glucose.

Human Chorionic Thryotrophin (HCT)

Extracts of the placenta yield a thyrotrophic hormone that has immunological properties relating it to the thyroid-stimulating hormone (TSH) of the adult pituitary. It reaches its highest level of concentration during the first two months and then declines progressively. Its role is also in doubt, although it may be responsible, in part, for the early development of the fetal thyroid gland, whose follicles develop and become functional two or three weeks before the fetal pituitary begins to secrete TSH.

Steroid Hormones

Although the trophic hormones discussed above are synthesized directly by the placenta, many of the steroid hormones synthesized during pregnancy require interplay between fetal and placental tissues. Progesterone is one exception to this and like the placental trophic hormones is synthesized independently of the fetal tissues other than those contributing to the placenta. The synthesis of other steroid hormones requires the functioning of what has been called the *fetoplacental unit* or *complex*. Many steroid hormones are formed during pregnancy, including estrogens, progestogens, androgens, and corticoids. We will consider only estrogens and progesterone.

Progesterone

Steroid synthesis in the placenta and the fetoplacental unit involves the same pathways as in the adult, starting with the 2-carbon *acetate* molecule to synthesize the 27-carbon *cholesterol* with its steroid configuration. Although cholesterol is found in the placenta, it has been shown that the placenta cannot synthesize this compound itself and must get it from the maternal circulation or from the fetus. The fetal liver rapidly converts acetate to cholesterol. In the placenta, cholesterol is converted into progesterone.

Estrogens

In the synthesis of the three main estrogens—*estrone, estradiol,* and *estriol*—some of the steps occur in the fetal liver and adrenal and some in the placenta. There is a back-and-forth transfer of compounds from fetus to placenta. In each location, a step or steps takes place until finally, through the mutual effort, the definitive compound is formed. Neither the fetus nor the placenta alone is capable of synthesizing the product.

There is a progressive rise in the urinary excretion of estrogens throughout pregnancy. Levels are low during the first trimester, increase after the 10th to 12th week, and show a sharp rise during the last 3 to 4 weeks. Some 20 different estrogens have been isolated from late pregnancy urine. Of these, estriol is the most abundant.

PARTURITION

After the fetus has developed to term, there remains still one final process, birth or *parturition*. Parturition has been extensively investigated and although a number of processes have been suggested as important precursors of this event, parturition has not been shown to be the result of any single causative agent or process. Rather, it is more probable that many processes may be involved. They lead by a series of interrelated events to the final common pathway, which is the contraction of the smooth muscle of the uterine wall resulting in the expulsion of the fetus.

Throughout gestation the mass of the fetus increases, and the purely mechanical stimulus of stretching the uterine walls that results may be a factor. However, more emphasis on biological factors, particularly hormonal levels, has been stressed. This is not to say that hormonal events are the only ones involved, although it is probable that they are the most important—and certainly the most interesting.

Analysis of changes in estrogen and progesterone levels late in gestation and the effects of these hormones on the response of the uterine muscle to the posterior pituitary hormone, *oxytocin,* have suggested a possible mechanism for the induction of labor. Throughout most of gestation, the uterus accommodates to the expanding fetus and remains relatively quiescent. During this time, the uterus is dominated by progesterone, and substances—such as oxytocin—which normally stimulate uterine muscular contraction, are prevented from doing so. At term, progesterone levels fall and estrogen levels peak, and now the uterus becomes estrogen-dominated and sensitive to muscle stimulants. Analysis of hormone levels in a number of different species, particularly the sheep and goat, shows that serum progesterone levels fall and estrogen levels rise just prior to the onset of labor and thus support his proposal. However, in the human, analysis of hormone levels has yielded controversial results, and evidence is not so satisfactory nor so conclusive as it is in other species.

An additional facet was introduced when it was suggested, mainly from work on the sheep, that the signal for the initiation of labor came from the fetus. The signal is a rise in *corticosteroids* secreted by the fetal adrenal. Experimental evidence shows that fetal hypophysectomy or adrenalectomy prolong pregnancy, while maternal hypophysectomy or adrenalectomy have no effect on the onset of labor. Fetal adrenocorticotrophic levels rise during the last half of pregnancy and the fetal adrenal cortex doubles in size during the last 10 days of pregnancy. Not only is labor preceded by a rise in fetal corticosteroids, but also injection of corticosteroids will induce labor. Liggins (1972) proposed that one function of the fetal corticosteroids in the initiation of labor could be to inhibit progesterone either by a direct inhibition of the progesterone effect on uterine muscle or by an inhibition of progesterone synthesis or metabolism. Increases in fetal corticosteroids would also increase the synthesis of estrogens. Again, the evidence on fetal hormone levels in humans, which is necessarily scant, is not conclusive and neither supports nor denies this hypothesis.

Prostaglandins present another link in the chain. In the sheep, the onset of labor is associated with an increase in PGF_{2a} in the maternal placenta, uterine myometrium, and uterine venous blood. The fetal adrenal may also be a factor in this event. Secretions from the fetal adrenal increase the rate of synthesis of prostaglandins in maternal tissues. Also, infusion of the pregnant ewe with prostaglandins will induce labor. The site of formation of the prostaglandins that may play a role in labor is not known, but the uterus and the maternal placenta are suggested as possibilities. Prostaglandins could function by increasing uterine muscle contractability by lowering the threshold of response to oxytocin. In line with the estrogen and progesterone changes at parturition, estrogen is known to stimulate prostaglandin release while progesterone has an inhibitory effect.

We can consider the initiation of labor as the result of a series of events leading to a final process, contraction of the uterine musculature. These events are not necessarily the same in all species. In any one species, a certain event or process may be more important than in another. It is possible to list events that have been described as occurring in some species, but not in all, in a sequence to suggest a possible chain of events leading up to parturition.

1. Throughout most of pregnancy, the uterus is under the influence of progesterone secreted by the placenta. Progesterone decreases uterine sensitivity to muscle stimulators and maintains the uterus in a quiescent state.

2. As pregnancy progresses, more and more ACTH is secreted by the fetal pituitary. The fetal adrenal cortex responds to this by showing an increase in mass and finally, near term, an increase in the output of corticosteroids.

3. Fetal corticosteroids decrease the synthesis, inhibit the action or change the metabolism of progesterone and increase the synthesis of estrogens and prostaglandins.

4. Fall in progesterone activity and rise in estrogens result in the release of the uterine muscle from progesterone inhibition. This allows the muscle to respond to muscle stimulants such as oxytocin.

5. Prostaglandins, also under progesterone and estrogen control,

are released, mainly from the maternal placenta, in increasing amounts; and they also act to lower the threshold of response to agents stimulating muscle contraction. The uterine muscle now begins the contractions characteristic of labor.

All of these events have been described in one species or another as occurring during or prior to parturition. They appear to be arranged in a logical time sequence, but whether or not they all occur in humans is not known. In this concept, the dramatic onset of labor, which we associate with the beginning of uterine contractions, is considered as only the final step of a gradual process taking place over the final weeks of pregnancy. It is not necessarily associated with sharp fluctuations in hormonal levels. It is characterized by gradual progressive change in the levels of a number of different hormones of the fetus and the placenta, occurring as a chain of interrelated events climaxing in the onset of uterine contractions.

MALE REPRODUCTIVE ACTIVITY

In nature, the basic pattern of reproductive activity in the male is also cyclic. Mature sperm are produced only during the breeding season. In domestic animals and in laboratory animals, spermatogenesis continues throughout the year, and mature sperm are always present in the testes and the epidiymis.

It was first demonstrated in 1927 by P. E. Smith, and has been repeatedly confirmed since, that both the spermatogenic and secretory functions of the tests are under the control of pituitary gonadotrophins. The same pituitary trophic hormones that are known to be active in the female are also found to be present in the male, with FSH functioning in the support of spermatogenic activity and LH, sometimes referred to as *interstitial cell-stimulating hormone* (ICSH), functioning in the support of secretory activity.

Control of Spermatogenesis

Hormonal Factors
Although spermatogonia are present in the testes of the newborn and undergo some mitotic activity in prepuberal males, the formation of mature sperm does not take place until the age of puberty— 12 to 15 years in man. In the mature testes, spermatogonial divisions and maturation to the prophase of the primary spermatocyte are independent of any hormonal control. Development from this stage through both meiotic divisions and the early and middle stages of spermatid maturation are dependent upon adequate levels

of testosterone, while the final stages of spermiogenesis require FSH. In the hypophysectomized male treated with LH, spermatogenesis will proceed through the early and middle stages of spermiogenesis because of the stimulatory effect of LH on the secretion of testosterone, but FSH must be supplied if the final stages are to be completed.

Nonhormonal Factors

The testes are normally found in the scrotal sacs outside of the body cavity. In some seasonal breeders the testes move out of the scrotal sacs and into the abdominal cavity during the nonbreeding season. When in this location, spermatogenic activity ceases. Positioning of the testes within the abdominal cavity (cryptorchidism) may be experimentally produced in laboratory animals. This operation results in a cessation of spermatogenic activity and, if the condition is prolonged, all of the epithelial cells of the seminiferous tubules, with the exception of the Sertoli cells, degenerate. The reason for this can be found in the rather small temperature difference (2.2°C) between the abdominal cavity and the scrotum. Testicular transplants to locations within the abdominal cavity results in a loss of spermatogenic activity, but transplants to the anterior chamber of the eye or to the scrotum function normally. Heat applied directly to the testes is also effective in inhibiting sperm development.

Dietary factors are also important. Inanition or protein depletion depress spermatogenic activity. This effect, however, is not direct but is mediated through a depression in gonadotrophin secretion. Vitamin A and E deficiencies also depress spermatogenesis, the depression in the case of vitamin A being reversible and that of vitamin E irreversible.

Other pituitary-mediated depressors of spermatogenesis are confinement and estrogen, the latter through its negative feedback effect. A number of nonsteroidal compounds are also known to inhibit gonadotrophin secretion.

Some disease organisms also have an adverse effect on the testes. One in particular is the causative agent of infectious mononucleosis, a disease quite common in college students. This disease has been known to result in a 10-fold reduction in the number of sperm per ejaculate as well as a marked increase in the percentage of abnormal sperm.

Concern about population growth has led to a search for chemical compounds that might be used to regulate spermatogenic activity and many compounds have been found which are effective in experimental animals. Compounds acting on almost every step in spermatogenesis have been tested. Alkylating agents, such as nitrogen mustard and esters of sulfonic acid, are radiomimetic drugs that inhibit mainly the division of the spermatogonia. Some heterocyclic compounds (nitrofurans, dinitropyrroles) have been shown to inhibit meiotic divisions, while others (diamines) exert their influence at the level of spermatid maturation. However, unfortunately, most of the tested compounds are active at levels close to toxic, and many of them produce undesired side effects, among them antibuse action. Although to date no satisfactory male "pill" has been produced, a number of these have found application as chemisterilants in insect, rodent, and parasite control.

Control of Secretory Activity

It has been known since "days of old," from castration experiments on man and animals, that the testis is responsible for the maintenance of the male reproductive tract and the male sexual characteristics. However, knowledge of the mechanisms of this control, the hormones involved, the cells responsible for the synthesis of these hormones, and the control of this synthesis has been only recently acquired.

The Leydig cells (interstitial cells) of the testis are the cells responsible for the secretion of the male hormone. These cells appear in clusters between the seminiferous tubules (Fig. 3–1). In the late 1920s it was established that the androgenic hormone secreted by the Leydig cells was testosterone and that these cells were under the trophic influence of the anterior pituitary gonadotrophin, LH. In hypophysectomized animals, LH will maintain the synthesis and secretion of testosterone by the Leydig cells; in this manner the sex ducts and accessories are also maintained.

REFERENCES

Diczfalusy, E. 1969. Steroid metabolism in the foetoplacental unit. Excerpta Med. Int. Congr. Ser. 183:65–109.

Gallagher, T. F. and F. C. Koch. 1929. The testicular hormone. J. Biol. Chem. 84:495–500.

Igarashi, M. and S. M. McConn. 1964. A hypothalamic follicle stimulating hormone-releasing factor. Endocrinology 74:446–456.

Ingram, D. L. 1953. The effect of hypophysectomy on the number of oocytes in the adult albino rat. J. Endocrinol. 9:307–311.

Klopper, A. 1974. The hormones of the placenta and their role in the onset of labour. MTP International Review of Science. Reproductive Physiology Series One, 8th ed. Ed., R. O. Greep.

Liggins, G. C. 1972. Endocrinology of the foeto-maternal unit. In: Human Reproductive Physiology, pp. 138–197. Ed., R. P. Shearman. London: Blackwell Scientific Publications.

Liggins, S. C. 1973. Endocrine Factors in Labour. Eds., A. Klopper and J. Gardner. Bristol: Cambridge University Press.

McConn, S. M., S. Taleisnik, and H. M. Friedman. 1960. LH-releasing activity in hypothalamic extracts. Proc. Soc. Exp. Biol. Med. 104: 432–434.

Schally, A. V., A. Arimura, A. J. Kastin, H. Matsuo, Y. Bara, T. W. Redding, R. M. G. Nair, L. Debelyuk, and W. F. White. 1971. Gonadotropin-releasing hormone: One polypeptide regulates secretion of lutenizing and follicle-stimulating hormones. Science 173:1087–1094.

Smith, P. E. 1927. The disabilities caused by hypophysectomy and their repair. J. Am. Med. Assoc. 88:158–161.

Steinberger, E. and A. Steinberger. 1974. Hormonal control of testicular function in mammals. In: Handbook of Physiology-Endocrinology, IV, Part 2, pp. 325–345. Eds., R. O. Greep and E. B. Astwood. Baltimore: Williams and Wilkins.

6

Fertilization

Fertilization is the process by which the sperm initiates and partici-pates in the development of the egg. Penetration of the egg by the sperm results in the initiation of a series of reactions that indicate the beginning of the development of the zygote. This phase of fertil-ization is known as *activation*. Following penetration and activa-tion of the egg, the male and female pronuclei approach each other and fuse to form the zygote nucleus. Fusion of the nuclei is termed *amphimixus* or *syngamy*. Although we may then ask whether we should consider the act of fertilization as occurring at the time the sperm penetrates the egg or at the time of amphimixus, it is best to consider all of the events starting with the approach of the sperm to the egg and ending with the fusion of the pronuclei under the head-ing of the fertilization process.

Fertilization has three distinct results. It activates the egg. It re-stores the diploid number and provides the male side of the genetic material to the system. In many species, it supplies the central body necessary for cell division, although there is some question whether or not this occurs in the mammal.

Fertilization may take place either inside or outside the body of the maternal parent. Interestingly, in those forms in which fertiliza-tion takes place outside of the body, we may correlate the number of eggs shed with the mating behavior of the parents. Where there is little close contact between the male and the female and the sperm are liberated merely in the general proximity of the ova, the female often releases many thousands of eggs. Such is the case in many in-vertebrates. Even a vertebrate such as the codfish sheds over a mil-lion eggs at a single ovulation. In other forms, the eggs may be de-posited in a specific location to await fertilization. Here the number of eggs may be reduced to one or two thousand. In species charac-terized by a more intimate relationship between the male and the female, the male clasps the female forcing the eggs out and fertiliz-ing them as they are shed, the number of eggs released may be a hundred or less. This type of behavior is seen in the Siamese fight-ing fish and in some amphibia.

For those forms that do not shed their eggs into an aquatic envi-ronment, internal fertilization is necessary. Following fertilization, the young may be carried within the mother and born at an ad-vanced stage of development, a process known as *viviparity*. On the other hand, the fertilized egg may be enclosed in protective envelopes and laid and allowed to develop outside of the mother, a process known as *oviparity*. Internal fertilization requires the development of a copulatory apparatus by means of which the sperm are deposited within the genital tract of the female. This process is termed *semination* and should not be confused with fertilization. Internal fertilization is characteristic of all forms above the amphibians, although it is not restricted to these species—as anyone who has raised tropical fish well knows.

EGG-SPERM INTERACTING SUBSTANCES

Since, by definition, fertilization begins with the approach of the sperm to the egg, we must first consider what is occurring at this time. This involves a study of the chemical substances that are carried or secreted by the eggs and the sperm and that play various roles in the fertilization process. The first comprehensive theory of fertilization involving the interplay of egg and sperm substances was introduced by F. R. Lillie (1919). He proposed a quite ingenious scheme with a major role assigned to an egg substance that he called *fertilizin*—thus labeling his theory as the *fertilizin theory*. The theory was based on his observations of the effect of "egg water"—obtained by allowing sea urchin eggs to stand in sea water—on sperm introduced into the water after the eggs were removed. Lillie proposed that egg water had three effects on sperm—attraction, activation, and agglutination. He postulated that fertilizin was a diffusible component of the egg surface and that fertilization was a species specific reaction between fertilizin in the egg and a complementary factor, *antifertilizin,* present in the sperm head.

Egg Substances—Attraction

Although attractive substances are often of importance in plants, particularly in ferns and mosses—where one such substance has been given the appropriate name of sirenin—there is considerable evidence that the eggs of most animals do not exert any attractive influence on the sperm. Anyone seeing the large numbers of sperm clustered around the egg has no difficulty understanding how someone could propose that eggs attract sperm. However, experimental results that have been advanced in support of attraction have proved to be inconclusive insofar as the eggs of most animals are concerned. In a number of species of *Hydrozoa,* however, the gonangia (the egg-containing organs) are known to secrete a chemical substance that both activates and attracts the sperm. Sperm in the vicinity of the gonangia—or in the vicinity of extracts of the gonangia—exhibit directional turning toward the attractive substance, which is a low molecular weight, heat-stable compound. Chemotaxis in these hydroids was at first thought to be species specific and therefore of possible importance in discouraging cross-fertilization, but was later shown not to be so.

Egg Substances—Activation

Sperm are normally active cells. Thus, an increase in activity as the result of exposure to egg substances is somehwat difficult to evaluate. However, there is little doubt that sperm activity is increased by egg secretions in many species. This becomes especially evident if sperm are allowed to age after their release before exposure to egg substances. Aged sperm are almost immotile, but when exposed to egg water, they show marked and easily noticeable increases in movement. Oxygen consumption may be used as an indication of increased activity and a fourfold increase in oxygen uptake has been reported in sea urchin sperm exposed to egg water. Again, increases in oxygen consumption are more apparent when aged sperm are used.

Attempts have been made to determine the chemical composition of the egg substance that increases sperm activity. The activating substance and the agglutinating substance are normally bound together but may be split by a number of physical and chemical methods. Good evidence suggests that these two substances are chemically different. Chemical analysis of fertilizins in general indicate that they are glycoproteins of high molecular weight which yield on hydrolysis a number of amino acids, one or a few monosaccharides, and considerable sulfate. Since the amino acids and the monosaccharides vary from species to species, we properly speak of fertilizins rather than a single compound, fertilizin.

Egg Substances—Agglutination

Although not of universal occurrence, sperm-agglutinating substances have been found in the eggs of a variety of species including echinoderms, molluscs, annelids, tunicates, and many vertebrates. When sperm are exposed to homologous egg water, they immediately lose their motility and clump together in groups, a reaction for which the agglutinating factor is responsible. In the sea urchin, agglutination reverses itself spontaneously. This has been explained on the basis of a mutual multivalence theory using concepts employed in antigen-antibody reactions. The reacting molecules are pictured as being multivalent with respect to their combining groups (Fig. 6–1). Large groups of sperm are thus built up as the fertilizin molecules combine with the sperm and bind them together (Fig. 6–1). Reversibility occurs as the result of the splitting of the multivalent agglutinin into univalent molecules attached to individual sperm (Fig. 6–1). After this spontaneous reversal, the sperm have their reacting groups occupied and as a result of this, although they are still motile, they have lost their fertilizing power and also cannot be agglutinated again by fresh egg water. In favor of this explanation is the fact that agglutinating egg water may be made nonagglutinating by treatment with heat, ultraviolet or x-rays, or proteolytic enzymes. Sperm exposed to egg water so treated, although they are not agglutinated and retain their motility, lose their fertilizing ability. The bonds in the fertilizin molecule broken by these treatments, which thus converts the compound into a univalent configuration, are assumed to be the same as those broken by the sperm, either mechanically or enzymatically, in spontaneous reversal.

Recently, it has been proposed that in the sea urchin. *Strongylocentrotus purpuratus,* agglutination is actually the swarming of freely moving sperm toward a common focus. The clusters containing motile sperm always remain spherical in shape even as more sperm join up, implying that the sperm are continually changing their positions. Sperm motility is necessary for this reaction and, if inhibitors of sperm motility are added, agglutination does not occur. However, this proposal is not supported by investigation in the starfish, *Asterias amurensis,* where antimotility agents have no effect on agglutination. Before the classical fertilizin-antifertilizin isoagglutination scheme—which is supported by a wealth of experimentation—can be questioned seriously, much more evidence must be introduced.

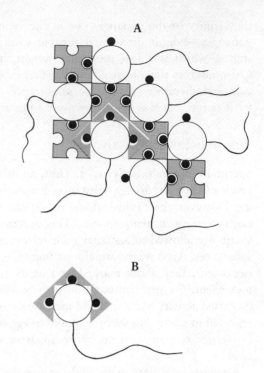

6–1 Reversible agglutination. A, multivalent fertilisin molecules agglutinate sperm; B, motile sperm with receptors covered by univalent agglutinin.

Sperm Substances—Antifertilizin

Antifertilizin, the sperm substance with which fertilizin reacts, can be assayed by its ability to neutralize the agglutinating action of fertilizin. Antifertilizin also has the capacity to agglutinate suspensions of eggs, and in this process a precipitation membrane is formed on the jelly coat. Chemical analysis of antifertilizin extracted from sperm show it to be an acidic protein of low molecular weight containing about 16 percent nitrogen.

Sperm Substances—Membrane-Penetrating Substances

Sperm have been shown to carry a number of substances other than antifertilizin. Many eggs are surrounded by tough membranes which, although they serve to protect the egg, also act as barriers to the penetration of the sperm. In order to reach the inside of the egg, sperm must have the means of overtaking these barriers. This is accomplished by a number of different kinds of penetrating agents carried by the sperm head.

Lytic Substances in Some Invertebrates

In general, the membranes of invertebrate eggs are not so complicated as those of the mammals and the sperm do not need to secrete lytic substances in order to penetrate through them to the surface of the egg. However, this is not true of all species. The keyhold limpet, *Megathura crenulata,* has a tough membrane that is resistant to strong acids but is broken down in seconds by lytic agents of the sperm. Sperm lysins have also been demonstrated in a number of other species including the mussel (*Mytilus*), the abalone (*Haliotis*), and the polychaete worm (*Hydroides*). In some species, the sperm leave distinct holes in the membranes after they have passed through. However, in other species—those of the echinoderms for example—the results are not so clear-cut and there is evidence both for and against the presence of lytic enzymes, which aid in sperm penetration.

Sperm Penetration in Mammals

As has been described in Chapter 4, the mammalian egg, after ovulation, is enclosed in its plasma membrane outside of which are found the noncellular zona pellucida and a number of layers of follicle cells forming the corona radiata and the cumulus oophorus. A sperm must pass through all three of these membranes, and it does so by virtue of three different enzymes that it carries. The outer follicle cells are interspersed in a ground substance that is a mucopolysaccharide containing considerable hyaluronic acid. Hyaluronic acid is a component of the ground substance of all connective tissue. It can be broken down by *hyaluronidase,* an enzyme similar to one found in snake venom. When carbon particles and hyaluronidase are injected into an animal subcutaneously, the carbon particles penetrate for considerably greater distances than when they are injected alone. For this reason, the term "spreading factor" has been applied to hyaluronidase. Hyaluronidase has been extracted from testicular tissue and has been localized on the head of the sperm, specifically in the acrosome. Release of hyaluronidase from the acrosome breaks down the intercellular connections of the cumulus cells and allows the sperm to penetrate between the cells to the corona layer.

Sperm, in turn, penetrate the corona radiata by releasing a second enzyme, called *corona-penetrating enzyme* (CPE). The mechanism

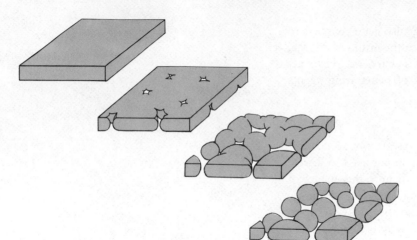

of penetration also involves an attack on the ground substance. Although CPE has not been chemically identified, there is no question that it is different from hyaluronidase.

The release of hyaluronidase and CPE occurs by means of a process called membrane vesiculation. It is accomplished by multiple fusions of two membranes situated in close apposition to each other. The process is diagrammed in Figure 6–2. Individual breakthroughs and fusions result in a fenestrated double-walled membrane and, as the process continues, the result is the development of individual separated double-walled vesicles. The membranes involved in the case of the sperm are the plasma membrane on the outside and the outer acrosomal membrane on the inside. Electron microscope studies have shown that sperm outside of the cumulus oophorus show no morphological difference from epididymal sperm. However, EM photographs of sperm penetrating the corona radiata and of sperm up against the zona pellucida show small individual vesicles over the anterior half of the sperm previously enclosed in the plasma and outer acrosomal membranes (Figs. 6–3, 4). At the equator of the sperm the outer acrosomal membrane becomes continuous with the plasma membrane; thus the sperm is still enclosed in a single continuous membrane. Over the posterior half of the head, posterior to the location of the broken-down acrosome, this membrane is the plasma membrane while over the anterior half it is the inner acrosomal membrane. Vesiculation and the formation of the composite sperm covering is illustrated diagrammatically in Figure 6–5. Vesiculation is considered to be a process that results in a slow progressive release of the acrosomal enzymes.

The final barrier is the zona pellucida. This calls into action an-

6–3 Vesiculation of the acrosomal membrane and the sperm plasma membrane over the anterior portion of the mouse sperm. Over the posterior region the membranes are still intact. (From J. M. Bedford, 1968. Am. J. Anat. 123, 329.)

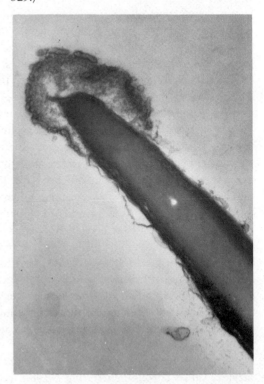

other enzyme, which is presumed to be located on the inner acrosomal membrane. Slits are seen in the zona pellucida after sperm penetration and are indicative of an enzymatic breakdown of the zona substance. This enzyme shows a close similarity to pancreatic trypsin as determined by inhibitor studies, amino acid analyses, and immunodiffusion tests, a quite remarkable finding in view of the different origins and functions of these enzymes. The enzyme has been called a number of different names including trypsinlike enzyme (TLE) and acrosin. The International Committee on Biochemical Nomenclature has proposed the use of the name *acrosomal proteinase,* which is indicative of both its origin and its proteolytic effect on the zona pellucida.

CAPACITATION

Penetration of the egg membranes thus occurs by means of the action of various enzymes released as the acrosome undergoes vesiculation. However, before the acrosomal reaction can occur, sperm must undergo a process known as *capacitation.* In most nonprimate mammals, mating is timed so that it takes place before ovulation and sperm are present in the uterine tubes for some time before the arrival of the ovum. This turns out to be a necessary condition of the fertilization process because, if animals are mated at the time of ovulation or if freshly ejaculated sperm are placed in the uterine tubes, fertilization does not occur. Capacitation represents a change in the sperm to make them capable of fertilizing the ovum. The length of time necessary for capacitation varies in different species, being one hour in the mouse, six hours in the rabbit, and seven hours in man.

The question then arises, "Why do sperm have to be capacitated?" The answer is related to the all-important acrosome reaction. Sperm that have not been capacitated will not undergo an acrosome reaction and are incapable of penetrating the egg membranes. In sperm that have not undergone capacitation, the breakdown of the acrosome does not occur because, as sperm pass through the male reproductive tract, they are exposed to what has been termed a *decapacitating factor* (DF). Decapacitating factor is found throughout the male reproductive tract and, in fact, capacitated sperm may become decapacitated when reexposed to DF in epididymal fluid or seminal plasm. Capacitation thus involves the removal or inactivation of a DF imposed on the sperm in the male reproductive tract.

Some physiological significance of decapacitation is seen in that it (1) prolongs life of the sperm, (2) prevents sperm from penetrating

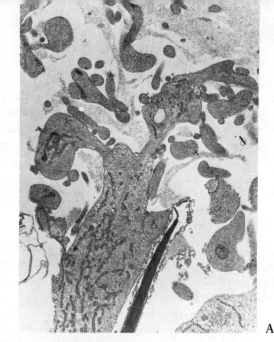

A

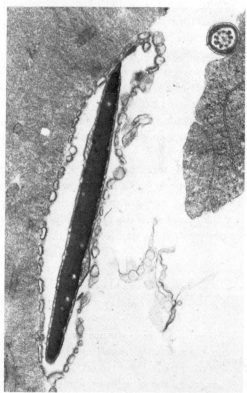

B

6-4 A, vesiculation of the anterior acrosomal cap of the rabbit sperm as it passes through the corona cells toward the zona pellucida; B, vesiculation of the acrosome of the rabbit sperm lying against the zona pellucida. (From J. M. Bedford, 1968 Am. J. Anat. 123, 329.)

the lining cells of the male and female reproductive tracts through which they pass, (3) prevents sperm agglutination, and (4) prevents phagocytosis of the sperm in the female reproductive tract.

It has also been shown that sperm must reside within the female reproductive tract in order to bring about the conversion of the enzymatically inactive proacrosin present in the ejaculated sperm to acrosin. Wineck et al. (1979) have demonstrated that the uterine factor which promotes this conversion is a glycosaminoglycan.

FUSION OF THE GAMETES

After the breakdown of the acrosome and the release of the enzymes contained therein have resulted in the sperm penetrating through the outer membranes of the egg down to the egg plasma membrane, the next step is the passage of the sperm through the plasma membrane into the egg cytoplasm. However, this does not involve a simple penetration of the sperm through the plasma membrane but rather a fusion of the sperm and the egg plasma membranes to form a common membrane. This is followed by the movement of the sperm nucleus, neck, and midpiece into the egg cytoplasm. Electron microscope studies of fertilization in the rodent show that a side-to-side contact is made (Fig. 6–6). The region that establishes and maintains contact is the postacrosomal part of the sperm. This is also the area where initial fusion of the sperm and the egg plasma membranes occurs, eventually enclosing the egg and the sperm in a single common mosaic membrane (Fig. 6–7).

Very soon after the sperm enters the egg cytoplasm its nuclear membrane disappears and its previously dense chromatin material begins to become loose in texture and filamentous in form. The entire sperm is incorporated into the egg cytoplasm (Fig. 6–8) but only the head forms the male pronucleus. The midpiece and the entire tail (with the possible exception of the centriole) degenerate.

MORPHOLOGICAL ASPECTS OF FERTILIZATION IN SOME INVERTEBRATES

Electron microscope studies of fertilization in many invertebrate species have given a somewhat different picture than that described for the mammal. The first accurate analysis of the structure of the acrosome and the morphology and significance of the acrosomal reaction were provided by the Colwins in the early 1960s in studies on two species of invertebrates, *Hydroides* (a marine annelid) and

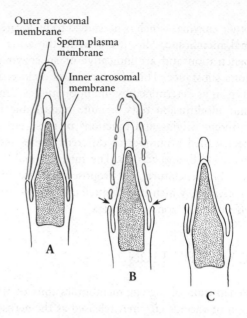

Outer acrosomal membrane
Sperm plasma membrane
Inner acrosomal membrane

A   B   C

6–5 Diagrammatic representation of vesiculation resulting in release of the acrosomal contents and exposure of the inner acrosomal membrane. At the arrow, fusion of outer acrosomal and sperm membranes.

6–6 Head of mouse sperm lying parallel to the surface of the egg. The rows of small vesicles are the remnants of the vesiculated sperm plasma membrane and the outer acrosomal membrane. (From M. Stefanini, C. Oura, and L. Zamboni, 1969. J. Submicrosc. Cytol. 1, 1.)

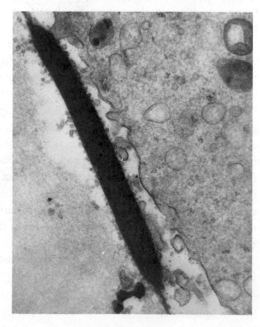

Saccoglossus (a hemichordate). Since then, numerous studies have shown that there is a similarity of acrosomal structure and function in a variety of invertebrates.

Fertilization in the Sand Dollar (*Echinarachnius parma*)

Acrosomal Structure

The acrosomal region (Figs. 6–9 A, 6–10 A) consists of a membrane-bound acrosomal vesicle and periacrosomal material. The acrosomal vesicle, the most anterior part of the sperm, lies just beneath the sperm plasma membrane. It is almost spherical but somewhat flattened posteriorly. Within the vesicle is a granule separated from the anterior half of the vesicle membrane by an EM lucid area but continuous with the basal part of the vesicle membrane through a more EM dense region. Periacrosomal material surrounds the vesicle, but the bulk is contained in a depression on the anterior surface of the nucleus.

The Acrosomal Reaction

The acrosomal reaction, induced by extracellular egg substances, takes place as the sperm approaches the egg. It may easily be induced by egg water. The reaction consists of a breakdown of both the sperm plasma membrane, and the acrosomal vesicle membrane and their fusion to each other in a circular area below the middle of the acrosomal vesicle (Figs. 6–9 B,C; 6–10). The region of this fusion, which the Colwins have termed the "rim of dehiscence," is evident in the unreacted sperm. In the process of this fusion, the anterior halves of both the sperm plasma membrane and the acrosomal vesicle membrane are lost, and the contents of the acrosomal vesicle are exposed. The basal part of the acrosomal vesicle membrane everts to begin the formation of an acrosomal tubule. This tubule elongates rapidly carrying with it the adherent acrosomal vesicle material (Figs. 6–9 C,D; 6–10 D,E).

Microfilaments at the base of the acrosomal tubule are apparent early in its formation. They have also been described in other invertebrates and found to contain the contractile protein, actin, as a principal component.

Attachment and Penetration

The acrosomal tubule penetrates through the egg jelly to reach the vitelline membrane. The acrosomal vesicle material adherent to the tubule is the first sperm product to reach the vitelline membrane, and it forms a morphological complex with this membrane, termed

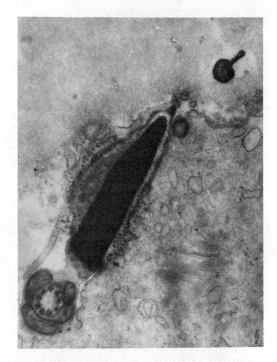

6–7 Fusion of the sperm and egg plasma membranes (arrows) establishing a continuity between the gametes. (From M. Stefanini, C. Oura, and L. Zamboni, 1969. J. Submicrosc. Cytol. 1, 1.)

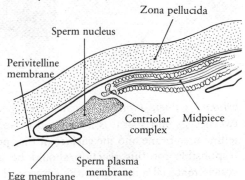

6–8 Diagram of a rabbit sperm nucleus and midpiece with mitochondrial spiral inside of the zona and egg vitelline membrane. (After D. Szöllösi and H. Ris, 1961. J. Biophys. Biochem. Cytol. 10, 275.)

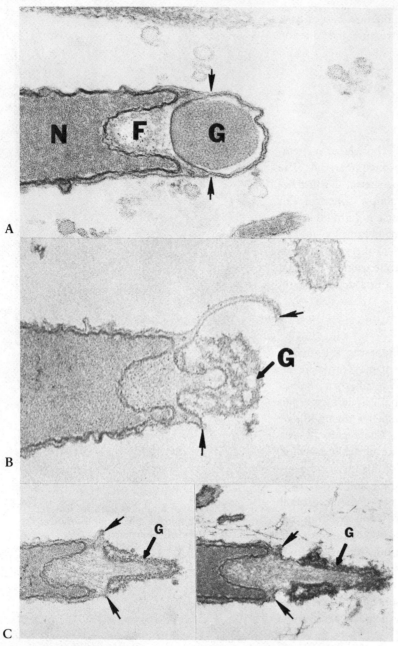

6–9 Electron micrographs of the unreacted acrosomal region and the acrosomal reaction of the sperm of *Echinarachnius parma*. A, unreacted acrosomal region. The acrosomal vesicle contains an acrosomal granule (G) enclosed in a complete acrosomal membrane. Periacrosomal material surrounds the vesicle with the bulk contained in a fossa (F) at the anterior end of the nucleus (N). Arrows show the region of future dehiscence and fusion of the sperm plasma membrane and the acrosomal vesicle membrane; B, fusion of the sperm plasma membrane and the acrosomal vesicle membrane; C, D, elongation of the acrosomal tubule with the former contents of the acrosomal vesicle adhering to it. (From R. G. Summers, B. L. Hylander, L. H. Colwin and A. L. Colwin, 1975. J. Biophys. Biochem. Cytol. 10, 275.)

primary gamete binding. Because the species specific reaction between eggs and sperm is a function of some component of the vitelline membrane and the surface of the sperm, the sperm substance responsible for this reaction should be a part of the acrosomal vesicle material adherent to the acrosomal tubule.

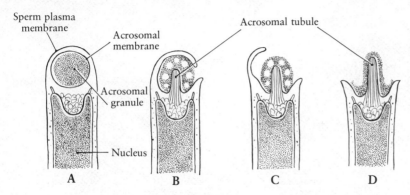

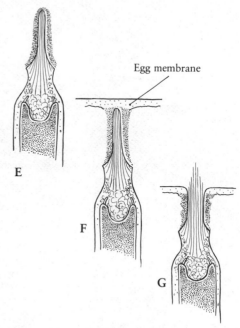

Membrane Fusion

Following primary gamete binding, a second and final step in the process of the movement of the sperm into the egg occurs. This is the fusion of the egg and sperm plasma membranes (Fig. 6–10 F,G). This fusion takes place between the egg plasma membrane and the acrosomal tubule. The acrosomal tubule consists partly of the acrosomal vesicle membrane and the sperm plasma membrane. The end result is the formation of a common egg–sperm plasma membrane, a system in which the egg and sperm nuclei now lie within the same covering. Following membrane fusion, egg cytoplasm may flow up around the sperm to form the classical fertilization cone.

The movement of the sperm nucleus into the main mass of the egg cytoplasm is not completely understood. It may be merely a passive event as when two droplets of water coalesce, or it may be due to contraction of actin filaments, or it may be due to movements of the fluid plasma membrane toward the point of egg–sperm membrane fusion.

Markedly similar series of events have been described in other species (Figs. 6–11, 6–12). Sperm and egg plasma membrane fusion, rather than penetration of the sperm through the egg plasma membrane, would appear to represent a widespread and fundamental pattern of fertilization.

6–10   Schematic representation of the unreacted acrosomal region in *Echinarachnius parma*, A, and the acrosomal reaction, B–G. B, C, the breakdown and fusion of the sperm plasma membrane and the acrosomal membrane and the beginning of the formation of the acrosomal tubules; D, E, the elongation of the acrosomal tubule with the adherent granule material; F, G, fusion of the egg and sperm membranes. (After R. G. Summers, B. L. Hylander, L. H. Colwin and A. L. Colwin, 1975. J. Biophys. Biochem. Cytol. 10, 275.)

RESPONSE OF THE EGG TO FERTILIZATION

From the description given in the preceding paragraphs, it is evident that successful penetration by the spermatozoon into the egg's cytoplasm requires a very specific interaction between the plasma membranes of the male and female gametes. The fusion of the plasmalemmas of the egg cell and the spermatozoon is a critical step in the fertilization process. First, it appears to be a prerequisite

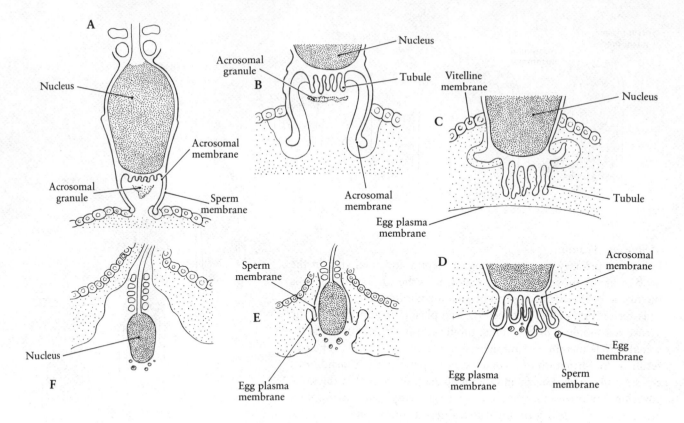

for the eventual incorporation of a functional sperm nucleus into the egg cytoplasm. Second, it typically results in the activation of the egg cell, thereby triggering the development of the embryo. *Egg activation* refers to the series of morphological, physiological, molecular, and metabolic changes that take place in the egg cell in response to contact with the spermatozoon. Some of these changes occur at the surface of the egg cell and result in rearrangements in the organization of the cortical granules and cortical cytoplasm. Other changes are expressed in the interior of the egg cell, such as the fusion of male and female nuclei to form the zygote nucleus. The absence of a successful interaction between egg and sperm results in death, since the unfertilized egg will soon degenerate.

Over the past several years, results from intensive investigations, primarily with sea urchins, have begun to shed light on the large number of changes in the egg that are evoked by its fusion with the sperm cell and the basis of the mechanism triggering all of these changes. For example, Epel (1977) indicates that the activation process in the West Coast sea urchin (*Strongylocentrotus purpuratus*) can be divided into a group of changes occurring within the first 60

6–11 Diagrams of the egg-sperm interaction in *Hydroides*. A, the dehiscence and fusion of the acromal membrane and the sperm plasma membrane as the sperm contacts the outer egg membrane. The acrosomal granule lies within the EM lucid cavity of the acrosomal vesicle; B, C, the eversion of the acrosomal membrane to form acrosomal tubules accompanied by the breakdown of the acrosomal granule; D, E, the acrosomal tubules pass through the vitelline membrane and interdigitate with the egg plasma membrane. The two membranes fuse and egg cytoplasm rises around the sperm nucleus to form the fertilization cone. Persisting acrosomal remnant marks the point of the sperm plasma membrane; F, the sperm moves into the egg cytoplasm. (From A. L. Colwin and A. L. Colwin, 1961. J. Biophys. Biochem. Cytol. 10, 211.)

seconds after sperm–egg contact and a group of changes beginning at about 5 minutes after activation (Fig. 6–13). The early responses of the egg include alterations in the intracellular concentrations of certain ions, the conversion of metabolically important coenzymes, and the release of stored enzymes into the cytoplasm. Late responses include the synthesis of proteins and DNA, both events being critical to embryonic development.

How the sperm cell triggers this vast array of activities within the egg cell is still unclear. Understanding the role of the sperm cell is complicated by the observation that the egg cells of echinoderms, as well as those of other animal species, can be experimentally activated (*experimental* or *artificial activation*) and stimulated to start development in the absence of the male gamete. An important clue to the mechanism underlying the early responses of the sea urchin egg was the observation by Mazia that the concentration of calcium ions increases shortly after fertilization. If sea urchin eggs are collected in calcium-free sea water and treated with special drugs (*ionophores*) that abolish the selective permeability of membranes to divalent cations within the cells, the eggs become activated and show a sequence of changes identical to those accompanying normal fertilization. The ionophore compound is a good artificial *parthenogenetic agent*. Similar observations using ionophorous antibiotics have been recorded on tunicates (*Ciona*), amphibians (*Xenopus*), and hamsters (*Mesocricetus*). It is suspected, therefore, that calcium ions, released from intracellular storage sites, act as the primary trigger of activation. One of the functions of the increased concentration of calcium may be to alter the surface of the egg to permit the influx of sodium ions and the release of acid (protons) from the egg. The release of acid from the *Strongylocentrotus* egg appears to be the essential mechanism underlying the activation of the late changes with the sudden shift in the pH of the cytoplasm turning on such processes as protein and DNA syntheses. An attractive hypothesis is that the transient increase in pH dissociates inhibitor molecules from critical proteins (such as enzymes), thus enabling them to function in key synthetic reactions.

There are a few cases, both among invertebrate and vertebrate animals, where the mature egg cell is spontaneously activated and develops into an adult organism in the absence of the male gamete. This condition, referred to as *natural parthenogenesis* or virginal reproduction, has been observed in rotifers, crustaceans, insects, and lizards. The adult organism produced by natural parthenogenesis has the haploid number of chromosomes. Domestically, a strain of turkey is currently available that regularly develops without a spermatozoon.

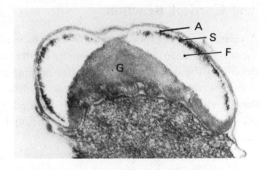

A

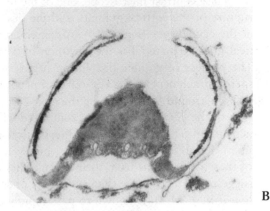

B

6–12 Electron micrograph of sections through a sperm of *Hydroides*. A, the unreacted sperm. The acrosomal membrane (A) and the sperm plasma membrane (S) are continuous around the rim of the opening. Fine granular material (F) lines the acrosomal membrane. An acrosomal granule (G) lies within the cavity of the acrosomal vesicle; B, stage comparable to Figure 6–11A. (From A. L. Colwin and L. H. Colwin 1961. J. Biophys. Biochem Cytol. 10, 231.)

The Cortical Reaction

A characteristic response of most eggs to penetration by a spermatozoon is a dramatic rearrangement of the cortical granules. Since details of the *cortical reaction* differ among animal species, we will first describe the nature of cortical granule alteration in echinoderms where it has been extensively studied by both light and electron microscopy, and then make additional observations for the same reaction in other animals.

When eggs of the sea urchin are inseminated and viewed under the phase contrast microscope, one of the first visible changes is the rupture of the cortical granules and the discharge of their contents at the egg surface (Fig. 6–14). A consequence of the released cortical granule material is the elevation of a membrane (Fig. 6–14). The process of granule dissolution begins at the site of successful sperm attachment to the egg cell and propagates itself in wavelike fashion around the egg during the next 20 to 30 seconds. The reaction of the cortical granules is completed within a minute or so of activation. The breakdown of the cortical granules is dependent upon the presence of calcium ions, but what stimulates the release of these critical ions from their storage sites is unclear. It has been suggested that a voltage change or wave of depolarization (*fertilization wave*), which is known to pass rapidly over the surface of the egg within seconds after fertilization (Fig. 6–13), may be instrumental in freeing calcium from its bound condition in the cytoplasm.

Structural details of the cortical reaction as revealed through the use of the electron microscope are summarized in Figures 6–15 and 6–16. Following activation there is an approximation and fusion of the cortical granule membrane and plasmalemma of the egg cell. A rupture or perforation, formed perhaps because of the digestive action of an enzyme within the cortical granule, subsequently develops at the site of fusion between these two membranes. As the cortical granule swells, the electron dense body is ejected through the rupture site and attaches itself to the vitelline membrane. Simultaneously, the vitelline membrane detaches from the plasmalemma of the egg cell because of the digestive action of a proteolytic enzyme (*delaminase*) released with the cortical granule material. The vitelline membrane with the attached electron dense material is approximately 500 to 800 Å thick and is known as the *fertilization membrane*. The space that appears between the egg surface and the fertilization membrane is the *perivitelline space*. Elevation of the fertilization membrane is related to the fluid pressure of the perivitelline space. Presumably, the fluid pressure is generated as a result of the colloidlike action exerted by the liquified, hydrophilic contents of the cortical granules within the perivitelline space.

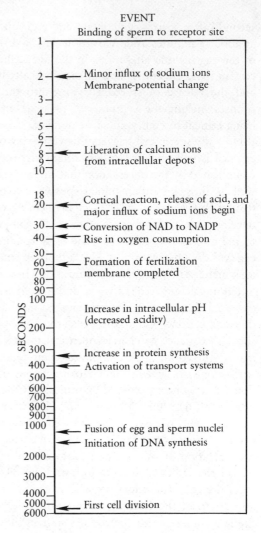

6–13 The temporal sequence of activities following fertilization in the egg of *Strongylocentrotus purpuratus* as reconstructed from studies by Epel and his colleagues. (From D. Epel, 1977. Sci. Am. 237, 129.)

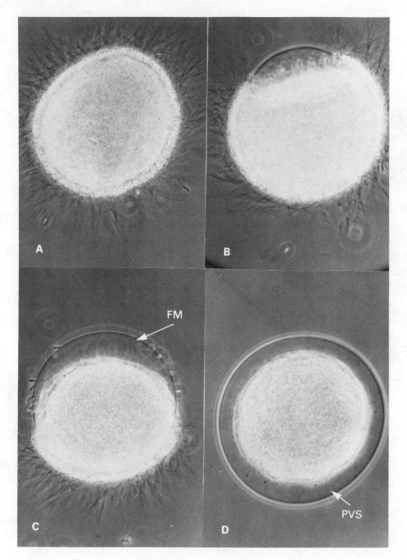

6–14 Eruption of cortical granules and elevation of the fertilization membrane (FM) as seen by light microscopy in eggs of *Lytechinus pictus* (echinoderm). A, 10 seconds after insemination the sperm are bound over the entire egg surface; B, 25 seconds after insemination; C, 35 seconds after insemination the cortical reaction begins to propagate over the egg; D, at 50 seconds the vitelline layer is completely elevated as the fertilization membrane. Note the cortical granule material in the pervitelline space (PVS). (From V. Vacquier, 1975. Exp. Cell Res. 82, 227.)

The hemispheric globules of each cortical granule are also released into the perivitelline space. This material joins together at the egg surface to form the viscous and transparent *hyaline layer*. Primarily composed of acid mucopolysaccharides, the hyaline layer probably serves to keep the cells of the cleaving embryo intact.

The limiting membranes of the cortical granules, by virtue of their fusion with the plasmalemma of the egg cell at the onset of the cortical reaction, appear to participate in the formation of the plasma membrane surrounding the fertilized egg cell. Hence, the surface of the one-celled embryo is a mosaic in which areas of the

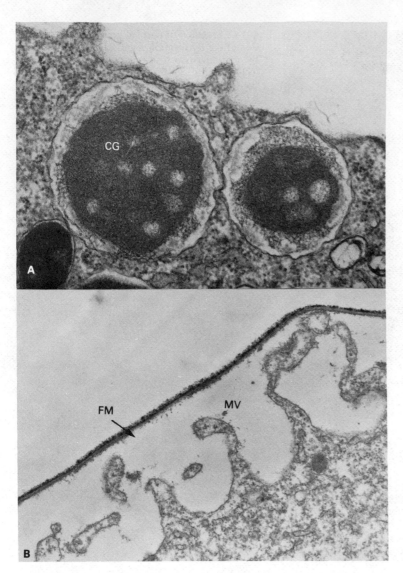

6–15 The echinoderm egg during the cortical reaction as seen in section. A, electron micrograph of the cortical granules (CG) of *Dendraster excentricus*. Note the dense material surrounded by less dense fibrous material in each granule; B, electron micrograph of the egg surface of *Dendraster* after breakdown of the cortical granules. The cortical granule contents have united with the vitelline layer of the egg to form the fertilization membrane (FM). Note that the surface of the egg is extended into microvilli (MV). (From V. Vacquier, 1975. Exp. Cell Res. 90, 465.)

original egg cell plasmalemma alternate with areas derived from limiting membranes of cortical granules.

The expulsion of cortical granule contents at the egg surface upon fertilization is found in many groups of animals, including frogs, teleost fishes, and some mammals. In the frog (*Rana*), extrusion of the cortical granules is initiated several minutes after fertilization (Fig. 6–17). The reaction is accompanied by the elevation of a vitelline membrane. As in the sea urchin, cortical granule contents are discharged into a perivitelline space. Cortical granule material joins with the vitelline membrane to form a fertilization membrane.

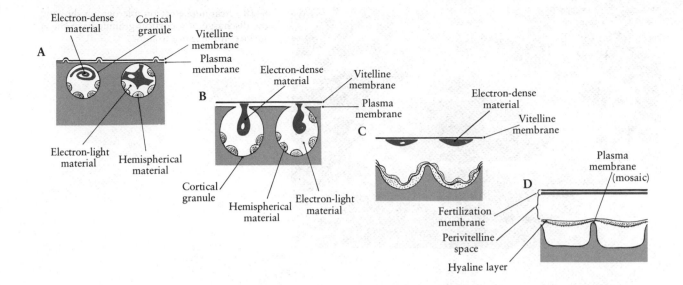

In teleost fishes, the spermatozoon enters the egg cytoplasm through a special opening, the *micropyle,* in the chorion at the animal pole. The cortical reaction begins at the micropyle and quickly passes around the cell. As in sea urchins and frogs, the chorion lifts off the egg surface in the wake of cortical granule breakdown. Surface views of the egg during the cortical reaction show that the central contents of the cortical granules are released intact into the perivitelline space (Fig. 6–18). They subsequently breakdown and their contents become part of the perivitelline fluid.

A cortical reaction is also observed in the fertilized eggs of many mammals, including rat, hamster, and man. The contents of the cortical granules are liberated into a preformed perivitelline space between the zona pellucida and the egg cell. No new membrane is elevated after fertilization as in sea urchins and frogs. The perivitelline space does gradually increase in volume, but this is probably due to the shrinkage of the egg itself following fertilization.

Although the release of cortical granule contents onto the egg surface during the cortical reaction might be considered typical in the animal kingdom, there are several animal species whose cortical granules show an unusual response with fertilization. For example, in the surf clam (*Spisula*) and the mussel (*Mytilus*), the cortical granules remain completely intact and undisturbed following fertilization. The cortical granules in the barnacle (*Barnea*) egg spontaneously breakdown, independently of fertilization, and their contents are liberated into the interior of the cell.

The variability in the response of the cortical granules to sperm penetration (or experimental activation) of the egg cell has made it

6–16 Diagrammatic summary of the formation of the fertilization membrane, the hyaline layer, and the plasma membrane of the fertilized egg in the sea urchin. (From Y. Endo, 1961. Exp. Cell Res. 25, 518.)

6–17 The extrusion of the contents of cortical granules in the frog's egg. The contents of some of the cortical granules have been liberated into the perivitelline space (PVS). Note the erupted cortical granule at the tip of the arrow. A large granule (CG) just before extrusion of its contents is seen to the left. The underside of the vitelline membrane (VM) appears to have a layer of diffuse material whose density is very much like that of the cortical granules. PG, pigment granule; YP, yolk platelet. (From N. Kemp and N. Istock, 1967. J. Cell Biol. 34, 111.)

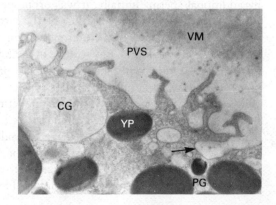

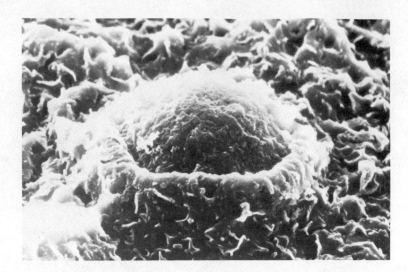

difficult to determine the significance of the cortical reaction in the developmental process. For those organisms in which the cortical granules release their contents at the egg surface upon activation, the cortical reaction has been implicated in prevention of multiple sperm entry into the egg cell at fertilization. Also, the cortical granules appear to contain a substance that hardens the fertilization membrane of echinoderms and the chorion of teleost fishes.

Finally it must be remembered that there are major groups of animals (insects, salamanders, birds) in which there are no cortical granules in their egg cells and hence no cortical reaction as a response to fertilization.

Blocks to Polyspermy

One of the most important physiological responses of the monospermic egg at fertilization is the reaction that prevents penetration by additional sperm. Initially, it was proposed that the cortical reaction, coupled with the elevation of the fertilization membrane, were important blocks to the entrance of many spermatozoa into the egg cell. However, the time course of the breakdown of the cortical granules and membrane elevation are probably too slow in many animals to account for complete protection. Studies by Rothschild and Schwann in the 1950s on echinoderm eggs suggested that the block to polyspermy was a diphasic (i.e., a two-step) process. The first step is postulated to occur very rapidly or within the first several seconds of activation. This reduces the receptivity of the egg to a second sperm by about 80 percent. The second step is attributable to the breakdown of the cortical granules with the subsequent elevation of the fertilization membrane. The experimental basis for this postulation is that inhibition of the cortical reaction typically results in the production of polyspermic eggs.

Since the interaction of egg and sperm is a surface phenomenon, a "sperm's-eye" view of the sequence of events at fertilization can be obtained using the scanning electron microscope. (SEM). Elegant studies by Tegner and Epel (1973) with SEM (Fig. 6–19) have demonstrated that hundreds of spermatozoa attach to the outer surface of the vitelline membrane within the first 25 seconds following insemination of *Strongylocentrotus* eggs. The sperm apparently bind chemically to an array of regularly spaced projections of the vitelline membrane. The cortical reaction is initiated 25 seconds after insemination. During the cortical reaction, there is a progressive detachment of the supernumerary spermatozoa from the vitelline membrane over an interval of time coincident with cortical granule breakdown. The detachment phase appears to result from the action of a protease (probably localized in the contents of the cortical granules) which digests the sperm–egg binding site. Artificial agents that induce polyspermy in the sea urchin, such as nicotine and soybean trypsin inhibitor, do so by interfering with the cortical reaction, specifically by inhibiting proteolytic activity and the wave of sperm detachment.

The cortical reaction in the sea urchin egg can only account for protection against polyspermy after 25 seconds following fertilization. Hence, other mechanisms must be operative to block multiple sperm entry prior to the onset of the cortical granule breakdown. It has been mentioned previously that the egg surface in the echinoderm shows a voltage shift within the first several seconds of the attachment of the first spermatozoon. The magnitude of membrane potential change is approximately 15 to 20 millivolts. Recently, Laurinda Jaffee (1976) has determined that this voltage change, generated as a result of the early influx of sodium ions into the cell, is probably the basis for the fast but incomplete block to polyspermy. When she artificially elevated the voltage across the egg membrane to a level comparable to that observed after fertilization and added sperm to the eggs, there was no evidence of fertilization.

Results with other animals suggest that similar processes operate to prevent polyspermy. In the hamster, for example, observations on artificially inseminated eggs indicate that many spermatozoa bind to the zona pellucida. Following the discharge of the cortical granules, the zona pellucida is conspicuously devoid of spermatozoa. The alteration of the zona pellucida to prevent penetration and further attachment by sperm is known as the *zona reaction*. It is mediated by a constituent of the cortical granules (a *protease*) whose properties are similar to those of the proteolytic enzyme

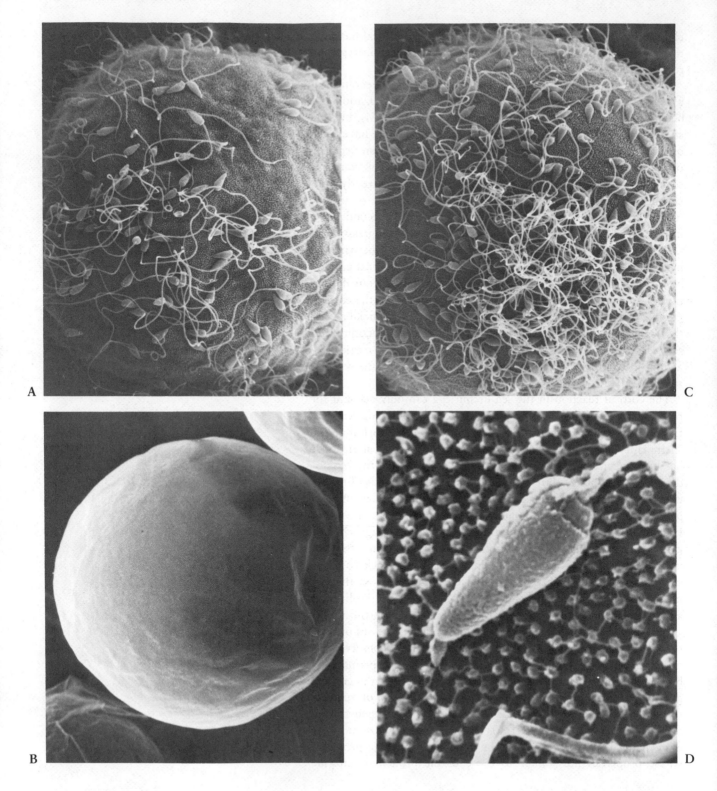

bringing about sperm detachment in the sea urchin. The zona reaction takes place over an interval of time of approximately two hours. However, the cortical reaction does not begin until some 20 to 25 minutes after insemination. Hence, several spermatozoa during this time interval penetrate the zona pellucida, pass through the perivitelline space, and join to the plasmalemma of the egg. Although details remain to be determined, there is presumably established at activation an alteration in the properties of the plasmalemma of the egg cell which assists in preventing polyspermy.

Recent studies by Longo and Anderson indicate that the egg cell and/or its accessory membranes may not be the only site preventing polyspermy. Brief exposure of *Spisula* sperm to egg water (i.e., sea water in which eggs have been sitting and then removed) severely reduces their ability to inseminate. A similar condition prevails in *Arbacia,* thus suggesting that mechanism(s) preventing polyspermy may reside within the spermatozoon as well as the egg cell.

In contrast to the examples cited above, the eggs of many insects, amphibians (salamanders), reptiles, and birds are normally entered by several spermatozoa at fertilization. Although these animals have avoided the difficulties of excluding extra sperm from penetrating the egg, mechanisms have been developed to prevent more than one sperm nucleus from joining with the female nucleus. A particularly interesting example is offered by the egg of the salamander. In the salamander (*Triturus*), as many as nine spermatozoa enter the egg cytoplasm at fertilization. For the first two hours and 20 minutes after insemination, the centriole of each sperm head enlarges into a conspicuous aster (Fig. 6–20 A). As soon as one sperm nucleus fuses with the nucleus of the egg, the remaining sperm nuclei begin to degenerate. Elegant experiments by Fankhauser and his colleagues with the egg of *Triturus* suggest that the newly formed zygote produces a substance that spreads throughout the cytoplasm and specifically acts to induce degeneration of the supernumerary nuclei (Fig. 6–20 B).

6-19 Scanning electron micrographs by Tegner and Epel of the sperm-attachment-detachment sequence on the surface of *Stronglyocentrotus purpuratus* eggs. The number of sperm bound to the egg surface increases until 25 seconds after insemination. The cortical reaction is then initiated and the sperm begin to detach. A, approximately 5 to 10 seconds after insemination; B, approximately 15 seconds after insemination; C, 3 minutes after insemination showing the hardened fertilization membrane; D, a spermatozoon having undergone the acrosome reaction and attached to the vitelline surface by an acrosomal process. Note the projections of the surface of the fertilization membrane. (From M. Tegner and D. Epel, 1973. Science 179, 685. Copyright 1973 by the American Association for the Advancement of Science.)

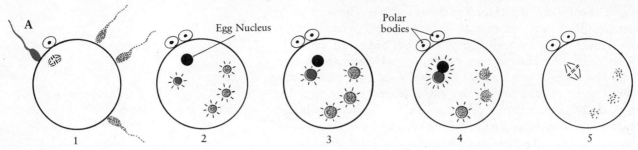

Reorganization of Constituents of the Egg Cell

With penetration of the spermatozoon into the cytoplasm of the egg cell, there are in many animal species dramatic shifts and noticeable changes in the organization of the cytoplasmic constituents. In some cases, it is evident that these changes have a profound influence upon the organization and future development of the embryo. The rearrangement of ooplasmic constituents at fertilization is best illustrated in those animal egg cells whose cytoplasm bears distinctive features or regional specializations (i.e., pigment granules). The amphibian egg cell, you will recall, is typically covered in its upper two-thirds by a heavily pigmented layer; the lower third of the egg cell is light in color. At fertilization in *Rana,* the spermatozoon enters the egg at a point 20 to 30 degrees from the midregion of the animal pole. Within 5 to 10 minutes, the pigmented, cortical cytoplasm opposite the site of sperm entrance moves upward toward the animal pole (Fig. 6–21 A). As a consequence of this cytoplasmic movement, a distinct zone of grayish-colored cytoplasm is revealed. This area is known as the *grey crescent* (Fig. 6–21 B).

The importance of this dramatic displacement and rearrangement of the cortical cytoplasm, which results in the expression of a structure not previously present (i.e., grey crescent), is severalfold. First, the position of the grey crescent marks the future dorsal side of the embryo and the site of the dorsal lip of the blastopore at gastrulation. The region opposite the grey crescent marks the future ventral side of the embryo. Second, the grey crescent establishes the axis of bilateral symmetry of the future embryo. Thus, the cleavage plane that bisects the grey crescent divides the embryo into right and left halves. In the majority of cases, this will be the first cleavage plane. It is interesting to note that the grey crescent also forms in the frog egg following artificial activation by pricking with a needle, but its expression bears no apparent relationship to the site of activation. Yet, studies of Roux in 1885 clearly showed that when the point of entry of sperm was controlled at the surface, the grey crescent consistently developed opposite the point of entry into the egg. He de-

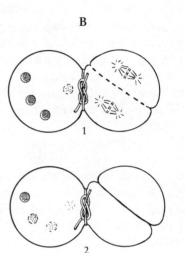

6–20 Polyspermy in the salamander egg. A, the spermatozoa enter the egg cell in the metaphase of the second meiotic division (1). The nuclei of all spermatozoa enlarge during the next 2 hours and 20 minutes (2,3). After fusion of the male nucleus with the female nucleus, the supernumerary sperm begin to regress (4). As the first cleavage division occurs, suppression of most supernumerary male nuclei is evident (5); B, the experiment of Fankhauser suggesting that the fused male and female nuclei release an inhibitory factor causing the destruction of accessory spermatozoa. The egg of *Triturus* was constricted before the beginning of cleavage (1). In the half on the right, the male and female nuclei have fused and cleavage initiated. Subsequently, in the left half of the egg, the nuclei of the sperm furthest from the constriction are still large; those nearest to the right half of the egg are degenerating. (After G. Fankhauser, 1948. Ann. N.Y. Acad. Sci. 49, 684.)

termined this by placing drops of sperm onto fine silk threads that were attached to selected sites in the animal hemisphere. We can conclude, therefore, that the action of the spermatozoon in part is to strengthen and accentuate one of several meridians of bilateral symmetry built into the unfertilized egg. In short, the main directional axes of the future amphibian embryo (dorsoventral; left-right), probably fixed in the cortical cytoplasm, are organized and determined by the site of sperm penetration. Similar observations on the relationship between fertilization and symmetrization have been made on the eggs of many molluscs and annelids. Third, the grey crescent appears to initiate the gastrulative process and to play a fundamental role in the determination of embryonic structures (Chapter 10).

The development of the urochordate (*Styela*) egg is another good example of fundamental change in cytoplasmic organization that becomes visible following fertilization. As seen from the surface, the unfertilized egg cell of *Styela* shows no evidence of bilateral organization. Its surface is covered by a layer of cortical cytoplasm containing yellow pigment granules. Following the entrance of the spermatozoon, there is a rapid movement of the yellowish cytoplasm toward the vegetal pole. Shortly, the yellowish cytoplasm reorganizes as a crescent-shaped area on the side of sperm entrance and just below the equator of the egg cell (Fig. 6–22). Subsequently, a light grey, crescent-shaped zone of cytoplasm develops opposite this yellow crescent. These cytoplasmic displacements give a distinct bilateral organization to the egg cell. Below the yellow and light grey crescents, the vegetal pole remains as the *vegetal cytoplasm* (slate grey in color). The transparent-appearing cytoplasm at the animal pole is known as the *animal plasm*. The relationships of these newly formed pigmented areas and their importance in giving rise to specific parts of the embryo will be discussed in a later chapter.

Metabolic and Synthetic Activities

The act of fertilization (or activation) transforms a physiologically and metabolically quiescent cell into one showing a series of complicated and rapid changes. The fertilized egg cell shows striking alterations in the permeability of its plasmalemma, in the viscosity of its cytoplasm, utilization of oxygen, activities of proteolytic and oxidative enzymes, and in the synthesis of proteins. The essence of fertilization lies in understanding why the unfertilized egg becomes metabolically "shut down" during late oogenesis and what mechanisms are invoked which suddenly "derepress" this inhibitory state.

An initial effort in characterizing the basis of egg activation was

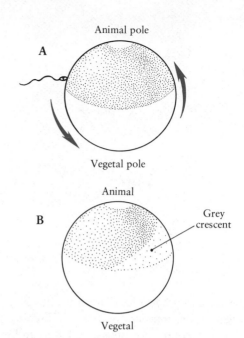

6–21 Formation of the grey crescent in the egg of the amphibian. A, the direction of cortical cytoplasmic movements (arrows); B, location of the grey crescent opposite to the site of sperm entry.

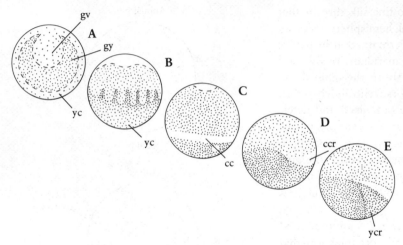

6–22 Reorganization of the cytoplasm in the egg of the tunicate, *Styela partita,* following fertilization. A, ripe, unfertilized egg showing germinal vesicle (gv), central mass of gray yolk (gy), and peripheral layer of yellow cytoplasm (yc); B, five minutes after fertilization showing streaming of yellow cytoplasm toward lower pole where sperm enters cell; C, consolidation of yellow cytoplasm at vegetal pole. Note the clear cytoplasm (cc) beneath yellow cap; D,E, later stages in the formation of the yellow crescent (ycr) and the clear cytoplasmic crescent (ccr). The yellow crescent marks the future posterior end of the embryo. (From E. G. Conklin, 1905. J. Acad. Nat. Sci. Philadelphia 13, 1.)

the discovery by Otto Warburg some 60 years ago that the rate of oxygen consumption in the sea urchin egg increased markedly within minutes of fertilization. Later studies by Lindahl and Holter with *Paracentrotus* (sea urchin) eggs confirmed this observation (Fig. 6–23). Shortly after the breakdown of the germinal vesicle, the rate of oxygen utilization sharply decreases and remains at a low level until fertilization. At this time it shows a precipitous rise. Similar changes in respiratory metabolism have been observed in teleost oocytes (Fig. 6–24). It would appear that an increase in oxygen consumption is a key reaction in the fertilization process. However, elevation in the rate of oxygen consumption upon fertilization is by no means a universal occurrence among animal species. Little change in the level of oxygen activity can be detected between unfertilized and fertilized eggs in the frog. In some marine annelids there actually appears to be a decrease in the rate of respiration in the fertilized egg. It is interesting to note that the direction and magnitude of respiratory change at the time of fertilization may be dependent upon the stage of nuclear maturation. Generally, only those eggs with reduction divisions completed will show an increase in respiration at the time of fertilization. Eggs of other species, penetrated by spermatozoa before completion of nuclear maturation, may not show any change in respiration until the process of maturation is terminated. It appears that the fertilized egg can regulate the rate of oxygen utilization, although the direction and magnitude of change vary with different animal species.

The intriguing question remains as to why the mature, unfertilized egg in so many animal species shows a low rate of respiration. Since oxygen is typically tied to the degradation of carbohydrates, it is possible that the physiological state of the unfertilized

6–23 Changes in the rate of oxygen consumption during maturation and at the time of fertilization in the egg of the echinoderm (*Paracentrotus*). (From P. Lindahl and H. Holtzer, 1941. C. R. Tra. Lab. Carlsberg, Ser. Chim. 24, 49.)

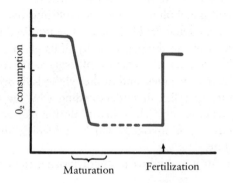

egg reflects a deficiency and/or inhibition of essential oxidative enzymes. Also, perhaps there are insufficient levels of oxidizable substrates in the cytoplasm. In both frogs and sea urchins, it has been established that carbohydrate metabolism in the egg consists of the Embden-Meyerhoff glycolytic pathway, the pentose phosphate shunt, the Krebs tricarboxylic acid cycle, and a cytochrome system. The unfertilized egg apparently contains all of the necessary enzymes to catalyze the step-by-step reactions during carbohydrate metabolism. Yet, in the echinoderm egg, oxidative enzymes associated with the pentose phosphate cycle, such as glucose-6-phosphate dehydrogenase and 6-phosphogluconate, rise sharply in activity following fertilization. There is also a rise in NAD kinase, an enzyme that is responsible for the phosphorylation of the coenzyme NAD (nicotinamide adenine dinucleotide) to NADP (nicotinamide adenine dinucleotide phosphate), and glycogen phosphorylase. The increase in glucose-6-phosphate dehydrogenase plus elevated levels of NADP and glucose-6-phosphate could account for the increased respiration of eggs. It is probable that during oogenesis many of these enzymes are prevented from interacting with their substrates because they become bound to either structural proteins or some cellular component of the egg cytoplasm. Several investigators have described the presence of proteolytic enzymes (proteases) in sea urchin eggs and observed marked increases in their activities following insemination. Such proteases might act in the presence of calcium to release these oxidative enzymes from their inactive states.

There is considerable increase in the synthesis of proteins within minutes of fertilization in a number of animal species (Fig. 6–25). The sudden shift in the rate of protein synthesis can be considered to mark the beginning of the transformation of the egg into the embryo. That these newly synthesized proteins are vital to the early development of the embryo can be confirmed by the use of inhibitors known to block the formation of proteins (*translational inhibitors*). The incubation of eggs in such translational inhibitors as *puromycin* or *cycloheximide* shortly after fertilization quickly arrests their further development.

The mechanism of the activation of the protein synthesizing machinery of the egg cell is still largely unclear, even in echinoderms, at which most of the attention has thus far been directed. In mature, unfertilized eggs of most sea urchins, the level of protein synthesis appears to be very low or negligible, demonstrated by the fact that the incorporation of radioactive amino acids into protein is small. By contrast, the rate of incorporation of labeled amino acids into protein increases sharply (as much as 100-fold) after insemination. Although the egg cell does become more permeable to protein precursors upon fertilization, these differences in amino acid uptake

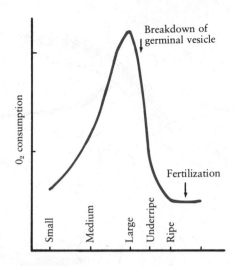

6–24 Rate of oxygen consumption in the course of the maturation and fertilization of teleost eggs (*Oryzias*). (From A. Monroy, 1965. Chemistry and Physiology of Fertilization. Holt, Rinehart and Winston, Inc., New York.)

6–25 Protein synthesis (measured by the uptake of ^{14}C-valine) in fertilized eggs of *Arbacia* without (control) and with (experimental) actinomycin D. Note that actinomycin D does not inhibit protein synthesis immediately after fertilization. (From P. Gross, L. Malkin and W. Moyer, 1964. Proc. Natl. Acad. Sci. U.S.A. 51, 407.)

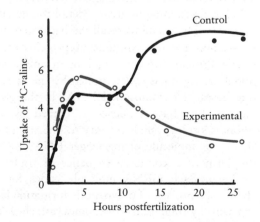

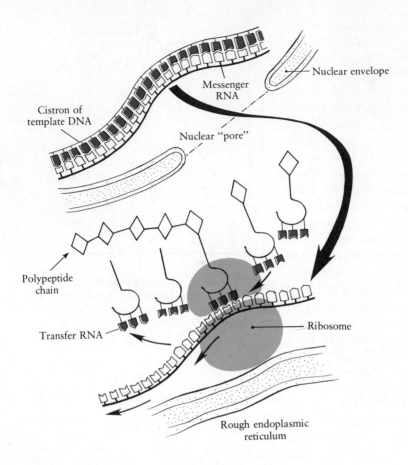

Nuclear envelope

Messenger RNA

Cistron of template DNA

Nuclear "pore"

Polypeptide chain

Transfer RNA

Ribosome

Rough endoplasmic reticulum

between unfertilized and fertilized eggs are not due to an increase in membrane permeability since similar results can be obtained using homogenates rather than whole cells. The unfertilized egg cell appears to produce less protein because of one or more blocks at some level in its protein-synthesizing machinery.

Before examining in greater detail the question of protein activation, it will be useful to recall the basic steps in the model proposed to account for the synthesis of proteins of eucaryotic cells (Fig. 6–26). Proteins are combinations of amino acids whose organizational arrangement is determined by the linear sequence of nucleotide bases of chromosomal DNA. In the presence of RNA polymerase, this base sequence is copied as a linear sequence of ribonucleotides complementary to one strand of DNA. The synthesis of this molecule of messenger RNA (mRNA) yields a chain in the form of a continual sequence of triplets of nucleotide bases (*codons*). Each mRNA molecule codes for a single polypeptide chain. The process of polypeptide formation is carried out in the cytoplasm by numerous ribosomes attached to the same mRNA strand. This complex of mRNA and the ribosomes is called a *polysome* or *polyribosome*. Apparently the ribosomes move along the mRNA chain, "reading" the code and building the polypeptide chain according to that information. Each amino acid is transported to the ribosome by a molecule of transfer RNA (tRNA). One end of the tRNA molecule is occupied by a base triplet sequence (*anticodon*) complementary to the specific codon of the mRNA molecule. The other end of the tRNA molecule carries the specific amino acid for which that mRNA triplet must code. The coupling of the amino acid to the tRNA molecule is a two-step process. First, each amino acid is activated or charged in the presence of ATP (adenosine triphosphate), with the reaction being catalyzed by a specific amino acid activating enzyme (an *aminoacyl synthetase*). These same aminoacyl synthetases catalyze the reaction, which then transfers each amino acid to its specific tRNA molecule.

There are, therefore, several possibilities by which the repression of the synthesis of proteins in the unfertilized egg might be explained. These include an absence or unavailability of mRNA molecules, an absence of functional ribosomes, or inaccessibility of the mRNA for proper complexing with the ribosomal population.

Initially, it was suspected that mRNA macromolecules were simply lacking in the unfertilized egg. This was based in part upon the observation that ribosomes from unfertilized eggs of sea urchins, by comparison with ribosomes from fertilized eggs, exhibited little ability to form protein when incubated with labeled amino acids. Nemer and Bard offered direct experimental data indicating that there was a major limitation on mRNA availability. They demonstrated that in vitro the unfertilized egg system actively synthesizes polyphenylalanine following the addition of polyuridylic acid (*Poly U;* a synthetic mRNA containing the UUU codon for the amino acid, phenylalanine). Since these experiments showed that the unfertilized egg had the necessary functional ribosomes to make protein, the low levels of protein synthesis prior to fertilization were due to an insufficiency of mRNA macromolecules. The fertilized egg cell provided the mRNA through transcription of its DNA, thereby accounting for the increase in protein synthesis.

However, additional studies by Gross and his colleagues (1964) with *Arbacia* eggs strongly indicate that protein synthesis does not require any RNA that might be transcribed at fertilization (Fig. 6–25). When eggs were treated with actinomycin D (an antibiotic that prevents the transcription of DNA-dependent RNA) and then inseminated, protein synthesis was initiated and increased steadily for about three hours. Similar *chemical enucleation* experiments carried out on the eggs of amphibians and teleost fishes show that early protein synthesis is unaffected by transcriptional inhibitors.

Also, when the unfertilized egg of the sea urchin is centrifuged under given experimental conditions, it can be divided into *anucleate* (without nucleus) and *nucleate* (with nucleus) halves. Neither half incorporates radioactive amino acids into protein. If artificially activated, however, both egg halves, including the one without a nucleus, actively form proteins. Puromycin effectively terminates all polypeptide formation in activated, anucleate, and nucleate halves.

It now appears that proteins synthesized following fertilization do so independently of any synthetic activities of the nucleus. Evidence from several studies now indicates that the templates for these early embryonic proteins are mRNA molecules transcribed from the maternal nucleus during oogenesis. Most of these maternal mRNAs are probably stored in an inactive form, presumably by being masked with a coating of protein. These particles of protein-coated RNA have been termed *informosomes*. In order to be available for protein synthesis, such particles must have their protein coats removed. Monroy and his colleagues (1965) have demonstrated that informosomes are indeed attached to ribosomes of the unfertilized sea urchin egg. They were able to stimulate both endogenous and Poly U-directed polypeptide synthesis in unfertilized egg ribosomes of *Paracentrotus* following treatment of preparations with trypsin. Presumably, the trypsin digests away the protein covering of the informosome, thus liberating the mRNA. In the intact egg cell, the mRNA is probably unmasked as a result of the transient activation of proteolytic calcium-dependent enzymes. However, the unmasking of mRNA in the egg's cytoplasm may not be the only step required to initiate protein synthesis.

Ribosomes present in the unfertilized eggs of *Paracentrotus* have a noticeable "stickiness," probably indicating the presence of a protein coat. Recently, there has been isolated from unfertilized eggs of *Paracentrotus* an extract of proteins which inhibits the binding of Poly U to ribosomes and also prevents the incorporation of amino acids into protein. Hence, the ribosomes of unfertilized eggs appear to contain an inhibitor of protein synthesis. This inhibitor is either removed or suppressed upon fertilization through proteolytic activity.

Can these observations on the suggested mechanism of the activation of protein synthesis in *Arbacia* and *Paracentrotus* (i.e., the unmasking of mRNA and/or the removal of a ribosomal inhibitor protein) be generalized to other egg cells? Unfortunately, it is still impossible to say. For example, Kedes and Stavy (1969) were not able to stimulate protein synthesis by trypsinizing egg ribosomes in the echinoderms *Strongylocentrotus* and *Lytechinus*. Also, ribosomes of *Strongylocentrotus* and *Arbacia* do not possess the "stickiness" suggestive of a ribosomal inhibitory protein. At present, the most likely resolution is that there are species differences in the mechanism of protein activation. Activation of protein synthesis in the unfertilized egg probably involves both an unmasking of stored mRNA as well as removal of an inhibitory ribosomal protein, but each of these to substantially different degrees in different species.

Whether the egg synthetases are a controlling factor in activating protein synthesis at fertilization also remains an open question. Although earlier studies tended to indicate that the aminoacyl synthetases show little change in activity from the unfertilized egg stage to cleavage, Ceccarini and his colleagues have shown that labeled valyl-tRNA synthetase from blastulas of *Paracentrotus* is twice as active in promoting protein synthesis in unfertilized eggs as valyl-tRNA synthetase from unfertilized eggs.

Shortly after the egg cell is activated, the chromosomal DNA begins to replicate itself. In the sea urchin, DNA synthesis, as measured by the incorporation of ³H-thymidine, occurs in both male and female nuclei within 20 minutes of fertilization. This is well in advance of the fusion of these two organelles to form the zygote nucleus.

Fusion of Pronuclei

The important structures of the spermatozoon that typically enter the egg cytoplasm are the nucleus, with its condensed chromatin material, and the centrosome (proximal and distal centrioles). In some animals, particularly the mammals, other constituents of the midpiece and/or the tail piece of the spermatozoon may also come to lie within the egg's cytoplasm. It is not known what role(s), if any, that the latter components of the spermatozoon play in the subsequent development of the egg cell. In mammals, electron microscope studies have shown that the mitochondria of the midpiece and the axial filaments of the tail piece undergo degeneration shortly after being incorporated into the egg's cytoplasm.

The nuclei of both male and female gametes undergo marked structural transformations after the incorporation of the spermatozoon into the egg's cytoplasm. These changes lead to the formation of the *male* and *female pronuclei*. The formation of the male pronucleus from the male nucleus begins with the breakdown of the sperm nuclear envelope and entails the reorganization of the sperm chromatin and the establishment of a pronuclear envelope. In the sea urchin, the spermatozoon, shortly after incorporation into the egg, rotates approximately 180 degrees and comes to lie lateral to its point of entrance. Concomitantly, the sperm nuclear envelope becomes vesicular and the chromatin material begins to disperse (Fig. 6–27 A). Subsequently, vesicles aggregate along the periphery

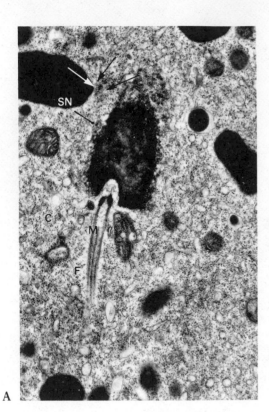

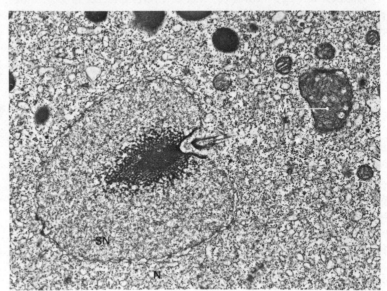

6–27 A, the beginning stage of the dispersal of sperm chromatin (arrows) in the sea urchin; B, the heart-shaped male pronucleus delimited by its own pronuclear envelope in the sea urchin; C, centriole; F, remains of spermatozoon flagellum; M, remains of mitochondrial body of male gamete; N, nuclear membrane; SN, nucleus of spermatozoon. (From F. Longo and E. Anderson, 1968. J. Cell Biol. 39, 339.)

of the dispersing chromatin and form the pronuclear envelope (Fig. 6–27 B). These structural changes occur very rapidly (within the first six minutes of insemination), leaving the male pronucleus considerably smaller than its counterpart, the female pronucleus (Fig. 6–28). Since meiosis is complete at the time of fertilization in echinoderms, the transformation of the egg nucleus into the female pronucleus occurs well in advance of the development of the male pronucleus. In organisms not having completed meiosis by the time of fertilization, development of the male pronucleus may or may not occur simultaneously with elaboration of the female pronucleus. For example, in the mussel, the dispersal of chromatin and the formation of the pronuclear envelope of the male pronucleus is completed within 18 minutes of insemination. This is well in advance of the completion of meiosis. By contrast, the fusion of vesicles along the margin of the dispersed chromatin material in the surf clam occurs at the completion of meiosis and at the onset of the development of the female pronucleus (approximately 40 minutes after insemination). Interestingly, both the female and male pronuclei are about of equal size. It has been suggested that the egg's cytoplasm

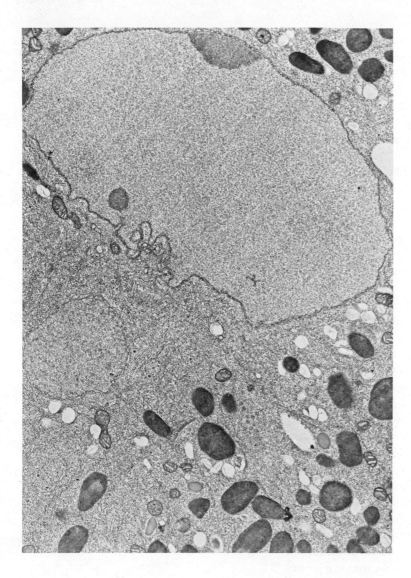

6–28 The approach of the male and female pronuclei in the fertilized egg of *Arbacia*. Note the cytoplasmic projections of the female pronucleus. (From F. Longo and E. Anderson, 1968. J. Cell Biol. 39, 339.)

contains some substance(s) that may regulate the synchronous development of male and female pronuclei in the surf clam.

Formation of the sperm *aster* accompanies the development of the male pronucleus. Generally, both the proximal and distal centrioles are incorporated into the egg. They tend to remain oriented at right angles to each other. The regions around each centriole gradually become packed with short, radiating microtubular fibers and endoplasmic vesicles of the smooth variety. The microtubules form the *astral rays,* yielding the sunburst arrangement characteristic of the aster. As the sperm aster continues to enlarge, the distal centriole becomes dissociated from the male pronucleus. The precise role of the sperm aster is still largely an unresolved problem. In forms such as the sea urchin and the frog, the sperm aster eventually divides to form the poles of the first *cleavage amphiaster*. It is assumed that the egg centrosome loses its capacity for division during the process of nuclear maturation. The ability, then, of the fertilized egg to undergo division is dependent upon the activities of the sperm aster. However, the fact that cleavage can follow parthenogenetic activation of eggs in several animal species supports the contention that elaboration of the first cleavage amphiaster is not always dependent upon a sperm centriole. Zamboni maintains that in the mammal, no centrioles are present at either pole of the first cleavage spindle. Hence, the sperm centriole either degenerates or simply does not participate in the first cleavage division.

The mechanism(s) by which female and male pronuclei move toward each other and exchange genetic material is poorly understood. In egg cells with small-to-moderate amounts of yolk, the two pronuclei are observed to move toward the center of the cell and probably only coincidently toward each other. The independence of the movements of the female pronucleus, for example, is demonstrated by the fact that it moves in artificially activated eggs just as it moves in naturally fertilized eggs. How the cytoplasm mediates these movements remains a mystery.

The actual process of fusion between female and male pronuclei varies considerably among animal species. In mammals (i.e., rabbit), the two pronuclei become tightly apposed to each other in the center of the egg cell. As they approach each other, numerous projections are elaborated on their proximal surfaces (Fig. 6–29). Some internuclear communication and exchange of material may result from contacts observed between adjacent projections of both pronuclei. Following vesiculation and fragmentation of the two pronuclear envelopes, the two groups of chromosomes move together and assume positions on the first cleavage spindle. No true zygote nucleus is produced. The stages of development of the fertilized rabbit egg between the approximation of pronuclei and the completion of the first cleavage division are shown in Figure 6–30. A similar pattern of pronuclear fusion is present in the rat, mussel, and surf clam.

By contrast, the envelopes of the two pronuclei actually fuse in the echinoderms (Fig. 6–31). Subsequently, there is a distinct mixing of nucleoplasmic contents. Following formation of this zygote nucleus, the male chromatin diffuses throughout the nucleoplasm and becomes indistinguishable from that of the female.

In summary, the sperm-egg contact transforms a metabolically repressed cell into one showing an array of morphological, physio-

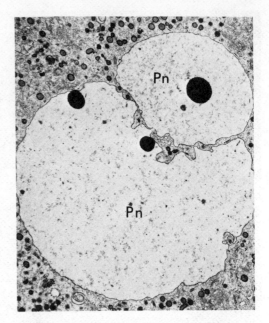

6–29   The approach of the male and female pronuclei in the rabbit. Note the irregularities in the adjacent pronuclear membranes. Pn, pronucleus. (From B. Gondos, 1972. J. Cell Sci. 10, 61.)

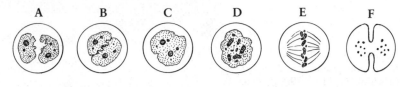

6–30   Stages in the development of the fertilized rabbit egg between 18 and 22 hours after mating. A, approach of male and female pronuclei; B, close association of pronuclei with flattening of opposing surfaces; C, communication between nuclei; D, breakdown of pronuclear membranes; E, metaphase spindle of first cleavage; F, first cleavage division. (After B. Gondos, 1972. J. Cell Sci. 10, 61.)

logical, and biochemical activities. The articulation of these activities, the definition of their sequence of appearance, and the interdependence of their expression are goals of the investigator examining the problem of fertilization. The egg of the sea urchin has contributed much to what we currently know about the program of fertilization. The activities comprising this program and their suggested relations are given in Figure 6–32.

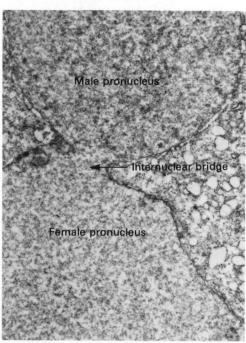

6–31   Fusion of the male and female pronuclei in the echinoderm egg. (From F. Longo and E. Anderson, 1968. J. Cell Biol. 39, 339.)

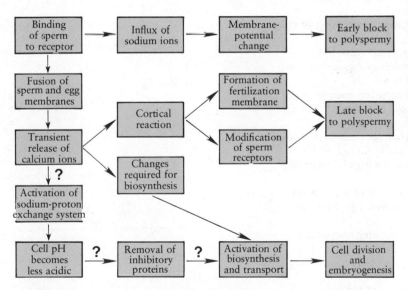

6–32   A flow diagram summarizing the suggested relationships among the early calcium-dependent changes and the late pH-dependent changes in the fertilized egg of *Strongylocentrotus*. A question mark indicates that the relationship between the activities is not well established. (From D. Epel, 1977. Sci. Am. 237, 129.)

REFERENCES

Anderson, E. 1968. Oocyte differentiation in sea urchin, *Arbacia punctulata*, with particular reference to the origin of cortical granules and their participation in the cortical reaction. J. Cell Biol. 37:514–539.

Austin, C. R. 1960. Capacitation and the release of hyaluronidase from spermatozoa. J. Reprod. Fertil. 1:310–311.

Austin, C. R. 1968. Ultrastructure of Fertilization. New York: Holt, Rinehart and Winston.

Barros, C. and C. R. Austin. 1967. *In vitro* fertilization and the sperm acrosome reaction in the hamster. J. Exp. Zool. 11:317–323.

Barros, C. and R. Yanagimachi. 1971. Induction of zona reaction in golden hamster eggs by cortical granule material. Nature (London) 233:268–269.

Bedford, J. M. 1968. Morphological aspects of sperm capacitation in mammals. In: Advances in Bioscience, 4. Ed., G. Raspe. New York: Pergamon Press.

Colwin, A. L. and L. H. Colwin. 1964. Role of gamete membranes in fertilization. In: Cellular Membranes in Development. 22nd Symposium of the Society for the Study of Development and Growth. Ed., M. Locke. New York: Academic Press.

Denny, P. and A. Tyler. 1964. Activation of protein biosynthesis in nonnucleate fragments of sea urchin eggs. Biochem. Biophys. Res. Commun. 14:245–259.

Endo, Y. 1961. Changes in the cortical layer of sea urchin eggs at fertilization as studied by the electron microscope. I. *Clypeaster japonicus*. Exp. Cell Res. 25:383–397.

Epel, D. 1975. The program of and the mechanism of fertilization in the echinoderm egg. Am. Zool. 15:507–522.

Epel, D. 1977. The program of fertilization. Sci. Am. 237:129–138.

Fankhauser, G. 1948. The organization of the amphibian egg during fertilization and cleavage. Ann. N.Y. Acad. Sci. 49:684–708.

Gondos, B., P. Bhiraleus, and L. Conner. 1972. Pronuclear membrane alterations during approximation of pronuclei and initiation of cleavage in the rabbit. J. Cell Sci. 10:61–78.

Gross, P., L. Malkin, and W. Moyer. 1964. Template for the first proteins of embryonic development. Proc. Nat. Acad. Sci. U.S.A. 51:407–414.

Jaffee, L. 1976. Fast block to polyspermy in sea urchin eggs is electrically mediated. Nature (London) 261:68–71.

Kedes, L. and L. Stavy. 1969. Structural and functional identity of ribosomes from eggs and embryos of sea urchins. J. Mol. Biol. 43:337–340.

Kemp, N. and N. Istock. 1967. Cortical changes in growing oocytes and in fertilized or pricked eggs of *Rana pipiens*. J. Cell Biol. 34:111–121.

Lillie, F. R. 1919. Problems of Fertilization. Chicago: University of Chicago Press.

Longo, F. and E. Anderson. 1969. Cytological aspects of fertilization in the lamellibranch, *Mytilus edulis*. II. Development of the male pronucleus and the association of the maternally and paternally derived chromosomes. J. Exp. Zool. 172:97–120.

Longo, F. and E. Anderson. 1970. An ultrastructural analysis of fertilization in the surf clam, *Spisula solidissima*. II. Development of the male pronucleus and the association of maternally and paternally derived chromosomes. J. Ultrastruct. Res. 33:515–527.

Metafora, S., L. Fellicetti, and R. Gambino. 1971. The mechanism of protein synthesis activation after fertilization of sea urchin eggs. Proc. Nat. Acad. Sci. U.S.A. 68:600–604.

Monroy, A. 1965. Chemistry and Physiology of Fertilization. New York: Holt, Rinehart and Winston.

Monroy, A., R. Maggio, and A. Rinaldi. 1965. Experimentally induced activation of the ribosomes of the unfertilized sea urchin egg. Proc. Nat. Acad. Sci. U.S.A. 54:107–111.

Nemer, M. and S. G. Bard. 1963. Polypeptide synthesis in sea urchin embryogenesis: An examination with synthetic polynucleotides. Science 140:664–666.

Stambaugh, R. and M. Smith. 1974. Amino acid content of rabbit acrosomes; proteinase and its similarity to human trypsin. Science 186:745–746.

Tegner, M. and D. Epel. 1973. Sea urchin sperm-egg interactions studied with scanning electron microscopy. Science 179:685–688.

Wineck, T. J., R. F. Parrish, and K. F. Polakoski. 1979. Fertilization: A uterine glycosaminoglycan stimulates the conversion of sperm proacrosin to acrosin. Science 203:553–554.

Zanewald, L. J. and W. L. Williams. 1970. A sperm enzyme that disperses the corona radiata and its inhibition by DF. Biol. Reprod. 2:363–368.

7

Cleavage and Blastulation

Soon after fertilization the zygote becomes rapidly converted into a population of cells. The series of cell divisions by which this transformation is achieved is known as *cleavage* or *segmentation*. The cells formed by this process are termed *cleavage cells* or *blastomeres*. The period of cleavage is considered to extend from fertilization to the time of the formation of a multicellular embryo known as the *blastula*. Generally, there is little evidence of growth during this time and the shape of the embryo does not visibly change.

Cleavage is a process that is easily observed in a variety of animal egg cells with the assistance of a microscope. The cleavages of the fertilized egg cell are typical animal cell divisions in that mitosis or *nuclear division* is immediately followed by *cytokinesis*. However, there are several characteristic differences between the cell divisions of cleavage and those found in later stages of embryonic development and in dividing tissues of the adult animal. The consecutive divisions of cleaving cells are not separated by intervening periods of growth. Hence, the total cytoplasmic volume of the embryo during this period of development remains approximately constant. As a consequence, the blastomeres of the embryo become smaller and smaller until each reaches a cell size characteristic of the species. The absence of a distinct growth phase between successive cleavages also gradually changes the ratio of nuclear to cytoplasmic volume. Segmentation begins with a cell that has a low nucleus-to-cytoplasmic volume when compared to the cells of the adult organism. In the mature sea urchin egg, the volume of nucleus/volume of cytoplasm is 1/500. By the 64-celled stage, this same ratio is 1/12. At the end of cleavage, the proportion is approximately 1/6.

The rate or rhythm of cleavage is measured by the time interval between two consecutive divisions (*generation time*). Eggs cleave at rates characteristic of the species, but this rate may be greatly influenced by temperature. Generation times at a given temperature are easily determined during early cleavage because the first several divisions of the egg tend to occur simultaneously in all blastomeres. Zebra fish eggs cleave about every 15 minutes at 26°C. The early cleavages of the killifish (*Fundulus*) are separated by an interval of about 45 to 60 minutes. By contrast, there may be 10 to 12 hours at 37°C between cleavages in young mouse embryos. It is interesting to note that forms like fishes and frogs reach the blastula stage at a lower temperature more rapidly than typical mammals at a higher temperature. Several studies, particularly those involving hybridization experiments between echinoderm species with different generation times at cleavage, have indicated that the cytoplasm of the fertilized egg cell carries a factor that is important in determining the rate at which cleavages occur.

PATTERNS OF CLEAVAGE

As pointed out in a previous chapter, animal egg cells may be quite different with respect to the amount and distribution of yolk or yolky cytoplasm. Indeed, from species to species the differences in the relative amounts of yolk and active cytoplasm influence the pattern by which the egg cell is progressively subdivided into daughter cells. The correlation between cleavage pattern and yolk was recognized by G. W. Balfour (1894) who observed that the rate at which the cleavage furrow passed through the egg was inversely proportional to the amount of yolk within the cell. Indeed, both mitosis and cytokinesis are progressively impeded with increasing amounts of yolky cytoplasm.

The egg cells of many annelids, molluscs, nematodes, echinoderms, cephalochordates, amphibians, and mammals contain small to moderate amounts of yolk. Such an egg cell is always divided into complete daughter cells, a pattern of cleavage that is termed *holoblastic.* In reptiles, birds, and elasmobranch and teleost fishes, the egg cell possesses a larger amount of yolk heavily concentrated at one pole. Only the active cytoplasm with the nucleus, never the yolk, undergoes cleavage. Such a pattern of cleavage is termed *meroblastic* or *discoidal.*

It is advisable at this time, as a basis for the understanding of later developmental events, to examine in detail selected animals that illustrate these cleavage patterns.

Cephalochordata—Amphioxus

The egg cell of *Amphioxus* at the time of fertilization is approximately 120 micrometers in diameter. The first cleavage appears as a furrow that completely encircles the cell some 60 to 90 minutes after insemination. The furrow subsequently divides the egg into two equal blastomeres along a meridional plane that extends from animal to vegetal pole (Fig. 7–1 A,B). This plane along which the egg is cleaved represents the axis of bilateral symmetry of the adult organism. The second cleavage occurs 45 minutes later and is also meridional, but at right angles to the first furrow (Fig. 7–1 C). The

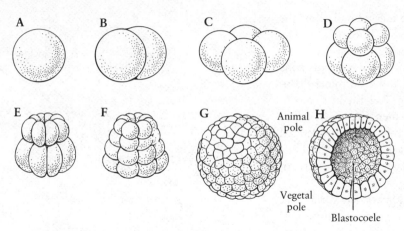

7–1 Cleavage and blastulation in the egg of *Amphioxus*. A, fertilized egg; B, 2-celled stage; C, 4-celled stage; D, 8-celled stage; E, 16-celled stage; F, 32-celled stage; G, blastula, surface view; H, blastula, hemisection. (From A. F. Huettner, 1972. Fundamentals of Comparative Embryology of the Vertebrates. Copyright 1949 by Macmillan Publishing Co., Inc., renewed by M. R. Huettner, R. A. Huettner, and R. J. Huettner.)

Animal pole

Vegetal pole

Blastocoele

two blastomeres are divided into four blastomeres. The third cleavage is horizontal, at right angles to the first two cleavage furrows, and slightly above the equators of the four blastomeres. Upon completion of the furrowing process, eight blastomeres are produced. Although the upper quartet of blastomeres is only slightly smaller than the lower quartet, the former are often called *micromeres* and the latter *macromeres* (Fig. 7–1 D). The fourth cleavage is meridional (Fig. 7–1 E). The fifth cleavage is horizontal, dividing the eight micromeres and eight macromeres simultaneously into a total of 32 blastomeres (Fig. 7–1 F). During succeeding cleavages, the larger macromeres in the vegetal hemisphere tend to divide more slowly than the smaller micromeres in the animal hemisphere. By the end of the period of cleavage, the cephalochordate embryo is organized as a hollow sphere or blastula whose cells enclose a fluid-filled cavity termed the *blastocoele* (Fig. 7–1 G). The 200 or so blastomeres are structured as a simple epithelium in which the larger cells are located in the vegetal hemisphere and the smaller cells in the animal hemisphere (Fig. 7–1 H).

Echinodermata—Sea Urchin

The fertilized egg of the sea urchin is approximately 90 to 100 micrometers in diameter and roughly spherical. The first cleavage generally occurs within 60 to 90 minutes of fertilization (Fig. 7–2 A,B). The furrow is meridional and cuts the egg cell into two equal-sized blastomeres. The second cleavage is meridional, but at right angles to the first. The third pair of cleavages is visible about three hours after fertilization. Each is horizontal and results in a cluster of four animal (upper) and four vegetal (lower) blastomeres (Fig. 7–2 D). The cleavages of the fourth division are quite unusual. The four blastomeres of the animal hemisphere divide meridionally, but the four blastomeres of the vegetal hemisphere divide horizontally. The result is a 16-celled embryo with the following layers: an upper zone of eight medium-sized blastomeres (*mesomeres*), a middle zone of four very large blastomeres (macromeres), and a bottom zone of four very small blastomeres (micromeres) (Fig. 7–2 E). In two subsequent cleavages, first the mesomeres and then the macromeres divide equatorially to form an embryo of 64 cells. A cavity, termed the blastocoele, appears very early in cleavage between the blastomeres. It continues to enlarge as the blastomeres increase in number and decrease in size.

Blastulation, or the process by which the blastocoele forms and the blastomeres become displaced into a tightly organized peripheral layer of cells, has received considerable attention in sea urchins. The formation of the blastocoele and its enlargement are probably related to an osmotic pressure exerted by the blastocoelic fluid. The uptake of water from the environment by the blastocoele forces the blastomeres outward where they attach to the hyaline layer. The adhesiveness of adjacent blastomeres and the increase in surface tension between dividing blastomeres act to maintain the peripheral position of the cells of the blastula. The sea urchin blastula consists of some 200 cells organized around a spacious, fluid-filled internal cavity (Fig. 7–2 G,H).

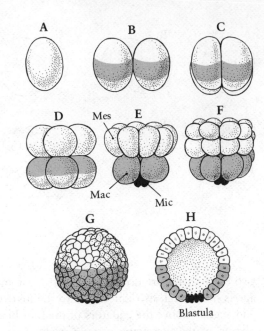

7–2 Cleavage and blastulation in the egg of the sea urchin, *Paracentrotus*. A, fertilized egg; B, 2-celled stage; C, 4-celled stage; D, 8-celled stage; E, 16-celled stage; F, 32-celled stage; G, blastula, surface view; H, blastula, hemisection. mes= mesomere; mac=macromere; mic=micromere.

Amphibia—Frog or Salamander

A good example showing the effect of the amount and distribution of yolk upon the pattern of segmentation is seen in the amphibian egg. Here the yolk is distributed along the animal–vegetal axis with the greatest concentration at the vegetal pole. Cleavage is initiated at the animal pole some two to three hours (temperature-dependent and species-dependent) after fertilization. The first two furrows are meridional and at right angles to each other, producing four cells of approximately equal size (Fig. 7–3 A–C). The first furrow generally passes through the grey crescent so that each of the resulting blastomeres contains a portion of this cytoplasm. Because of the unequal distribution of the yolk within the egg, the third pair of cleavages is displaced markedly toward the animal pole (Fig. 7–3 D). The larger blastomeres or macromeres produced by this division are confined to the vegetal hemisphere and the smaller blastomeres or micromeres to the animal hemisphere of the embryo. After about the fourth or fifth cleavages, the regularity of the segmentation process is lost and blastomeres tend to divide at different rates. Blastomeres containing yolk-laden platelets tend to divide more slowly than those with less yolk. For a short period of time, the blas-

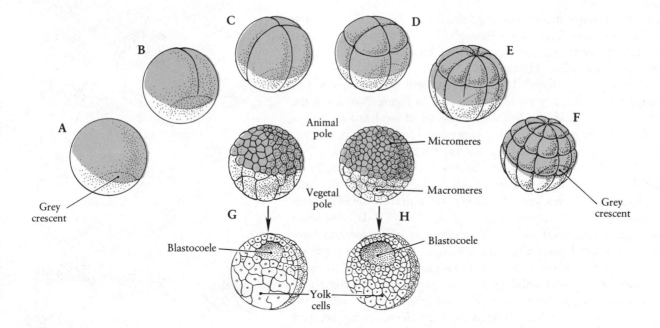

Grey crescent

A

B

C

D

E

F

Animal pole

Vegetal pole

Micromeres

Macromeres

Grey crescent

Blastocoele

G

H

Blastocoele

Yolk cells

tomeres are packed together and the embryo takes on the appearance of a cluster of mulberries. Such a configuration is referred to as a *morula stage*. Narrow spaces appear between the blastomeres. These gradually coalesce into a single cavity or blastocoele. As with *Amphioxus* and the sea urchin, there emerges with continued cleavages a hollow, spherically shaped ball of cells, the blastula (Fig. 7–3 G). A hemisection through the late blastula shows the blastocoele eccentrically displaced toward the animal pole (Fig. 7–3 H). The cells of the animal hemisphere are small and organized into two or more layers; they form the roof of the blastocoele. The cells of the vegetal hemisphere are large, yolk laden, and form the floor of the blastocoele. The pattern of cleavage in amphibians is often termed *unequal holoblastic*, a phrase that recognizes the noticeable contrast in the size of the blastomeres of the blastula.

Osteichthyes—Bony Fishes

The egg cells of bony fishes have more yolk than those of the amphibians, and consequently the active cytoplasm along with the nucleus tends to be located at the animal pole. Representative species within this group of vertebrates show a range in cleavage pattern from incomplete holoblastic to meroblastic. In a primitive bony fish such as *Amia* (the bowfin), meridional cleavages start at the animal pole, but they are greatly retarded in their efforts to reach the vegetal pole because of the large yolk mass (Fig. 7–4 A).

7–3 Cleavage and blastulation in the egg of a typical amphibian. A, fertilized egg; B, beginning of 2-celled stage; C, 4-celled stage; D, 8-celled stage; E, 16-celled stage; F, 32-celled stage; G, blastula, surface view; H, blastula, hemisection. (From A. F. Huettner, 1972. Fundamentals of Comparative Embryology of the Vertebrates. Copyright 1949 by Macmillan Publishing Co., Inc., renewed by M. R. Huettner, R. A. Huettner, and R. J. Huettner.)

Indeed, subsequent divisions are initiated in the animal pole well before preceding furrows cut through the yolk toward the vegetal pole. As in the frog and the salamander, however, the whole egg is divided into daughter blastomeres.

More typical in higher bony fishes (as well as in elasmobranch fishes) is the cleavage pattern illustrated in Figure 7–4 B for the zebrafish (*Brachydanio*). Within 25 minutes of fertilization, the cytoplasm of the egg cell is entirely segregated from the yolk and appears as a distinct cap or *blastodisc* at the animal pole (Figs. 7–4 B,1; 7–5 A). Only the blastodisc becomes cellularized during cleavage. Initially, the cleavages are meridional or vertical and all of the resultant blastomeres lie in the same plane with their lower surfaces formed by the yolk below (Figs. 7–4 B,2–4; 7–5 B–D). The sixth cleavage is horizontal and yields an upper set of blastomeres completely separated from neighboring blastomeres while the lower set of blastomeres retains a connection with the yolk mass. Continued divisions in the horizontal plane add more cells with completed boundaries. Within four hours of fertilization in the zebrafish, the blastula stage is reached. Termed the *blastoderm,* it appears as a compact mass of small blastomeres elevated above the yolk mass (Fig. 7–4 B,6). A hemisection through the blastoderm shows the presence of a blastocoele (Fig. 7–4 B,7). Although the blastocoele is largely lined by distinct blastomeres, its floor is formed by a syncytial cytoplasm in which numerous nuclei can be detected. This layer, known as the *periblast,* is formed as follows. At the end of cleavage, the lowermost blastomeres, produced as a result of horizontal divisions, are still continuous with the yolk mass (i.e., they lack lower boundaries). The lateral boundaries between these blastomeres disappear and their cytoplasms and nuclei join together to form a distinct layer on top of the yolk mass.

Aves—The Bird

Segregation of the active cytoplasm from the yolk in the bird is completed by the end of oogenesis. Therefore, the whitish-colored blastodisc, approximately three millimeters in diameter, is already organized at the time of fertilization. With successful fertilization of the ovum in the oviduct, the first cleavage furrow appears some three to five hours after ovulation. The first cleavage furrow is considered to be meridional; it bisects the blastodisc into two partially separated blastomeres (Fig. 7–6 A,G). The second cleavage consists of two meridional furrows, each one of which is at a right angle to the first cleavage furrow (Fig. 7–6 B). The third set of cleavages are also vertical and tend to be variable in position, but typically are parallel to the plane of the first cleavage furrow. The fourth set of

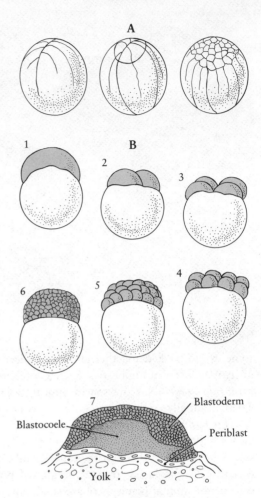

7–4 Patterns of cleavage in bony fishes. A, holoblastic cleavage in a primitive bony fish such as *Amia.* (From E. Korschelt, 1936. Vergleichende Entwicklungsgeschichte der Tiere. G. Fischer, Jena); B, meroblastic cleavage in advanced bony fish such as *Brachydanio.* (1) egg 25 minutes after fertilization; (2) two-celled stage; (3) four-celled stage; (4) eight-celled stage; (5) late cleavage; (6) blastula, lateral view; (7) blastula, hemisection. (After K. Hisaoka and H. Battle, 1958. J. Morphol. 102, 311.)

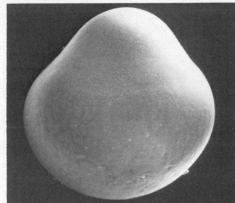

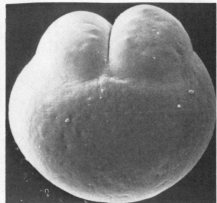

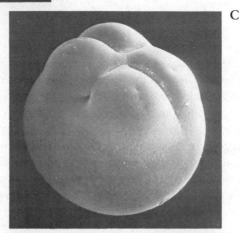

C

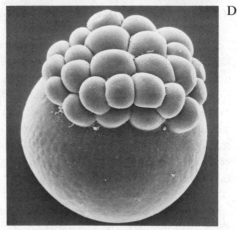

D

cleavages are considered to be vertical and occur in such a fashion that eight *central cells* are separated from eight *marginal cells* (Fig. 7–6 D). The centrally located cells have upper and lateral surfaces, but, lacking a lower surface, are continuous with the yolk below (Fig. 7–6 H). The marginal cells are incomplete peripherally since the furrows do not extend to the margins of the blastodisc; they lack a lower surface and therefore possess only a pair of lateral surfaces (Fig. 7–6 D,H). From this point onward, the succession of cleavages becomes asynchronous and irregular. Three types of furrows are evident: (1) vertical furrows that extend peripherad toward the margin of the blastodisc; (2) vertical furrows that cut across the inner ends of radiating furrows, thereby producing peripheral boundaries to marginal cells; these blastomeres then become part of the centrally located cells; (3) horizontal furrows that occur below the surface (and parallel to it) and establish lower boundaries to the cells. Horizontal cleavages begin sometime after the 32-celled stage.

By the time the embryo or blastoderm consists of 60 to 100 cells (Fig. 7–6 I), it is organized as a mass of centrally located cells, actively dividing, which lie over a fluid-filled cavity. Beyond the centrally located cells, vertical cleavages continue to add more central cells, thereby advancing peripherally the segmentation of the blastodisc. Horizontal cleavages progress centrifugally and establish lower boundaries for the more peripherally located cells. Some of the nuclei formed by these horizontal divisions have been observed to wander yolkward and peripherally into uncleaved portions of the cytoplasm. This nucleated cytoplasm becomes evident below the blastoderm. It forms the periblast. Eventually, the periblast beneath the margins of the blastoderm becomes cellularized and further adds to the expanding population of blastomeres with completed boundaries.

7–5   Scanning electron micrographs of the blastodisc stage (A), 2-celled stage (B), 4-celled stage (C), and 32-celled stage in *Brachydanio*. (From H. Beams and R. Kessel, 1976. Am. Sci. 64, 279. Reprinted by permission of American Scientist, Journal of Sigma Xi, The Scientific Research Society.)

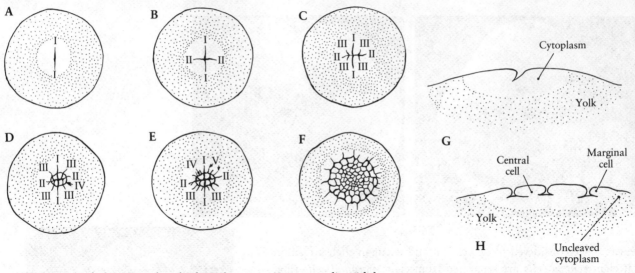

At the end of cleavage, the chick embryo appears as a discoidal cap of cells atop the yolk (Fig. 7–6 J). This blastoderm is five to six cells thick in the center but only one to two cells deep at the periphery. With transmitted light under the microscope, the blastoderm can be divided into two recognizable regions. There is a central region or *area pellucida;* it appears translucent because its blastomeres are separated from the yolk by a fluid-filled cavity. By contrast, the peripheral part of the blastoderm lies against the yolk, thus rendering it more opaque (*area opaca*). Only the cells of the area pellucida will contribute to the construction of the embryo.

Mammalia—The Pig and Monkey

With the exception of the eggs of primitive mammals (i.e., duckbill platypus and spiny anteater), which have a large amount of yolk and divide in meroblastic fashion, the ova of marsupial and placental mammals are exceedingly small. Their size reflects the scanty amount of yolk that is manufactured and stored during oogenesis. The ovum is only about 70 micrometers in diameter in the mouse and approximately 120 micrometers in the dog. As one might expect, the segmentation of the fertilized egg is holoblastic and all blastomeres are more or less of equal size (Fig. 7–7).

Cleavage of the mammalian egg is initiated in the upper end of the oviduct some 24 to 25 hours after insemination. In the mouse, rabbit, and monkey, the first cleavage furrow appears to be meridional, extending along an imaginary axis from animal to vegetal pole. By contrast to the oligolecithal eggs of other invertebrate and chordate organisms, the mammalian egg lacks synchronization of mitoses of blastomeres from the two-celled stage onward. Con-

7–6 Cleavage and blastulation in the egg of the bird. A, 2-celled stage, polar view; B, 4-celled stage, polar view; C, 8-celled stage, polar view; D, 16-celled stage, polar view; E, 32-celled stage, polar view; F, early morula, polar view; G, 2-celled stage, hemisection; H, 8-celled stage, hemisection; I, early blastula, hemisection; J, advanced blastula, hemisection. I–V, temporal sequence of cleavage furrows. (A–F, from Foundations of Embryology by B. Patten and B. Carlson. Copyright © 1974 by McGraw-Hill Inc. Used with permission of McGraw-Hill Book Company; H–J, after A. F. Huettner, 1972. Fundamentals of Comparative Embryology of the Vertebrates. Copyright 1949 by Macmillan Publishing Co., Inc., renewed by M. R. Huettner, R. A. Huettner, and R. J. Huettner.)

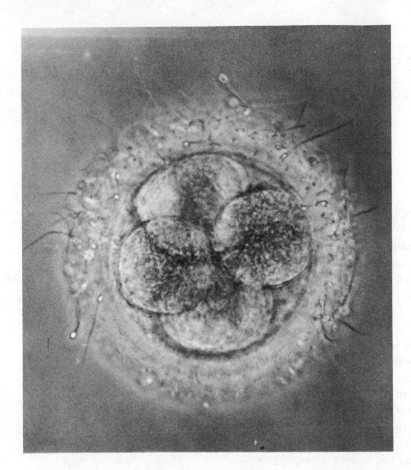

7–7   Human egg at the four-celled stage. Note the spermatozoa in the zona pellucida. (From R. Edwards and R. Fowler, 1970. Sci. Am. 223, 44.)

sequently, it is not unusual to find three-celled, five-celled, and seven-celled stages in the mammalian embryo (Figs. 7–8, 7–9). Examine carefully the sequence of cleavage and blastulation in the egg of the pig (Fig. 7–9). Note that one of the first two blastomeres is more precocious than the other in the onset of the second cleavage, thus giving rise to a three-celled stage. From this stage onward, one can divide the embryo into a part that divides more rapidly and a part that divides more slowly (Fig. 7–9 C-I). If the fates of the cells comprising these two areas are traced into the blastula stage, it can be shown that the more rapidly dividing cells will contribute to the *trophoblast* and the more slowly dividing cells into the *formative* or *inner mass cells*.

The result of the segmentation of the fertilized egg is the production of a solid sphere of cells or morula. In such forms as the bat, the superficial cells are organized at this stage into a loose epithelial layer (Fig. 7–10 A). This outer layer of trophoblast will contribute to the formation of the extraembryonic membranes of the embryo,

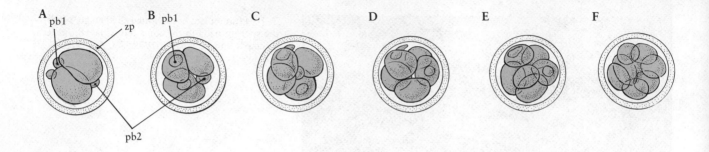

7–8 Early cleavage of the egg of the monkey, *Macacus rhesus*. A, two-celled stage; B, three-celled stage; C, four-celled stage; D, five-celled stage; E, six-celled stage; F, seven-celled stage. pb1, pb2, polar bodies 1 and 2; zp, zona pellucida. (After W. Lewis and C. Hartmann, 1933. Carnegie Contributions to Embryology 24, 189.)

make contact with the uterine wall during implantation, and mediate the supply of nourishment to the embryo from the maternal body by way of the placenta. The cells lying in the interior constitute the inner cell mass. The inner cell mass contributes directly to the construction of the various parts of the embryo proper.

Before entrance into the uterine portion of the oviduct, the morula gradually becomes transformed into the blastocyst (Fig. 7–10 B). Crevices increasingly appear between the inner cell mass and most of the cells of the overlying trophoblast. As the fluid-filled spaces progressively coalesce, a large cavity or blastocoele is formed with displacement of the inner cell mass toward the future dorsal side of the embryo. At this site, the inner cell mass remains connected to the inner surface of the trophoblast. Continued uptake of water and of fluids from the oviduct into the blastocoele noticeably increases the volume of the blastocyst. Under these conditions, the zona pellucida is greatly stretched. Eventually, this membrane ruptures and the blastocyst is set free in preparation for implantation into the wall of the uterus.

THE CLEAVING CELL

The cleavage of a blastomere involves a mitosis or nuclear division followed immediately by cytokinesis or physical separation into two daughter cells. In holoblastic organisms, each blastomere tends to round up just prior to division so that its surface area is minimal (Fig. 7–11). By the late anaphase stage of mitosis, the blastomere elongates in a plane parallel to the mitotic spindle apparatus. Consequently, the surface at the equator of the dividing blastomere is noticeably flattened. This condition is exaggerated in telophase when the diameter of the blastomere actively decreases with the formation of the cleavage furrow.

When one spherical blastomere divides into two daughter cells with a similar shape, the combined diameters and surface areas of

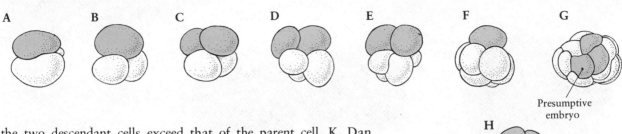

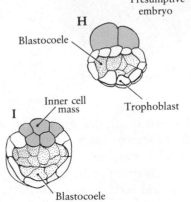

7–9 Cleavage and blastulation of the egg of the pig based upon models reconstructed in wax. A, two-celled stage; B, three-celled stage; C, four-celled stage; D, five-celled stage; E, six-celled stage; F, eight-celled stage; G, morula stage; H, formation of the blastocoele; I, early blastocyst. (After C. Heuser and G. Streeter, 1929. Carnegie Contributions to Embryology 20, 1.)

the two descendant cells exceed that of the parent cell. K. Dan (1937) has estimated that the surface area increases by about 26 percent in a divided echinoderm blastomere. The process of segmentation, therefore, is always accompanied by the formation of additional surface membrane.

Because of their size, shape, and transparency (particularly invertebrate eggs), cleaving eggs have been viewed as ideal subjects for the study of the fundamental processes of cell division. Investigators have been particularly interested in the role(s) of the visible parts of the blastomeres in the cleavage process and in the physicochemical basis for the separation of one cell into two cells.

The most visible structural component of the cleaving cell is the mitotic apparatus (Fig. 7–12). This complex includes the chromosomes, spindles, asters, and centrioles. Under the light microscope, each centriole appears as a rod-shaped particle embedded in a clear area of cytoplasm, the *centrosome*. With the electron microscope, each centriole is, in fact, a pair of hollow cylinders with the long axis of one being at right angles to the long axis of the other. A typical cylinder consists of nine peripherally arranged fibrils, each of which is a triplet of microtubules. Although the precise mechanism remains unclear, centrioles are believed to self-duplicate from precursor molecules in the cytoplasm just prior to the onset of a cleavage. Each centriole serves as a site for the organization of protein subunits into a linear array of microtubules and vesicular elements that comprise the spindle and astral fibers. Chromosomes engaged by the spindle fibers are drawn toward the centrioles during the mitotic phase of the cell division cycle. The size of the mitotic apparatus varies among different animal species. In general, the size of the mitotic apparatus is proportional to the volume of cytoplasm that it occupies.

The location of the mitotic apparatus within the cytoplasm of a dividing blastomere appears to determine both the position of the cleavage furrow as well as the time of its appearance. When the mitotic apparatus is in the center of a spherical blastomere, the furrow tends to appear simultaneously throughout the circumference of the cell. However, if the mitotic apparatus is naturally or experimentally displaced to one side of the blastomere, the furrow appears first in the nearest surface and then in the more distant sur-

7–10 The inner cell mass and trophoblast at the morula (A) and early blastocyst (B) stages of the bat. (From J. Brachet, 1935. Traité d'embryologie des vertebres, 2nd ed. Revised by A. Dalcq and P. Gerard. Masson, Paris.)

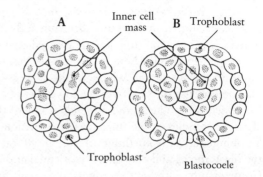

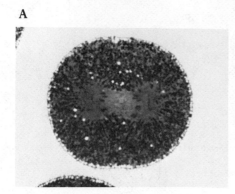

A

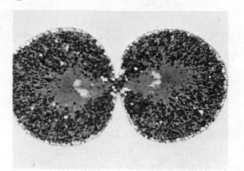

B

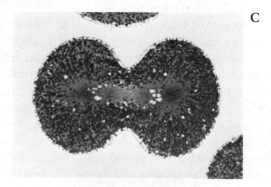

C

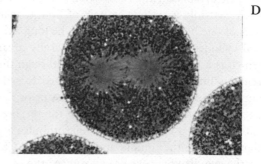

D

face. The types of cleavage found among invertebrate and vertebrate organisms clearly demonstrate that the furrowing of the cytoplasm in dividing blastomeres bears a structural relationship to the orientation of the mitotic apparatus. In forms like echinoderms, amphibians, and urochordates, the cleavage spindles of the mitotic apparatus tend to be oriented with their long axes perpendicular or parallel to the axes of cell polarity. The plane of furrowing is always perpendicular to the axis of the mitotic spindle. Such a division is said to be *meridional* or *radial* because the resultant blastomeres are organized in a radially symmetrical pattern around a polar axis (Fig. 7–13 A). A peculiarity of the radial type of cleavage is seen in many vertebrates. Here a distinct left-sideness and right-sideness are imparted to the embryo with the first and succeeding divisions of the egg cell. In frogs, for example, the mitotic spindle is oriented in such a way that the first cleavage furrow coincides with the median plane of the embryo. The first two blastomeres are mirror images of each other, but with one representing the left side of the embryo and the other the right side. Cleavage of this type is referred to as being *bilaterally symmetrical.*

An entirely different relationship between the orientation of the mitotic spindle and the axis of cell polarity is visible in the dividing eggs of many molluscs, annelids, and nemertean worms (Fig. 7–13 B). After three divisions, it is noted that the upper quartet of blastomeres is shifted in the same direction such that each upper blastomere lies over the junction of two adjacent blastomeres of the lower quartet of cells. Note that this is in sharp contrast to the condition in the sea urchin where, at the same stage, the upper tier of blastomeres lies directly over the lower tier of blastomeres. This arrangement in molluscs and annelids is due to the fact that the four cleavage spindles of the third cleavage division tend to be tipped at an oblique angle (something other than 90° or 180°) to the axes of the blastomeres and coordinately oriented in the pattern of a spiral. Consequently, although the division furrows are at right angles to

7–11 Cleavage in sea urchin eggs. Midlongitudinal sections (1μ) of a cleaving *Strongylocentrotus purpuratus* egg with fertilization membranes and hyaline layers removed. The dark cytoplasmic granules are yolk granules. The yolk-free zone contains the mitotic apparatus. A, metaphase: chromosomes are condensed (dark) and lined up at the equator; B, early telophase: chromosomes have separated and furrowing has commenced; C, midtelophase; D, late telophase: cleavage is nearly complete. Cleavage is complete within 15 minutes. (Courtesy of C. Asnes and T. Schroeder.)

the axes of the mitotic apparatus, the resulting upper tier of blastomeres comes off in spiral fashion. This *spiral type* of cleavage is continued with subsequent divisions. If the blastomeres appear to rotate in a clockwise direction, the spiral is *dextral;* if the blastomeres appear to rotate in a counterclockwise direction, the spiral is *sinistral*. The coiling, either dextral or sinistral, of the shells of snails reflects the spiral pattern of cleavage.

The events of mitosis and cytokinesis overlap in the cell cycle. Hence, there has always been intense interest in the possibility that the form and arrangement of the mitotic spindle and asters might function in the direct physical separation of a blastomere into two daughter cells. There is now an abundance of experimental evidence which indicates that these visible structures of the blastomere do not play an important physical role in cleavage. Y. Hiramoto (1965) removed the entire mitotic apparatus by aspiration with a micropipette shortly after metaphase in an echinoderm cleaving egg (Fig. 7–14 A–C). The division of the experimental cell was unaffected by this manipulation. Even if the mitotic apparatus was displaced by removal of part of the egg cytoplasm, the cleavage furrow still appeared in its normal position (Fig. 7–14 D–F). Two conclusions can be drawn from these observations. First, the position of the cleavage furrow is fixed by anaphase of the cell cycle. Second, furrowing is independent of the mitotic apparatus. R. Rappaport (1966) demonstrated that division continues following the initial appearance of a cleavage furrow even if the cytoplasm between the mitotic apparatus and cell surface is stirred vigorously or if the cell contents are displaced by alternate compression at the subpolar regions of the cell. It would appear, therefore, that after metaphase the division of the blastomere is independent of any subsurface organization.

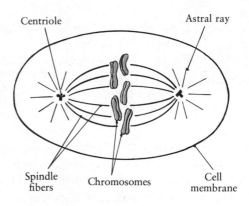

7–12 The most visible structural component of the cleaving cell is the mitotic apparatus. The mitotic apparatus includes the chromosomes, spindles, asters, and centrioles.

THE MECHANISM OF CLEAVAGE

The capacity of a cleavage furrow to continue its activities despite isolation from and disruption of subsurface structures clearly suggests that the site of the division mechanism resides in the surface of the blastomere. Within recent years, several theories have been proposed to account for the ability of a blastomere to divide itself into two halves at a highly predictable time and in a precisely predictable pattern. These theories include: the *polar expansion theory*, the *contractile ring theory*, and the *polar relaxation theory*. The polar expansion concept explains segmentation as due to the active growth and expansion of the polar regions of the blastomere, resulting in the passive inward dipping (i.e., furrowing) of the equa-

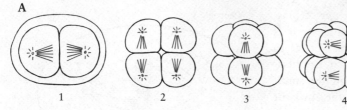

A

1 2 3 4 5

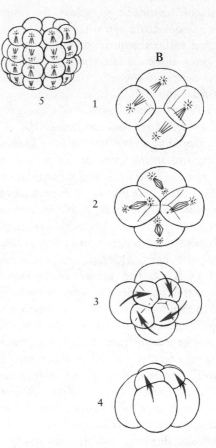

B

1

2

3

4

torial surface. The polar relaxation theory proposes that segmentation occurs because the polar surfaces of the blastomere relax, allowing the equatorial surface of the cell to actively contract. The contractile ring (or *equatorial constriction*) concept states that a blastomere divides because of the presence of a band of contractile material at the equator of the cell.

All three theories recognize that cleavage is a rather brief event with furrowing itself being preceded by dramatic changes in the physical and/or chemical properties of the cell surface. In the polar relaxation and equatorial constriction theories, it is additionally recognized that the entire cell surface or cortical cytoplasm becomes contractile just before the onset of furrowing. Eventually, the contractility is heightened at the equator of the cell, either through an increase at the equator of the cell (contractile ring) or a decrease at the poles of the cell (polar relaxation).

Most current data best supports the hypothesis that the cleaving cell divides because of the development of a specialized equatorial ring of contractile material located in the cortical cytoplasm. Observations with the electron microscope reveal the presence of an electron-dense, microfilamentous band at the base of cleavage furrows in a variety of animals, including squids, salamanders, jellyfish, echinoderms, and mammals (Fig. 7–15). In echinoderms, this band, about 0.1 micrometers thick and 10 micrometers wide, consists of numerous microfilaments, each of which is about 50 to 70 Å in diameter. All filaments are oriented parallel to the equatorial surface and parallel to the plane of the cleavage furrow. These microfilaments are presumed to be the visible expression of the contractile ring that cuts the blastomere into two daughter cells. Support for this interpretation comes from the correlation between the appearance of the furrow and the presence of the specialized microfilamentous bands. Also, *cytochalasin B,* an antibiotic from molds known to dissolve microfilaments, severely disturbs cytokinesis. Eggs treated with cytochalasin B before cleavage will show nuclear division but no physical separation into daughter cells. Eggs treated with cytochalasin B after physical division is initiated show either arrest or reversal of the furrowing process.

7–13 A, an example of radial cleavage as seen in an echinoderm. Note the orientation of the cleavage furrow to the mitotic apparatus. (1) 2-celled stage; (2) 4-celled stage (viewed from animal pole); (3) 8-celled stage (lateral view); (4) 16-celled stage (lateral view); (5) 32-celled stage (lateral view); B, an example of spiral cleavage as seen in a mollusc. (1) 4-celled stage with spindles of second division still visible; (2) 4-celled stage with metaphase spindles in place for the third division; (3) 8-celled stage (animal pole view); (4) 8-celled stage (lateral view). Arrows indicate direction of spiral. (From E. Korschelt, 1936. Vergleichende Entwicklungsgeschichte der Tiere. G. Fischer, Jena.)

The precise mechanism by which contraction of the microfilamentous band is achieved and translated into a furrow is not known. It has been suggested that contraction may occur by the filaments sliding past each other, much as in the actomyosin filament model proposed to account for the shortening of vertebrate skeletal muscle. An actomyosin basis for the cleavage contractile mechanism is supported by several lines of evidence. Actinoid or actinlike proteins have been isolated from the cortical cytoplasm of sea urchin eggs. When combined with rabbit muscle myosin, the complexed protein has many of the properties of ordinary actomyosin extracted from voluntary muscle tissue. The diameter of the furrow microfilaments is very similar to that recorded for actin threads. Also, Rappaport (1967) has determined that the microfilamentous band in echinodern cleaving eggs has a capacity for isometric contraction of approximately 1.25 to $2.4 - \times 10^5$ dynes/cm². Actomyosin threads during isometric contraction exert a tension of about 2.45×10^5 dynes/cm². The tension developed during cytokinesis is clearly visible in the appearance of the cleavage furrow (Fig. 7–16).

H. Sakai (1968) has offered an alternative hypothesis to explain the chemical basis for the cleavage contractile mechanism. He has isolated a KC1-soluble protein from a water-insoluble residue of homogenized sea urchin eggs. This protein can be made to form threads that contract and relax in the presence of certain metal ions, such as calcium. Since these same threads also contract and relax in the presence of oxidants of -SH groups, Sakai believes that cortical contraction occurs in the cleaving cell because of the oxidation of -SH containing proteins in the cortical cytoplasm.

How are the changes initiated which lead to the required modifications in the equatorial surface of the cleaving cell? What is the nature of the stimulus and the stimulation process? Rappaport (1967) and others are convinced that the functional differentiation of the surface required for furrow formation is a consequence of stimulation by the asters of the mitotic apparatus. Assessment of the role of the asters and other components of the mitotic apparatus has been accomplished by the geometrical alteration of the blastomere before metaphase (Fig. 7–17). When an echinoderm egg is converted into a torus-shaped structure by a glass bead, the first cleavage produces a horseshoe-shaped binucleate cell (Fig. 7–17 A,B). Two mitotic apparatuses form in the arms of the horseshoe-shaped cell in anticipation of the second cleavage division (Fig. 7–17 C). Only the astral rays are present at the bend of the torus-shaped cell. Successive cleavages appear not only at right angles to the mitotic apparatuses but also across the asters at the horseshoe bend to produce uninu-

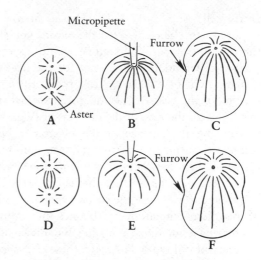

7–14 A–C, Successive stages of cleavage when the mitotic apparatus is removed by aspiration. A, before the spindle is removed; B, spindle removed; C, furrow still appears in predetermined position; D–F, successive stages of cleavage when the mitotic spindle is displaced by removing part of the egg protoplasm; D, before displacement; E, after displacement; F, furrow still appears at predetermined position. (From Y. Hiramoto, 1956. Exp. Cell Res. 11, 630.)

7–15 Microfilaments form a band in the furrow plane between two forming blastomeres in a rat egg. (After D. Szöllösi, 1970. J. Cell Biol. 44, 192.)

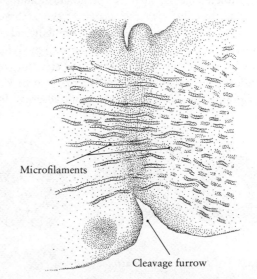

cleate cells (Fig. 7–17 C,D). Hence, furrow formation does not require the presence of either the mitotic spindle or chromosomes in the division plane. Asters alone would appear to bring about the surface differentiation necessary for the development of a furrow. When asters of a cleaving cell form, their rays penetrate to all regions of the cell. At the equatorial surface, the rays of one aster overlap with the rays of the other aster (Fig. 7–18). The astral rays, penetrating the surface of the blastomere, probably subject the equatorial surface to greater influence or stimulatory activity because of their overlapping configuration at this site. It would be convenient to propose that the astral fibers conduct one or more substances that induce the surface changes leading to the formation of the microfilamentous band. Since the 1930s, a number of investigators have identified centrifugable, division-related substances in a variety of cell types. However, these *cleavage-initiating substances* (CIS) appear to play more of a role in nuclear division than cytoplasmic division. It remains to be determined whether astral fibers function by transporting some critical substance or by inducing changes in the molecular configuration of the cortical cytoplasm.

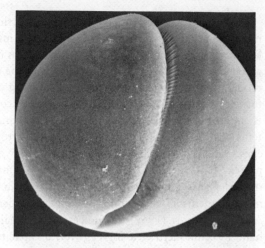

7–16 A scanning electron micrograph of the first cleavage in the egg of a frog to show the tension lines in the furrow. (From H. Beams and R. Kessel, 1976. Am. Sci. 64, 279. Reprinted by permission of American Scientist, Journal of Sigma Xi, The Scientific Research Society.)

THE SIGNIFICANCE OF CLEAVAGE

The period of cleavage is a time during which the fertilized egg becomes transformed into a multicellular embryo. During this time the nuclear to cytoplasmic volume is adjusted to that characteristic of the adult somatic cell. Since DNA synthesis and cell division are prominent features of cleavage, this developmental period is particularly susceptible to exogenous agents that damage chromosomes and nucleic acids, such as x-irradiation and ultraviolet radiation.

Additionally, cleavage provides the embryo with sufficient cell numbers to permit systematic movement and rearrangement of cells during the next major phase of development (gastrulation) in anticipation of the complex multilayered structure of the adult organism. Indeed, the blastula (or blastoderm) can be visualized as consisting of populations of cells of presumptive organ-forming areas that are

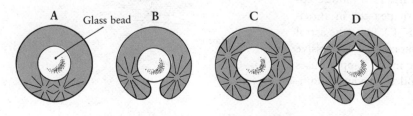

7–17 Cleavage of a torus-shaped echinoderm egg. A, before the first cleavage; B, after the first cleavage; C, before the second cleavage to show a mitotic apparatus in each arm of the binucleate cell; D, beginning of third cleavage to show that a furrow has formed between two asters not joined by a spindle, resulting in uninucleate cells. (From R. Rappaport, 1971. Int. Rev. Cytol. 31, 169.)

topographically organized into distinct zones. These presumptive organ-forming areas will be considered in greater detail in subsequent chapters.

REFERENCES

Arnold, J. 1969. Cleavage furrow formation in a telolecithal egg (*Loligo pealii*). I. Filaments in early furrow formation. J. Cell Biol. 41:893–904.

Dan, K., T. Yanigata, and M. Sugiyama 1937. Behavior of the cell surface during cleavage. I. Protoplasma. 28:66–81.

Hiramoto, Y. 1965. Further studies on cell division without mitotic apparatus in sea urchin egg. J. Cell Biol. 25:161–167.

Perry, M., H. John, and N. Thomas. 1971. Actin-like filaments in the cleavage furrow of the newt egg. Exp. Cell Res. 65:249–253.

Rappaport, R. 1961. Experiments concerning the cleavage stimulus in sand dollar eggs. J. Exp. Zool. 148:81–89.

Rappaport, R. 1966. Experiments concerning the cleavage furrow in invertebrate eggs. J. Exp. Zool. 161:1–8.

Rappaport, R. 1967. Cell division: Direct measurement of maximum tension exerted by furrow of echinoderm eggs. Science 156: 1241–1243.

Rappaport, R. 1971. Cytokinesis in animal cells. Int. Rev. Cytol. 31:169–213.

Sakai, H. 1968. Contractile properties of protein threads from sea urchin eggs in relation to cell division. Int. Rev. Cytol. 23:89–112.

Szollosi, D. 1970. Cortical cytoplasmic filaments of cleaving eggs: A structural element corresponding to the contractile ring. J. Cell Biol. 44:192–209.

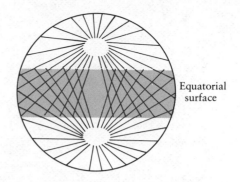

7–18 The equatorial stimulation pattern of cleavage as proposed by Rappaport. The equatorial surface of a cleaving cell is subjected to greater stimulatory activity because of the overlapping of the astral rays at this site. (From R. Rappaport, 1971. Int. Rev. Cytol. 31, 169.)

8

Gastrulation

We have described cleavage and blastulation as processes that offer little in the way of morphological differentiation but serve to provide the building blocks for future tissue and organ construction. Gastrulation is the period in development concerned with the sorting out and movement of these building blocks to the various regions of the embryo where they will be used. The blastula is a mass of cells showing little or no axiate pattern, and the arrangement of the cells bears no apparent relationship to the body plan of the future organism. Gastrulation involves a dynamic series of orderly morphogenetic movements that rearrange and reorganize large groups of cells into patterns in which they can take part in the formation of the various tissues and organs of the body. Following gastrulation the axiate pattern of the organism is easily recognizable.

Gastrulation also results in the formation of a multilayered embryo. In some species, such as *Amphioxus,* gastrulation results in the formation of a two-layered embryo. In others, such as the frog, a three-layered condition results. However, in those forms in which a two-layered condition is the initial consequence of gastrulation, reorganization of the inner layer soon takes place and results in the formation of a three-layered embryo. These three layers are known as the primary germ layers: ectoderm, endoderm, and mesoderm. The presumptive endoderm and mesoderm, located on the surface of the egg in the blastula, are moved to the inside of the gastrula. The result is essentially an outer tube of ectoderm surrounding an inner tube of endoderm with a tube of mesoderm placed between them, a structure characteristic of the general vertebrate body plan. Each of these layers will develop into specific parts of the organism. The ectoderm differentiates into epidermis and neural tissue, the endoderm into the lining of the gastrointestinal tract and the respiratory system, and the mesoderm into urogenital structures, circulatory system, connective tissue, and muscle.

THE CELL MOVEMENTS OF GASTRULATION

Certain general types of cell movements occur during gastrulation. To a large extent the amount of yolk influences the type and amount of movement and not all types are seen in all eggs. *Invagination* is the major movement in most eggs with small amounts of yolk. Invagination is the inpushing or inpocketing of an unbroken sheet of cells at one region of the blastula. It has been compared to placing the thumbs on the surface of a hollow rubber ball and pushing in with sufficient force to obliterate the original cavity (the blastocoele) establishing a new cavity (the gastrocoele). This movement is best exemplified in the sea urchin and in *Amphioxus*. The term invagination has also been applied to the movement of the cells through the primitive streak of the chick embryo. *Involution* is the rolling in of cells over a rim. The cells that involute are replaced by cells on the surface, which move toward the point of involution so that a continual stream of cells passes over the rim into the interior. This is the type of movement characteristic of eggs with moderate amounts of yolk such as those of the amphibians. However, if we consider the rubber ball analogy, it is apparent that involution must necessarily also accompany invagination. A third major movement is that of the cells on the surface of the blastula. This is called *epiboly*. Cells move over the surface toward the region of invagination or involution. At the completion of gastrulation, the epibolic movements have resulted in the spread of the presumptive ectoderm over the entire surface of the embryo. In most embryos the region at which the cells move into the inside is limited to a small part of the embryo. Thus, as cells from outlying areas approach this region they must show a considerable amount of *convergence*. Conversely, once inside, the cells move away from the point of entry, a movement of *divergence*. The region where cells move to the inside is known as the *blastopore* in *Amphioxus* and the amphibians. In avian species it is known as the *primitive streak*.

GASTRULATION IN AMPHIOXUS

Gastrulation at its simplest occurs in those species in which cellular movements are not restricted by the presence of large amounts of inert yolk. Such is the case in *Amphioxus*. The blastula of *Amphioxus* has been described in Chapter 7 as a single layer of columnar cells surrounding a large cavity, the blastocoele (Fig. 8–1 A). An animal and a vegetal pole may be recognized on the basis of the larger cells at the vegetal pole. The first indication of gastrulation is a flattening of the blastula at the vegetal pole (Fig. 8–1 B). This flattened plate of cells, presumptive endoderm, then gradually folds inwards, invaginating into the blastocoele converting the spherical blastula into a cup-shaped gastrula (Fig. 8–1 C,F). The invaginated cells move toward the surface ectodermal cells at the animal pole

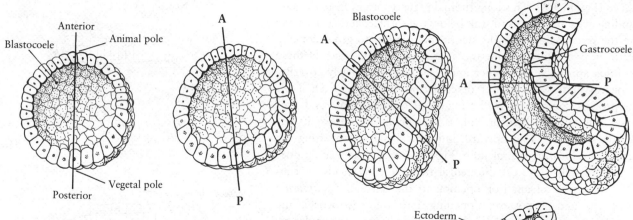

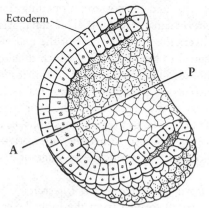

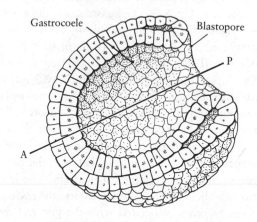

gradually obliterating the blastocoele and forming a new cavity, the *gastrocoele* or *archenteron*. The gastrocoele opens to the outside by way of the *blastopore,* an opening which becomes progressively smaller as gastrulation and neurulation continue (Fig. 8–1,2). The gastrula has a double-layered wall, the two layers being continuous with each other at the lips of the blastopore. The inner layer will form endoderm, mesoderm, and notochord, while the outer layer will form epidermis and neural tissue. During the formation of the gastrula, the embryo rotates through an arc of about 120 degrees.

The cup-shaped gastrula now undergoes elongation in the cranio-caudal axis. One region of the elongated embryo develops a flattened surface marking the dorsal side (Fig. 8–2). A cross section through the gastrula at this time (Fig. 8–3 A) shows an outer layer of cells flattened at one side surrounding an inner layer of larger cells arranged around a cavity, the gastrocoele. The flattened dorsal region of the outer layer marks the site of the formation of the nervous system. The inner layer is made up mostly of presumptive endoderm but contains a middorsal strip of presumptive notochord bounded on either side by strips of presumptive mesoderm (Fig. 8–3 A,B).

Development of the Organ Rudiments

Further development involves the differentiation of the primary organ rudiments by local proliferation and folding of particular regions of the inner and outer layer of cells.

The Nervous System
The presumptive nervous system is in the form of a flattened longitudinal plate of cells, the *neural plate,* on the dorsal surface of the

8–1   Gastrulation in *Amphioxus* showing change in polarity. Cells at the posterior pole flatten and invaginate toward the animal pole eventually obliterating the blastocoele and replacing it with a new cavity, the gastrocoele. (From A. F. Huettner, 1972. Comparative Embryology of the Vertebrates. Copyright 1949 by Macmillan Publishing Co., Inc. Renewed 1977 by M. R. Huettner, R. A. Huettner and R. J. Huettner.)

embryo (Fig. 8–3 A). This longitudinal plate separates from the surrounding cells and begins to sink below the surface, and at the same time the cells that border the neural plate begin to grow dorsally over it as two folds of epidermis (Fig. 8–3 B). The edges of these two folds approach each other and then fuse, completely covering the neural plate with a sheet of epidermis (Figs. 8–3 C,D; 8–4). This process commences in the region of the blastopore and progresses cranially. As the neural plate sinks below the surface, its lateral edges begin to fold upward and join dorsally, converting the neural plate into the neural tube (Figs. 8–3 E,F). The folding does not immediately close off the neural tube either cranially or caudally but leaves an anterior opening to the outside, the *anterior neuropore*, and a posterior opening into the gastrocoele, the *neurenteric* canal (Fig. 8–4). This canal arises because the epidermis that covers the posterior part of the neural tube is derived from tissue ventral to the blastopore, which thus not only covers the neural tube but also the blastopore. The epidermis shuts off the opening of the gastrocoele to the outside but leaves it in communication with the cavity of the neural tube. The neurenteric canal persists for only a short time. The gastrocoele reestablishes an opening to the outside posteriorly and also forms one anteriorly—the anal and oral openings—but only at a much later stage of development.

Notochord, Mesoderm, and Intestine

These are all formed from the inner layer of cells surrounding the gastrocoele (Fig. 8–3). The gastrocoele develops three longitudinally running outpocketings, one along the midline and the other two dorsolaterally on either side of the first. When these are completely pinched off, the result is the formation of four tubelike structures (Fig. 8–3 E,F). The middorsal tube will form the notochord, the two dorsolateral tubes will form the mesoderm, and the tube remaining after the others have pinched off will become the alimentary tract. The mesodermal bands soon show transverse divisions forming segmentally arranged somites. From the somites, mesoderm extends laterally and ventrally between the gut and the overlying ectoderm forming the lateral mesoderm. The lateral mesoderm splits into two sheets surrounding a cavity, the *coelom*. The inner of these sheets becomes associated with the gut and the outer with the ectoderm. They are named the *splanchnic* and the *somatic* mesoderm. The combined endoderm and mesoderm is called the *splanchnopleure,* and the combined ectoderm and mesoderm is called the *somatopleure.*

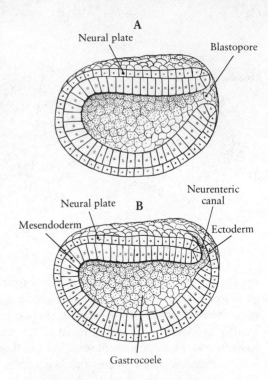

8–2 Gastrulae of *Amphioxus*. A, elongation in a craniocaudal direction, the blastopore representing the future caudal end of the embryo; B, ectoderm growing over the blastopore as the neural tube develops. Cavity of the neural tube is connected to the gastrocoele by way of the neurenteric canal. (From A. F. Huettner, 1972. Comparative Embryology of the Vertebrates. Copyright 1949 by Macmillan Publishing Co., Inc. Renewed 1977 by M. R. Huettner, R. A. Huettner, and R. J. Huettner.)

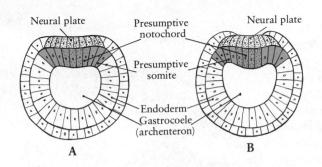

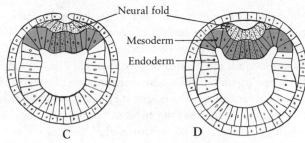

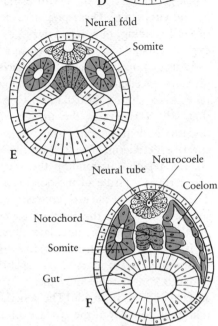

GASTRULATION IN AMPHIBIANS

The end result of gastrulation in the amphibians is the same as it is in *Amphioxus*—the conversion of an undifferentiated blastula into a trilaminar gastrula in which the inner sheets of cells are destined to form endodermal and mesodermal structures and the outer layer of cells is destined to form ectodermal derivatives. However, because of the large amount of yolk in the amphibian egg, the movements by which these events are brought about differ from the relatively simple type of gastrulation in *Amphioxus*.

The first indication of gastrulation is the appearance of a small groove on the surface of the blastula just ventral to the position of the grey crescent (Fig. 8–5 A). This slit is the beginning of the blastopore and represents the area where the surface cells are beginning to move into the inside. The slit-shaped blastopore increases in length and becomes sickle-shaped, then semicircular, then horseshoe-shaped, and finally the ends of the horseshoe met to form a circular blastopore surrounding a plug of endodermal material, the *yolk plug* (Fig. 8–5 B–F). The region where the blastopore first forms is called the *dorsal lip* of the blastopore, and the region of the completion of the circular blastopore is the *ventral lip* of the blastopore. Between them, around the periphery, are the *lateral lips*.

An extensive series of vital stain studies by W. Vogt (1929) presented a comprehensive and coherent study of the complicated cellular movements that occur during amphibian gastrulation. Reference to presumptive fate maps and to the figures representing the results of vital staining experiments is essential to the understanding of gastrulation in the amphibians. However, the results of the vital staining experiments should not be misinterpreted. Because particular areas on the surface of the blastula may be shown to undergo specific movements that result in their becoming a part of certain tissues or organs does not mean that the blastula is a mosaic of discrete regions differing from one another morphologically. These

8–3 Transverse sections through the *Amphioxus* embryo during the early differentiation of the embryonic axis showing the formation of the neural tube from the outer layer of cells and the endoderm, notochord, and mesoderm from the inner layer of cells. (From A. F. Huettner, 1972. Comparative Embryology of the Vertebrates. Copyright 1949 by Macmillan Publishing Co., Inc. Renewed 1977 by M. R. Huettner, R. A. Huettner, and R. J. Huettner.)

experiments merely reveal that under normal conditions of undisturbed development certain regions of the blastula will develop in accordance with their position within the whole. These regions have a certain fate. However, the blastula is not a mosaic of predetermined organs. Vital stains reveal nothing of the intrinsic properties or potencies of the regions they mark, and the vast majority of the regions of the blastula have the potency to differentiate into a much greater variety of structures than the particular fate indicated by the vital stain. These potencies, not revealed by the techhnique of vital staining, may be analyzed by transplantation and isolation experiments as will be described in a later chapter.

Examination of an amphibian presumptive fate map (Fig. 8–6) gives an excellent indication of the general type of movement that takes place during gastrulation. One important line on the map is that which separates the invaginating material, prospective endoderm and mesoderm, from the noninvaginating material, prospective ectoderm. The prospective endoderm is seen as a disc-shaped region surrounding the vegetal pole. Between it and the ectoderm is a girdle of mesoderm, often called the *marginal zone.* The mesoderm of the grey crescent region is mostly presumptive notochord. Lateral to the presumptive notochord in the marginal zone are the presumptive somite, lateral, and tail mesoderm, respectively. It is quite obvious from the location of the blastopore that the presumptive areas marked out on the surface of the blastula must undergo considerable movement during gastrulation, both on the surface and on the inside. The general pattern of convergence of the marginal zone over the surface of the blastula toward the blastopore and its elongation underneath the surface is illustrated in Figure 8–7. Of particular interest are those structures that, at the end of gastrulation, are oriented along the craniocaudal axis, particularly the notochord and the nervous system. In the early blastula, they have a mediolateral orientation, perpendicular to the future craniocaudal axis (Fig. 8–8).

Movements of the Presumptive Mesoderm

Separation of the mesoderm from the endoderm follows somewhat different patterns in the anurans and the urodeles. In the anurans, the mesoderm does not split off from the endoderm until late in gastrulation, after invagination, whereas, in the urodeles this separation occurs during invagination and the two germ layers move into the interior of the gastrula as separate units. The gastrular movements associated with the formation of the mesoderm and the endoderm described in this section refer primarily to those occurring in the urodeles as originally presented in Vogt's comprehensive vital staining studies.

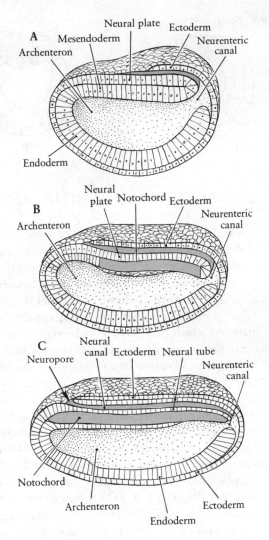

8–4 Midsagittal sections of *Amphioxus* during the formation of the neural tube. These diagrams should be used in conjunction with the transverse sections in Figure 8–3. (From A. F. Huettner 1972. Comparative Embryology of the Vertebrates. Copyright 1949 by Macmillan Publishing Co., Inc. Renewed 1977 by M. R. Huettner, R. A. Huettner, and R. J. Huettner.)

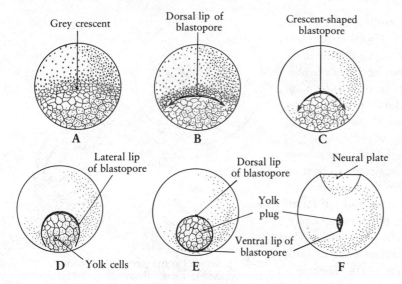

Grey crescent | Dorsal lip of blastopore | Crescent-shaped blastopore

A | B | C

Lateral lip of blastopore | Dorsal lip of blastopore | Neural plate

Yolk plug

Ventral lip of blastopore

D | Yolk cells | E | F

8–5 Diagram of the development of the blastopore in the frog seen from the caudal aspect.

Two important facts in regard to the formation of the blastopore have already been presented. First, the blastopore develops in the region of the presumptive endoderm; and second, it shows a definite sequential growth pattern progressing from an original slit-shaped structure through stages to a circular structure.

The first statement indicates that the presumptive endoderm must be the first material to involute over the dorsal lip of the slit-shaped blastopore (Fig. 8–6). It is followed by the cells lying just below the presumptive notochord, which next involute over the dorsal lip and move cranially to form the *prechordal plate*. This is the first mesoderm to involute and it is, in turn, followed by the presumptive notochord.

The second statement about the development of the blastopore indicates that there is a time sequence in the involution of the presumptive areas corresponding to the stepwise formation of the blastopore. That is, the first mesoderm to move into the interior is that which involutes over the dorsal lip at the beginning of the formation of the blastopore to form prechordal plate and notochord. As the lateral lips develop, somite material moves over the surface and involutes over the lateral lips and is followed by lateral mesoderm. Finally, tail mesoderm involutes over the ventral lip at late stages in gastrulation. The smaller amount of material involuting over the lateral, and particularly the ventral, lips is indicated by the narrowness of the marginal zone in the region of these presumptive areas (Fig. 8–6).

It may help to visualize the cell movements during gastrulation by reference to the results obtained by marking regions of the blas-

8–6 Generalized presumptive fate map of the amphibian showing the position of the presumptive areas on the surface of the early gastrula at the time of the first appearance of the blastopore. A, caudal view; B, lateral view.

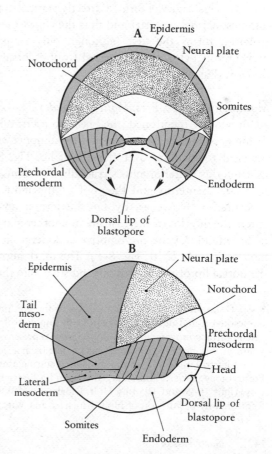

A

Epidermis

Neural plate

Notochord

Somites

Prechordal mesoderm

Endoderm

Dorsal lip of blastopore

B

Epidermis

Neural plate

Notochord

Tail mesoderm

Prechordal mesoderm

Head

Lateral mesoderm

Dorsal lip of blastopore

Somites

Endoderm

tula with vital stains. A mark applied to the midline area in the region of the presumptive notochord (Mark 5, Fig. 8–9 A) illustrates the elongation and movement toward the dorsal lip, the involution and then the elongation and cranial movement once inside. This circular mark ends up on an elongated group of cells forming the roof of the archenteron (Fig. 8–9 C). Marks placed on the presumptive somite material (Mark s, Fig. 8–9 D) also converge toward the dorsal lip, involute, and continue to converge slightly as they move cranially. A single small circular mark will stain adjoining regions of a number of somites, indicating again the elongation that takes place in this material, particularly after it involutes.

Although we consider notochord, somite, lateral, and tail mesoderm as separate presumptive regions, they are, of course, not physically separated from each other during gastrular movements. The entire mass of mesoderm involutes as a continuous sheet of cells, which may be called the mesodermal mantle (Fig. 8–10). The mesodermal mantle shows its greatest development and undergoes its largest movements in the presumptive notochord and somite regions.

As gastrulation continues, the gastrocoele replaces the blastocoele. This cavity is formed directly ventral to the earliest involuting mesodermal material and thus the chordamesoderm during gastrulation forms the first (although only temporary) roof of the archenteron before it is replaced by the dorsal growth of the endoderm (Figs. 8–11, 8–12).

Movements of the Presumptive Endoderm

As previously mentioned, the blastopore first appears in the region of the presumptive endoderm and presumptive endoderm is the first material to involute over the dorsal lip (Fig. 8–6). Inside of the gastrula this material moves cranially and forms the floor and walls of the archenteron and the roof of the most cranial end of the archenteron. However, by far the largest amount of endoderm enters the interior of the gastrula in another manner. A mark placed in the middle of the presumptive endoderm illustrates this type of movement (Mark 10, Fig. 8–9). The mark approaches the area of the dorsal lip of the blastopore and sinks into the interior below the

8–8   Diagram of the changes in shape of the presumptive chordamesoderm and neural plate regions during gastrulation. Solid lines represent surface movements and dotted lines represent movements after involution. For both regions there is a change from a side-to-side orientation before gastrulation to a craniocaudal orientation after gastrulation. (From Embryology, revised and enlarged edition by Lester George Barth. Copyright 1949 and 1953 by Holt, Rinehart and Winston, Inc. Reprinted by permission of Holt, Rinehart and Winston.)

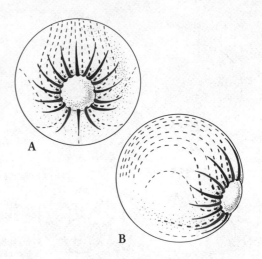

8–7   Scheme of convergence of the mesoderm toward the blastopore (heavy lines) and its elongation in a craniocaudal direction (dotted lines) once it has involuted. (After W. Vogt, 1929.)

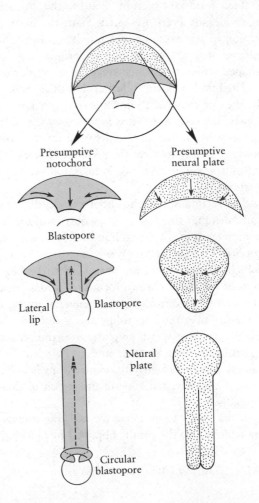

Presumptive notochord

Presumptive neural plate

Blastopore

Lateral lip

Blastopore

Neural plate

Circular blastopore

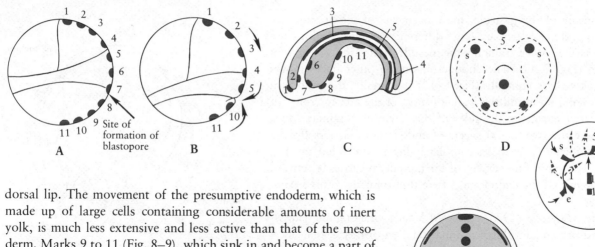

dorsal lip. The movement of the presumptive endoderm, which is made up of large cells containing considerable amounts of inert yolk, is much less extensive and less active than that of the mesoderm. Marks 9 to 11 (Fig. 8–9), which sink in and become a part of the floor of the archenteron, show considerably less stretching than their counterparts (Marks 4 and 5), which form the temporary roof of the archenteron.

The marks placed along a semicircular line through the middle of the grey crescent in Figure 8–9 A stain a continuous line of tissue on the surface of the blastula. When the blastopore forms between Marks 7 and 8, these areas reach the interior through different routes: Mark 7 involuting over the dorsal lip, Mark 8 sinking in below the dorsal lip. Nevertheless, these marks still stain a continuous line of tissue on the interior of the gastrula. The prechordal plate and the notochord also involute over the dorsal lip, trailing behind Mark 7, while Marks 9 to 11 follow behind Mark 8. Inside of the gastrula they still form a continuous sheet of tissue, a part of which forms the roof of the archenteron—the presumptive chordamesoderm—and a part of which forms the floor of the archenteron—the presumptive endoderm. Figure 8–11 also illustrates the movements of the presumptive chordamesoderm and endoderm, as seen in midsagittal section, and diagrams the replacement of the blastocoele by the gastrocoele. A careful study of Figure 8–11 should give a clear indication of the cellular movements that are taking place in the regions of the dorsal and ventral lips of the blastopore.

A mark placed exactly where the lateral lip of the blastopore will develop (Mark e; Fig. 8–9 D) illustrates the manner in which the endoderm and the mesoderm are separated at the time they pass into the interior of the gastrula. Half of the mark will involute over the lateral lip of the blastopore as a part of the mesodermal mantle to form the lateral mesoderm, but the other half will invaginate with the endodermal mass to form a part of the wall of the archenteron. Regions that are in contact with each other on the surface of the blastula may thus have very different presumptive fates.

8–9 Vital staining experiments on anuran gastrulae. A–C, movements of marks placed along the middorsal region of the embryo running from the animal to the vegetal pole and passing through the middle of the presumptive chordamesoderm (refer to presumptive fate map, Fig. 8–6). A, before gastrulation; B, midgastrula—marks 6–9 have passed over the rim of the blastopore; C, completion of gastrulation; D, E, movement of marks placed on presumptive mesoderm and presumptive endodermal material seen from the caudal aspect; F, G, surface movements of marks placed on presumptive neural plate tissue. (From V. Hamburger, 1960. A Manual of Experimental Embryology. The University of Chicago Press.)

Once inside of the gastrula, the movements of the presumptive endoderm and mesoderm are quite different. Although both tissues elongate as they move cranially, the mesoderm also shows a ventral migration (Fig. 8–12). The endoderm, on the other hand, moves dorsally as well as cranially (Fig. 8–12). Originally, the endoderm forms only the floor and the walls of most of the archenteron, but its dorsal movement up the sides of this cavity is continuecd to a point where the two lateral sheets of endoderm meet dorsally and thus the archenteron becomes completely lined with endoderm (Fig. 8–12 B). The ventral movement of the mesoderm carries it between the ectoderm and the endoderm, where it also finally forms a complete layer.

Recently, Løvtrup (1975) reviewed Vogt's vital staining experiments and presented a different interpretation of their significance. He proposed that the material on the surface of the blastula below the limit of invagination consists only of the notochord and endoderm and these should be the only features show on fate maps referring to the superficial layer. He concluded that the presumptive mesoderm was located in the same area pictured by Vogt but was represented by a ring of small spherical cells beneath the surface. His contention was that when presumptive mesoderm cells were stained, the stain had actually marked these cells below the surface layer. Keller (1976) has reported vital staining experiments on *Xenopus*. He also concludes that only presumptive endoderm is located on the surface of the blastula below the limit of invagination and that all of the presumptive mesoderm and also the notochord are located in a deeper layer below the surface.

Movements of the Prospective Ectoderm

Although all of the ectoderm always remains on the surface of the gastrula, this tissue also undergoes extensive movement during gastrulation. As the mesodermal mantle passes to the inside, the ectoderm remaining in contact with it also moved over the surface of the gastrula toward the blastopore. And also, as the mesoderm converges toward the midline, so does the ectoderm. Marks on the surface in the midline of the presumptive neural plate move toward the dorsal lip and undergo elongation as they do so (Marks m,n, Fig. 8–9 F,G). They remain in the midline. Marks on the lateral wings of the presumptive neural plate show movements of both elongation and convergence (Fig. 8–9 F,G).

The remainder of the ectoderm, the presumptive epidermis, also undergoes extensive movement, retaining its contacts with the presumptive neural plate and with the presumptive mesoderm and moving in conformity with these contacts. Its type of movement could be compared with the opening of a fan.

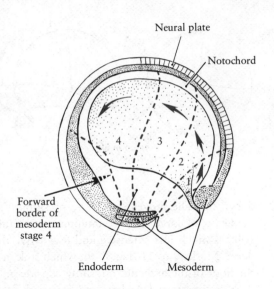

8–10   Movement of the mesodermal mantle after involution. Arrows represent direction of movement and dotted lines represent the location of the leading edge of the mantle at four successive stages. (From V. Hamburger, 1960. A Manual of Experimental Embryology. The University of Chicago Press.)

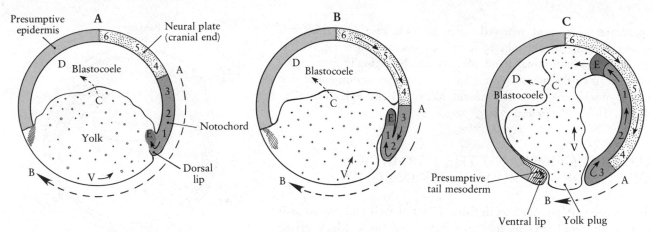

Formation of Organ Rudiments

The chordamesoderm develops into notochord and mesoderm. A middorsal rod of cells separates from the remainder of the mesoderm to form the primordium of the notochord (Figs. 8–12; 8–13). The portion of the mesoderm adjacent to the notochord develops a series of transverse fissures which forms it into longitudinally oriented bands of somites, one band on either side of the notochord (Fig. 8–12; 8–13). The transverse separations occur only in the most dorsal part of the mesoderm, the more lateral and ventral regions remaining unsegmented. Adjoining the somites, between them and the lateral mesoderm, the intermediate mesoderm, which is presumptive nephrogenous tissue, develops. Lateral to the intermediate mesoderm, the mesoderm separates into somatic and splanchnic layers surrounding a cavity, the embryonic coelom (Fig. 8–13 B).

The presumptive neural plate at the end of gastrulation is an elongated oval area overlying the cranial end of the archenteron, the prechordal plate, the notochord, and the somites. Soon the edges of the plate thicken and are raised above the surface of the embryo to form the neural folds (Fig. 8–13 B). As the neural folds continue to elevate they meet in the middorsal line to form the neural tube (Fig. 8–13 C), which will form the brain anteriorly and the spinal cord posteriorly. The cavity of the neural tube is the primordium of the ventricular system of the brain and the central canal of the spinal cord.

Fusion of the neural folds occurs first in the region of the future hindbrain and progresses cranially and caudally. The neural plate is much broader in the head region; and at the time of the formation of the neural folds, the cranial end can be recognized by its greater size and earlier differentiation (Fig. 8–13).

As the neural folds elevate, they carry with them the adjacent

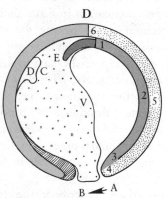

8–11 Diagram of midsagittal sections of anuran embryos from the time of the first appearance of the blastopore to the yolk-plug stage. Groups of cells are differentiated and marked so that their movements may be followed. (From Embryology, revised and enlarged edition by Lester George Barth. Copyright 1949 and 1953 by Holt, Rinehart and Winston, Inc. Reprinted by permission of Holt, Rinehart and Winston.)

epidermal cells; and when the neural folds fuse, the epidermis grows over the neural tube to form its epidermal covering. As this occurs, the longitudinal band of cells which originally formed the outer limit of the neural plate is cut off and appears on either side in the pocket between the neural folds and the epidermis (Fig. 8–13). This is the *neural crest*.

GASTRULATION AND THE FORMATION OF THE ORGAN RUDIMENTS IN FISHES

The process of gastrulation in fishes is not as well understood as it is in such vertebrates as the amphibians and birds. Many of the studies on gastrulation in fishes date back to the 1930s and 1940s when techniques for tracing the movements of cells were based solely upon the use of vital dyes.

In primitive bony fishes and in the lungfishes, where the fertilized egg cleaves completely, gastrulation appears to follow the pattern observed in the amphibians (i.e., endoderm and chordamesoderm are invaginated through a blastopore). By contrast, in teleost and elasmobranch fishes, where cleavage is restricted to a disc of cytoplasm at the animal pole of the fertilized egg, gastrulation appears to be complex and quite different from that observed in other vertebrates.

As previously described, the late stage blastoderm of elasmobranch and teleost fishes consists of a cellularized mass lying upon a syncytial layer of cytoplasm or periblast (Fig. 8–14). The periblast is closely associated with the uncleaved yolk. Analysis of the blastoderm shows that it consists of a superficial layer of enveloping blastomeres, tightly joined to each other, and deeper-lying blastomeres (Fig. 8–14). Only the blastoderm is responsible for the formation of the various parts of the embryo. The periblast, the yolk, and the cytoplasm surrounding the yolk are extraembryonic since they make little, if any, contribution to the formation of the embryo.

Our knowledge of the potencies or fate of the cells of the late stage blastoderm in these fishes is scarce and, in the specific case of teleosts, a matter of considerable controversy. For example, until recently only two fate maps had been published for all teleost fishes. The early studies by Oppenheimer on *Fundulus* (killifish) and Pasteels (1937) on *Salmo* (trout), in which spots of vital dye placed upon the surface of the pregastrular embryo were traced during gastrulation, assumed that the endoderm and the mesoderm were originally on the surface of the late stage blastula (i.e., as commonly shown in the fate map of an amphibian embryo). They hypothe-

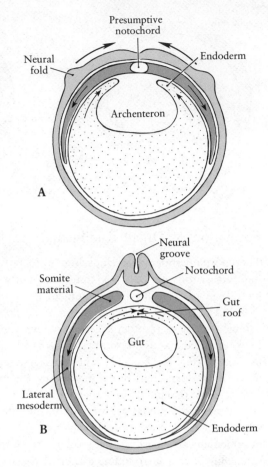

8–12 Diagrams showing the progressive movement of the mesoderm and endoderm inside the amphibian gastrula. A, the chordamesoderm forms the temporary roof of the archenteron. The ventral movement of the mesoderm and the dorsal movement of the endoderm are indicated by the dotted arrows; B, the dorsal movement of the endoderm has resulted in the formation of a gut cavity completely surrounded by endoderm. (From Embryology, revised and enlarged edition by Lester George Barth. Copyright 1949 and 1953 by Holt, Rinehart and Winston, Inc. Reprinted by permission of Holt, Rinehart and Winston.)

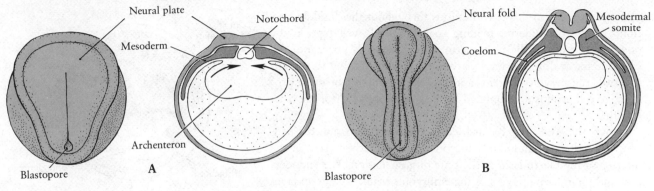

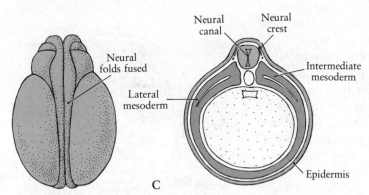

8–13 Three stages in neurulation in the amphibian embryo. The drawings on the left in A, B, and C represent dorsal views of whole embryos at successively later stages. The drawings on the right represent cross sections of the embryos on the left.

sized that the prospective endoderm and mesoderm were wheeled into place in the interior by a movement of invagination along the *germ ring,* the latter being a thickening of the entire outer edge of the blastoderm, which forms as the time of gastrulation approaches. In other words, the edge of the blastoderm acts as a blastopore through which the cells of the endoderm and chordamesoderm are invaginated, much as in the frog and salamander.

More recent investigations on *Salmo,* particularly those by Ballard (1973), have challenged the traditional view that the germ layers are formed during gastrulation as a result of invagination. Using the technique of implanting chalk particles at selected sites on the surface and in the deeper portions of the blastoderm, Ballard has traced the movements of cells during gastrulation. A fate map based upon his observations is shown in Figure 8–15. It is clear from the tracing studies that the fate map is three-dimensional, with areas of cells overlapping and at various depths in the blastoderm. Analysis of the fate map shows that the cellular envelope which covers the entire surface of the blastoderm will give rise to the ectoderm. A broad sheet of cells forms the prospective mesoderm and will contribute to the somites of the trunk and tail, to the lateral

8–14 Diagram of the blastoderm of a typical bony fish (*Fundulus*). (After T. Lentz and J. P. Trinkaus, 1967 J. Cell Biol. 32, 121.)

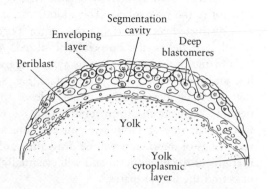

plates, and the heart. It is continuous throughout the "middle portion" of the blastoderm, tending to be the only cell type in the nonaxial portion of the blastoderm. Along the axial portion of the blastoderm, at different levels, are the cells contributing to the notochord, the nervous system, and the endoderm. All of these prospective cell groups are confined to the "posterior" half of the blastoderm.

Hence, the studies of Ballard led to the conclusion that the prospective endoderm and chordamesoderm are already present in the interior of the blastoderm at the time of gastrulation. The endodermal and mesodermal layers of the embryonic trunk (i.e., germ layer formation) are assembled by the rearrangement and convergence of blastomeres from these presumptive areas in the interior of the blastoderm.

At what will become the posterior edge of the blastoderm, the presumptive endodermal and mesodermal cells move and converge to form a cresent-shaped structure known as the *embryonic shield* (Fig. 8–16 A). It is within the embryonic shield that the primary organs are laid down, including the neural tube, the notochord, and the somites (Fig. 8–16 B,C). Simultaneously with the period of primary organ formation, the germ ring or the margin of the blastoderm spreads by epiboly over the surface of the yolk sphere. Participating in this overgrowth are the ectoderm, the mesoderm, and the periblast. Hence, these three tissues form a complete envelope that gradually encloses the unsegmented yolk, thereby bringing it within the confines of the developing embryo. Just before the complete enclosure of the yolk, a yolk plug can be seen between the constricted edges of the blastoderm (Fig. 8–16 D).

The body of the fish embryo, with its primary organ rudiments, differentiates in an anterior-to-posterior sequence (Fig. 8–16). Shortly after the onset of gastrulation, the notochordal cells converge and concentrate as an axial strand in the sagittal plane of the embryonic shield. Their complete separation from adjacent mesodermal cells occurs when the germ ring is approximately at the equator of the yolk sphere. The endodermal cells gradually organize as a distinct sheet underlying the central portion of the embryonic shield, just below the notochordal strand. Above the notochord, cells of the presumptive nervous system aggregate toward the midline and form a thickened neural plate (Fig. 8–16 B). Subsequently, the sheets of mesoderm to either side of the notochordal strand begin to segment and form somites (Fig. 8–16 C). They form in the trout at the rate of about one pair per hour at 10°C. The more lateral wings of mesoderm will be drawn toward the midline from the margins of the blastoderm and will eventually contribute to the kidneys and the lateral plates.

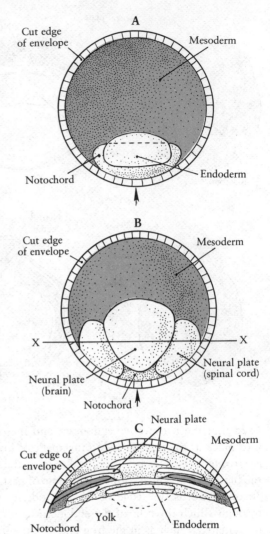

8–15 Three-dimensional fate map of the trout blastoderm as shown (A) from below and (B) from above. The arrow marks the axis of symmetry. A, the area of prospective notochord underlies the general mesodermal sheet, and is itself underlaid by the area of prospective endoderm; B, the neural areas overlie the general mesodermal sheet. The cellular envelope lies superficial to all other areas but is only shown at the margin of the blastoderm; C, a typical transverse section through the posterior end of the blastoderm at level of X in (B). (After W. Ballard, 1973. J. Exp. Zool. 184, 49.)

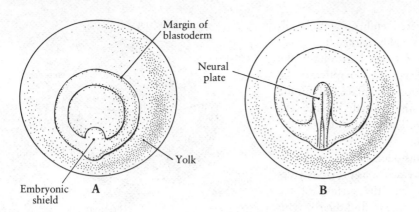

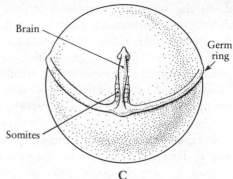

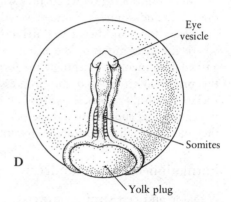

8–16 Stages in the development of the trout (*Salmo*). A, beginning of gastrulation and formation of the embryonic shield; B, formation of the neural plate; C, formation of neural tube and somites; D, overgrowth of the yolk by germ ring nearly completed. (From B. I. Balinsky, 1975. An Introduction to Embryology, 4th edition. W. B. Saunders Company, Philadelphia.)

The process of neurulation in bony fishes differs in many details from the neural fold methods of most vertebrate organisms. In the trout, for example, the neural plate is observed to form a thickened, elongated *neural keel* or ridge along the middorsal axis of the embryo. The neural keel loses its association with the overlying enveloping layer of the blastoderm and sinks into the underlying tissue. Anteriorly, the presumptive brain portion of the neural keel presses down against the yolk syncytium. The ventricles of the brain and the central canal of the spinal cord are subsequently formed by the separation of cells within the neural keel.

Gastrulation and the formation of primary organ rudiments in the elasmobranch fishes is often described as following the same pattern as that observed in bony fishes. However, the recent investigations by Ballard raise serious questions regarding the similarity in the process of gastrulation between the two major groups of modern fishes. Using the shark, *Scyllium,* as an example, it is generally presumed that the presumptive organ-forming areas are laid out on the surface of the blastoderm (Fig. 8–17 A). The notochord, mesoderm, and much of the endoderm involute over the posterior margin of the blastoderm during gastrulation. In essence, the posterior edge of the blastoderm acts as a dorsal-lip area. The result of gastrulation is the production of an embryo, with the germ layers arranged as shown in Figure 8–17 B. Similar to the amphibian and the amniote, the neural plate is rolled into a neural tube.

GASTRULATION AND THE FORMATION OF THE ORGAN RUDIMENTS IN BIRDS

Gastrulation in birds involves the same processes that take place during gastrulation in *Amphioxus* and the amphibians and produces the same end results—a multilayered embryo with well-defined organ primordia. However, in the highly telolecithal avian egg, in which the active cytoplasm is limited to the blastoderm, the yolk plays no part in gastrulation—except to complicate the process—and all of the events of grastrulation take place only in the blastoderm. Only in later stages does the growth of the extraembryonic membranes encompass the yolk and make it available for the nutrition of the developing embryo.

Integrated cellular movements of the blastoderm cells are the essential elements of gastrulation. These movements, as previously described, involve the progression of cells over the surface of the blastula toward a region where they will be able to find their way to the inside and establish a three-layered embryo in which the organ primordia form and begin to differentiate. In the chick, the region where the cells move to the inside is the primitive streak; avian gastrulation involves essentially the formation and the regression of the primitive streak and the progressive movements of cells associated with these processes. It is now widely accepted that all of the embryonic endoderm and mesoderm is of gastrular origin (i.e., they pass through the primitive streak).

Formation of the Endoderm

A major and persistent controversy in chick embryology involves the formation of the endoderm. Various factors have contributed to this controversy, not the least of which is the fact that at the time of laying the egg is already a two-layered system with an outer layer of cells, termed the *epiblast,* underlain, at least in its future posterior region, by an inner layer of cells termed the *hypoblast.* It has been proposed that the epiblast is presumptive ectoderm and mesoderm and that the hypoblast is presumptive endoderm—thus denying the involvement of the primitive streak in the formation of the endoderm. The controversy concerns two points: (1) the origin and movement of the inner layer of cells, and (2) the prospective fate of the inner layer of cells, mainly its role in the formation of the embryonic endoderm.

Origin and Movement of the Inner Layer of Cells

Over a number of years, many investigators have proposed and supported the formation of the hypoblast simply by a separation of the deeper yolk laden cells from the superficial cells of the blastoderm, the separation beginning mainly at the future posterior end of the embryo and moving anteriorly. Whether this separation is by a cutting off or delaminating of a more or less continuous sheet of cells (Fig. 8–18 C) or by a separating of individual cells and their

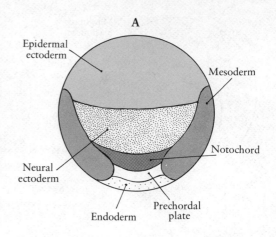

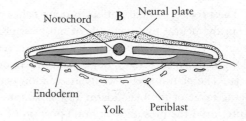

8–17 A, presumptive organ-forming areas in the blastoderm of the shark (*Scyllium*) embryo. Top view; B, section through the shark embryo at the end of gastrulation. (From Comparative Embryology of the Vertebrates by O. E. Nelson. Copyright © 1953 The Blakiston Co., Inc. Used with permission of McGraw-Hill Book Company.)

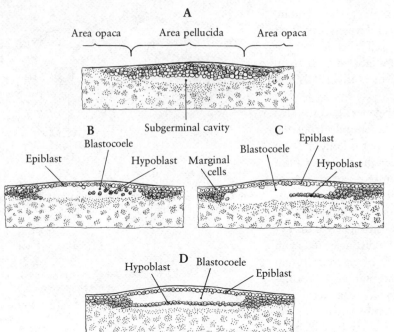

A

Area opaca   Area pellucida   Area opaca

Subgerminal cavity

B

Blastocoele

Epiblast   Hypoblast   Marginal cells

C

Epiblast

Blastocoele

Hypoblast

D   Blastocoele

Hypoblast   Epiblast

8–18   Two proposed methods of formation of the hypoblast. A, cross section through the blastoderm before the separation of the hypoblast (shaded) cells from the epiblast cells by B, polyinvagination or C, delamination. Both methods result in the formation of a two-layered embryo, D.

subsequent joining to form a continuous hypoblast layer (Fig. 8–18 B)—a process sometimes termed *polyinvagination*—the result is essentially the same: the formation of a two-layered embryo (8–18 D). Before the formation of the hypoblast, a cavity develops below the blastoderm, a cavity best referred to as the *subgerminal cavity* (Fig. 8–18 A). After the appearance of the hypoblast, the cavity between the epiblast and the hypoblast is usually termed the blastocoele, although whether it is homologous to the amphibian blastocoele is a matter of question.

In regard to the question about the origin of the endoderm, it is appropriate to consider the techniques that have been and are being used to solve this problem. Methods of investigation are varied and technical difficulties are always present. Early investigators attempted to predict directions of cell migration from histological sections by using cell position and shape as clues, an obviously difficult piece of detective work. Later, vital staining and the application of carbon or other particles were used to mark cells and follow morphogenetic movements. Marking procedures may be done in ova or in vitro, using a number of different methods of explantation and orientation of the blastoderm. Difficulties arise because vital stains often tend to diffuse; particles may not remain associated with the same group of cells to which they are applied; larger particles may behave differently than smaller; morphogenetic movements may be restricted depending upon the method of transplant, the medium, and the layer in contact with the substrate; and development itself may be inhibited in transplanted blastoderms. Cell labeling with radioisotopes and subsequent transplantation of a labeled graft to an unlabeled host (Fig. 8–19) was introduced in the early 1950s and has proved to be a highly valuable technique.

On the basis of a number of studies it is now generally concluded that the presumptive endoderm does not come entirely from the separation of a hypoblast from an epiblast layer but is built up from cells from two different sources. The first is from the posterior germ wall in the area opaca in the region of the future posterior end of the embryo. Cells spread out from this point of origin in a fan-shaped pattern (Fig. 8–20). These cells are destined to form only the extraembryonic endoderm. Some investigators call this layer the *endophyll*. The endophyll (or hypoblast) should be distinguished from the second source of endoderm cells, which are of gastrular origin and will form the embryonic endoderm. At the time of the formation of the endophyll, these presumptive embryonic endoderm cells are still a part of the surface layer of cells, the epiblast. In conjunction with the term endophyll, the surface layer may be called *ectophyll*. The formation of the embryonic endoderm will be described in relation to the formation and function of the primitive streak.

Development of the Primitive Streak

Morphogenetic movements that are concerned with the formation of the primitive streak appear within a few hours after incubation and probably begin as soon as the temperature of the blastoderm cells reaches the normal level for growth (38.5°C). After three to four hours of incubation, a thickening on one quadrant of the area pellucida, the future posterior quadrant, represents the beginning of the formation of the primitive streak (Fig. 8–21 A). Within a few hours after its first indication, the thickening becomes more pronounced and begins to show an elongation in the future craniocaudal axis (Fig. 8–21 B). By the end of the first half day of incubation, the rather indefinite caudal thickening has developed into a well-defined fingerlike process that extends about half way across the area pellucida. This may be called the intermediate streak stage (Fig. 8–21 C). During the time the primitive streak is developing, the area pellucida is increasing in size as the blastoderm cells begin to spread over the yolk. At the intermediate streak stage, the enlarging area pellucida is no longer circular but shows a posterior projection. By 18 to 19 hours of incubation, the streak has reached its maximum length, extending about three quarters of the way across the area pellucida. It ends anteriorly in a depression, the *primitive*

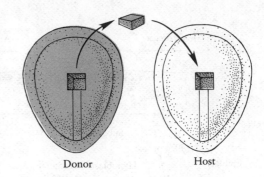

8–19 Diagram illustrating the method of tracing cell movements by transplanting grafts from embryos labeled with tritiated thymidine (stippled) into an unlabeled host.

8–20 Diagram to show the fanlike cell movements of the hypoblast away from its point of origin. The solid arrows represent endoderm cell movements and the dotted arrows show the expansion of the area pellucida and the area opaca. (After N. T. Spratt, Jr. and H. Haas, 1960. J. Exp. Zool. 144, 139.)

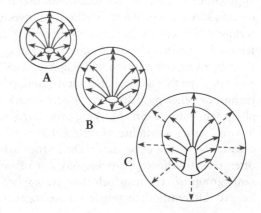

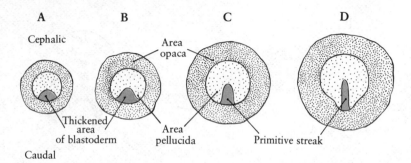

A — Cephalic

B — Area opaca

Thickened area of blastoderm — Area pellucida

C — Primitive streak

D

Caudal

8–21 Chick embryos showing the early development of the primitive streak. A, 3 to 4 hours of incubation; B, 7 to 8 hours of incubation (early streak); C, 10 to 12 hours of incubation (mid-streak); D, 18 to 19 hours of incubation (definitive streak). These diagrams cover Hamburger and Harrison stages one to four. (After V. Hamburger and H. L. Hamilton, 1951. J. Morphol. 88, 49.)

pit, which is surrounded by an elevated area, *Hensen's node* (Fig. 8–21 D).

The increase in thickness of the caudal end of the blastoderm, which is the first indication of the formation of the primitive streak, is the result of an active migration of cells toward this region. Marking studies have not produced uniform results, but it appears that the part of the blastoderm that contributes to the primitive streak is rather small, probably not more than the posterior quarter of the area pellucida. A presumptive fate map of the prestreak blastoderm indicates that all of the material to be invaginated through the primitive streak occupies a relatively small area in the posterior region of the blastoderm (Fig. 8–22). The movement of the cells of the posterior half of the blastoderm as determined by marking experiments is illustrated in Figure 8–23. Here it is seen that a mark placed approximately in the middle of the blastoderm at six hours of incubation moves away from the developing streak, is never incorporated into the streak, and never invaginates (Fig. 8–23 A). A transverse mark across the blastoderm, just posterior to the midline, illustrates that the surface cells in the center of the blastoderm, just posterior to the midline, move away from the developing streak (Fig. 8–23 B). Marks slightly posterior to the midline but lateral to the developing streak also move away from the streak. The more lateral one goes, the less the movement; the most lateral regions show little, if any, displacement. Only when a transverse mark is placed at some distance posterior to the midline do we find that these cells move toward and become incorporated into the primitive streak (Fig. 8–23 C) before they invaginate to form mesoderm. The marks still on the surface at 17 hours represent presumptive mesoderm moving toward the primitive streak prior to invaginating.

As the primitive streak develops, the area pellucida continues to increase in size by overgrowing the yolk in all directions. However, it grows more rapidly in a posterior direction and soon assumes a pear-shaped configuration (Fig. 8–24). During this time the primitive streak continues to elongate until it reaches its maximum

8–22 Presumptive fate map of the two to three-hour incubation stage. White crescent, neural material; vertical lines, chorda; horizontal lines, head mesoderm; inclined lines, somite mesoderm; dots, lateral mesoderm (From M. E. Milan, 1953. Arch. Biol. 64, 143.)

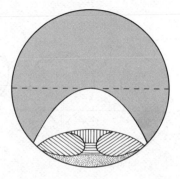

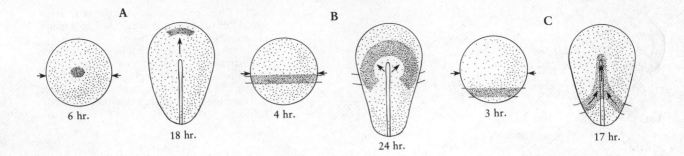

6 hr.   4 hr.   3 hr.

18 hr.   24 hr.   17 hr.

length. It has been suggested that the elongation of the primitive streak is due to the incorporation of new material at both its anterior and posterior ends. Recent marking experiments do not confirm this hypothesis. Not only do marks placed on the blastoderm anterior to the developing streak never become incorporated into the streak, but marks placed on either the posterior or anterior ends of the streak remain in these areas as the streak elongates. These facts point to an elongation of the primitive streak as a stretching of the streak at about its midpoint, at an area where it first appears between the area pellucida and the area opaca. This concept is illustrated in Figure 8–24, indicating that the point of origin of the primitive streak ends up in the middle of the early streak and remains in this site. This concept very nicely gives an understanding of how the primitive streak elongates and how the area pellucida gradually changes from a circular to a pear-shaped structure.

Function of the Primitive Streak

The primitive streak is an invagination area (Fig. 8–25). Although it has been suggested that it acts as a blastema (a group of rapidly dividing undifferentiated cells that will develop into differentiated structures), there is convincing evidence to the contrary: (1) the mitotic index is no higher in the primitive streak than in other areas of the blastema; (2) staining and marking experiments show that cells

8–23 Marking experiments showing the movement of the cells of the epiblast during the early development of the primitive streak. A, a mark in the middle of the blastodisc at the beginning of primitive streak formation does not become incorporated into the definitive primitive streak; B, a transverse mark posterior to the midline shows the incorporation of only a small amount of material into Hensen's node; C, a transverse mark near the posterior end of the area pellucida at three hours colors almost all of the primitive streak at 17 hours. (From M. E. Milan, 1953. Arch. Biol. 64, 143.)

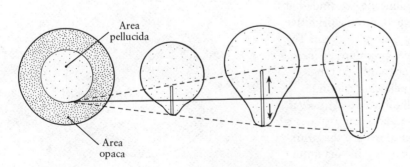

Area pellucida

Area opaca

8–24 Diagram of the formation and elongation of the primitive streak. The primitive streak is considered to originate at the posterior border of the area pellucida and the area opaca. This region then becomes the middle of the primitive streak in later stages as elongation takes place in both directions from the midpoint. (From L. Vakaet, 1962. J. Embryol. Exp. Morphol. 10, 33.)

move into the primitive streak, move to the inside, and then move away from the streak; and (3) cells implanted into the primitive streak move quickly out of the streak and then are replaced. Marking experiments indicate that invagination takes place mainly at the sides of the streak, with very little occurring at either extremity. Invagination at the two ends occurs most actively during the formation of the streak, ceases at the node region at the definitive streak stage (18–19 hours of incubation), and ceases in the posterior part of the streak at the headfold stage (23–25 hours of incubation).

Cellular Movements During Gastrulation

Lower Layer
The lowest layer is derived from two sources. One of these has already been described as being laid down before the formation of the primitive streak, originating from the posterior germ wall and forming the extraembryonic endoderm.

The process of invagination through the primitive streak involves a coordinated movement of surface cells toward the primitive streak and a downward (inward) movement of these cells at the primitive streak, which is followed by lateral and anterior movement away from the streak underneath the surface cells (Fig. 8–25). The lips of the primitive streak, the same as those of the blastopore of the amphibian egg, are occupied by a continually changing population of cells that remain in the primitive streak only temporarily as they move into the inside and then move away from the streak region. The movement of the surface cells toward the streak and their movement once inside are diagrammed in Figure 8–25 B.

Both marking and transplant experiments have given evidence that presumptive embryonic endoderm cells have a gastrular origin and are invaginated through the anterior part of the early streak. The cells that are to form the embryonic endoderm penetrate into the lower layer of cells, the hypoblast (endophyll), and push these cells laterally and anteriorly, replacing them. Thus, the deep layer of cells in the region of the anterior part of the streak is now made up of cells of gastrular origin. Figure 8–26 illustrates the position of the presumptive embryonic endoderm around the anterior end of the primitive streak during the early stages of streak formation and its disappearance from the surface layer by the time the streak reaches its maximum length. The embryonic endoderm and the endoderm of germ wall origin form a continuous sheet of cells.

The Mesoderm Layer
The entire middle layer, which includes the mesoderm and the notochord, is invaginated through the primitive streak. The process

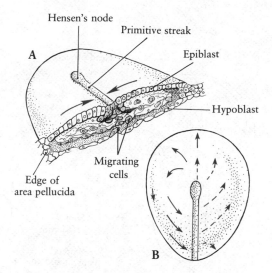

8–25 The function of the primitive streak. A, cells reach the primitive streak and move inward, leaving the surface layer. Some of these cells replace cells of the already present hypoblast (endophyll) and some migrate away from the streak area between the epiblast and the hypoblast to form the mesoderm; B, movements of the surface cells on the left side (solid lines) and movements of the inner cells invaginated over the primitive streak (dotted lines) on the right side.

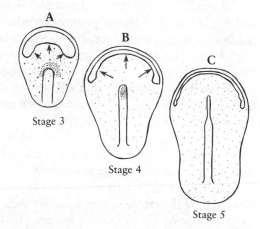

8–26 Gastrular origin of the embryonic endoderm. A, at stage 3, some of the endoderm has invaginated and moved laterally and anteriorly (fine dots), some is in the process of invaginating (closely spaced fine dots), and some is still on the surface as part of the epiblast (heavy dots); B, at stage 4, the endoderm has spread under the surface in all directions, and a small amount is still in the process of invagination. At this stage there is no longer any endoderm on the surface. C, at stage 5. (From G. Nicolet, 1971. Adv. Morphog. 9, 234.)

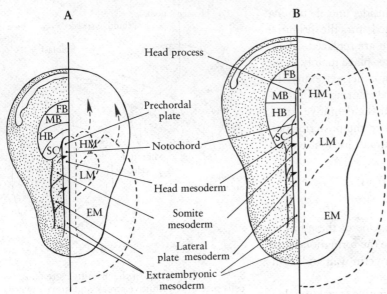

A

B

Head process

Prechordal
plate

Notochord

Head mesoderm

Somite
mesoderm

Lateral
plate mesoderm

Extraembryonic
mesoderm

8–27 Fate map at the primitive streak stage. Surface material is shown on the left as solid lines and invaginated material on the right as dotted lines. The order in which the mesoderm invaginates is seen to be prechordal plate, notochord, head mesoderm (HM), somite mesoderm, lateral plate mesoderm (LM), and extraembryonic mesoderm (EM). Forebrain (FB), midbrain (MB), hindbrain (HB), and spinal cord (SC) are formed from the ectoderm around the anterior end of the primitive streak. B, at the head process stage. (From G. Nicolet, 1970. J. Embryol. Exp. Morphol. 23, 79.)

begins as the streak first forms and continues during its regression. At the time of the maximum development of the primitive streak, most of the extraembryonic mesoderm, the prechordal plate, the head mesoderm, and the presumptive cardiac vesicles have moved to the inside. The notochordal material is condensed in the node and the somite and lateral plate mesoderm, and some of the extraembryonic mesoderm, are still on the surface of the blastoderm (Fig. 8–27). During the formation of the head process and the regression of the primitive streak, the notochordal material condensed in the node is laid down and the somite, lateral plate, and extraembryonic mesoderm invaginate in succession. Comparing this fate map (Fig. 8–27) with that of the amphibian (Fig. 8–6) shows that the presumptive areas are similarly arranged although there is a wide lateral dispersion of the areas in the amphibian and a marked restriction of the areas close to the primitive streak in the chick. In the chick egg a large part of the mesoderm is concerned with the formation of the extraembryonic membranes. The chronology of invagination is similar in the two species: (1) the invagination of the foregut and prechordal plate precedes that of the notochord; (2) the notochord forms a large part of the node, as it does of the dorsal lip of the blastopore, which is considered to be the homologue of the node; and (3) the anterior somite, posterior somite, and lateral plate mesoderm invaginate in succession. The cells, which then remain on the surface, will form neural and epidermal tissues.

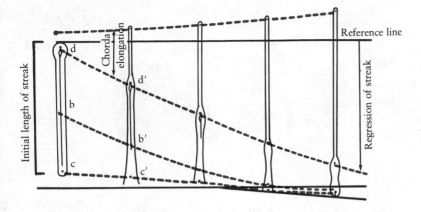

8–28 Graphic representation of the regression of the primitive streak and the increase in the length of the notochord. (From N. T. Spratt, Jr., 1947. J. Exp. Zool. 104, 69.)

Regression of the Primitive Streak and the Formation of the Organ Rudiments

The laying down of the organs of the embryonic axis takes place during the regression of the primitive streak. Streak regression takes place shortly after it reaches its maximum development. A graphic summary of streak regression is shown in Figure 8–28. Transverse marks placed across the area pellucida during streak regression indicate that the entire area pellucida caudal to Hensen's node undergoes regression, although it is much more rapid in the area of the primitive streak (Fig. 8–29). The most posterior end of the streak does not contribute anything to embryonic structures.

The anterior end of the streak consists of presumptive prechordal plate and notchcord, which are laid down as the streak regresses (Fig. 8–30). During this regression cells leave Hensen's node and the primitive streak immediately posterior to it and condense to form the tissue of the notochord. The presumptive neural material, located in front of and lateral to the node, elongates and stretches in a craniocaudal direction, and the lateral parts converge toward the midline. Neurulation and organ formation take place in a craniocaudal sequence. As the node retreats, the neural plate, underlain by the notochord, develops in front of it (Fig. 8–30 C).

Formation of the Somites

Laterad of the developing notochord, the mesoderm can be divided into two populations of cells. One, the most medial, represents presumptive somite material. The cells form a loosely arranged columnar epithelium attached to the basal lamina of the overlying epiblast in a region that is coextensive with the developing neural plate. The cells are joined to each other at their basal ends. A more

8–29 Marking experiments on the regression of the primitive streak. The greatest regression is seen in the midline but there is a regression of lateral areas also. The posterior end of the streak (mark 3) does not form any part of the embryo. (From G. Nicolet, 1971. J. Embryol. Exp. Morphol. 23, 79.)

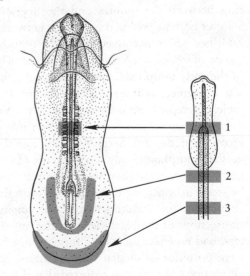

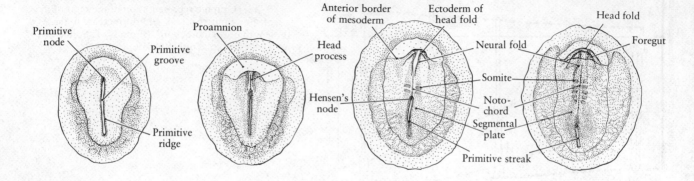

Primitive node • Primitive groove • Primitive ridge • Proamnion • Anterior border of mesoderm • Head process • Hensen's node • Ectoderm of head fold • Neural fold • Somite • Noto-chord • Segmental plate • Primitive streak • Head fold • Foregut

8–30 Formation of the embryonic axis anterior to the regressing primitive streak. A, definitive streak, 18–19 hours, stage 4; B, head process, 19–22 hours, stage 5; C, beginning of somite formation, 23–24 hours, stage 7+; D, four-somite stage.

lateral, loosely arranged group of cells presents the flattened appearance of typical mesenchyme, which do not form cellular junctions either to the overlying presumptive epidermis nor between themselves. They will form the lateral mesoderm.

As the neural plate condenses toward the midline, so do the presumptive somite cells below it. As they do so, they lose their loose arrangement and become tightly opposed virtually eliminating the intercellular spaces. New intercellular junctions are formed at the apical ends of the cells. At intervals along this group of cells, the *segmental plate,* gaps appear between the plate and the overlying neural plate. These gaps are the beginning of the formation of the intersomitic furrows and occur at regularly spaced intervals running in a craniocaudal direction where the somite cells break their connections with and are "released" from the neural plate cells (Fig. 8–30 C,D).

As the neural plate folds up to form the neural tube, all connection between the somites and the neural tube is lost. Later, the somites become enclosed in a loose network of fibers which also establishes a fibrous connection to the notochord.

The mechanism of somite formation. The mechanisms involved in the early morphogenesis of the chick somites have been the subject of numerous investigations. In the 1950s, Spratt presented a widely accepted explanation which proposed that two "somite-forming centers" develop in a region just posterior and lateral to Hensen's node (Fig. 8–31 A). Although they could not be distinguished morphologically, on the basis of extirpation and transplantation experiments they were pictured as two small areas of the blastoderm which, as they regressed with the primitive streak, were responsible for the induction of the somites. Spratt reported that transections of the blastoderm, either anterior or lateral to the centers, had no effect on somite formation, whereas if the transections were posterior or medial to the centers, no somites were formed. Other investigators also reported that if the somite centers were removed by excising the entire anterior end of the primitive streak, then the somites did not develop. However, it was also shown that if the somite centers and not the primitive streak were removed (Fig. 8–31 B), or if the anterior part of the streak and the centers were removed and a Hensen's node implanted at the anterior end of the cut streak (Fig. 8–31 C), then the somites developed normally. The existence of somite-forming centers is thus questionable, and other mechanisms for somite formation must be sought out. A number have been proposed, including induction by the overlying neural plate or by the notochord or some influence brought about by the regression of the primitive streak.

Recently, a series of experiments by Lipton and Jacobson (1974) has presented a comprehensive view of somite formation which, in fact, implicates the neural plate, the regression of the primitive streak, and the notochord as all playing a role in the process. In one experiment, the blastoderm was cut longitudinally so that one part contained all of the primitive streak as well as Spratt's proposed somite-forming centers (Fig. 8–32 A). In a second, they removed a wedge-shaped section of the blastoderm containing the anterior end of the primitive streak and the adjacent somite centers (Fig. 8–32 B); and in a third, they removed the same wedge-shaped piece as in the second and then extended a cut posteriorly through the middle of the primitive streak (Fig. 8–32 C). In a high percentage of cases in all three experiments, the pieces lacking the anterior end of the primitive streak and the somite-forming centers developed somites. In examining the blastoderms cultured after the above-mentioned operations were performed, four important observations were made. First, there was no notochordal tissue in any of the cultures, since Hensen's node was completely removed in all of the experiments. Second, the fragments that formed somites always contained some neural plate material. Third, only those embryos in the second experiment which ended up showing a U-shaped configuration as the result of the formation of a longitudinal split down the middle, after the wedge was removed, formed somites. Fourth, although somites developed after 10 hours of incubation, over the next 14 to 20 hours most of them broke down, dispersing laterally. Based on these four observations, we may reach four conclusions. From the first, neither Hensen's node, the notochord, nor the somite-forming centers are necessary for somite formation. From the second, neural plate material is necessary. From the third, a longitudinal splitting of the embryo is important. From the fourth, the presence of the notochord may be necessary for the stabilization of the somites once they are formed.

Thus, we are presented with the following view of somite formation. As the presumptive somite cells migrate laterally away from

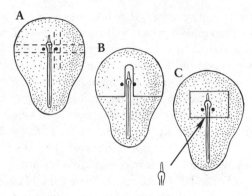

8–31 Diagrams of three experiments on the role of the somite centers. A, (Spratt, 1954), if the blastoderm is cut either anterior or lateral to the somite centers (asterisks), somite development is normal. If the cut is posterior or medial to the centers, no somites develop; B, (Bellairs, 1963), the somite centers are removed but the entire primitive streak and Hensen's node are retained. Although lacking somite centers, somite development is normal; C, (Nicolet, 1970), the entire anterior end of the primitive streak is removed. No somites will develop. However, if a portion of Hensen's node is implanted at the anterior end of the cut streak, somites will develop. (From B. H. Lipton and A. G. Jacobson, 1974. Dev. Biol. 38, 91.)

8–32 Diagrams of three studies by Lipton and Jacobson on the mechanism of somite formation. For explanation, see text. (From B. H. Lipton and A. G. Jacobson 1974. Dev. Biol. 38, 91.)

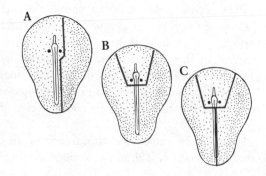

the primitive streak, they become closely associated with that region of the epiblast which will form the neural plate and, through this association, are imprinted with a prepattern of segmentation. This segmentation, however, is only realized when the primitive streak regresses and splits the mesoderm into right and left halves. This shearing action of the regressing primitive streak can be simulated by mechanically cutting the mesoderm longitudinally. Interestingly, in normal somite formation, as the streak regresses, the somites appear at some distance in front of Hensen's node, at the level where the notochord is developing, and they are formed progressively in a craniocaudal sequence. Yet, when the blastoderm is split mechanically, the entire length of the mesoderm is divided into right and left halves simultaneously and, following this, all of the somites along the length of the split form at the same time. Finally, recalling that the somites develop fibrous connections to the notochord, we may postulate that, although the notochord has no function in somite formation, it may be necessary for the stabilization of the somites once they are formed. Lacking these connections the somites tend to disperse laterally.

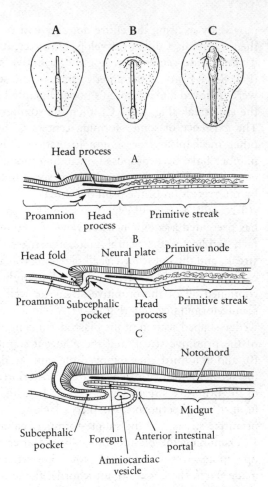

8–33 Diagrams of midsagittal sections of the chick embryo during the formation of the embryonic axis. Arrows indicate foldings that lead to the formation of the head fold and the foregut. A, head process, 20–22 hours; B, head fold, 23–24 hours. C, 28–29 hours.

Establishment of the Fore-, Mid-, and Hindgut

While the neural folds are developing, an elevation of the entire blastoderm at the cranial end of the embryo appears. This forms a process that extends forward over the underlying ectoderm. This is the *head fold* (Fig. 8–30 C,D; 8–33). The pocketlike recess between the head fold and the ectoderm is the *subcephalic pocket*. Craniad of the head fold, the blastoderm contains no mesodermal layer in a region known as the *proamnion*. Since the entire thickness of the blastoderm is included in the head fold, the endoderm is elevated also and is pushed into the elevation as a shallow pocket beneath the neural plate. This finger-shaped pocket is the foregut, and the opening leading into it is the *anterior intestinal portal* (Fig. 8–33 C). A hindgut and a *posterior intestinal portal* develop at a later time (60–70 hours) in conjunction with the formation of the tail fold. Between the foregut and the hindgut, the median sheet of endoderm, lying underneath the notochord and the somites and on the top of the yolk, is the roof of the open midgut. As development proceeds, continued downward and inward folding of the endoderm of the midgut area, accompanied by cranial and caudal growth of the head fold and the tail fold, increases the size of the fore- and hindgut regions and progressively decreases the size of the open midgut, which retains its connection to the yolk sac by a narrow stalk.

Figure 8–34 shows the appearance of an embryo during early somite formation. The cross sections illustrate the connection be-

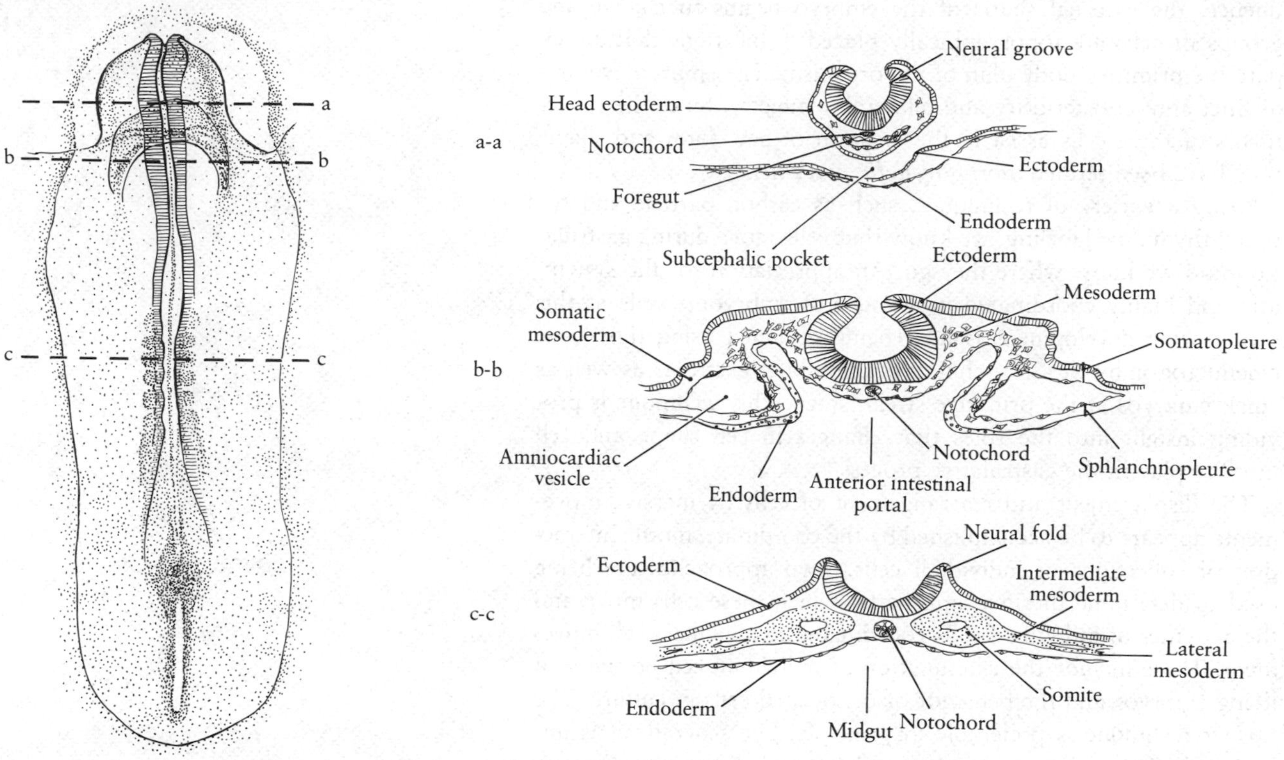
a
b
b
c
c
a-a
Neural groove
Head ectoderm
Notochord
Ectoderm
Foregut
Endoderm
Subcephalic pocket
b-b
Ectoderm
Mesoderm
Somatic mesoderm
Somatopleure
Amniocardiac vesicle
Notochord
Sphlanchnopleure
Endoderm
Anterior intestinal portal
c-c
Neural fold
Ectoderm
Intermediate mesoderm
Lateral mesoderm
Somite
Endoderm
Midgut
Notochord

tween the closed foregut and the open midgut by way of the anterior intestinal portal. The mesoderm is differentiating into somite and lateral mesoderm between which the intermediate mesoderm is seen.

8–34 Whole mount of a five-somite embryo with transverse sections pictured at the levels indicated. A, through the head fold showing the closed foregut and subcephalic pocket; B, through the anterior intestinal portal; C, through a pair of somites.

THE MECHANISMS OF GASTRULATION

Morphogenetic Cell Movements

Gastrulation is a developmental event that involves the massive translocation of embryonic cells after the blastular stage is completed. The future primordia of mesodermal and endodermal structures, such as muscle and gut, are removed from the surface to new positions within the embryo. Their place at the surface of the embryo is taken by an actively spreading population of cells (ectodermal), which will contribute to the skin, nervous system, and sense organs. Hence, this crucial phase of development is characterized by movements of cells that involve the whole embryo. As a consequence, the external shape of the embryo begins to change and groups of cells are topographically placed in locations that anticipate the primitive body plan of the organism. The embryo acquires distinct anteroposteriority and bilateral symmetry. Since the movements of these cells assist in the creation of new form and shape, they have been termed *morphogenetic movements*.

Using a variety of techniques, such as carbon particle and tritiated thymidine labeling, we know that cells move during gastrulation and we know where they go. An appreciation for the systematic and highly coordinated movement of embryonic cells at this time during development is now being obtained using time-lapse cinemicrography of sea urchin and amphibian gastrulas as well as chick embryos at the primitive streak stage. This technique is providing insight into the roles that changes in cell shape and cell motility play in the gastrulative process.

The displacement and rearrangement of cells by massive movements appears to be accomplished by the coordinate, motile interaction of collections of individual cells. Two approaches are being used to determine the mechanisms by which these cells move and the activities of individual cells coordinated to give mass cell movement. These include the examination of individual cell behavior in living embryos and the behavior of dissociated cells in culture. The former technique is preferable in principle, but generally it is impractical since embryos are often opaque and difficult to observe. Much of what is currently known regarding the mechanisms of cell locomotion comes from the tissue culture of cells. However, when cells of gastrulating embryos are disrupted and subsequently cultured for study, it must be remembered that modes of behavior may be generated in vitro that have no consequence for normal gastrulation.

The small, transparent holoblastic eggs of echinoderms have been particularly useful in studying the mechanics of the cellular activities responsible for the rearrangement of cells and the changes in form during gastrulation. At about 12 hours after the start of development in the sea urchin, some 40 cells (micromeres) migrate from the vegetal pole into the hollow, fluid-filled blastocoele (Fig. 8–35 A,B). Movement is accomplished by means of numerous, long, *pseudopodia,* some up to 30 micrometers in length, being thrown out from the cell surfaces into the interior of the blastula. When these pseudopodia contact and adhere to the inner wall (ectoderm) of the blastula, shortening or contraction of these thin processes pulls the cell body toward the point of attachment (Fig. 8–35 C). Electron micrographs through these migratory cells, destined to become the primary mesenchyme cells, show large numbers of microtubules distributed parallel to their long axes, thus indicating

A
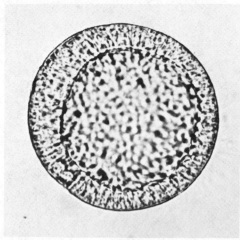

B
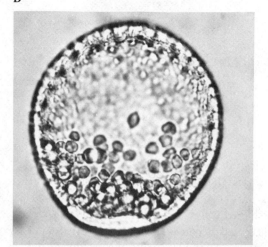

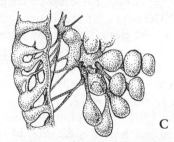
C

that microtubules are probably responsible for the development and activity of the pseudopodia. The primary mesenchyme cells will later lay down the skeletal system of the embryo.

Gastrulation begins by a small flattening of the columnar-shaped cells of the vegetal plate, which gradually extends into the blastocoele as the archenteron (Fig. 8–35 D). Just prior to this infolding, the cells of the vegetal plate lose contact with their neighbors, round up at their inner ends, and show strong pulsatory activity. This pulsatory activity causes the initial invagination, which brings the tip of the infolded cellular layer about one third of the way across the blastocoele. The second phase of gastrulation begins, after a pause, with the appearance of intense pseudopodial activity of the cells at the tip of the archenteron. Thin, long, pseudopodia, shot out from these cells, form stable contacts with the inner surface of the gastrular wall. Subsequent contraction of the pseudopodia pulls the archenteron further into the interior of the embryo. The attachment of the pseudopodia to the inner wall also appears to be important in maintaining the structural integrity of the archenteron during gastrulation. If the pseudopodia are detached experimentally, the archenteron everts to the outside so that the embryo becomes an exogastrula.

Amphibian embryos have also been particularly popular material for a variety of investigations on the gastrulative process. Their cells are large and the movements of cells are more clearly visible than in most other vertebrate embryos. The onset of gastrulation in frogs or salamanders is marked by an infolding of the presumptive endodermal cells on the borderline of the vegetal region just below the center of the grey crescent area. The upper rim of the groove represents the dorsal lip of the developing blastopore. The cells that initi-

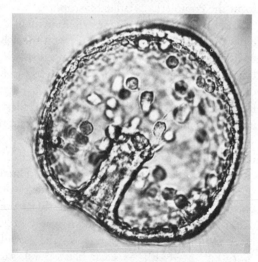
D

8–35 A late blastula of the sea urchin (A) is shown just before the migration of primary mesenchyme cells into the blastocoele (B). A sketch of the attachment of the pseudopods of the primary mesenchyme to the thickened ectoderm is shown in C. Gastrulation involves the flattening and invagination of cells of the vegetal plate (D). Note the secondary mesenchyme cells at the tip of the gut. (A,B, and D from G. Karp, 1974. Dev. Biol. 41, 110; C, after T. Gustafson and L. Wolpert, 1967. Biol. Rev. 42, 442.)

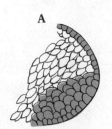 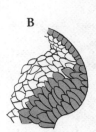 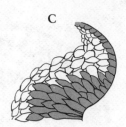 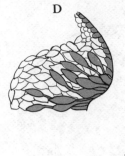

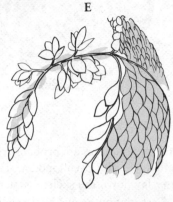

ate the formation of the blastopore are observed to change dramatically in shape, which causes them to sink to the inside. As it approaches and becomes part of the blastopore each cell is transformed from a cuboidal-shaped cell to a *flask* or *bottle-shaped cell* (Fig. 8–36 A-D). The flask cell becomes progressively attenuated until the bulk of the cell is moved completely into the interior of the embryo. Deepening of the blastopore is reflected in the gradual stretching and elongating of the bottle cells, with some attaining lengths of 200 micrometers. During the invagination process, the outer surfaces of these migratory cells always maintain firm connections with neighboring cells on the surface of the embryo despite being greatly stretched. Although studied extensively by Holtfreter (1943a,b; 1944) it is not known what initially stimulates bottle-cell formation and how the activities of these cells are coordinated to form the complete, circular blastopore.

The changes in the shapes of individual cells at the blastopore have been studied for many years with the light microscope because of their apparent involvement with cell translocation during gastrulation. Holtfreter in particular has made significant contributions to our understanding of the structure and migration of presumptive mesodermal and endodermal cells at the blastopore in the amphibian. The salient features of his hypothesis regarding this subject should be briefly mentioned. He postulated that the driving force initiating the formation of the blastopore is located within the presumptive bottle cells of the endoderm. Initially, the inner ends of these cells migrate inward in response to the alkaline pH of the blastocoelic fluid, thus creating the blastoporal invagination. The distal ends of these cells remain firmly attached to a specialized layer of material on the surface of the gastrula, termed the *surface coat* (Fig. 8–36 E). As each blastoporal cell moves inward, it is drawn out into the shape of a flask. The presumptive notochordal and mesodermal cells are drawn over the lips of the blastopore in sheetlike fashion because the flask cells exert a pulling force on these cells by way of the surface coat. Hence, the tightly joined endodermal, notochordal, and mesodermal cells at the surface func-

8–36 A–D, successive changes in the shape of blastoporal cells during gastrulation in the amphibian as seen with the light microscope (After J. Holtfreter, 1943. J. Exp. Zool. 94, 261); E, a part of the dorsal lip of the blastopore showing cells held together by the surface coat as proposed by Holtfreter. (After J. Holtfreter, 1943. J. Exp. Zool. 93, 251.)

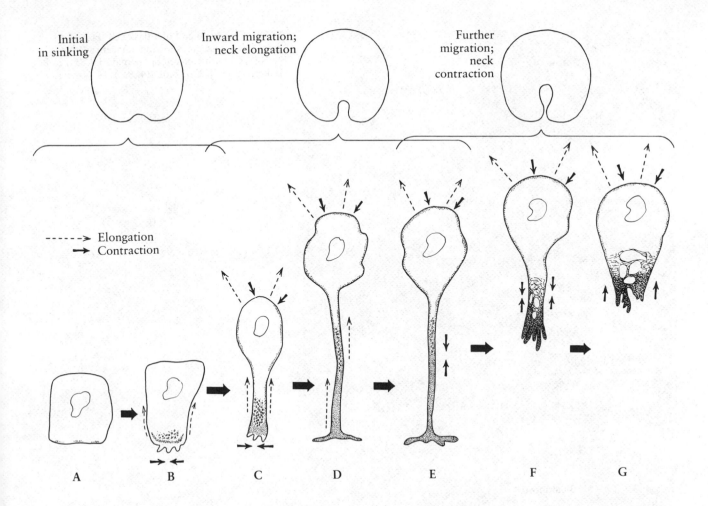

Initial
in sinking

Inward migration;
neck elongation

Further
migration;
neck
contraction

----> Elongation
—→ Contraction

A B C D E F G

tion to integrate into a coordinated system the pulling activities of the independently migrating bottle cells.

Since the surface coat is essential to Holtfreter's theory of gastrulation, various investigators have attempted to verify its existence. Positive and incontrovertible evidence for the presence of such a coat or covering of elastized material remains to be forthcoming. Electron microscopic studies have not generally supported the notion that there is a continuous extracellular covering for the young amphibian embryo.

Based largely upon electron microscopic studies, Baker (1965) has proposed a plausible model for the general mechanism of bottle cell formation and cell movement through the blastopore (Fig. 8–37). According to Baker, each cell moving through the blastopore passes through a sequence of shapes that resemble a cube, a wedge,

8–37 Theoretical scheme for the transformation of a blastoporal cell during gastrulation as proposed by Baker. A, the cell as it appears prior to gastrulation; B, the distal end of the cell contracts causing an initial insinking and formation of the blastoporal groove. Note the shape (wedge) of the cell; C–D, the proximal surface of the cell migrates inward, deepening the blastoporal groove. The distal end of the cell continues to contract and the neck of the cell elongates; E–G, the neck of the cell contracts after maximum elongation of the cell is reached. Note that this shortening furthers invagination and pulls adjacent cells into the groove. (From P. Baker, 1965. J. Cell Biol. 24, 95.)

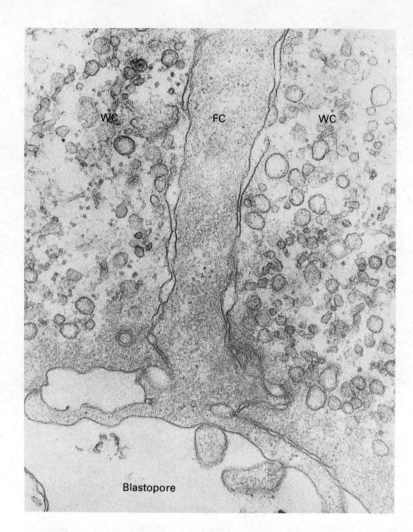

WC   FC   WC

Blastopore

8–38   The distal end of a flask cell (FC) of an amphibian gastrula, showing adjacent wedge cells (WC) with areas of dense material. (From P. Baker, 1965. J. Cell Biol. 24, 95.)

and a flask (Figs. 8–38; 8–39). The distal ends of cells invaginating over the blastopore are observed to contain a layer of electron-opaque material which has a filamentous appearance, suggestive of a contractile function (Fig. 8–39). It is proposed that alternate shortening (contraction) and elongating (expansion) of this dense layer in the distal ends of these cells accounts for their transformation into flask-shaped cells and their consequent movement through the blastopore (Fig. 8–37). Some contractile activities in the neck regions of flask cells may also be partially responsible for cell movement. As invaginating cells contract distally and migrate inward, neighboring cells are drawn in behind. Temporary bonds or junctions between adjacent cells of the blastopore appear to coordinate the movements of invagination. The cells, then, appear to move as a

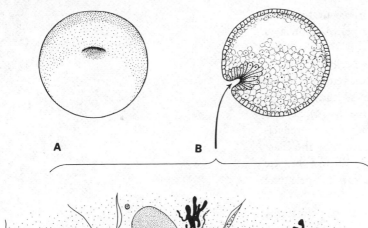

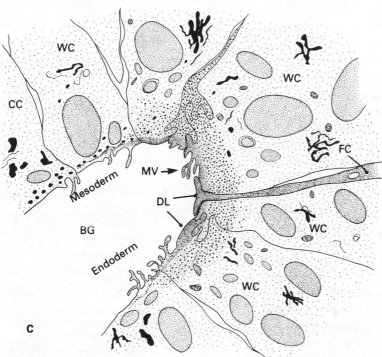

8–39 A, early gastrula of the frog with blastoporal lip just beginning to form; B, a sagittal section through the blastoporal groove showing wedge and flask cells; C, a reconstruction from electron micrographs of a parasagittal section through the blastoporal groove at a stage represented by B. Note the flask (FC), wedge (WC), and cuboidal (CC) cells that line the groove. The distal surfaces of these invaginating cells contain a dense layer (DL). BG, blastoporal groove; MV, microvilli. (From P. Baker, 1965. J. Cell Biol. 24, 95.)

supercellular unit into the interior in great measure because of the pulling activities of the bottle cells. Other factors may also be involved in the orderly, integrated involution of the chordamesodermal cells. Among these are the inherent tendency for chordamesodermal cells to stretch in an anteroposterior direction.

Because their eggs are often transparent, teleost fishes have been used in analyzing morphogenetic movements at gastrulation. Following cleavage, the blastoderm flattens and, because of an intrinsic capacity to spread, moves by epiboly over the yolk sphere toward the vegetal pole. Three separate structures appear to participate in the spreading movements: the enveloping layer of the blastoderm or the cohesive epithelium that forms the outer surface of the blastoderm, the deep cells of the blastoderm, and the periblast or layer of syncytial cytoplasm, which sits atop the fluid yolk (Fig. 8–14).

With the onset of gastrulation in *Fundulus,* the periblast tissue is observed to spread over the yolk prior to the movements of the cellular blastoderm. Subsequently, the blastoderm spreads over the periblast until it reaches the margin of the latter (Fig. 8–14). Several types of experiments, including the complete removal of the enveloping layer and deep cells, point to the conclusion that the blastoderm acquires the intrinsic capacity for epiboly during the late blastula stage and that the blastoderm requires for its spreading movements a natural substratum, the expanding periblast.

By forming firm adhesive connections with the periblast, the marginal cells of the enveloping layer appear to be the prime movers in epiboly. During spreading movements these marginal cells show exceedingly thin, fan like extensions (5 μm–10 μm wide) known as *ruffled membranes*. Time-lapse cinemicrography indicates that the contacts of the ruffled membranes with the periblast are alternatively being broken and remade continuously as the cells move over the periblast. Hence, ruffled membranes appear to be the locomotory organs of the enveloping layer; their waves of adhesive contact with the periblast produce a gliding movement whose thrust is transferred to the nonmarginal cells of the blastoderm. If these marginal connections are severed during epiboly, the blastoderm promptly retracts, clearly indicating that the latter is under tension during the spreading process. What keeps the enveloping layer intact during this stretching process? Studies by Trinkaus and Lentz with the electron microscope show that the cells of the enveloping layer are bound together by *tight junctions* in which the outer leaflets of opposing plasmalemmas are fused by primitive *demosomes*. Cell contact is also seen in the interdigitation of fingerlike cytoplasmic projections of adjacent enveloping layer cells (Fig. 8–40).

In contrast to the cells of the enveloping layer, which spread as an epithelial sheet, the deep blastomeres of the blastoderm appear to translocate by an entirely different mechanism. Prior to the onset of gastrulation, both time-lapse cinemicrographic and ultrastructure studies show that the deep blastomeres change shape constantly, although no actual movement is in evidence. Each cell forms protruding, rounded and transparent bulges known as *lobopodia* (Fig. 8–41). With the onset of epiboly, however, the lobopodia begin to form adhesive contacts with other deep cells as well as with cells of the overlying enveloping layer. As this occurs, each lobopodium becomes stretched into a thin cytoplasmic projection or *filopodium*. A firm contact with another cell apparently provides traction, for, when the filopodium shortens, the cell is pulled in the direction of

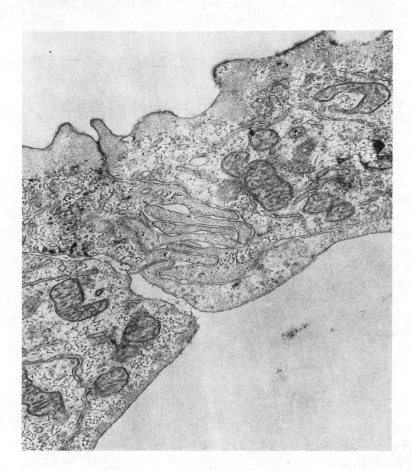

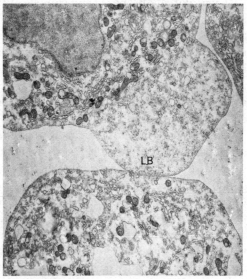

8–40 Enveloping layer cells of *Fundulus* showing several cytoplasmic projections interdigitating with one another. (From J. Trinkaus and T. Lentz, 1967. J. Cell Biol. 32, 139.)

the adhesion. Hence, the deep blastomeres appear to move as individual units by crawling over each other. Although their movements are initially random, they subsequently migrate in unidirectional fashion toward the margins of the blastoderm to participate in the formation of the germ ring. Eventually they converge dorsally and posteriorly to form the embryonic shield. It should be pointed out at this time that the deep cells, which give rise to the tissues of the teleost embryo, do not appear to play an important role in epiboly.

The key to our complete understanding of the mechanisms underlying epibolic cellular movements in teleost fishes resides in the periblast. It is this layer of the gastrulating embryo which serves as a specific substratum for the spreading blastoderm. It is also this layer that appears to control the rate at which the blastoderm moves down around the yolk. Yet, the mechanism by which the periblast itself spreads is simply not known. Ultrastructure studies have confirmed that the periblast is continuous with a thinner layer of cytoplasm lying on the surface of the yolk proper (Fig. 8–14). It

8–41 A deep cell of the early *Fundulus* gastrula showing contact with another blastomere by its lobopodium (LP). (From J. Trinkaus and T. Lentz, 1967. J. Cell Biol. 32, 139.)

has been proposed that movement of the periblast may involve some type of controlled and complex flow of cytoplasm into the yolk cytoplasmic layer.

Studies of the mechanisms of morphogenetic movements during gastrulation and early embryogenesis in the chick have been directed in great measure at the spreading of the area opaca, the immigration or invagination of the chordamesoderm and endoderm through the primitive streak, and the expansion of the hypoblast.

The area opaca of the chick blastoderm, which is composed of extraembryonic ectoderm, mesoderm, and endodern, spreads as an epithelial sheet beneath the vitelline membrane to encompass the yolk during the first several days following incubation. It is well known that the chick blastoderm fails to spread normally if removed from the yolk and cultured on an agar or a plasma clot. New has demonstrated (1959) that spreading of the area opaca in vitro is perfectly normal when the blastoderm is cultured with its own vitelline membrane (Fig. 8–42). Other experiments by New have given clear evidence that the cells at the margin of the area opaca use the inner surface of the vitelline membrane as a substratum upon which to move. Although the area opaca in vitro will adhere to the outer surface of the vitelline membrane, expansion is only possible upon the inner surface of the vitelline membrane, suggesting that the latter is constructed in such a fashion as to promote movement.

It was initially proposed the epiboly of the blastoderm was due to centrally located sites of intense cellular proliferation which effected a "push from behind." Although there is cell division within the blastoderm during epiboly, principally near the margins of the blastoderm, there is little experimental evidence to support such a proposal. For example, the area opaca will continue to spread upon the vitelline membrane when blastoderms are cultured in the presence of known mitotic inhibitors.

An alternative proposal, namely that the marginal cells of the area opaca act by pulling the rest of the blastoderm over the yolk, is supported by evidence from investigations with the electron microscope. In contrast to the other cells of the chick blastoderm, only the marginal cells are observed to form long, thin processes or filopodia (as long as 500 μm) during spreading activity. Presumably, these processes serve as locomotory organs and contract, thereby pulling the marginal cells with them. Hence, the marginal cells appear to advance as an epithelial sheet with the nonmarginal cells being pulled along in rather passive fashion. The pull created by the marginal cells puts the rest of the cells of the blastoderm under tension during movement. As with the enveloping layer of cells in the teleost blastoderm, specialized junctional complexes be-

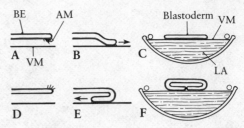

8–42 When the chick blastoderm is explanted normally onto its vitelline membrane (A), its adhesive margin (AM) attaches to the inner surface of the vitelline membrane (B). Normal expansion of the blastoderm then follows (C). If the blastoderm is inverted and placed on the vitelline membrane (D), the adhesive surface of the blastoderm curls under to bring it into contact with the vitelline membrane (E). Expansion in this case leads to the formation of the hollow vesicle (F). BE, blastoderm edge; LA, liquid albumin; VM, vitelline membrane. (After D.A.T. New, 1959. J. Embryol. Exp. Morphol. 7, 149.)

tween the nonmarginal cells keep these cells together as a tight cohesive sheet. This prevents their being pulled apart under the tension of epiboly.

The morphogenetic movements of cells leading to the formation of the primitive streak are initiated shortly after the incubation temperature reaches 38.5°C. As pointed out previously, the directions in which cells of the epiblast migrate during the formation of the primitive streak are known, chiefly through the carbon and carmine particle tracing studies of Spratt and Haas (1965). However, the mechanism by which the cells of the epiblast converge toward the streak remains a mystery. That the presumptive endodermal and chordamesodermal cells migrate as an epithelial sheet is supported by the fine structure studies, which indicate the presence of numerous points of apparent fusion between surfaces of adjacent cells.

The primitive streak is an invagination center. It is not surprising, therefore, to find that movement of epiblast cells through the streak appears to be very similar to that described for the movement of chordamesodermal and endodermal cells through the blastopore of the gastrulating amphibian embryo. Bottle or flask-shaped cells are identifiable at all levels of the primitive streak, suggesting that the changes in cell shape that accompany the invagination process may be brought about by the contraction of an electron-dense material found in the cytoplasm of these cells. Whether microtubules, also observed in cells of the primitive streak, play any role in the movement of cells through the streak awaits further experimental proof.

The movement of chordamesodermal and endodermal cells from the base of the primitive streak outward beneath the epiblast in lateral and anterior directions is a steady and continuous process. In the case of mesodermal cells, there is a distinct change in shape as each cell leaves the primitive streak. At first flask-shaped, each quickly becomes transformed into a stellate-shaped cell whose leading edge bears numerous filopodia. Broader cytoplasmic projections (ruffled membranes?) also mark the advancing edges of these mesodermal cells. The filopodia extend into and adhere to the adjacent epithelial surfaces of the overlying epiblast and the underlying hypoblast (Fig. 8–43). The filamentous appearance of the filopodia offers evidence that these organs may be contractile and hence effect movement by pulling. Since all mesodermal cells are connected to each other as well as to cells of the primitive streak by a variety of junctional complexes, one is left with the impression that movement away from the primitive streak is in the form of a loosely arranged network of interconnected cells.

The hypoblast of the late-stage chick blastoderm is presumptive to the extraembryonic endoderm of the yolk sac. Its cells are loosely packed and show signs of movement well in advance of the

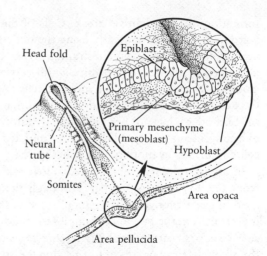

8–43   Diagram of the gastrulating chick embryo at the four-somite stage. The embryo consists of head fold, open neural groove and neural folds, somites, and primitive streak. A transverse section through the primitive streak shows the cells of the area pellucida and the area opaca. The inset shows the cells of the epiblast and the laterally migrating mesoderm. The hypoblast is a thin epithelium below the mesoderm. (From E. Hay, 1968. Epithelial-Mesenchymal Interactions. R. Fleishmajer and R. E. Billingham, eds. Williams and Wilkins, Baltimore. Copyright © 1968, Williams and Wilkins Company, Baltimore.)

formation of the primitive streak. Cells of the hypoblast move forward and radially, apparently using the undersurface of the overlying epiblast as a specific substratum. What causes this migration and whether it is active or passive is still very much a source of controversy. The proposal that hypoblast cells are pushed passively by the action of a center of rapid cell division in the posterior part of the blastoderm has not been adequately tested. It is equally possible that movements of hypoblast cells are initiated with changes in such cell parameters as motility and adhesiveness.

In all gastrulating embryos, cells move with precision and order from one location to another. Although the mechanisms of most morphogenetic movements accomplishing this task are still obscure, it is clear from the previous examples that such properites of cells as surface adhesiveness, the ability to change shape (deformation), and the ability to form organs of locomotion (i.e., ruffled membranes and filopodia) are important to the event of translocation. It is extremely important for the reader to appreciate that movements, and, indeed, the larger picture of gastrulation, involve the interplay of cell motility, cell shape, and cell contact behavior. For example, we have seen several cases in which a cell must adhere to a substratum before it can move from one place to another. For the cell to leave one location, it must be free of contacts with adjacent cells (i.e., lose surface adhesiveness). The formation of filopodia in cells that move as individual units, or the formation of ruffled membranes at the margins of cell masses moving as epithelial sheets, necessitates contact with a substratum and consequent changes in cell shape.

Unfortunately, many fundamental questions can be raised about morphogenetic movements at gastrulation. Why do cells move in their particular directions? Do cells of the gastrula have a capacity to read and respond to some chemical and/or molecular "road map" to guide them? What signals initiate and terminate such changes in cell properties as adhesiveness, motility, and others? Recent advances in cell membrane structure and in the surface chemistry of adult cells may point the way to answering these questions on gastrulating embryos.

Cellular Rearrangement and Cellular Segregation

The transformation of the fertilized egg into a multicellular system in which groups of cells are shifted into arrangements that foreshadow the tissue patterns of the adult organism occurs principally between the blastula and neurula stages. Irrespective of whether the postgastrula embryo is round (frog) or flat (chick), the primary germ layers are always arranged such that the mesoderm

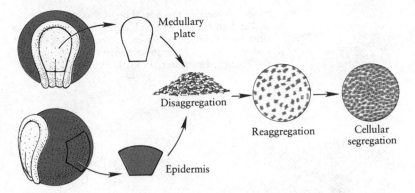

8–44   A diagrammatic summary of the technique for the disaggregation of embryonic tissues (medullary plate and epidermis) and their reaggregation for studies designed to examine cellular segregation. (From P. Townes and J. Holtfreter, 1955. J. Exp. Zool. 128, 53.)

occupies a position between the outer ectoderm and the inner endoderm.

Much of the history of embryology has been concerned with the nature of the mechanisms controlling the rearrangement and segregation of groups of cells that result from morphogenetic movements not only during gastrulation but also during the period of organ formation. For example, why do the mesodermal cells, which form a loosely packed association, stay together after gastrulation as a homogeneous layer insinuated between ectoderm and endoderm? Are the germ layers of the postgastrular embryo organized the way they are because of special properties of their constituent cells, or are they passively channeled into their topographical positions because of some overriding influence of the whole embryo? The rearrangement of cells and the sorting out or segregation of cells into specific tissues or organs are inextricably related to changes in cell shape, cell contact behavior, and cell motility.

Unfortunately, our current understanding of the roles of cell shapes, cell contact behavior, and cell motility in the organization of germ layers and in the construction of tissues is based largely upon observations using artificial or in vitro techniques. Fragments of embryos or reaggregated suspensions of isolated embryonic cells are allowed to first interact in a culture medium and then observed. A routine procedure is illustrated for amphibian cells in Figure 8–44. A fragment from the embryo is excised with glass needles and placed into a potassium hydroxide solution (pH 9.6–9.8). At this pH, the tissue fragment disaggregates or dissociates into individual, single cells. Treatment of similar fragments with trypsin or solutions containing EDTA (ethylenediaminetetraacetic acid, a chelating agent) without calcium and magnesium ions will also bring about *disaggregation*. Cells prepared in this way from a variety of embryonic tissues (i.e., gastrular ectoderm, endoderm, mesoderm; neural plate) are then brought together in selected combinations in a cul-

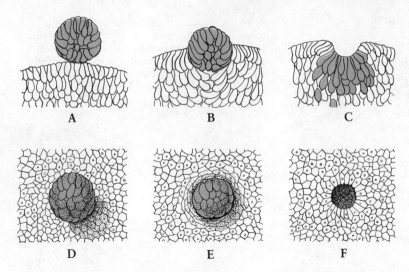

8–45 A piece of the dorsal lip of the blastopore will sink into a piece of endoderm, forming a distinct invagination. A, B, and C are cross sections; D, E, and F are surface views of A, B, and C. (From J. Holtfreter, 1944. J. Exp. Zool. 95, 171.)

ture medium at a pH of 8.0. The cells are then observed to reaggregate.

Early studies by Holtfreter pioneered and elucidated much of the basis of current views on the rearrangement and self-isolation of embryonic cells. Experiments by Holtfreter using fragments of embryos, individual cells in culture, and reaggregated suspensions of embryonic cells led him to believe that inherent associative properties of cells and cell clusters provide a partial explanation for what goes on during the gastrulative process. For example, when he isolated a fragment of presumptive endoderm from a frog embryo at the blastula stage, it rounded up into a compact aggregate and then spread on the bottom of the culture dish. An isolated dorsal lip of the blastopore, when added to a fragment of endoderm, formed a distinctive invagination (Fig. 8–45). Based upon an extensive series of experiments utilizing various combinations of embryo fragments and disaggregated cells, it gradually became apparent that tissues and group of cells recognized and adhered to only like tissues and cells. Holtfreter introduced the concept of *selective cellular affinities* to explain these patterns of cell behavior.

When ectodermal and endodermal cells of the gastrula are dissociated and combined in vitro, there is initially random movement and indiscriminate union between diverse cell types. Gradually, however, there is sorting out and self-isolation in the reaggregate, leading to the formation of homogeneous layers of superficial ectoderm and internal endoderm (Fig. 8–46 A). Although both germ layers are capable of forming an epithelium, a permanent association between the two layers is lacking. A mosaic of cells is seen during the first 10 hours in an aggregate formed by the recombination

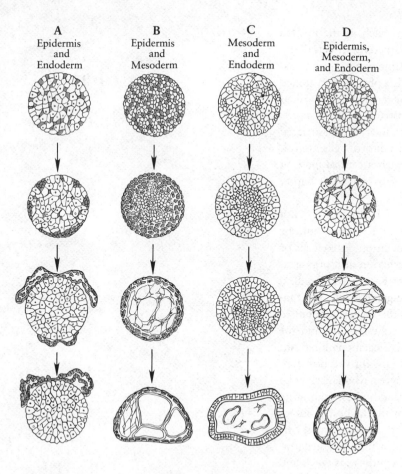

A	B	C	D
Epidermis and Endoderm	Epidermis and Mesoderm	Mesoderm and Endoderm	Epidermis, Mesoderm, and Endoderm

8–46 Rearrangement and segregation of disaggregated and reaggregated embryonic cells (amphibian). A, combined epidermal and endodermal cells; B, combined epidermal and mesodermal cells; C, combined mesodermal and endodermal cells; D, combined epidermal, mesodermal, and endodermal cells. (From P. Townes and J. Holtfreter, 1955. J. Exp. Zool. 128, 53.)

of ectoderm and mesoderm. The mesodermal cells then slip to the interior of the aggregate to become surrounded by a thick layer of ectoderm (Fig. 8–46 B). The inner mesodermal tissue may then differentiate into blood vessels, mesenchyme, and so on while the outer ectodermal tissue becomes a thin epidermis. When endoderm and mesoderm are combined as single cells, the reaggregate shows that the endoderm forms an external covering to the entire preparation (Fig. 8–46 C). This pattern of cell segregation, contrary to the normal topographical arrangements of these two layers, resembles that of a total exogastrula. If all three germ layers are dissociated into single cells and then mixed, an aggregate forms in which the mesoderm holds together the ectoderm at the surface and the endoderm at the interior (Fig. 8–46 D). As with other cell combinations, the rearrangement of germ cells in this aggregate involves the segregation and association of like cells and their placement into topographic relationships similar to those produced by the normal movements of ectoderm, mesoderm, and endoderm at gastrulation.

The sorting out process features cell motility, such as the inward movements of mesoderm and the outward spreading of ectoderm, and the adhesion of like cell types to yield histologically specific tissue layers. This pattern of cell behavior is also observed in mixed aggregates of embryonic cells taken from other species as well as from embryos considerably older than the gastrula–neurula stages. If two or more organs, such as chick heart and liver, are dissociated and the cell suspensions mixed, random movements of cells are followed by segregation and self-assembly in which a central mass of heart cells becomes surrounded by a layer of liver cells (Chapter 13).

Although the experimental investigations of Holtfreter did not reveal the basis for cellular rearrangement and sorting out, he clearly demonstrated that the preferential association of like cells or groups of cells was important to tissue construction and organization. Since his observations, several hypotheses have been advanced to explain the phenomena of cellular rearrangement and segregation. We will consider briefly only those hypotheses that attempt to account for the adhesion of like cells into a cohesive unit and the positioning of these units in patterns peculiar to each combination.

Chemotaxis has often been invoked to account for cell positioning and cell self-assembly. Might not cells segregate themselves in response to differential concentrations of metabolites, migrating along a gradient either toward or away from the highest point of concentration? For example, certain cells in an aggregate might be attracted toward the periphery in response to a higher concentration of oxygen. The evidence to support this hypothesis is weak and unconvincing, primarily because the behavior of cells in an aggregate does not generally conform to that dictated by the principle of chemotaxis.

Curtis (1961) postulates that the sorting out of vertebrate cells is primarily due to differences in the time (*timing hypothesis*) at which diverse cell types become adhesive and hence can be joined together. He assumes that the cell surface becomes modified by the process of dissociation. Each cell loses its adhesiveness and become migratory. Diverse cell types within an aggregate gradually reacquire their adhesive qualities, but at different times. The combined effects of random movements, rising adhesiveness, and reduced shear (i.e., a force produced by cells moving over each other, which tends to promote motility; its effects are least at the surface of an aggregate) trap cells at the surface of an aggregate. In this manner, all cells of one type become trapped at the surface with other less adhesive cells being herded toward the center of the aggregate. Some evidence is available to support the timing hypothesis. Experiments have been conducted in which the position of the germ layers in an aggregate can be altered by varying the times at which they are dissociated before being recombined in culture. A strong argument against the hypothesis is that it requires an artifactual effect (i.e., loss of adhesiveness owing to dissociation) to explain the normal topographical relationships of cells in a mixed aggregate.

Spreading and sorting out of trypsin-dissociated embryonic tissues in mixed aggregates have been studied extensively by both Steinberg (1964) and Moscona (1968). Steinberg observed that there appears to be a hierarchy of "preference" for the external or internal position of like cells in combinations of tissues. The hierarchy predicts topographical relationships between cell types and follows a transitive rule: if cell type A surrounds B and cell type B surrounds C, then cell type A will surround C. Random motility and quantitiative differences in the general adhesiveness of cells (*differential adhesiveness hypothesis*) play central roles in the self-isolation and organization of cells into functional units.

Steinberg believes that an aggregate may be treated as if it were a multiple-phase system of immiscible liquids. When a cell touches other cells in culture, it may remain in contact with that cell(s) or move away to make contact with other cells. What determines how the cell responds to its initial contact with another cell? Suppose that an aggregate is composed of two cell types, A and B, and that A cells cohere more strongly than B cells. When cell A adheres to cell A (or cell B), it is said to possess a certain amount of free energy, which is used to make and maintain the contact. For the aggregate to achieve thermodynamic stability or equilibrium, the free energy of A and B cells must be at a minimum. This can only be obtained when there is maximum adhesion of cell surfaces (i.e., when the adhesive contacts on the cell surface are used to a maximum extent). Hence, cells will tend to exchange weaker for stronger bonds of adhesion. If A-B adhesions are intermediate in strength between A-A and B-B adhesions, but weaker than the average of the two, then there will be a continual exchange of A-B adhesions for A-A adhesions until most of the A cells cohere. Since cells tend to maximize their contracts over as much of their surface as possible, the more adhesive A cells will move to the interior of the aggregate, thereby excluding the less adhesive B cells to the surface of the aggregate. Hence, the more cohesive A cells will form the internal component of the aggregate, surrounded by and embedded in a continuous layer of less cohesive B cells. Since the B cells at the surface of the aggregate do not use their adhesiveness to maximal capacity, the requirements of a thermodynamically stable system dictate the reduction of surface area of the aggregate to a minimum (i.e., a sphere).

There is experimental evidence to support the Steinberg hypothesis that the sorting out of cells in embryonic systems, including gastrulation, requires random cell movement and differences in the frequency of adhesive sites on cell surfaces. Direct measurements of the interfacial free energies of adhesion for several embryonic tissues of the chick tend to support the concept that quantitative differences in cellular adhesiveness do exist. However, studies by Moscona suggest that selective cell adhesions are probably related to specific *cell ligands* or carbohydrate-containing molecules located on or near to the outer surface of cells. He believes that cell recognition and sorting out are probably due to qualitative differences between embryonic cells in their surface chemical composition. Plasma membrane constituents commonly include monosaccharide sugars linked to proteins (glycoproteins) and lipids (glycolipids). Side chains of sugars of variable lengths are envisioned as projecting from the glycoproteins into the environment of the cell. The glycoproteins of the cell surface are free to interact with constituents of the extracellular environment, including enzymes and other cells. When cells are treated with enzymes that digest specific carbohydrates, such as betagalactosidase, their surfaces become altered and there is less specificity in reaggregation behavior. Roth and his colleagues (1971) have shown that glycosyltransferases, enzymes that catalyze the addition of activated sugars to glycoproteins, are present on the surfaces of embryonic cells. The basis for the adhesion between embryonic cells and the control for altering intercellular adhesion may relate to complementary reactions between carbohydrate-containing molecules and glycosyltransferases of cell surfaces. Closer examination of the chemical composition of cell surfaces will undoubtedly provide a better understanding of gastrulation.

In analyzing gastrulation of amphibians, Holtfreter demonstrated that the mesoderm becomes surrounded by endoderm, thus indicating the greater cohesiveness of the mesoderm. Also, the endodermal tissue generally takes up an internal position in combination with ectoderm. Thus, there appears to be a hierarchy of cohesiveness between germ layers (from greatest to least): mesoderm, endoderm, and ectoderm. How does one account for the fact that the relationship between the endoderm and mesoderm in reaggregate experiments is exactly the reverse of the relationship of these two germ layers in the intact, gastrulating embryo? In studying the results of recombination experiments, one should remember that the relationship of endoderm and mesoderm occurs with cells obtained from the germ layers *after* the latter have achieved their normal topographical relationships in the intact embryo. Hence, it is likely that there are changes in the cellular adhesiveness of endoderm and mesoderm during gastrulation (i.e., the cellular adhesiveness of mesoderm increases). It can also be concluded that an ectodermal covering is required for the normal shifting of the mesoderm over the endoderm. In the absence of an ectodermal covering, the mesoderm will exhibit its "abnormal" behavior of invaginating into the endodermal mass.

REFERENCES

Baker, J. 1965. Fine structure and morphogenetic movements in the gastrula of the tree frog, *Hyla regilla*. J. Cell Biol. 24:95–116.

Ballard, W. 1973. A new fate map for *Salmo gairdneri*. J. Exp. Zool. 184:49–75.

Ballard, W. W. 1976. Problems of gastrulation: Real and verbal. Biol. Sci. 26:36–39.

Curtis, A. S. G. 1961. Timing mechanisms in the specific adhesions of cells. Ex. Cell Res. Suppl. 8:107–122.

Gustafson, T. and L. Wolpert. 1967. Cellular movement and contact in sea urchin morphogenesis. Biol. Rev. 42:442–498.

Hamburger, V. 1942. A Manual of Experimental Embryology, pp. 43–55. Chicago: University of Chicago Press.

Hamburger, V. and H. L. Hamilton. 1951. A series of normal stages in the development of the chick embryo. J. Morphol. 88:49–92.

Holtfreter, J. 1943a. A study of the mechanics of gastrulation. Part I. J. Exp. Zool. 94:261–318.

Holtfreter, J. 1943b. Properties and functions of the surface coat in amphibian embryos. J. Exp. Zool. 93:251–323.

Holtfreter, J. 1944. A study of the mechanics of gastrulation. Part II. J. Exp. Zool. 95:171–212.

Johnson, K. 1970. The role of changes in cell contact behavior in amphibian gastrulation. J. Exp. Zool. 175:391–428.

Keller, R. E. 1976. Vital dye mapping of the gastrula and neurula of *Xenopus laevis*. II. Prospective areas and morphogenetic movements of the deep layer. Dev. Biol. 51:118–137.

Lentz, T. and J. Trinkaus. 1967. A fine structural study of cytodifferentiation during cleavage, blastula, and gastrula stages of *Fundulus heteroclitus*. J. Cell Biol. 32:121–138.

Lipton, B. H. and A. G. Jacobson. 1974. Experimental analysis of the mechanisms of somite formation. Dev. Biol. 38:91–103.

Løvtrup, S. 1975. Fate maps and gastrulation in amphibia—a critique of current views. Can. J. Zool. 53:473–479.

Malan, M. E. 1953. The elongation of the primitive streak and the localization of the presumptive chordamesoderm of the early chick blastoderm studied by means of coloured marks with Nile blue sulphate. Arch. Biol. 64:149–182.

Moscona, A. A. 1968. Cell aggregation: Properties of specific cell-ligands and their role in the formation of multicellular systems. Dev. Biol. 18:250–277.

New, D. A. T. 1959. Adhesive properties and expansion of the chick blastoderm. J. Embryol. Exp. Morphol. 7:146–164.

Nicolet, G. 1971. Avian gastrulation. Adv. Morphog. 9:231–261.

Pasteels, J. J. 1937. Etudes sur la gastrulation des vertébrates méroblastiques. III. Oiseaux. IV. Conclusions générales. Arch. Biol. 48:381–488.

Peter, K. 1938. Die Engwicklung des Endoderms beim Hühnchen. Z. Mikrosk-Anat. Forsch. 43:362–415.

Roth, S. 1968. Studies on intercellular adhesive selectivity. Dev. Biol. 16:602–613.

Roth, S., E. McGuire, and S. Roseman. 1971. Evidence for cell-surface glycosyltransferases: Their potential role in cellular recognition. J. Cell Biol. 51:536–547.

Spratt, N. T., Jr. and H. Haas. 1965. Germ layer formation and the role of the primitive streak in the chick. I. Basic architecture and morphogenetic tissue movements. J. Exp. Zool. 158:8–38.

Steinberg, M. 1964. The problem of adhesive selectivity in cellular interactions. In: Cellular Membranes in Development, pp. 321–366. Ed., M. Locke. New York: Academic Press.

Townes, P. and J. Holtfreter. 1955. Directed movements and selective adhesion of embryonic amphibian cells. J. Exp. Zool. 128:53–120.

Trinkaus, J. and T. Lentz. 1967. Surface specializations of *Fundulus* cells and their relation to cell movements during gastrulation. J. Cell Biol. 32:139–153.

Vakaet, L. 1962. Some new data concerning the formation of the definitive endoblast in the chick embryo. J. Embryol. Exp. Morphol. 10:38–57.

Vogt, W. 1929. Gestaltinganalyse am Amphibienkern mit ortlicher Vitalfarbung. Vorwort euber Wege Zeil. I. Methodik und Wirkungweise der ortlicher Vitalfarbung mit Agar als Farbtrager. Wilhelm Roux' Arch. Entwicklungomech. Org. 120:385–706.

9

Organization of the Early Embryo

PREFORMATION AND EPIGENESIS

Each living organism can be viewed as consisting of a series of systems in which fundamental parts and processes are arranged in an orderly temporospatial pattern. The tissues and organs of these systems in turn have their own characteristic structure and function. If the history of each organism is traced back through time, we know that this structural and functional complexity that organisms demonstrate originates with the fertilized egg, a deceptively simple and apparently unstructured cell. The visible steps by which the fertilized egg becomes transformed into the embryonic and adult stages, and the processes underlying these gradual transformations, constitute a meaning for the term development. Generally, multicellular animals with sexual reproduction show remarkable similarity in the broad steps by which these transformations occur (i.e., fertilization, cleavage, gastrulation, etc.).

Humans in general, and the scientist in particular, have always been interested in the forces or mechanisms underlying the precise, predictable, and ordered expressions of development. Historically, two theories have been invoked to explain the events of development: *preformation* and *epigenesis*. Prior to the late 1800s, each theory was based primarily on comparative and descriptive observations of embryos. The theory of preformation denied that development resulted in an increased level of order and postulated instead that the complexity associated with embryogenesis represented the gradual growth and enlargement of preexisting organization. The preformationists of the 17th and 18th centuries held that the complete adult organism was present in each egg (these people were called ovists) or sperm (these people were called animaculists or spermists), but in miniaturized state. Development was simply a matter of an increase in size.

The alternative theory was that of epigenesis, proposed initially on the basis of observations by Kaspar Friedrich Wolff (1733–1794) on plants and animals. Using the chick for study, he (1759) concluded that the egg contained no future parts of the embryo. He saw only the relatively simple, unstructured material that we know as protoplasm. Hence, the order and complexity associated with the development of the embryo must emerge gradually from a simple, formless cell by formative and synthetic processes.

With improvement in optical equipment and perfection of the light microscope in the 19th century, it became obvious that the organism did not exist in miniaturized form in either the egg or the sperm. As originally proposed, therefore, the theory of preformation was abandoned. However, the concept itself did not die. August Weismann (1834–1914) proposed that the various parts and organs of the body of the embryo (1880) were represented by linearly arranged *particles* or *determinants* in the nucleus of the fertilized egg. He envisaged development as an expression of these invisible, but performed elements, with each one determining a specific part of the embryo.

During the last half of the 19th century, it gradually became apparent that simple observations on how an embryo developed were inadequate to allow for a choice between the theories of preformation and epigenesis. Wilhelm Roux (1850–1924) dramatically changed the approach to embryogenesis by shifting the emphasis from an observational or descriptive to an experimental one. He founded the discipline of *analytical embryology* (developmental mechanics). Assuming that the concept of preformation as postulated by August Weismann was correct, he reasoned (1888) that destruction of one of the first two blastomeres of an embryo should produce an individual lacking certain parts and organs. Roux performed the simple experiment of destroying with a hot needle one of the first two blastomeres of the egg of the frog (*Rana*) (Fig. 9–1 A). The surviving blastomere developed as a half-embryo, thus suggesting that each cell at the two-celled stage possessed half of the parts necessary to form a complete embryo. Although these conclusions of Roux have been repeated and shown to be erroneous, his experimentation pointed toward a new direction for embryological thought.

Hans Driesch (1867–1941) followed up the work of Roux by studying the development of the early cleaving blastomeres in echinoderms. By vigorous shaking, he was able (1892) to completely separate the first two blastomeres of the *Echinus* egg (Fig. 9–1 B). Each blastomere subsequently formed a ciliated blastula that gastrulated and developed into a pluteus larva somewhat smaller in size than normal. The ability of each blastomere to form a whole embryo led Driesch to view the developing egg as a "harmonious equipotential system"; that is, parts of the egg, represented by the two blastomeres, had an equal ability to reorganize and form a whole embryo. The results by Driesch emphasized the epigenetic aspect of early development. Driesch failed to understand the basis for

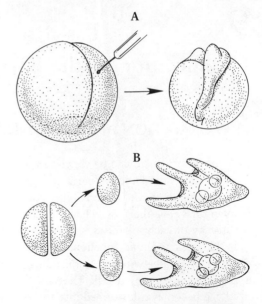

9–1 Preformation and epigenesis. A, half embryo produced in experiments by W. Roux following destruction of one blastomere with a hot needle at the two-celled stage in the frog. B, development of two normal-appearing embryos (plutei larvae) in the sea urchin produced by H. Driesch following separation of the first two blastomeres by shaking in sea water.

epigenesis, and in later life invoked the *principle of vitalism* to explain the totipotency of the mature egg cell.

Where do we stand today concerning preformation and epigensis? The gradual transformation of the egg and the emergence of the embryo appear to require the utilization of both of these opposing concepts. The information for the total development of an organism is present in the fertilized egg cell in the form of its genetic material. More specifically, the nucleotide sequences of the chains of DNA form an invisible, but preformed code. This code is the blueprint for development. The problem faced by the embryo is essentially that of decoding this information at the proper time in the proper place. Development of the embryo is epigenetic in the sense that the cytoplasm with its constituents as well as the cortex of the egg becomes fashioned into recognizable parts under the direction of the DNA code. How these various components of the fertilized egg cell interact to produce an organism with its various tissues and organ systems will be discussed here and in chapters to follow.

NUCLEIC ACID AND PROTEIN SYNTHESES

Through gastrulation, there is little change in the mass of the embryo and little to indicate the future shape of the embryo. Yet the early embryo is confronted with many tasks as it anticipates transformation into parts with specific structures and specific functions. These tasks are accomplished in a predictable and systematic series of steps.

As described in the chapter on cleavage, there is a rapid increase in cell numbers shortly after fertilization. Every nuclear division requires an increase in DNA and an increase in those proteins associated with the DNA of the chromosome. Each nuclear division also requires the assembly of protein subunits to construct the mitotic apparatus.

In all cleaving cells, the synthesis of DNA occurs during the S (synthetic) phase of the cell cycle. Typically, the frequency of DNA synthesis or the number of times per unit time that the genome is replicated tends to decrease through gastrulation (i.e., the length of the cell cycle increases). The genome of midcleavage frog nuclei is replicated approximately once per hour. By gastrulation, however, the genome is replicated only about once per day. In early cleavage stages of the sea urchin, the number of nuclei doubles every one to two hours and the DNA, amounting to 1.8×10^{-12} grams per diploid nucleus, doubles during an S period lasting 10 to 12 minutes at 16°C. This rate of DNA synthesis is about 60 times greater than

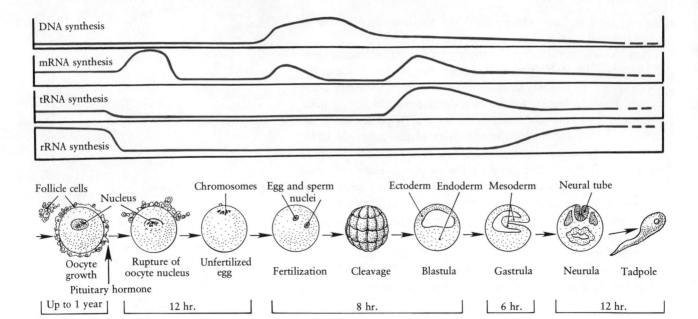

DNA synthesis

mRNA synthesis

tRNA synthesis

rRNA synthesis

Follicle cells | Nucleus | Chromosomes | Egg and sperm nuclei | Ectoderm Endoderm Mesoderm | Neural tube

Oocyte growth — Pituitary hormone | Rupture of oocyte nucleus | Unfertilized egg | Fertilization | Cleavage | Blastula | Gastrula | Neurula | Tadpole

Up to 1 year | 12 hr. | 8 hr. | 6 hr. | 12 hr.

that in most other eucaryotic cells. The duration of the S phase in the frog is about 15 minutes at midcleavage. This lengthens to approximately six hours during gastrulation. Generally, then, it is at the end of cleavage that mitotic activity of the embryo decreases and permits a typical cell cycle to become detectable. The general pattern of change in the synthesis of DNA during oogenesis and the early development of the frog embryo is summarized in Figure 9–2.

Cleaving eggs appear to be capable of synthesizing DNA at a rapid rate because the precursors for this acid, as well as the essential catalyzing enzymes, are already present in the cytoplasm of the fertilized egg. *DNA polymerase,* the enzyme that promotes the construction of the new polynucleotide chain on the existing DNA template, is present in substantial amounts in the egg's cytoplasm. In the sea urchin, it has been shown that the egg starts with a large amount of DNA polymerase. The localization of the polymerase gradually changes as it becomes progressively concentrated in the nucleus with each successive division cycle. How this polymerase migration occurs remains an unanswered question.

The sources of the precursors for the DNA molecule have been postulated to be severalfold. In the sea urchin, thymidine is probably provided as a result of the transformation and breakdown of ribonucleotides in the cytoplasm of the egg. *Ribonucleotide reductase,* an enzyme that converts ribonucleotides into deoxyribonucleotides, is known to be present in substantial amounts in the cytoplasm of developing sea urchin eggs. There is also evidence in

9–2 Changes in nucleic acid syntheses during oogenesis and early development of the frog embryo. (From J. Gurdon, 1968. Essays Biochem. 4, 25.)

both sea urchins and frogs that DNA can be synthesized from low molecular weight precursors. When glycine, an amino acid that can be used for the synthesis of purine groups in the DNA molecule, is labeled (^{14}C-glycine) and the eggs of sea urchins (or frogs) exposed to it, the radioactive carbon atoms are actively incorporated into DNA in the eggs.

Activity at the level of the nucleus is also expressed during early embryogenesis in the synthesis of ribonucleic acid or RNA. The formation of RNA in the early embryo is generally described as rather weak and limited by comparison to later stages of development. Still, the active incorporation of radioactively labeled precursors of RNA, such as ^{3}H-uridine, has been shown to occur in most animals by gastrulation (Fig. 9–2). Of the three major species of RNA, ribosomal RNA (rRNA) is not detectable in the embryos of sea urchins and frogs until gastrulation. The onset of this type of RNA synthesis at this particular time can be correlated with the appearance of visible nucleoli within the nucleoplasm of embryonic cells. Emerson and Humphreys (1970) are of the opinion, however, that rRNA synthesis occurs much earlier in the sea urchin, but that DNA-like RNA (probably messenger RNA [mRNA]) accumulates so rapidly during cleavage that the rRNA cannot be detected. The atypical morphology of nucleoli, which is often visible at this time, is ascribed to the rapid cell division occurring during cleavage. The cleaving cells of both sea urchins and frogs apparently utilize the huge stockpile of ribosomes built up in the cytoplasm during oogenesis. By contrast, rRNA synthesis is detected much earlier in development (early cleavage stages) in the mammalian embryo because there are so few ribosomes packaged in the cytoplasm of the ovum.

Most of the RNA formed in the embryo before the onset of gastrulation appears to be DNA-like or mRNA. In sea urchins, activation of the DNA-like RNA synthesizing machinery is not apparent until the embryo is at the two- to four-celled stage. Between the 8- and 16-celled stages, there is a dramatic increase in mRNA output. Some of these messengers or transcripts appear to have base sequences that are identical to the base sequences of stable mRNAs synthesized during oogenesis. Other messengers have base sequences complementary to DNA segments not previously transcribed. The onset of mRNA synthesis appears to be slightly later in the amphibian embryo with transcription being detected at about the midblastula stage (Fig. 9–2).

The third species of RNA is transfer RNA (tRNA). In most organisms, it can be detected after the initiation of mRNA synthesis and just before the onset of gastrulation.

The appearance of different species of RNA at different times during early embryogenesis probably indicates that the genes directing their formation are being independently activated and controlled. Presumably, the stage at which each type of RNA appears is in some way related to the needs of the embryo.

Although the synthesis of RNA begins shortly after the activation of the egg, transcription of the embryonic genome does not appear essential for development prior to the stage of gastrulation. For example, eggs exposed to *actinomycin D,* an agent that is known to block transcription, continue to show all outward signs of being able to develop in normal fashion. Presumably, the mRNAs formed during cleavage are coated or masked in some fashion to prevent their translation until a later time in development. In both frogs and sea urchins, embryos in which transcription has been blocked will develop to the blastula stage. At this time further development of the embryos is arrested (i.e., actinomycin-treated embryos will not gastrulate). These experiments using actinomycin-treated embryos permit several conclusions. First, the early development of embryos through cleavage and blastulation is not dependent upon newly synthesized RNA. Second, gastrulation is arrested in the absence of transcription of RNA from the embryonic genome.

It has already been pointed out that in echinoderms there is a marked elevation in the synthesis of proteins following fertilization of the egg cell (Chapter 6). The rate of polypeptide formation climbs sharply through early cleavage and then levels off. Indeed, within minutes of fertilization, it has been estimated that in the sea urchin the rate of protein synthesis is as much as 70 times that of the unfertilized egg cell. Just prior to gastrulation, there is a second surge in polypeptide formation. In other animals, such as frogs, the change in the rate of protein synthesis after insemination is not so dramatic as in echinoderms. However, in most organisms studied there is a burst of intense protein formation during gastrulation. Based upon the elevated levels of RNA and protein syntheses, it appears, therefore, that gastrulation is a period of large-scale synthetic activities.

As one might expect, the normal development of the early embryo requires a continual input of newly synthesized proteins. Treatment of embryos after fertilization with the classical inhibitors of protein synthesis, such as *puromycin* and *cycloheximide,* immediately interrupts cell division and brings development to a standstill. Hence, it is apparent that these proteins are essential to normal embryogenesis. A number of questions can be raised regarding these early embryonic proteins. What is the nature or amino acid composition of these proteins? Are they fashioned from mRNAs produced during oogenesis (maternal RNA) or from mRNAs produced after fertilization (early embryonic RNA)? What roles do these proteins play during early embryogenesis?

The sea urchin has been a favorite subject for the analysis of such questions concerning proteins during the early stages of development. The rise in the synthesis of proteins after fertilization is accompanied by a corresponding increase in the number of polyribosomes. Each polyribosome consists of three to seven ribosomes per strand of mRNA. By the blastula stage, the number of polyribosomes within the cytoplasm of the constituent blastomeres increases dramatically. Analysis of this population of polyribosomes shows that two classes of polyribosomes are present: *heavy polyribosomes,* with an average of 23 ribosomes per mRNA and *light polyribosomes,* with an average of 9 ribosomes per mRNA strand. Both the heavy and light polyribosomes are active in the incorporation of labeled amino acids into protein. The light or *s-polyribosomes* appear to be totally responsible for the manufacture of *histones.* Histones are low molecular weight basic proteins that are associated with the DNA of the chromatin material. Not unexpectedly, the pattern of histone synthesis parallels the pattern of DNA synthesis during early embryogenesis. Approximately 50 percent of the proteins formed during cleavage appear to be histones. As the synthesis of DNA declines, approximately 10 hours after fertilization in the sea urchin, so also does the rate of histone synthesis. Histones are probably formed on maternal, preformed mRNA templates as well as on newly synthesized embryonic mRNA templates. For example, if sea urchin embryos are treated with actinomycin D before fertilization and the polyribosome population analyzed at selected intervals after insemination, it can be shown that there is a considerable reduction in the number of s-polyribosomes and in the synthesis of histones. Presumably, the reduction in histones indicates that newly synthesized DNA-like RNA is being utilized to make these nuclear proteins. However, the fact that histones are produced in actinomycin-treated embryos is strong evidence that a portion of these special proteins is being made with maternal RNA as a template. It has been estimated that approximately two-thirds of the histones formed during cleavage are translated from the maternal templates. Following their formation, the histones migrate from the cytoplasm of the blastomere into the nucleus.

There are other proteins synthesized after fertilization that appear to utilize preformed, maternal RNA templates. These include the *tubulin proteins* that participate in the formation of the mitotic apparatus of the cleaving cell, *ribonucleotide reductase,* and *hatching enzyme.* Hatching enzyme appears in homogenates of sea urchins at the midblastula stage and apparently serves to digest away the fertilization membrane, thus setting free the swimming larva. There is some evidence to suggest that the tubulin proteins are also present in large amounts in the unfertilized egg. Several studies also suggest that tubulin may be synthesized at the direction of mRNA molecules transcribed from the embryonic genome.

The embryo prior to gastrulation is primarily concerned with chromosomal replication, cell division, and protein synthesis, utilizing as a primary informational source many of the mRNAs manufactured during oogenesis and stored within the egg cell. At selected periods of time following fertilization, specific mRNA molecules are selected for translation into proteins. These proteins are vital to the construction of DNA and cell membrane. Gradually, the stockpile of maternal mRNAs is replaced by an increasing population of messengers transcribed from the embryo's own genome.

THE EQUIVALENCE OF NUCLEI

Development of the embryo begins with the rapid conversation of the single, fertilized egg into a population of cells. Although the cells of the early embryo are initially alike, they gradually diverge phenotypically and give rise to specialized cell types with very specific properties. By the end of gastrulation, the cells are broadly fixed or determined with respect to their fate or specific destiny. Some cells will become ectodermal cells, some endodermal cells, and others mesodermal cells. In this connection, one might propose that the origin of the differences between these cells of the early embryo could be attributed to differences in either the nuclei or cytoplasm distributed to the blastomeres during the process of cleavage.

In his germ plasm theory, A. F. L. Weismann postulated that every part of the embryo was represented by a separate *determinant* or *particle* located on the chromosomes of the nucleus of the sex cell. These determinants were then distributed to different blastomeres during cleavage, thus accounting for the fate of the various blastomeres. Differentiation of a given blastomere could only take place in accordance with the type of determinants present. Although we now know that Weismann's proposal is untenable from a genetic point of view, it is still important to ask whether the cells of the early embryo, and hence the structures of the embryo fashioned from them, become different because of differences in their nuclei. That is, might not the early specialization of cells involve the selective elimination of genes and/or the differential distribution of genetic material to blastomeres during segmentation of the fertilized egg?

Several lines of evidence suggest that all cells of the embryo possess nuclei containing all of the genetic information necessary

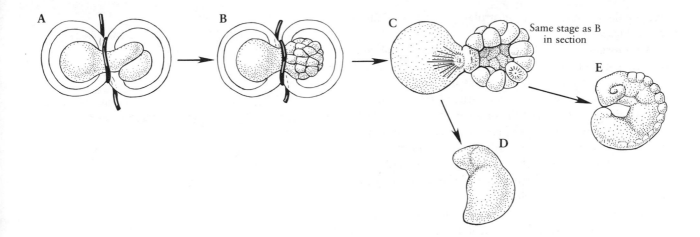

A   B   C   Same stage as B in section   E   D

for normal cell differentiation and expression. The studies by Driesch on isolated blastomeres of the sea urchin, the experiments by Spemann on delayed nuclear supply in the egg of *Triturus,* and the nuclear transfer studies of Briggs and King, as well as by Gurdon and colleagues, support this concept.

The view by Weismann that blastomere specialization resulted from the selective distribution of determinants during cleavage was initially, as we previously noted (page 182), contradicted by the studies of Driesch. Development of complete but slightly smaller than normal embryos from isolated blastomeres of the two-celled and four-celled stages of sea urchin and frog eggs indicated that the cells of the very early embryo, at least, have all of the information necessary to support total development.

To investigate more fully the characteristics and potentialities of cleavage nuclei, Spemann (1928) devised the elegant technique of *delayed nuclear implantation* or supply (Fig. 9–3). Using the fertilized egg of *Triturus,* he constricted the fertilized cell into two halves with a specially designed hair loop just prior to cleavage. By constricting the egg still further through tightening of the loop, the zygote nucleus was displaced toward one pole of the egg. A thin cytoplasmic bridge remained as the only connection to the nonnucleated portion of the cell (Fig. 9–3 A). Cleavage occurred but was restricted entirely to the nucleated portion of the egg (Fig. 9–3 A). After approximately the fourth division, the nuclei were quite small in size. One of these nuclei crossed the cytoplasmic bridge into the non-segmented portion of the original egg (Fig. 9–3 B,C). Immediately, this half of the egg began to cleave. When Spemann then tightened the hair loop, the original fertilized egg was separated into two distinct cleaving halves. In most cases, each

9–3   The delayed nuclear implantation experiment of Spemann. A, a hair loop placed around the fertilized egg of the salamander (*Triturus*)—cleavage has begun in the nucleated half of the egg; B, a nucleus has passed across the cytoplasmic bridge into the undivided portion of the egg; C, same as in B, but in section; D–E, normal-appearing embryos develop from the half with the zygote nucleus and the half with the delayed nuclear supply. (From H. Spemann, 1938. Embryonic Development and Induction. Yale University Press, New Haven.)

cleaving half was observed to gastrulate and develop into a normal embryo (Fig. 9–3 D,E).

It is important to point out that both types of embryos initially possessed about one half of the original egg cytoplasm. Yet, the development of one type of embryo was directed by only $1/16$ of the original egg nucleus, while development of the second type of embryo was directed by $15/16$ of the original egg nucleus. Spemann was one of the first investigators to provide experimental support for the concept that the nuclei of the early cleaving embryo are equivalent to each other as well as to the nucleus of the fertilized egg. That is, these nuclei contain all of the nuclear information required for the achievement of normal development.

A more direct method for testing the genetic equivalence of the nuclei of cleaving blastomeres and, indeed, of cells in general has been that of *nuclear transplantation*. The objective of a nuclear transplant is to insert the nucleus of a blastomere or specialized cell type into an unfertilized, but activated egg whose nucleus has been removed. The first successful transplant of a nucleus into an animal egg cell (*Rana pipiens*) was achieved by Robert W. Briggs and Thomas J. King of the Institute of Cancer Research in Philadelphia. The technique basically involves three steps, which are summarized in Figure 9–4. The first step involves the removal of the egg nucleus. A mature egg cell is artificially activated by pricking with a drawn glass needle. With the aid of a dissecting microscope, the female nucleus can then be observed as it approaches the cell surface to complete the second maturation division. It is then flipped out of the cell with a second glass needle. The second step requires the preparation of the nucleus to be transplanted (*donor nucleus*). A cell, a blastomere for example, is dissociated from its neighbors in a medium typically lacking calcium or magnesium ions. The most difficult step is the placement of the donor nucleus into the enucleated egg. This requires a high level of manual skill and endless patience. Briggs and King discovered that the nuclear transplantation is best accomplished by sucking a single donor cell into a micropipette whose bore is slightly smaller than the diameter of the cell. As the cell is drawn into the micropipette, the cell membrane ruptures, thus liberating the nucleus. The nucleus with a halo of its own cytoplasm is then injected into the cytoplasm of the enucleated or recipient cell. If the membrane of the donor cell fails to break in the transplant process, the donor nucleus will not respond to the cytoplasm of the egg.

To determine if the nuclei remain equivalent to one another during the course of development. Briggs and King used donor nuclei from various stages of development of the leopard frog, *Rana pipiens*. Nuclei transplanted from blastula cells resulted in about 80

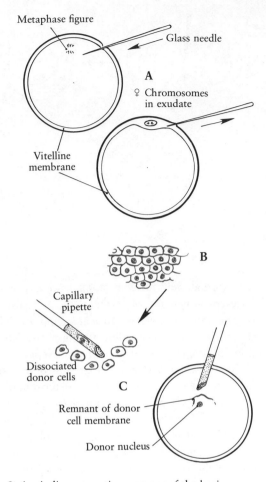

9–4 A diagrammatic summary of the basic steps involved in nuclear transplantation. A, activation and removal of the nucleus of the ripe egg cell; B, aspiration into a capillary pipette of a dissociated donor cell; C, injection of the donor nucleus and donor cell debris into the enucleated egg.

percent of the transfer embryos undergoing cleavage, with the majority of these continuing to develop into tadpoles. However, when the donor nuclei were obtained from progressively later stages, the resulting transfers showed increased disturbances in development with fewer transfers reaching the tadpole stage. For example, only about 65 percent of the transfers reach the blastula stage when the donor nucleus (endodermal) is contributed by a late gastrula embryo. This figure drops to about 33 percent when the donor nucleus (endodermal) is supplied by an embryo in the neurula stage. Additionally, many of these transplant embryos subsequently become arrested in gastrula or prehatching stages. These experiments with *Rana* suggest that nuclei do gradually become modified and apparently restricted in their capacity to promote normal development.

Wishing to test the permanence and stability of the presumed changes in the nucleus, Briggs and King undertook the difficult and tedious task of cloning nuclei (*serial nuclear transplantation*). In a serial transplant, a donor nucleus is isolated from an abnormal or arrested embryo and injected into an enucleated egg. At the blastula stage, nuclei are again isolated from blastomeres and injected into a new population of enucleated eggs. This procedure can be repeated several times, the result being a group of individuals all having an identical set of genes in their nuclei. Figure 9–5 summarizes in diagrammatic fashion the basic steps in serial transplantation as carried out in amphibians.

With the leopard frog, it has been shown that the original recipient eggs, injected with nuclei isolated from the endoderm of late gastrula embryos, developed into a variety of embryo types, ranging from arrested gastrulas to normal embryos (Fig. 9–5). However, when one blastula of the original recipient generation served as a donor for transfers to a new group of enucleated eggs, the new clone of embryos displayed a very uniform type of development. Most of the embryos of this generation gastrulated normally but later showed marked morphological deficiencies, particularly in ectodermal structures. Continued serial transplantation of blastular nuclei from the original recipient generation showed no change in the type of deficiencies produced. The nuclear alterations appeared to be stable and specific. Hence, these nuclear cloning experiments support the hypothesis that some of the nuclei had experienced a stable, reproducible change, expressed in the inability of these nuclei to support normal development of an enucleated egg cell (i.e., ectodermal differentiation).

Does the observation that *Rana* nuclei appear to become irreversibly altered during the course of development, expressed in a failure to support total development, mean that the nuclei have experi-

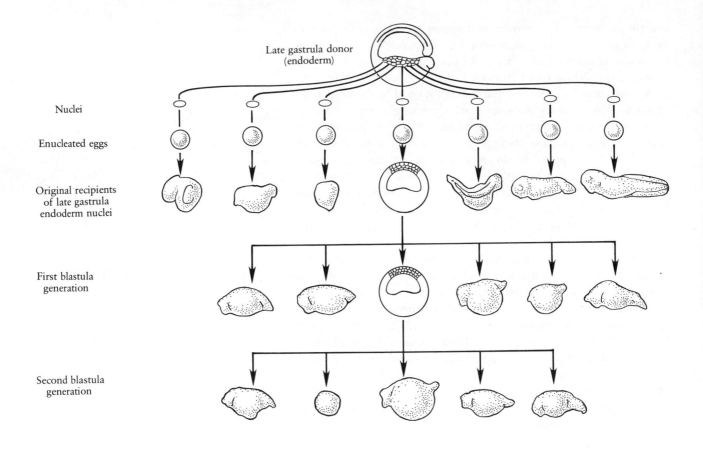

Late gastrula donor
(endoderm)

Nuclei

Enucleated eggs

Original recipients
of late gastrula
endoderm nuclei

First blastula
generation

Second blastula
generation

enced gene loss or elimination? Not at all. Indeed, the failure of later stage embryonic nuclei to promote and sustain total development is probably related to chromosomal damage precipitated by an incompatibility between the donor nucleus and the host cytoplasm. It must be remembered that donor nuclei from gastrular and neurular stages of development, for example, are being isolated from cells with significantly reduced rates of mitosis. Sudden transfer of such a nucleus into the cytoplasm of an egg, which is programmed for rapid division, can produce physical damage to chromosomes and subsequent embryonic deficiencies because of its failure to divide rapidly enough.

Although the nuclei from later developmental stages of *Rana pipiens* appear to show severe restrictions after transplantation, experiments carried out by Gurdon and his colleagues using *Xenopus* (African clawed frog) have yielded different interpretations (Fig. 9–6). A particularly useful feature in *Xenopus* is that a mutant strain exists which possesses one nucleolus per nucleus while the

9–5 Diagram illustrating the basic steps involved in the serial transplantation of endodermal nuclei. Donor nuclei are initially obtained from the presumptive anterior midgut region of the late gastrula. They promote the various types of development shown for the "original recipients" following transplantation into enucleated eggs. One of the original recipients, sacrificed at the blastula stage, provides nuclei for a single clone of individuals (first and second blastula generations). The first and second blastula generations show more uniform types of development. (After T. King and R. Briggs, 1956. Cold Spring Harbor Symp. Quant. Biol. 21, 271.)

normal, wild-type strain has two nucleoli per nucleus. When the mutant strain is used as a source of donor nuclei, one can always distinguish the division products of the transplanted nucleus.

Gurdon and his colleagues have concentrated on testing the capacity of nuclei from fully differentiated cells to support total development. When nuclei of fully differentiated larval intestinal epithelial cells from the mutant strain of *Xenopus* are used as donors, approximately 1.5 percent of the total number of transfers develop into normal, adult frogs. All cells in these embryos possess a single nucleolus in their nuclei. Indeed, both female and male *Xenopus* frogs, fertile and completely normal, have been raised from eggs into which intestinal nuclei had been placed. It would appear, then, that many of the transplanted nuclei retain all the genetic information required for the development of all cell types. About 20 percent of the transfers reach the stage at which there are distinct neuromuscular responses, demonstrating that intestinal nuclei retain the genes required for the differentiation of several very specific cell types (nerve and muscle). Donor nuclei from cultured adult skin cells also have the capacity to support the differentiation of many cell types. Gurdon and his colleagues argue that no irreversible changes occur in the nucleus during development because some transfers always show *totipotency*.

The inability of some transplanted nuclei to support normal development does appear to increase as the cells from which they are taken become differentiated. However, Marie DiBerardino of the Institute for Cancer Research has determined that there are marked disturbances in the number and shape of the chromosomes in these nuclear transplant embryos. In other words, the failure of many nuclear transplants to develop into more complete embryos may be limited by the nuclear transplant technique itself. The origin of these chromosomal abnormalities in *Xenopus* is attributable to an incompatibility between the very slow rate of division of differentiating cells (serving as donor nuclei) and the rapid rate of division of the egg (recipient cell).

Although there are differences in the results of nuclear transfer experiments with *Rana* and *Xenopus*, it is known that the nuclei of both organisms become smaller, divide more slowly, and may be susceptible to greater damage by injection as development progresses. Whether nuclei do, in fact, experience stable and irreversible changes during embryogenesis remains an open question. However, because nuclei from fully differentiated tissues have been shown in several experiments to sustain normal development, the conclusion appears to be warranted that nuclei are totipotent and contain a full gene complement. Certainly, none of the nuclear

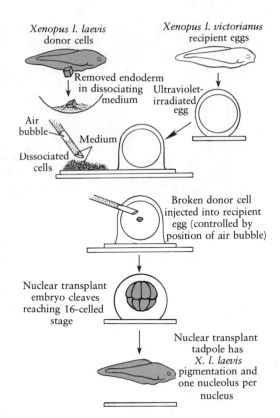

9–6   The principal stages involved in the transplantation of nuclei in the amphibian, *Xenopus laevis*. Donor nuclei are obtained from a strain of subspecies, *Xenopus laevis laevis,* which has only one nucleolus per nucleus. The young tadpoles of this species have many pigment cells in their bodies. Recipient eggs are from another subspecies, *Xenopus laevis victorianus.* The nuclei of diploid cells in this subspecies have two nucleoli and the tadpoles have no body pigment. The nuclear-transplant tadpoles have the characteristics of the nuclear, not the cytoplasmic, parent. (From J. Gurdon, 1966. Endeavor 25, 95.)

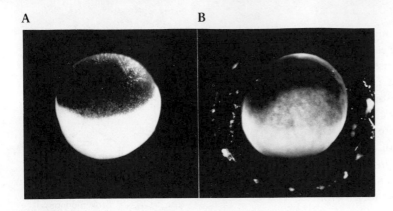

9–7   Formation of the grey crescent in *Xenopus laevis*. A, mature egg following isolation from the ovary; B, same egg after fertilization showing the grey crescent and the fertilization membrane. (Courtesy of J. Brachet.)

transfer experiments supports the hypothesis that blastomeres and the specialized cell types derived from them become different because of selective gene loss.

SIGNIFICANCE OF THE EGG CYTOPLASM AND THE EGG CORTEX

Studies employing techniques of nuclear transplantation, primarily with amphibian eggs, have given a rather clear indication that the basis for differences in the destinies of cells of the early embryo cannot be ascribed to differences in their nuclei. By logic, then, one must examine the possibility that the fate of a blastomere and its descendant cells is somehow related to the nature of the cytoplasm received by it during the cleavage process. In other words, the type of differentiation that a blastomere will undergo is probably related to the nature of the egg cytoplasm it receives during segmentation of the egg. The significance of cytoplasmic substances during early embryogenesis can be demonstrated with several examples.

You will recall that shortly after fertilization in the egg of the frog a distinct, crescent-shaped zone of grey colored cytoplasm appears at the lower margin of the animal hemisphere approximately opposite to the site of sperm penetration (Fig. 9–7). This grey crescent can also be identified in the uncleaved eggs of salamanders. The first cleavage furrow usually passes through the center of the grey crescent and thus each of the first two blastomeres receives approximately half of the crescent material. Spemann noted that if he placed a hair ligature on the fertilized egg in such a way that constriction divided the grey crescent in half, the resulting two blastomeres when isolated and cultured, developed into two normal embryos (Fig. 9–8). However, if the ligature was placed and tightened so that only one blastomere received grey crescent material, the results were quite different. The blastomere with the grey cres-

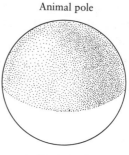

Animal pole

Vegetal pole

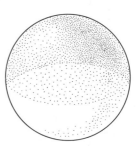

cent developed into a normal embryo; however, the blastomere
lacking grey crescent produced only an epithelial ball of cells with
little visible differentiation. Spemann showed that these differences
were not dependent upon which blastomere received the original
egg nucleus and thus whatever controls the future differentiation of
the embryo must be associated with some cytoplasmic material contained in the grey crescent of the fertilized egg. More recently,
Curtis (1962) demonstrated that excision of the grey crescent at fer
tilization in *Xenopus* does not affect cleavage, but there is an absence of gastrulation and failure in the differentiation of cell types.

The importance of the distribution of cytoplasmic substances of
the egg for the differentiation of parts of the early embryo is well illustrated in the development of a variety of protochordates and invertebrates, particularly annelids and molluscs.

The eggs of some protochordates, such as the tunicate *Styela*,
show dramatic regional differences in the appearance of the cytoplasm. Recall that before the onset of furrow formation, the
fertilized egg displays four areas of recognizable plasms. The animal
hemisphere is characterized by clear, transparent cytoplasm while
the vegetal hemisphere cytoplasm is slaty grey in color and packed
with coarse yolk granules. Just below the equator of the cell, there
is a light grey, crescent-shaped zone of cytoplasm and a yellow,
crescent-shaped zone of cytoplasm (Fig. 9–9). This "yellow plasm"
is characterized by an abundance of yellow pigment granules and
numerous mitochondria. The visible distinctions between these
plasms permit an observer to trace the fate of these particular
regions of the egg cell during cleavage and gastrulation. The clear
cytoplasm of the animal hemisphere becomes segregated in the ectodermal cells of the embryo; the slaty grey cytoplasm gives rise to
cells of the endoderm; the light grey cytoplasm becomes localized in
the cells of the nervous system and the notochord; and the yellow
plasm is distributed to cells producing muscle tissue and mesenchyme.

The arrangement of these four cytoplasmic areas defines a distinct bilateral organization for the uncleaved egg. The first cleavage
furrow always divides the egg cell along the plane of bilateral symmetry, thus providing portions of the four plasms to the first two
blastomeres (Fig. 9–9 A). If the first two blastomeres are isolated
and cultured, each blastomere develops as a half-embryo. By the
eight-celled stage, the yellow plasm is specifically confined to the
posterior pair of the lower quartet of blastomeres (Fig. 9–9 B).
These two blastomeres will give rise to the muscle and mesenchyme
cells of the embryo.

The apparent relationship between the yellow plasm and the expression of muscle tissue in *Styela* suggests a cause-and-effect inter-

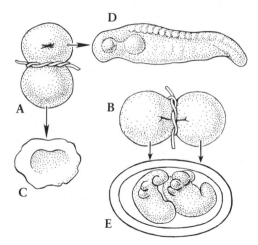

9–8   Experiments of Spemann involving constriction of the salamander's egg in the frontal
(A) and medial (B) planes. After frontal constriction, only the egg half containing the grey crescent cytoplasm developed into a complete embryo (D); the half lacking the grey crescent
developed abnormally (C). After medial constriction (B), both halves, each of which contains grey
crescent cytoplasm, developed into complete embryos (E). (From H. Spemann, 1938. Embryonic
Development and Induction. Yale University
Press, New Haven.)

9–9   Localization of various pigmented plasms
in the ascidian *Styela partita* at the 2-celled (A),
8-celled (B), and 64-celled stages (C). cc = clear
cytoplasm representing ectodermal cells; dg =
dark grey cytoplasm representing endodermal
cells; lg = light grey cytoplasm representing
neural plate (NP) and notochord (N); yc = yellow
cytoplasm representing muscle cells (M) and
mesenchymal cells (ME). (After E. G. Conklin,
1905. J. Acad. Nat. Sci. Philadelphia 13, 1.)

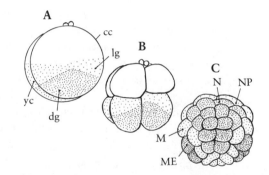

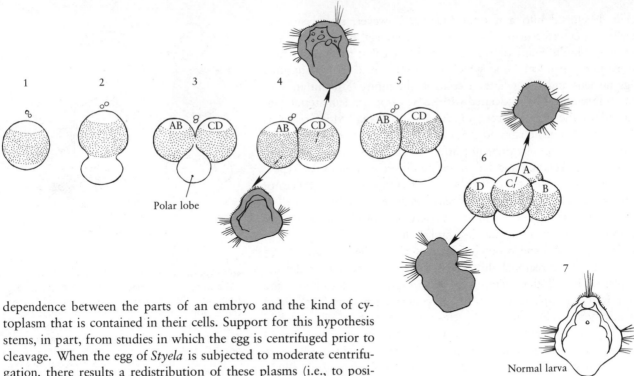

Polar lobe

Normal larva

9–10 Cleavage of the mollusc egg (*Dentalium*) and the larvae that develop from isolated blastomeres. Only those blastomeres receiving polar lobe material develop normally. The letters indicate the blastomere from which each larva develops. (From E. B. Wilson, 1904. J. Exp. Zool. 1, 1.)

dependence between the parts of an embryo and the kind of cytoplasm that is contained in their cells. Support for this hypothesis stems, in part, from studies in which the egg is centrifuged prior to cleavage. When the egg of *Styela* is subjected to moderate centrifugation, there results a redistribution of these plasms (i.e., to positions that are abnormal). Larvae may develop from these centrifuged eggs, but there are atypical distributions of muscle, nerve, and endodermal cells. Interestingly, the muscle cells, for example, develop in that position where the yellow plasm comes to lie as a result of the centrifugation. These experiments with the ascidian egg suggest that there is a close correlation between prelocalization in the egg cytoplasm and the subsequent expression of tissue and organ rudiments.

The eggs of many molluscs, including those of *Dentalium* and *Ilyanassa*, are also distinguished by having visible regional differences in their cytoplasm. In *Dentalium*, for example, three zones of plasm can be recognized: a clear layer of cytoplasm at the animal pole, a broad granular layer at the equator of the cell, and a transparent layer of cytoplasm at the vegetal pole (Fig. 9–10 1). Just prior to the first cleavage division, the vegetal cytoplasm becomes localized as a large protrusion from the vegetal hemisphere. This is known as the *polar lobe* of the first cleavage division (Fig. 9–10 2). During the first division of the egg, the polar lobe remains connected to the egg by a thin bridge of cytoplasm. At the two-celled stage, it is observed that the polar lobe becomes localized into one of the daughter cells (the CD blastomere) (Fig. 9–10 3). A second polar lobe forms in similar fashion from the vegetal region of the CD blastomere just prior to the second cleavage division. At the four-celled stage, the polar lobe plasm is localized in only one of the daughter cells (the D blastomere). Hence, in the mollusc egg, a distinct cytoplasmic region of the fertilized egg is unequally distributed to the first four blastomeres.

Since polar lobe formation is characteristic of several annelid and mollusc species, a variety of experiments have been conducted to determine the role of the polar lobe with its plasm during early embryogenesis. If the AB and CD blastomeres of *Dentalium* are separated and cultured, only the cell containing the polar plasm (CD blastomere) yields a complete *trochophore larva*. The AB blastomere forms a defective larva that typically lacks structures of mesodermal origin (Fig. 9–10 4). At the four-celled stage, only the D blastomere is able to develop as a complete, though smaller-than-normal larva (Fig. 9–10 6). That the polar plasm is related to the differentiation of several adult structures, particularly those of mesodermal origin, is additionally supported by experiments in which the polar lobe is severed from the egg prior to furrow formation. Removal of the polar lobe at the first cleavage in *Dentalium* and *Ilyanassa* produces a larva that lacks an apical tuft of cilia and such structures as a velum, foot, shell, heart, and intestine. If the vegetal 60 percent of the lobe is extirpated, an apical tuft still appears in the larva, suggesting that the cytoplasm required for its expression is located in the "animal region" of the polar lobe. Removal of the vegetal one-third of an unfertilized egg yields results similar to those produced by removal of the polar lobe at the first cleavage division. Hence, the cytoplasmic structures or determinants responsible for the expression of lobe-dependent structures are set aside as early as the unfertilized egg stage.

It is proposed that the polar lobe of annelids and molluscs probably contains several cytoplasmic substances that become progressively segregated during cleavage until each reaches its own target embryonic cell. The nature of these components of the cytoplasm is currently being investigated using various histochemical and electron microscopic techniques. Dohmen and Verdonk (1974) have demonstrated that the polar lobe of *Bithynia* (a gastropod), comprising less than 1 percent of the total egg volume, contains a dense body, the *vegetal body,* which consists of vesicles with electron-dense particles (Fig. 9–11). They suggest that the vegetal body may be responsible for the morphogenetic expression of the polar lobe. The development of *Bithynia* embryos lacking the vegetal body (i.e., lobeless) is consistent with results reported for lobeless embryos of *Dentalium* and *Ilyanassa*. These embryos will cleave and gastrulate in the same way as in lobed embryos. However, after gastrulation, the embryos swell into balloonlike structures with the endodermal tissue lying against the superficial ectodermal cells. Some of the en-

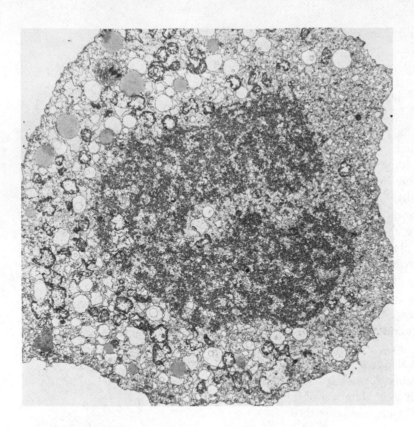

9–11 Electron micrograph of the first polar lobe with the vegetal body in *Bithynia tentaculata* (gastropod). (From M. Dohmen and N. Verdonk, 1974. J. Embryol. Exp. Morphol. 31, 423.)

9–12 Sketch of an 11-day-old living lobeless embryo showing partial exogastrulation. (After J. Cather and N. Verdonk, 1974. J. Embryol. Exp. Morphol. 31, 415.)

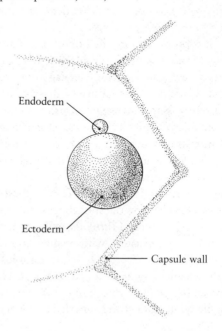

doderm may even project to the exterior (Fig. 9–12). However, no mesodermal tissue is observed in these lobeless embryos.

The sequestering of cytoplasmic substances or *morphogenetic determinants* within blastomeres during the period of cleavage appears to be essential for the normal expression of adult tissues and organs. Primarily on the basis of experiments designed to displace through centrifugation the various constituents of the egg cytoplasm, it also appears that the *egg cortex* in many animal species may be the site where cytoplasmic factors affecting embryogenesis are located. In other words, the regional differences in the egg cytoplasm that we can see and trace into given blastomeres may not be, per se, directly involved in specifying parts of the embryo. Rather, these special plasms are probably expressions of topographical accumulations that become localized under the influence of morphogenetic information in the periphery of the egg cell.

When an egg cell, such as that of the sea urchin (*Arbacia*), is centrifuged at moderate speeds for several minutes, the constituents of the fluid cytoplasm separate into layers according to their specific gravities, but the gellike, viscous peripheral cytoplasm or cortical cytoplasm, approximately three micrometers in thickness, is unaffected by the centrifugal field. Generally, the pigment and yolk granules accumulate as distinct layers at the centrifugal pole (the point farthest from the axis of the centrifuge rotor) of the cell while the lipid droplets gather in a layer at the centripetal pole (Fig. 9–13 A). The transparent cytoplasm and nucleus organize between these other stratifications. It was Morgan who first demonstrated that, independently of this rearrangement of egg cytoplasm and pigment distribution, the centrifuged eggs of the sea urchin will cleave in accord with their original axiate pattern, gastrulate by invagination in the region where the micromeres form (which marks the vegetal pole), and develop into quite normal larvae (Fig. 9–13 B).

Similarly, the lobe plasm of the vegetal hemisphere and the clear plasm of the animal hemisphere of the uncleaved egg of *Ilyanassa* can be forced "to exchange positions" through centrifugation (Fig. 9–14). Despite this redistribution, a polar lobe will form in the vegetal hemisphere, though it contains hyaline cytoplasm derived from the animal pole of the egg cell. Clement (1976) has shown that these eggs continue to develop and may form lobe-dependent structures (such as an apical tuft), indicating that substances responsible for organ expression are not contained in the bulk of the cytoplasm. In *Dentalium,* if the polar lobe is removed after centrifugation, the resulting embryo lacks an apical tuft. This is clear evidence that the determinant for apical tuft formation is not displaced by centrifugation.

Suppose that eggs of forms like *Lymnaea* (snail), *Styela,* and *Arbacia* are permitted to stand after disruption of their normal organization through moderate centrifugation. It is observed that the cytoplasmic substances and inclusions do not remain in their new positions, but rather reorganize throughout the egg, tending toward a restoration of their normal arrangement. Hence, it follows that the fluid cytoplasm with its regional variations is probably organized in relation to local differences in the immovable portion of the cell or egg cortex.

More direct proof of the involvement of the cortical cytoplasm in controlling early events of embryogenesis has been demonstrated using the grey crescent of amphibian eggs. Classical experiments of Brachet and of Pasteels pointed out that localized destructions of the grey crescent in frog's eggs are followed by abnormalities of such axial structures as the neural tube, notochord, and somites. Experiments by Curtis on *Xenopus* (1962) have shown that removal of the cortex of the grey crescent (approximately 0.5–3.0 μm in thickness) will not disturb mitosis or cytokinesis of the fertilized egg, but it will prevent formation of the blastopore and the development of axial structures (Fig. 9–15 A). After perfecting a technique for the isolation of cortical cytoplasm material, he transplanted grey

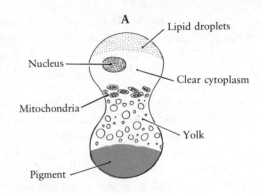

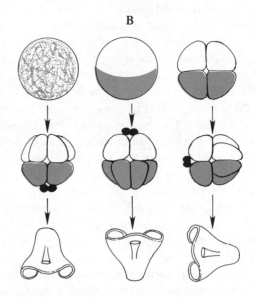

9–13   A, stratification of the sea urchin (*Arbacia*) whole egg following moderate centrifugation (From E. Harvey, 1936. Biol. Bull. 71. 101); B, centrifuged eggs will develop normally despite the dislocation of cytoplasmic constituents. (After T. Morgan, 1927. Experimental Embryology. Columbia University Press, New York.)

crescent cortex to the ventral side of a second or host egg cell. When the grey cresent was obtained from the eight-celled or younger stages, the resulting embryo developed with two sets of axial structures (Fig. 9–15 B). An egg cell receiving a transplant of cytoplasm taken from beneath the grey crescent developed into a normal embryo with only a single set of axial structures. Interestingly, the eight-celled *Xenopus* embryo no longer responds to a transplant of additional crescent taken from a younger stage (Fig. 9–15 C). Also, extirpation of the grey crescent at this stage no longer interrupts the process of gastrulation (Fig. 9–15 D). These results suggest that a change in cortical organization occurs during the second or third cleavages.

The cortical material in the amphibian egg appears to have morphogenetic properties that play a leading role in the initiation of gastrulation and in the expression of different cell types. A number of questions remain about the cortical cytoplasm as a source of developmental information. How widespread in the animal kingdom is the cortical control of embryogenesis? What is the nature of specific morphogenetic substances or determinants, and what is their pattern of organization in the egg cortex? Attempts to isolate and identify chemically active morphogenetic determinants in the egg cytoplasm in general has been a difficult and unrewarding task. Horstadius and his colleagues (1967) have made efforts in this direction using unfertilized egg homogenates of the sea urchin (see the following section). Investigators at the Zoological Laboratory of the University of Utrecht have identified Feulgen-positive granules (DNA?) in the cortical region of the vegetal pole where the first polar lobe will form in *Dentalium*. These granules may have a template function, specifying those morphogenetic determinants responsible for the formation of the apical tuft and mesodermal structures. More recently, Malacinski has isolated an axial-specific determinant from the germinal vesicle of unfertilized eggs of frogs, which he suggests becomes part of the grey crescent following germinal vesicle breakdown (see Chapter 10).

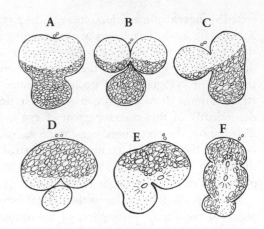

9–14 A–C, normal cleavage of the egg of the mollusc, *Ilyanassa;* D–F, cleavage in the centrifuged eggs of *Ilyanassa.* Note that centrifugation displaces the yolk-rich vegetal plasm to the animal pole. (From T. Morgan, 1927. Experimental Embryology. Columbia University Press, New York.)

CYTOPLASMIC GRADIENTS AND MORPHOGENETIC SUBSTANCES—SEA URCHIN

It would be convenient to view the differentiation of the tissues and organ rudiments of the early embryo as being controlled solely by an organized system of morphogenetic determinants that exhibit a certain spatial configuration and become segregated into different blastomeres. Yet the experiments of Driesch on isolated sea urchin blastomeres clearly indicate that regional peculiarities in the egg cytoplasm and its cortex are only some of the factors required for development. Isolated sea urchin blastomeres from two- and four-celled stages possess an ability to regulate and organize themselves to form whole embryos. Hence, each blastomere in isolation gives rise to structures not normally part of its expression in the intact embryo. We refer to these blastomeres as being totipotent. How these blastomeres regulate their activities to differentiate into structures they would not normally become has been analyzed in the sea urchin.

You will recall from the chapter on cleavage that the fertilized egg of the sea urchin divides in holoblastic fashion (Fig. 9–16). The embryo at the 16-celled stage consists of eight mesomeres in the animal hemisphere and eight blastomeres in the vegetal hemisphere, four of which are very large (macromeres) and four of which are small (micromeres) (Fig. 9–16 D). By the 64-celled stage, the eight mesomeres have proliferated into two tiers of 16 cells each. These are termed the An_1 and An_2 (animal) layers. Below the animal hemisphere, there are three recognizable layers of cells: Veg_1 (8 cells), Veg_2 (8 cells), and Mic (micromeres, 16 cells) (Fig. 9–16 F). Continued division of cells yields a ciliated blastula some six hours after fertilization. At approximately 10 hours after fertilization, the blastula is released from the confines of the fertilization membrane and the embryo becomes free-swimming. Long, stiff cilia make up the apical tuft and mark the animal pole of the blastula. Just prior to gastrulation, certain cells at the vegetal pole, termed the *primary mesenchyme,* migrate into the interior of the blastocoele (Fig. 9–16 I). They are descendants of the micromeres and will form the skeletal system. Gastrulation occurs by the invagination of cells largely derived from Veg_2. The gastrula subsequently produces *secondary mesenchyme* from the tip of the gut (Fig. 9–16 J). Following the formation of the gut, skeletal system, and the mouth, the free-swimming organism is known as the *pluteus larva.*

If the different layers of blastomeres are followed through gastrulation, a specific fate can be assigned to each (Fig. 9–16). The An_1, An_2, and Veg_1 cells form the ectoderm of the larva, contributing also to the apical tuft, mouth, ciliary bands, and anal arms. The Veg_2 cells form the endodermal lining of the gastrointestinal tract or *archenteron.* The Mic cells form primary mesenchyme, the major derivative of which is the skeletal system with its calcareous spicules.

Since the first two cleavages in the sea urchin are radial, each resultant blastomere receives all the major regions of the egg cytoplasm (i.e., presumptive ectoderm, endoderm, and mesoderm or

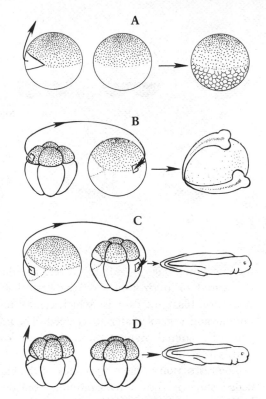

9–15 Grey crescent transplantation experiments of Curtis in *Xenopus*. A, uncleaved egg from which cortical grey crescent has been excised fails to gastrulate; B, transplant of cortical grey crescent from eight-celled stage onto ventral side of a second egg produces an embryo with two sets of axial structures; C, transplant of cortical grey crescent from uncleaved egg to eight-celled embryo does not result in the induction of a second embryonic axis; D, extirpation of cortical grey crescent at eight-celled stage produces a normal embryo. (From A. Curtis, 1962. J. Embryol. Exp. Morphol. 10, 410.)

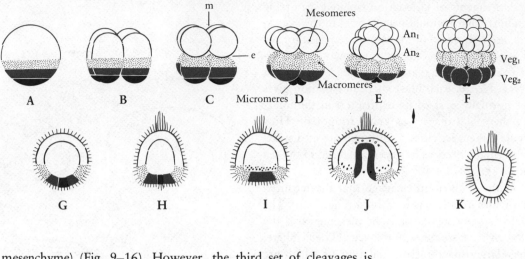

mesenchyme) (Fig. 9–16). However, the third set of cleavages is equatorial or horizontal. For the first time during development, therefore, blastomeres exist which clearly reflect differences in the animal and vegetal material received. The upper four cells contain primarily animal material, and the four lower cells contain primarily vegetal material.

The restriction in the totipotency of the blastomeres by the eight-celled stage is shown by examining the development of isolated half-embryos. If the upper quartet of blastomeres at the eight-celled stage is isolated by an equatorial separation (Fig. 9–16 C; along plane e) and subsequently cultured, the result is the production of a ciliated, hollow ball of cells known as a *dauerblastula* (Fig. 9–16 K). Neither an archenteron nor a skeleton is formed in the dauerblastula and development does not proceed beyond the blastulalike stage. Such an embryo is said to be *animalized*. The vegetal four cells yielded by the equatorial separation differentiate as an ovoid-shaped embryo with a disproportionately large archenteron, few spicules, and little ectodermal specialization (i.e., mouth, cilia). Often, the gut cavity is evaginated outward rather than inward, a condition known as *exogastrulation* (Fig. 9–16 L). Such an embryo is said to be *vegetalized*. By contrast, if the eight-celled embryo is separated into two four-celled halves by a meridional divison (Fig. 9–16 C; along plane m), each half develops into a complete, though slightly smaller than normal larva.

These same patterns of expression are also evident in the manipulated, unfertilized egg. The unfertilized egg can be cut equatorially into upper and lower halves with a glass needle and each half can subsequently be fertilized. Each egg fragment cleaves, but the upper fragment develops as a dauerblastula while the lower fragment develops as a vegetalized embryo. In short, the unfertilized egg ap-

9–16 Diagram of the normal development of the sea urchin, *Paracentrotus lividus*. A, uncleaved egg; B, 4-celled stage; C, 8-celled stage; D, 16-celled stage; E, 32-celled stage; F, 64-celled stage; G, young blastula; H, later blastula with apical tuft; I, blastula after migration of primary mesenchyme; J, gastrula with archenteron or gut cavity; K, dauerblastula produced by isolation of the four animal cells at the 8-celled stage; L, exogastrula produced by the isolation of the four vegetal cells at the 8-celled stage. An_1, animal layer 1; An_2, animal layer 2; Veg_1, vegetal layer 1; Veg_2, vegetal layer 2. (From S. Horstadius, 1939. Biol Rev. 14, 132.)

pears to consist of two halves, one animal and one vegetal, each of which possesses properties that the other lacks.

The interpretation of the early development of the sea urchin egg, as advanced in extensive studies by Horstadius, Needham, and Runnström, is that the direction in which a blastomere develops is under the influence of two mutually, antagonistic gradients in the cytoplasm. Each gradient is viewed as having an organizational center. One gradient exerts a maximum influence at the animal pole; the other gradient exerts a maximum influence at the vegetal pole. Each gradient diminishes in influence from its organizational center. The differentiation of the various parts of the embryo is directly related to an interaction between these animal-vegetal and vegetal-animal gradients. Defects and anomalies in embryonic development can be traced to naturally or artificially induced disturbances in the balance of these gradients.

Support for the paired gradient concept derives from several types of experiments, including the microsurgical separation and culturing of blastomeres, the production of differential reduction gradients by dyes, the alteration of patterns of carbohydrate and protein metabolism, and the isolation of morphogenetic agents from unfertilized egg cells. Presently, the interrelationships between the proposed cytoplasmic gradients, the metabolism of the egg itself, and the presence of morphogenetic determinants in the cytoplasm are unclear.

Horstadius (1939) found that the sea urchin egg is particularly well-suited to examining a variety of developmental problems, including questions relating to the existence of cytoplasmic gradients. By using fine glass needles and very narrow diameter pipettes in conjunction with a calcium-free surgical medium, Horstadius was able to separate blastomeres at selected stages of development (particularly at the 32- and 64-celled stages). He then combined specific groups of blastomeres and observed their development in a small depression of celluloid. If the double gradient hypothesis is correct, then differentiation of various combinations of blastomeres should be predictable on the basis of the relative amounts of animal and vegetal components. In other words, if a proper balance of animal and vegetal material is the main requirement for normal development, then it would be possible to bring about this state by using novel combinations of blastomeres.

The influence of Veg_1, Veg_2, and the micromeres upon the differentiation of isolated animal embryo halves is shown in Figure 9–17. As previously noted, an isolated animal embryo half (i.e., $An_1 + An_2$ blastomeres) develops into a hollow, ciliated ball of cells often with an enlarged apical tuft (Fig. 9–17 A). If a layer of Veg_2 cells is added to the animal half, the result is a blastula with cilia, an apical tuft, archenteron, and mouth cavity. A perfect pluteus larva is obtained from this combination of blastomeres (Fig. 9–17 C). The Veg_2 cells have the ability to check apical tuft size and stimulate differentiation of a ciliated band and mouth cavity. Additionally, the presence of Veg_2 cells causes the differentiation of skeletal tissue, the latter being normally produced by the micromeres. An animal half to which has been added a layer of Veg_1 cells produces an imperfect pluteus larva (Fig. 9–17 B). However, a normal larva can be obtained if only four micromeres are combined with the animal half, thus showing the greater vegetalizing influence of the micromeres (Fig. 9–17 E). The micromeres provide the required vegetal influence to balance the animal half, thus restoring the balance between animal and vegetal ratios compatible with normal development. *Regulation* is evident in the sense that structures normally derived from Veg_1 and Veg_2 blastomeres are formed from animal cells under the vegetalizing influence of micromere material.

Additional evidence that normal sea urchin development requires a balance of animal and vegetal factors or substances comes from experiments in which various numbers of micromeres are cultured with other cellular layers (Fig. 9–18). One or two micromeres added to a layer of An_1 cells reduces the animalizing influence, but does not permit a normal pluteus larva to develop. However, the addition of four micromeres to the An_1 layer results in a normal pluteus larva. If An_2 cells are used, fewer micromeres must be added to achieve normal development. Micromeres added to Veg_1 and Veg_2 layers, as expected, tend to exaggerate vegetal characteristics.

In experiments first done by Ernest F. G. Herbst dating back to 1893, it has been demonstrated that a wide range of chemical treatments can modify the direction of the development of sea urchin embryos. When lithium chloride is added to the medium surrounding fertilized eggs, the resultant embryos show signs of excessive gut development and exogastrulation. Such agents, which cause an embryo to develop as if it were an isolated vegetal half-embryo, are referred to as *vegetalizing agents*. Other vegetalizing agents include certain amino acids (valine and tyrosine) and metabolic inhibitors such as dinitrophenol and chloramphenicol. On the other hand, trypsin, chymotrysin, and sodium thiocyanate cause fertilized eggs to develop as dauerblastulas, thus acting as *animalizing agents*. In view of the heterogeneity of these animalizing and vegetalizing agents, some investigators have suggested that these substances act by upsetting biochemical equilibriums in the egg.

There is also evidence to indicate that the proposed pair of cytoplasmic gradients may be closely linked to the metabolism of the sea urchin egg. When embryos (blastulas or gastrulas) are placed in

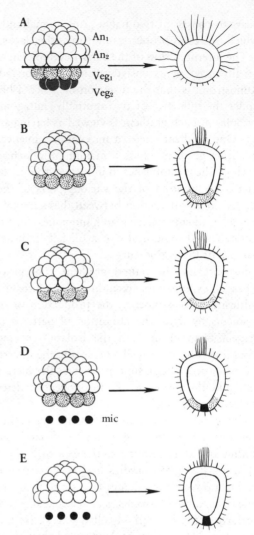

9–17 Diagram of the influence of Veg_1, Veg_2, and the micromeres on the differentiation of isolated animal halves in *Paracentrotus*. A, isolated animal half; B, animal half + Veg_1; C, animal half + Veg_2; D, animal half + Veg_1 + micromeres; E, animal half + micromeres. (From S. Horstadius, 1939. Biol. Rev. 14, 132.)

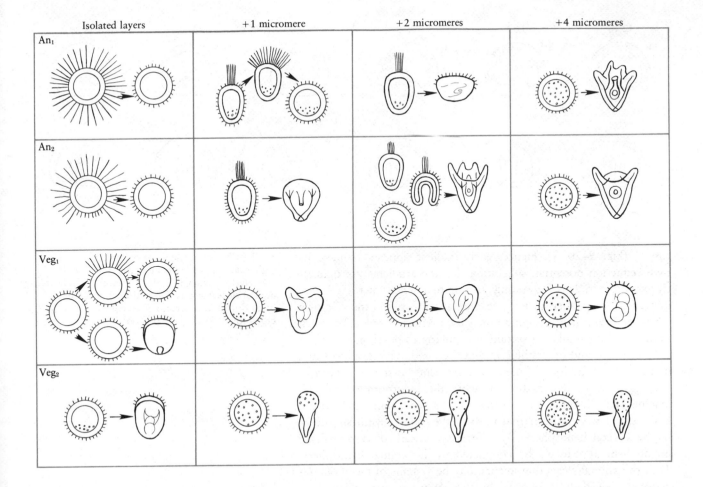

	Isolated layers	+1 micromere	+2 micromeres	+4 micromeres

9–18 Diagram of the development of the layers An₁, An₂, Veg₁, and Veg₂ following isolation (left column) and the addition of one, two, and four micromeres. (From S. Horstadius, 1939. Biol. Rev. 14, 132.)

a chamber with Janus green dye and sealed from an external source of oxygen, the oxygen of the sea water is gradually exhausted. The Janus green then acts as an acceptor of electrons from oxidative phosphorylation and becomes reduced. As it does so, the dye progressively changes in color from grayish-blue to red and then to colorless. The pattern of reduction of the dye in late blastulas begins near the vegetal pole and spreads laterally and toward the equator of the embryos (Fig. 9–19). When the advancing border of the reduced dye reaches the equator, a second reduction front appears at the animal pole and proceeds toward the vegetal hemisphere. When the same experiments are conducted using isolated vegetal halves (Fig. 9–20 B), an early and intense reduction center is noted at the vegetal pole; it then moves toward the animal hemisphere. However, no secondary gradient is visible in the animal end of the embryo. A similar observation has been made on animal halves (i.e., no second reduction front appears after the first one

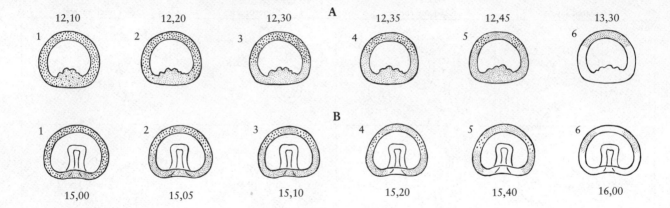

A

| 12,10 | 12,20 | 12,30 | 12,35 | 12,45 | 13,30 |

B

| 15,00 | 15,05 | 15,10 | 15,20 | 15,40 | 16,00 |

forms) (Fig. 9–20 A). Hence, each gradient appears to have its own reduction potential, suggesting that the gradients are qualitatively different. It is interesting to note that when micromeres are implanted into either an isolated animal half or into the side of a whole embryo, they precipitate their own center of reduction. Such implants also stimulate a second archenteron to develop.

Runnström and others believe that these reduction gradients are, in fact, manifestations of metabolic gradients in the cytoplasm of the egg. Studies designed to measure the incorporation of ^{14}C-leucine and ^{14}C-valine into protein in isolated animal and vegetal sea urchin halves indicate that most of the protein synthesis occurs in the vegetal hemisphere. By contrast, the bulk of carbohydrate metabolism appears to be conducted in the animal hemisphere. That the animal–vegetal gradients may be systems of metabolic reactions tends to be supported by the actions of vegetalizing and animalizing agents. Lithium chloride, a vegetalizing agent, disturbs the respiration of the embryo by either uncoupling the oxidative phosphorylating reactions or inhibiting the actions of certain glycolytic enzymes. Dinitrophenol appears to act in a similar fashion. Vegetalization, then, is essentially a suppression or disturbance in the oxidative processes of the embryo (i.e., the animalizing influence of the animal hemisphere is affected). Why structures developing at the animal pole are more sensitive to these agents than structures derived from the vegetal pole remains unknown.

Animalizing agents, such as trypsin and polysulfonated organic compounds (Evans blue), appear to interfere with the formation of functional proteins. Although the mechanism by which they act is not understood, it is suggested that acidic groups of some of these compounds immobilize the proteins by joining to functional side groups. The exaggeration of ectodermal structures under the influ-

9–19 Change in the color of Janus green showing reduction gradients in a later blastula (A, 1–6) and a gastrula (B, 1–6). Numbers indicate time of observations. Large dots, blue color; small dots, red color; no dots, colorless. (From S. Horstadius, 1952. J. Exp. Zool. 120, 421.)

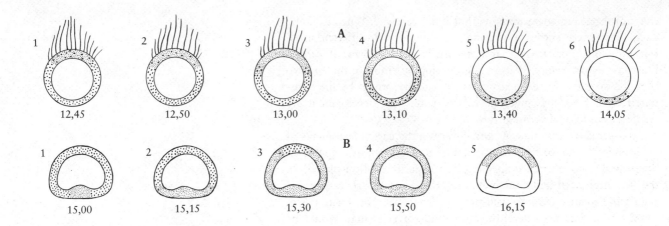

A

| 1 | 2 | 3 | 4 | 5 | 6 |
| 12,45 | 12,50 | 13,00 | 13,10 | 13,40 | 14,05 |

B

| 1 | 2 | 3 | 4 | 5 |
| 15,00 | 15,15 | 15,30 | 15,50 | 16,15 |

ence of these agents appears to be due to disturbances in the vegetal–animal gradient.

Treatment of sea urchin embryos with various chemical compounds has been helpful in establishing the presence of gradients and probable biochemical basis for their existence. A much more fundamental question can now be asked. What is the chemical basis, if any, for the determination of animal and vegetal properties? Are there chemical substances in the sea urchin egg with animal and vegetal properties that act as morphogenetic determinants? Horstadius, Josefsson, and Runnström in a series of papers (1967, 1969) have reported on their efforts to isolate and identify animalizing and vegetalizing substances in unfertilized egg and early cleavage stages of the sea urchin. By using sophisticated techniques of centrifugation and column chromatography, some fractions were obtained which exhibited strong animalization of whole eggs and vegetal embryo halves. Other fractions vegetalized animal halves but failed to affect whole eggs. Absorption curves of animalizing fractions using ultraviolet light indicated that there may be several animalizing agents. One fraction strongly resembled the amino acid tryptophan while another fraction resembled a nucleotide structure.

REGULATIVE AND MOSAIC DEVELOPMENTS

Our discussion of molluscs, tunicates, sea urchins, and frogs tends to suggest that there are two broad patterns controlling early embryogenesis among animals. In most molluscs, annelids, and tunicates, the fate of early blastomeres is typically fixed or determined by the onset of segmentation. Cleavage parcels out to various blastomeres the morphogenetic substances localized in patchwork fashion in the egg. Each blastomere can only express itself in terms of

9–20 Reduction of Janus green in isolated animal (A, 1–6) and vegetal (B, 1–5) halves of the sea urchin embryo. Numbers indicate time of observations. Symbols as in Figure 9–19. (From S. Horstadius, 1952. J. Exp. Zool. 120, 421.)

the morphogenetic determinants that it has received. When isolated, each blastomere shows a striking capacity for self-differentiation, but only into structures that it normally would form. If certain blastomeres are removed from the developing embryo, the embryo remains deficient in those structures normally formed by the extirpated cells. Eggs that give rise to this pattern of development are termed *mosaic* or *determinate*.

By contrast to mosaic eggs and embryos, the early blastomeres of echinoderms and vertebrates are labile and totipotent, capable of developing into normal embryos when experimentally isolated. In the sea urchin, meridional halves of the blastula are capable of regulating themselves into well-proportioned embryos. Each meridional half forms considerably more kinds of cells than would be normally expected. Eggs that give rise to this pattern of development are termed *regulative* or *indeterminate*.

The distinction between mosaic and regulative development is by no means clear-cut and absolute. Two examples can be used to illustrate this point. Horstadius has shown that the various layers of the 16-celled stage of *Cerebratulus* (nemertean worm), when isolated, form only what is expected. Combinations of blastomeres show no signs of interaction between animal and vegetal components as in the sea urchin. In short, the embryo behaves as a mosaic. Yet a nucleated fragment of the unfertilized egg, following insemination, develops into a normal embryo. This is indicative of regulative development. Recall that each of the first two blastomeres of the frog's egg can in isolation compensate for the loss of the other blastomere and subsequently form a whole embryo. By contrast, at the four-celled stage, only the two blastomeres containing grey crescent material can yield normal embryos. Since the grey crescent represents an area of localized morphogenetic substance, the egg can be considered mosaic.

Differences between mosaic and regulative patterns of development are probably indicative of differences in the time at which events involved in the determination of parts of the embryo occur. In some organisms the localization of cytoplasmic determinants that control the direction of later development takes place by fertilization. In other organisms it may not occur until after several cleavages. It is likely that all developing organisms at some stage possess the power of regulation.

REFERENCES

Arnold, J. and L. Williams-Arnold. 1974. Cortical-nuclear interactions in cephalopod development: Cytochalasin B effects on the informational pattern in the cell surface. J. Embryol. Exp. Morphol. 31:1–25.

Brachet, J. and E. Hubert. 1972. Studies on nucleocytoplasmic interactions during early amphibian development. I. Localized destruction of the egg cortex. J. Embryol. Exp. Morphol. 27:121–145.

Briggs, R. and T. J. King. 1952. Transplantation of living nuclei from blastula cells into enucleated frogs' eggs. Proc. Nat. Acad. Sci. U.S.A. 38:455–463.

Cather, J. and N. Verdonk. 1974. The development of *Bithynia tentaculata* (Prosobranchia, Gastropoda) after removal of the polar lobe. J. Embryol. Exp. Morphol. 31:415–422.

Clement, A. C. 1976. Cell determination and organogenesis in molluscan development: A reappraisal based on deletion experiments in *Ilyanassa*. Am. Zool. 16:447–453.

Curtis, A. S. G. 1962. Morphogenetic interactions before gastrulation in the amphibian *Xenopus laevis*—the cortical field. J. Embryol. Exp. Morphol. 10:410–422.

Curtis, A. S. G. 1963. The cell cortex. Endeavor 22:134–137.

DiBerardino, M. A. and N. Hoffner. 1970. Origin of the chromosomal abnormalities in nuclear transplants, a revaluation of nuclear differentiation and nuclear equivalence in amphibians. Dev. Biol. 23:185–209.

Dohmen, M. and N. H. Verdonk. 1974. The structure of a morphogenetic cytoplasm present in the polar lobe of *Bithynia tentaculata* (Gastropoda, Prosobranchia). J. Embryol. Exp. Morphol. 31:423–433.

Driesch, H. 1892. The potency of the first two cleavage cells in echinoderm development. Experimental production of partial and double formations. In: Foundations of Experimental Embryology, pp. 38–50. Eds., B. H. Willier and J. M. Oppenheimer. Englewood Cliffs, N.J.: Prentice-Hall.

Emerson, C. P. and T. Humphreys. 1970. Regulation of DNA-like RNA and the apparent activation of ribosomal RNA synthesis in sea urchin embryos: Quantitative measurements of newly synthesized RNA. Dev. Biol. 23:86–112.

Geilenkirchen, W., N. H. Verdonk, and L. Timmermans. 1970. Experimental studies on morphogenetic factors localized in the first and second polar lobe of *Dentalium* eggs. J. Embryol. Exp. Morphol. 23:237–243.

Gurdon, J. B. 1968. Transplanted nuclei and cell differentiation. Sci. Am. 219:24–35.

Horstadius, S. 1939. The mechanics of sea urchin development, studied by operative methods. Biol. Rev. 14:132–179.

Horstadius, S. 1952. Induction and inhibition of reduction gradients by the micromeres in the sea urchin egg. J. Exp. Zool. 120:421–436.

Horstadius, S., L. Josefsson, and J. Runnström. 1967. Morphogenetic agents from unfertilized eggs of the sea urchin, *Paracentrotus lividus*. Dev. Biol. 16:189–202.

Josefsson, L. and S. Horstadius. 1969. Morphogenetic substances from sea urchin eggs. Isolation of animalizing and vegetalizing substances from unfertilized eggs of *Paracentrotus lividus*. Dev. Biol. 20:481–500.

Kobel, H., R. Brun, and M. Fischberg. 1973. Nuclear transplantation with melanophores, ciliated epidermal cells, and the established cell-line A-8 in *Xenopus laevis*. J. Embryol. Exp. Morphol. 29:539–547.

Malacinski, G. 1974. Biological properties of a presumptive morphogenetic determinant from the amphibian oocyte germinal vesicle nucleus. Cell Differ. 3:31–44.

Raven, C. P. 1970. The cortical and subcortical cytoplasm of *Lymnaea* egg. Int. Rev. Cytol. 28:1–44.

Roux, W. 1888. Contributions to the developmental mechanics of the embryo. On the artificial production of half-embryos by destruction of one of the first two blastomeres, and the later development (postgeneration) of the missing half of the body. In: Foundations of Experimental Embryology, pp. 2–37. Eds., B. H. Willier and J. M. Oppenheimer. Englewood Cliffs, N.J.: Prentice-Hall.

Timmermans, L., W. Geilenkirchen, and N. H. Verdonk. 1970. Local accumulation of Feulgen-positive granules in the egg cortex of *Dentalium dentale L.* J. Embryol. Exp. Morphol. 23:245–252.

Verdonk, N. H., W. Geilenkirchen, and L. Timmermans. 1971. The localization of morphogenetic factors in uncleaved eggs of *Dentalium*. J. Embryol. Exp. Morphol. 25:57–63.

10

Neurulation and
Embryonic Induction

Gastrulation is a developmental process that involves the movement of the primordia of presumptive internal structures from the surface to specific positions in the interior of the embryo. These morphogenetic movements and the subsequent events of neurulation are responsible for the first visible signs of a distinct embryonic axis and the organization of the basic body plan of the embryo. The expression of the ectoderm, mesoderm, and endoderm by the end of gastrulation, as well as the subsequent development of the neural tube and neural crest, constitute an early building plan of the embryo which requires dramatic changes in the physical and chemical properties of embryonic cells. The nuclear transplantation experiments discussed in the previous chapter provide evidence that the same genetic material is present in all embryonic cells throughout the course of development. Hence, the initial changes in embryonic cells which lead to the formation of cell types such as ectoderm, mesoderm, and endoderm can be regarded as due to the differential expression of the same genome.

On the basis of various microsurgical and tissue culture techniques, it is known that the fate of individual embryonic cells is controlled, in part, by extrinsic factors. These factors include the changing fluid microenvironment of the cells and intimate associations with adjacent or neighboring populations of cells. The interdependent relationship between adjacent populations of cells, which is the basis for the early differentiation of most tissues and organs, is best illustrated in vivo by removing portions of the embryo. When this is done, remaining intact areas of the embryo may fail to differentiate properly or be abnormally expressed. In contrast to earlier developmental stages in which embryonic cells are remarkably adaptable, these same cells show more limited capacities of expression by the end of gastrulation. The production of different cell types is one of the immediate consequences of the ordered, morphogenetic movements of gastrulation.

NEURULATION AND THE EVENT OF NEURAL INDUCTION

One of the key interactions between cells of vertebrate gastrulas that has occupied the attention of embryologists for many years, perhaps longer than any other event in development, is that of neural induction. In this process, the chordamesoderm, with passage through the blastopore or primitive streak, acts upon the overlying adjacent ectoderm to stimulate the latter to form a thickened plate of cells, the *neural plate*. Failure of the chordamesoderm to migrate properly into a position adjacent to the cells that respond to its influence leads to defects in the central nervous system. The dependence of one group of cells (ectoderm) upon another group of cells (chordamesoderm) for the expression of the differentiated state (neural tissue) is an example of an *embryonic induction*. The cell group that is the source of the stimulation or influence is the *inductor* or *inducer*.

Since the discovery of the importance of the chordamesoderm or dorsal lip of the blastopore in the tissue differentiations of the early embryo by Hans Spemann and his colleagues between 1916 and 1925, the succeeding decades have seen numerous efforts at establishing the physicochemical basis for neural induction and the subsequent morphogenesis of the central nervous system. Although the event of neural induction has been for many years the most extensively studied of tissue interactions, its mechanism still eludes us. It may be used here to illustrate some of the basic problems associated with the study of inductive tissue interactions in general. We shall in the following pages review the famous grafting studies of Spemann and give consideration to some of the approaches currently being employed to examine the mechanics of neural induction. Before doing this, the event of neurulation itself should be examined in greater detail.

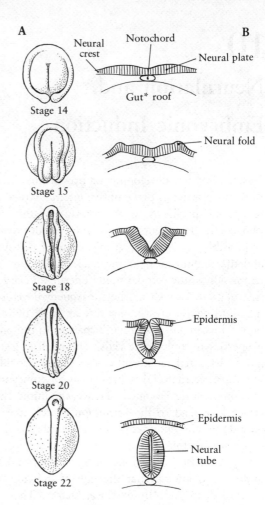

10–1   A, the sequence of stages in the neurulation of an amphibian such as *Ambystoma;* B, diagrammatic cross sections of stages shown in A. (After B. Kallen, 1965. Organogenesis. R. H. DeHaan and H. Ursprung, eds. Holt, Rinehart and Winston. New York.)

NEURULATION, MICROTUBULES, AND MICROFILAMENTS

Neurulation is the process whereby the neural or medullary plate becomes transformed into the dorsal, hollow neural tube. During this time the primordia of brain, spinal cord, and neural crest become internalized and completely segregated from the rest of the surface ectoderm. In forms such as the frog and the salamander, the neural tube is completed throughout its length at much the same time (Fig. 10–1). By contrast, neural tube formation in amniote embryos, beginning in advance of the completion of the gastrula-

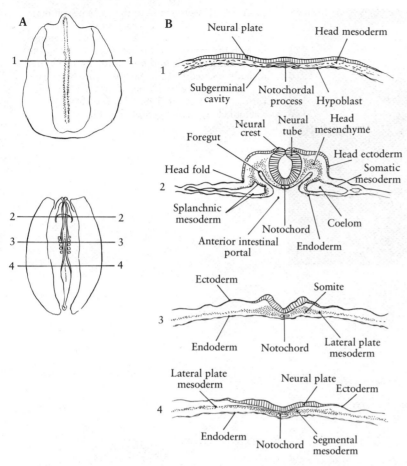

A

1 —— 1

2 —— 2
3 —— 3
4 —— 4

B

1

Neural plate   Head mesoderm

Subgerminal   Notochordal   Hypoblast
cavity   process

2

Foregut   Neural   Neural   Head
               crest   tube   mesenchyme

                                   Head ectoderm
                                   Somatic
                                   mesoderm
Head fold

Splanchnic
mesoderm
               Notochord   Coelom
Anterior intestinal   Endoderm
portal

3

Ectoderm   Somite

Endoderm   Notochord   Lateral plate
                         mesoderm

4

Lateral plate   Neural plate
mesoderm   Ectoderm

Endoderm   Notochord   Segmental
                         mesoderm

10–2   A, the sequence of stages in the neurulation of the chick embryo; B, diagrammatic cross sections of stages shown in A. (Reprinted with permission of Macmillan Publishing Company, from Atlas of Descriptive Embryology by W. W. Mathews. Copyright © 1972 by Willis W. Mathews.)

tion process, occurs by the sequential, anterior-to-posterior fusion of the neural folds in the wake of primitive streak regression (Fig. 10–2). Despite this visible difference among vertebrate embryos, the mechanics of the transformation of a flattened plate of neural cells into a tube appear to be essentially the same. Changes in the shape and size of neural plate cells apparently play an important role in the morphogenetic movements required in the conversion of plate to tube.

Of all the vertebrates, it is the amphibian that has been the most extensively studied with respect to neurulation. As much as 50 percent of the outer ectodermal layer contributes to the formation of the neural plate in amphibian embryos. Figure 10–3 A shows a surface view of the neural plate at about the time of neural fold formation. The neural plate is distinctly keel shaped, being wider anteriorly, and is readily distinguished from the adjacent ectodermal cells. A transverse section through the early neural plate shows that

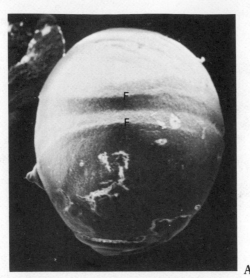

A

10–3   A, survey picture of the early neural plate stage of *Xenopus;* B, cross section through the early neural plate stage of *Xenopus;* C, a section through the same neural plate showing subapical microfilaments (mf) and microtubules (mt) in the medially located cells. F, neural folds; M, muscle; NP, neural plate; N, notochord. (A, from D. Tarin, 1971. J. Anat. 109, 535; B,C, from P. Karfunkel, 1971. Dev. Biol. 25, 30.)

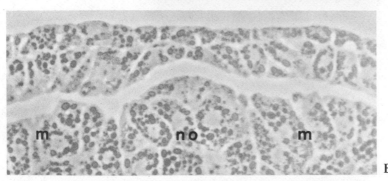

B

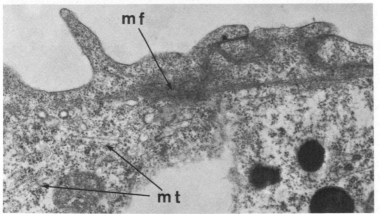

C

it consists of either a single layer (*Triturus*) or several layers (*Xenopus*) of cuboidal-shaped cells (Fig. 10–3 B). In *Xenopus,* as the margins of the neural plate rise and the neural folds become prominent (Fig. 10–4), dramatic changes are observed in the shape of the

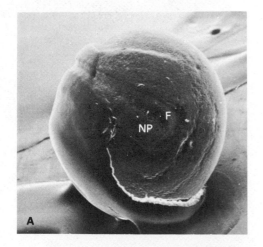

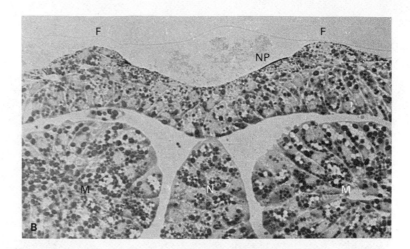

neural plate cells. The medially situated cells of the upper layer become taller and wedge shaped, their narrowed ends abutting upon the neurocoele. The cells of the lower layer become more columnar in shape with their long axes oriented in a dorsoventral plane. Upon the approximation and fusion of the neural folds in the middorsal line (Fig. 10–5), the long axes of the deep cells are always radially positioned with respect to the lumen of the neural tube. The changes in the orientation and shape of the neural cells during neurulation in *Xenopus* are diagrammatically summarized in Figure 10–6.

The elongation and stretching of neural plate cells appear to be intrinsic properties. In other words, the changes in cell shape probably occur independently of forces such as those that may be generated by movements of the epidermal ectoderm toward the midline during neurulation. Holtfreter for example, has shown that isolated neural plate cells retain their columnar shape and even continue to elongate when cultured.

Electron microscopic observations show that cell elongation during amphibian neurulation correlates with the presence of both microtubules and microfilaments (Figs. 10–3 C; 10–6). Schroeder (1973), Karfunkel (1971, 1972), and others have noted that the cells of the early neural plate contain numerous microtubules, approximately 240 Å in diameter and randomly oriented in the cytoplasm. Those of the median superficial cells of the neural plate in *Xenopus* become arranged parallel to the axis of cell elongation during neural fold formation (Fig. 10–6). Microfilaments initially appear in the upper cells of the neural plate as a dense band just below the exposed surface of each cell (Fig. 10–6). As the neural plate becomes tubelike, most cells are oriented radially to the neurocoele and possess microtubules arranged with the elongating

10–4 A, survey picture, viewed from the anterior end, of the neural folds (F) and the remainder of the neural plate (NP) during early neurulation in *Xenopus;* B, cross section through the early neural fold (F) stage of *Xenopus*. M, muscle; N, notochord. (A, from D. Tarin, 1971. J. Anat. 109, 535; B, from P. Karfunkel, 1971. Dev. Biol. 25, 30.)

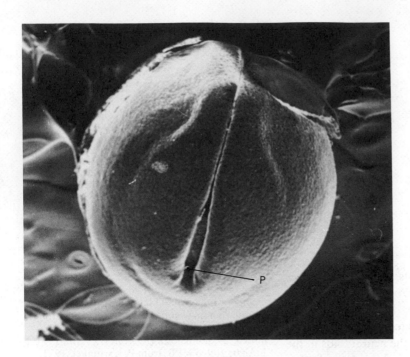

10–5 Survey picture, viewed from the anterior end, showing approximation of the neural folds in *Xenopus*. P, anterior neuropore. (From D. Tarin, 1972. J. Anat. 111, 1.)

axis of the cells. Microfilaments are generally absent from the apical or inner ends of the cells, which form the floor of the lumen of the neural tube. They persist, however, in the cells forming the dorsal aspect of the neural tube (Fig. 10–6).

You will recall that microtubules and microfilaments have been previously associated with morphogenetic events involving changes in cell shape and cell movement (i.e., blastopore and primitive streak formation; cytokinesis of cleaving blastomeres). Although both microtubules and microfilaments can be correlated with changes in cell shape during amphibian neurulation, it is still not clear how these cytoskeletal elements generate cell shape changes. It has been proposed that the microfilaments, initially arranged in circumferential bundles parallel to the neural plate cell surfaces, act by virtue of contracting, thereby narrowing the apical ends of the simple neural epithelium in the salamander or the median superficial layer of cells in *Xenopus*. The consequence of this contractile activity is a progressive change in the shape of each cell (i.e., from cuboidal, to wedge, to flask), the result of which is an imposition of curvature on the previously flattened neural plate. Since the basal or lower surfaces of the cells are less constricted than the apical surfaces, the effect is a rolling upward and inward of the margins of the neural plate. This rolling of the neural plate into the neural tube has been likened to drawing tight the strings of a purse.

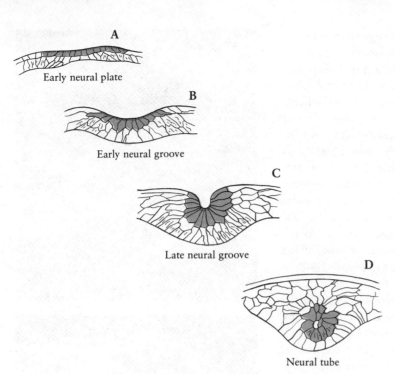

A

Early neural plate

B

Early neural groove

C

Late neural groove

D

Neural tube

10–6 Tracings of shapes of neural plate cells during neurulation in *Xenopus*. Note that only the superficial, medial cells form the boundary of the neurocoele. The dots in the cells represent microfilaments. Straight lines inside cells indicate microtubules. Note their orientation during tube formation. (After P. Karfunkel, 1971. Dev. Biol. 25, 30.)

The microtubules appear to be responsible for the first step in neurulation or the elongation of ectodermal cells to form the flat neural plate. The formation of elongated cells might be due to either an extension of the microtubules by the directional addition and polymerization of subunits or by the sliding of microtubules away from each other. In either case, the effect would be to elongate the cell by pushing out on its apical and basal ends.

That changes in cell shape are critical to the neurulation process has been shown by treating amphibian embryos with various agents or drugs whose actions are known to interfere with the assembly or maintenance of microfilaments and microtubules. For example, if frog embryos are exposed at the early neural plate stage (i.e., prior to cell elongation) with vinblastine, a compound that precipitates microtubular protein and thus destroys the integrity of microtubules, wedge-shaped and flask-shaped cells never appear, and neural folds fail to form. If the cells are treated after elongation, they fail to maintain their shape, thus offering direct experimental proof that microtubules are responsible for the elongation of cells of the neural plate. Vinblastine also disrupts microfilaments. It not only prevents the apical ends of cells of the neural plate from contracting, but it also causes them to lose their constricted state if treatment is initiated after tube formation. The drug cytochalasin B, a fungal metabolite, also interferes with microfilament formation. Treatment of amphibian embryos during neurulation with this drug causes an opening up and subsequent flattening of the neural tube.

The active role of both microtubules (cell elongation) and microfilaments (cell contraction) during neural tube formation is also supported by observations on and experimental manipulations with chick neurulas. During the transformation of the neural plate into prominent neural folds (Fig. 10–7), the cells lying along the neural groove become elongate and wedge shaped, their apices appearing narrower and more convex. Bundles of microfilaments are quite prominent in the subapical cytoplasm of these cells. As in the case of amphibian embryos, microtubules are arranged parallel to the long axes of neural cells. The changes in the shape of cells during neurulation in the chick embryo are summarized in Figure 10–8.

That the elongation of neural cells is due to the presence of microtubules has been demonstrated by culturing chick embryos at the neural fold stage with either colchicine or colcemid. The cells of the neural folds round up and subsequently the neural folds fall back toward the yolk. Similarly, if cells of the neural plate are treated with cytochalasin B prior to becoming apically constricted, these same cells fail to contract and the neural folds fail to elevate.

It may be concluded, at least in amphibian and chick embryos, that the curvature of the neural plate and the elevation and approximation of the neural folds during neurulation is a two-step process dependent upon the presence of microtubules and microfilaments (Fig. 10–9). First, the ectodermal cells undergo elongation to form a neural plate with an active role played by microtubules. Second, constriction of the neural plate cells at their apical ends is microfilament mediated, resulting in the initial invagination of the neural plate and the subsequent formation of the neural tube. Fusion of the neural folds and their separation from the adjacent cells of the ectoderm produces the neural tube. Whether the correlation between the presence of the cytoskeletal organelles and the transformation of the neural epithelial cells into a tube applies to other vertebrate embryos remains to be established.

The induction of the neural plate in the chick embryo appears to involve the de novo formation of microtubules and microfilaments because neither of these are present prior to neural plate formation. It has not been determined whether the formation of these cytoskeletal structures is due to the polymerization of preformed subunits or the synthesis and polymerization of new subunits.

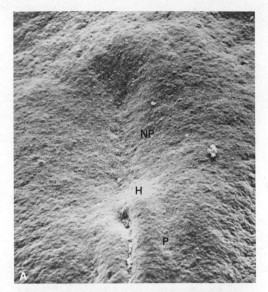

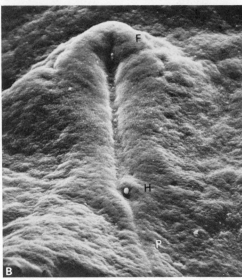

10–7 A, survey picture showing the late neural plate (NP) stage of the chick; B, formation of the neural folds in the chick. F, neural folds; H, Hensen's node; P, lateral folds of primitive streak. (From P. Portch and A. Barson, 1974. J. Anat. 117, 341.)

DETERMINATION AND SPEMANN'S PRIMARY ORGANIZER

The techniques of transplantation or tissue grafting and culturing of embryos have been successfully employed in examining several of the fundamental questions relating to the significance of cellular rearrangements and the differentiation of tissue and organ primordia in the early embryo. Small pieces of tissue may be surgically removed from preselected sites of embryos at various stages of development and inserted into prepared cuts or wounds on the same or different embryos. If the graft is placed on the same embryo from which it is excised, the transplant is referred to as being *autoplastic*. Grafts can as easily be made between individuals of the same species (*homoplastic transplant*) or between different species of the same genus (*heteroplastic transplant*). The embryo providing the graft is the *donor;* the embryo receiving the graft is the *host*.

It is important to know in a transplantation experiment which tissues of the embryo are derived from the graft and which tissues are from the host. An induction, for example, can be said to occur under the influence of a graft if host cells participate in the formation of structures not normally formed by them. A distinction is readily made if donor and host cells are sufficiently different from each other. Heteroplastic transplants are often used because differences in cell size, cell-staining properties, or cell inclusions (i.e., pigment granules) commonly exist between donor and host cells, thus facilitating interpretation of transplant experiments.

In the early 1920s Spemann investigated the question of when specific areas of the vertebrate embryo become firmly committed to specific developmental pathways. Using embryos of the salamander (*Triturus taeniatus*), he placed a small piece of presumptive ectoderm from an early gastrula stage into the presumptive neural plate area of another embryo of the same stage of development (Fig. 10–10 A). The result was that the graft developed in accordance with the cells around it and gave rise to the neural plate cells of the host (Fig. 10–10 A). The reciprocal transplant, or graft of presumptive neural plate cells placed into the anteroventral ectodermal (epidermal) area (Fig. 10–10 B), also developed in conformity with the surrounding cells and contributed to the integumentary cells of the host (Fig. 10–10 B). If ectodermal or presumptive neural plate tissue was grafted to the marginal or chordamesodermal area of the early gastrula, Spemann observed that the transplant moved through the blastopore with the morphogenetic movements of the host embryo and differentiated in accordance with its new mesodermal environment, giving rise to such mesodermal derivatives as no-

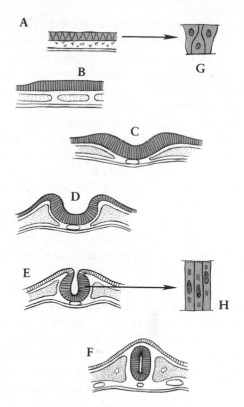

10–8 Diagrammatic drawings of the cells of the chick neural plate, neural folds, and neural tube during neurulation. A, the preplate blastoderm; B, the neural plate; C, early neural fold formation; D, the early neural groove; E, the late neural groove; F, the neural tube; G, the appearance of individual cells of the preplate blastoderm; H, the cells of the neural groove are elongate with microtubules arranged parallel to the cells' long axes and microfilaments (dots) at the apices of cells. (After P. Karfunkel, 1972. J. Exp. Zool. 181, 289.)

tochord, somites, and kidney tubules. Heteroplastic transplants between *Triturus cristatus* and *Triturus taeniatus* embryos at the early gastrula stage have yielded similar results (Fig. 10–11).

From reciprocal transplants between ectoderm and neural plate areas, as well as those involving the grafting of chordamesoderm and endoderm to other embryonic areas, it can be concluded that the cells of the early gastrula possess the ability to differentiate into a variety of cell types. The presumptive neural cell can develop into a skin or somite cell when placed in the appropriate environment. Presumptive somite cells can differentiate into skin cells. We refer to this lability or capacity to differentiate in several directions of an early embryonic cell as being its *prospective potency*. The normal or expected fate of a cell is its *prospective significance*.

Suppose reciprocal transplants between epidermal ectoderm and presumptive neural plate areas are executed using late stage gastrulas as tissue donors. The results are very different when compared to those with early stage gastrulas as tissue donors. In all cases, the grafts from late gastrulas differentiate in accordance with the presumptive areas from which they were excised before transplantation. For example, a transplanted piece of neural plate when placed into a cut in the skin ectoderm of an early gastrula will sink beneath the surface and form recognizable neural structures (Fig. 10–10 C). A graft of epidermal tissue when placed into the presumptive neural area will differentiate as epidermis only. These results serve to establish that the neural plate and the epidermis have lost their abilities to develop into any derivatives other than neural and integumentary structures, respectively.

Hence, by the end of gastrulation, the potencies of presumptive epidermal and neural cells become restricted to their expected fate or prospective significance. This restriction of cell lability or channeling of developmental potential is known as the process of *determination*. We speak of the nervous system or the epidermis as being determined by the end of gastrulation. Similarly, chordamesodermal and endodermal cells also become broadly determined or limited with respect to cell type. The expression of further change within these areas (i.e., the determination of individual structures and parts within the ectoderm, neural plate, chordamesoderm, and endoderm) is dependent upon subsequent and successive determinative steps.

The early grafting experiments of Spemann provided strong evidence that determination of the epidermal and neural tissues was related to the rearrangement of cells brought about by the process of gastrulation. Hilde Mangold, a student of Spemann's, carried out a variety of heteroplastic transplant experiments in an effort to define the exact times of determination of the different parts of the

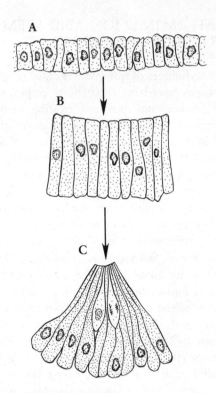

10–9 Neurulation is a two-step process dependent upon the transformation of a plate of cells (A) into elongate neural cells by microtubules (B) and their apical constriction by microfilaments to convert into a tube (C).

gastrula. Her efforts (1924) established that the chordamesoderm (mainly notochord and paraxial or somitic mesoderm), which shifts forward beneath the ectoderm with the morphogenetic movements of gastrulation, plays a decisive role in the determination of the epidermal and neural areas. She excised a piece of the dorsal lip of the blastopore from an early gastrula of *Triturus cristatus* and placed it onto the lateral lip of the blastopore of an early gastrula of *Triturus taeniatus* (Fig. 10–12 A). The transplanted tissue was subsequently incorporated into the interior of the host embryo. When the host embryo developed further, there was found a nearly complete second set of organs, giving to the host the appearance of conjoint twins (Fig. 10–12 B,C). Sections through the host showed that the secondary embryo lacked the anterior part of the head. There was, however, a neural tube on either side of which were somites and kidney tubules. A notochord and gut tube were identified beneath the neural tube (Fig. 10–12 D). Based upon differences in pigmentation of cells between the two species in the heteroplastic transplant (i.e., *T. taeniatus* cells contain dark pigment granules), Mangold determined that most of the neural tube, part of the somites, the kidney tubules, and the inner ear primordia of the secondary embryo were derived from host tissues. The notochord apparently differentiated solely from graft cells, thus demonstrating the self-differentiation properties of this part of the dorsal lip. Hence, the ventral ectoderm of *T. taeniatus* had been altered by an interaction with the dorsal lip graft and had differentiated as neural tissue rather than skin.

Because of the ability of the dorsal lip of the blastopore (or the roof of the primitive archenteron) to stimulate from host cells the development of a nearly whole secondary embryo after transplantation, Spemann termed the dorsal lip of the blastopore the *primary organizer* (or simply organizer). Under the influence of the organizer, a secondary embryo, possessing the essential features of axial organization, can be induced to form from tissues normally having distinctly different prospective fates. For example, the transplanted dorsal lip induced presumptive epidermis of the host to form a neural plate. It also influences the mesoderm and endoderm, stimulating the formation of structures from host tissues as a result of inductions. Spemann assigned two properties to the dorsal lip: induc-

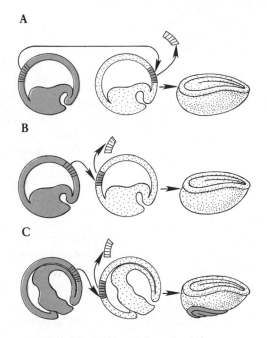

10–10 A, transplant of presumptive ectoderm (epidermis) from early newt gastrula placed into presumptive neural plate of another early newt gastrula will develop in accordance with its new surroundings (i.e., neural plate); B, transplant of presumptive neural plate from early newt gastrula placed into presumptive ectoderm (epidermis) of another early newt gastrula will develop in accordance with its new surroundings (i.e., epidermis); C, the transplant of neural plate from late newt gastrula placed into presumptive ectoderm (epidermis) of early newt gastrula develops in its new surroundings in accordance with its expected fate (i.e., neural plate).

10–11 A cross section through the anterior end of a *Triturus taeniatus* embryo formed from a graft with presumptive epidermis from *T. cristatus* placed into the neural plate region. The region of the forebrain (shown between the asterisks) of *T. taeniatus* has developed from *T. cristatus* presumptive epidermis. (From H. Spemann, 1938. Embryonic Development and Induction. Yale University Press, New Haven.)

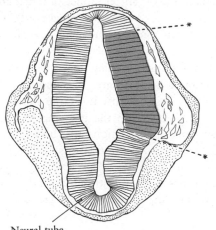

Neural tube

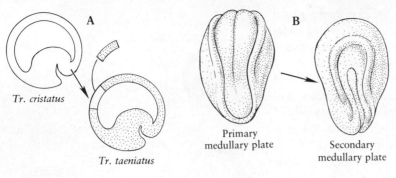

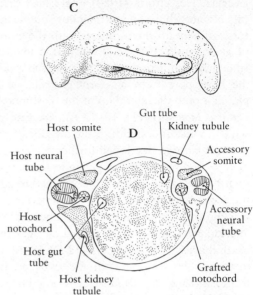

tion of the overlying ectoderm to form a neural plate and tube, and self-differentiation by the notochord into the major embryonic axis.

The organizer or primary embryonic inductor can be traced to that region of the fertilized egg previously identified as the grey crescent. Complete extirpation of the grey crescent at the time of fertilization results in an embryo lacking neural and mesodermal structures. Destruction of the grey crescent by controlled exposure to ultraviolet irradiation produces results similar to those by extirpation. By contrast, transplantation of the cortex of the grey crescent onto the ventral side of a second normal egg will yield an embryo with a second set of axial organs (Fig. 9–15). We are able to conclude from these experiments that the phenomenon of primary determination, at least in the amphibian, can be related to the early cytoplasmic localization of some substance(s) in the grey crescent. The formation of the main axis of the embryo is thus foreshadowed in the early organization of the egg cell itself.

In the amphibian blastula and early gastrula, the region that has inducing capabilities appears to coincide spatially with the region of cells that becomes invaginated and internalized during gastrulation. This is a rather large region and it might be expected that different regions of the organizer induce different structures along the axis of the embryo (i.e., brain and spinal cord).

Recall that the portion of the organizer which is first to become invaginated at the rim of the dorsal lip of the blastopore will reach furthest forward, coming to lie beneath the anterior end of the presumptive neural plate. The posterior region of the organizer is temporally last to turn in at the dorsal lip of the blastopore. It comes to lie beneath the presumptive spinal cord of the embryo. These temporal relationships between different regions of the organizer or chordamesoderm and the overlying ectoderm are summarized in Figure 10–13. By excising pieces of the dorsal lip at different times during gastrulation and transplanting them into cuts prepared on the surface of early gastrulas, it is possible to determine

10–12 A, diagram of Mangold's experiment in which dorsal lip of the early gastrula of *Triturus cristatus* was placed onto the lateral aspect of an early gastrulating embryo of *T. taeniatus;* B, the host embryo is induced by the dorsal lip transplant to form a secondary neural plate; C, subsequently, the host embryo shows a secondary embryo on its belly which includes ear vesicle, neural tube, and somites; D, transverse section through *Triturus* embryo showing structures of host and secondary embryo. (From H. Spemann, 1938. Embryonic Development and Induction. Yale University Press, New Haven.)

if regional or topographical differences exist in the organizer with respect to inductive capacities. When the dorsal lip of the early gastrula is transplanted, it acts primarily as a *head inductor*. It induces in the host embryo only head structures such as the formation of brain, eyes, and nose rudiments (Fig. 10–14 A). If the dorsal lip of the late gastrula is used as a donor graft, only trunk and tail structures are induced (Fig. 10–14 B). The graft acts as a *spinocaudal inductor*. Further experimental analysis of the head inductor indicates that it can be divided into an *archencephalic inductor* (stimulating formation of forebrain, optic cups, and nose primordia) and a *deuterencephalic inductor* (stimulating formation of hindbrain and inner ear vesicles).

The inducing capacity of the dorsal lip thus changes during gastrulation as the chordamesoderm invaginates. Consequently, the organizer is viewed as having regions that induce only certain parts or structures of the embryo. The presence of inductor tissue, however, does not assure that an induction will take place in host tissues. Several studies have demonstrated that the reacting cells, or those cells being induced, must be in a particular physiological state in order to differentiate under the influence of the inductor. This state of receptiveness to determinative stimuli is referred to as *competence*. Under the influence of the chordamesoderm, the differentiation of the neural tissues is an expression of the primary competence of the ectoderm. The ectoderm gradually loses its capacity to react to the inductive influence of the chordamesoderm between the gastrula and neurula stages of development. This can be demonstrated by transplanting the dorsal lip beneath the flank ectoderm of successively later stages of amphibian embryos. The decrease in neural competence with aging of the ectoderm has also been tested by isolating fragments of gastrula ectoderm, maintaining them for given intervals of time in culture, and then exposing each fragment to a strong inductor. Ectoderm that is not exposed to a chordamesodermal influence, or ectoderm exposed to the inductor at a very late stage of gastrulation, will differentiate as epidermis.

The loss of neural competence by the ectoderm with time does not prevent responsiveness by this germ layer to new and different inductive stimuli. Although the postgastrular ectoderm cannot be stimulated to form neural tissue, it does become competent to respond to other inductors. For example, the primary optic vesicle of the forebrain and the hindbrain induce the overlying ectoderm to form the eye lenses and the inner ear vesicles, respectively. Hence, the gradual and progressive elaborations of embryonic structures in all germ layers would appear to require successive states of competence along with a succession of inductors.

The inductive processes observed by Spemann and others in the

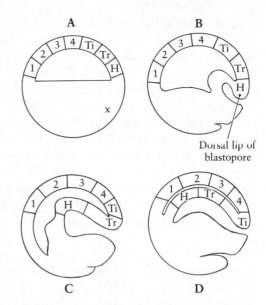

10–13 Diagram to show in longitudinal section the relative positions of the inductors within the chordamesoderm during different stages of amphibian development. A, late blastula; B, early gastrula; C, midgastrula; D, late gastrula. 1–4, different regions of the ectoderm; H, head inductor; Tr, trunk inductor; Ti, tail inductor; X, future position of the dorsal lip of the blastopore. By transplanting the dorsal lip of the blastopore at different times during gastrulation, the regional specificity of the chordamesoderm can be demonstrated.

10–14 A, if a transplant is made of dorsal lip at the early gastrula stage (*Triturus*), the host develops a second head; B, if the transplant of the dorsal lip is taken from a late gastrula, the host embryo develops an accessory tail. (After H. Mangold, 1932. Naturwissenschaften 20, 371.)

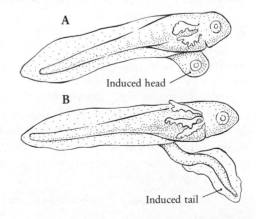

embryogenesis of the amphibian appear to be essentially the same in other anamniote and amniote embryos. The inducing action of the chordamesoderm has been experimentally tested in several vertebrate groups, including the cyclostomes, bony fishes, birds, and mammals. Waddington and his collaborators have succeeded in inserting grafts of the anterior half of the primitive streak of the chick, which includes Hensen's node, beneath a prepared cut in the ectoderm of the area pellucida (Fig. 10–15). This part of the primitive streak induces a secondary embryonic axis consisting of neural tube, notochord, and somites (Fig. 10–15). The posterior half of the primitive streak lacks the ability to stimulate neural plate formation in host ectoderm, presumably because the prospective fate of the cells migrating through this part of the streak is that of extraembryonic mesoderm. As with the dorsal lip of the amphibian gastrula, the anterior end of the primitive streak shows regional specificity with respect to inductive capacities. This has been demonstrated by removing Hensen's node at progressively later stages of primitive streak regression and transplanting it beneath host ectoderm.

The organizing action of the bird primitive streak does not appear to be species specific. The anterior end of the primitive streak of the duck can be isolated and grafted beneath the ectoderm of a chick embryo at a comparable stage of development (Fig. 10–16). The duck graft induces the host ectoderm to form a secondary neural tube (Fig. 10–16).

Very inadequate information is currently available on the chordamesoderm and its influence upon the overlying ectoderm in embryos of reptiles and mammals. Presumably, the ectoderm undergoes a spatial and temporal determination upon stimulation by the chordamesoderm cells, following the latter's displacement through the primitive streak, and becomes specified into different regions of the neural tube. Some work done with rabbit embryos shows that the ectoderm is competent to form neural tissue.

The fact that the primary organizer or chodamesoderm is capable of inducing the overlying ectoderm to form a neural plate explains several additional observations. We now know why there is a correlation between the width of the neural plate and the width of the primitive gut roof in different groups of vertebrates. Also, our understanding of the role of the organizer in primary determination has served to explain the basis for a number of teratological or abnormally developed types known as anterior, posterior, and cross-doubled embryos (*duplicitas anterior, duplicitas posterior,* and *duplicitas cruciata,* respectively). If the egg of a salamander is partially constricted with a hair loop along the plane of bilateral symmetry during the period of gastrulation, the invaginating chordamesoderm

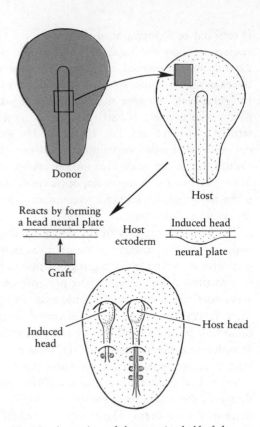

10–15 A portion of the anterior half of the primitive streak of the chick when transplanted beneath host ectoderm of a second embryo will induce an accessory head.

becomes split into two tongues of tissue upon contact with the strand of hair. Each finger-shaped piece of chordamesoderm then pushes forward on either side of the constriction at the blastopore. The resulting Y-shaped chordamesodermal sheet induces a pair of neural folds anteriorly. The resulting embryo appears to be doubled with two more or less perfectly formed anterior ends joined to a single posterior end. Doubling of both anterior and posterior ends of an embryo can also be obtained by grafting halves of gastrulas together in such a way that their organizers either converge or diverge anteriorly. If the Y-shaped chordamesoderm converges anteriorly, the embryo will be doubled at its posterior end.

The production of crossed-doubled embryos experimentally is particularly interesting. Two gastrula halves, each having a dorsal lip, are brought together with their sites of invagination opposite to each other (Fig. 10–17 A). The chordamesoderm of each gastrula-half moves in through its own blastopore. As the primitive archenteron of one gastrula meets the primitive archenteron of the other gastrula, each diverges to either side. The whole chordamesodermal complex takes on the appearance of a cross (Fig. 10–17 B). The portions of the cross at right angles to the plane of chordamesodermal migration are actually composites of the organizers of both gastrulas. Neural folds arise in the ectoderm over the cross-shaped organizer complex, producing a double embryo whose two heads and brains are at right angles to the axis of the trunks (Fig. 10–17 C). Each half-gastrula produces a posterior trunk region with spinal cord. However, each head and each brain are partly formed from both gastrulas.

INDUCTION—A CHEMICAL PROCESS

The discovery of the organizer-inductor property of the dorsal lip of the amphibian blastopore, and later of the anterior half of the primitive streak, provided a tremendous impetus to the discipline of experimental embryology. Particularly in the 1930s and 1940s, there was a frantic rush to uncover the nature and basis for neural induction. Questions regarding the interaction between cells of the chordamesoderm and cells of the overlying ectoderm were numerous. Was contact between the chordamesoderm and the ectoderm required in order for a successful induction to occur? Was it necessary for the chordamesodermal tissue to be viable and intact? Was the inductor a chemical substance, and, if so, could it be isolated and characterized? Where was the inductor located? What was the minimum period of time required for the inductor to stimulate the ectoderm to form neural tissue? The organizer concept of

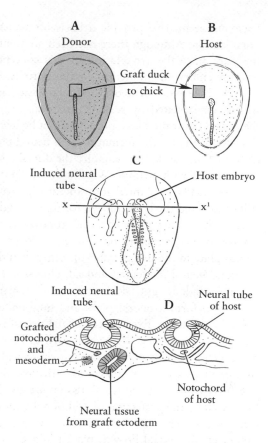

10–16 Diagrammatic drawing to show the induction of an accessory neural tube as a result of grafting notochordal tissue (Hensen's node) from a duck donor to a chick host. A, duck showing the location of the graft; B, chick host showing the site of the graft transplant; C, chick host showing induced accessory neural tube after 31.5 hours following graft transplant; D, section (transverse) at the level of X–X' in C to show induced neural tube. (From Foundations of Embryology by B. Patten and B. Carlson. Copyright © 1974 by McGraw-Hill, Inc. Used with permission of McGraw-Hill Book Company.)

Spemann seemed to provide a basis for understanding embryonic organization. Although there has been an accumulation of substantial data since the articulation of this concept, the mechanism of primary embryonic induction continues to be elusive.

The whole issue of neural induction was, and to a large extent still is, complicated by several rather surprising discoveries. First, the dorsal lip of the blastopore need not be living and its cells intact in order to induce the formation of a neural plate in the amphibian embryo. One can kill or denature the dorsal lip by heating, freezing, or treatment with alcohol. When a dorsal lip treated in this fashion is subsequently implanted into an early gastrula, neural induction still occurs and the host embryo forms a secondary embryonic axis.

Second, a wide variety of tissues (known as abnormal, foreign, or heterogeneous inductors because they do not actually induce the neural plate in the living embryo), other than the chordamesoderm, are good neural inductors. Indeed, almost any adult tissue, including liver, kidney, gut, skin, and so on, can induce competent ectoderm to form a neural plate and tube under the proper experimental conditions. Even pieces of the neural plate and neural tube are effective inducers. We are thus led to believe that the inductive principle or agent is nonspecific and either widely distributed in tissues or that various substances are effective inducing agents.

Efforts at determining which tissues are good inductors have been facilitated by the perfection of additional grafting techniques. In the original transplantation experiments by Spemann with the primary organizer, the dorsal lip was placed in a wound cut on the surface of the host embryo. Owing to its innate tendency to undergo invagination, the graft slips beneath the surface to become located in a position to influence the ectoderm (Fig. 10–18 A). Unfortunately, adult tissues do not possess the capacity for self-invagination. Mangold, therefore, developed a method whereby the tissue to be tested is placed directly into the blastocoele through a cut made in the roof of a late blastula or early gastrula (Fig. 10–18 B). As gastrulation progresses, the implanted tissue is pressed against the inner surface of the ectoderm by the invaginating chordamesoderm and endoderm. This method makes it possible to test the action of tissues older than the host and to determine the action of killed inductors. Subsequently, Holtfreter developed the *sandwich* or *explantation method* for the study of the inductive activity of various tissues. The inductor to be tested, often in the form of a centrifuged tissue homogenate, is placed between two strips of competent ectoderm excised from the animal hemisphere of a late blastula or early gastrula (Fig. 10–18 C). The free edges of the ectoderm fuse together, thus completely enclosing the inductor material.

Third, inductions can be experimentally produced with tissues

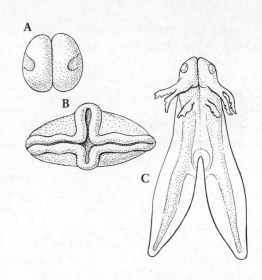

10–17 A, two dorsal gastrula halves of a salamander grafted together so that the directions of invagination of their blastopores are opposed; B, the cross-shaped appearance of the chordamesoderm following invaginations of the two gastrula halves; C, the resulting embryo showing crossed-doubling or duplicitas cruciata. Each half-gastrula has produced a posterior trunk region with spinal cord, but two heads and brains are formed at right angles to the axis of the trunks, each formed partly from both half-gastrulae. (After J. Huxley and G. DeBeer, 1934. Elements of Experimental Embryology. The Cambridge University Press, New York.)

from phylogenetically distant species. For example, tissues from *Hydra* and the guinea pig serve as effective inductors of neural plate in the salamander embryo.

Fourth, strong acids and alkalies, as well as salt and weak organic dyestuff solutions, can induce isolated, competent amphibian ectoderm to form neural tubes. It goes without saying that neural induction in vivo is clearly not initiated by sharp fluctuations in the pH of either the ectoderm or the chordamesoderm. However, since such diverse substances have inductive capacities, with many acting upon the reacting tissue by sublethal cytolysis (i.e., they cause cell injury through the destruction of cell membranes), some investigators believe that the key to understanding primary induction lies in the ectoderm. They argue that the process of neural induction involves the unmasking of some preexisting, inactive substance in the ectoderm, which then triggers the specific program of neural differentiation. Induction as an event of *evocation* will be examined in a later section of this chapter.

There are now several lines of evidence to indicate that neural differentiation is induced by substances that are chemical in nature and diffusible. Definition of the properties and characteristics of these chemical substances that function as inductive messengers during primary determination is largely based on *foreign inductors*. The diffusion hypothesis was originally set forth by Mangold. Whether direct cell contact between ectoderm and chordamesoderm layers, as initially proposed by Weiss in 1950, plays any role in primary embryonic induction is still a matter of question. Support for the diffusion hypothesis has come from a variety of studies in which filters of known porosity and thickness were inserted between inducer tissue and competent ectoderm. Gallera observed that neural induction occurred in the chick when a Millipore filter, 0.8 micrometers pore size and 20 micrometers in thickness, was inserted between the chordamesodermal inductor and competent ectoderm, thus indicating that the inducing stimulus must be soluble in order to pass through the filter. With the electron microscope, it was further seen that microvilli from the chordamesodermal cells had penetrated into the filter, but there was no evidence of cytoplasmic contact with the ectoderm. In a similar study with *Xenopus*, Nyholm and colleagues showed that filters as thick as 20 to 25 micrometers did not prevent induction. Although no fine, cellular processes were detected in the filters, a granular material apparently originating from the chordamesoderm was seen to a depth of two to four micrometers in the filter pores. These experiments indicate that at least the early stages of neural induction do not require cell-to-cell contact.

It is particularly interesting to note that recent studies by Kelly

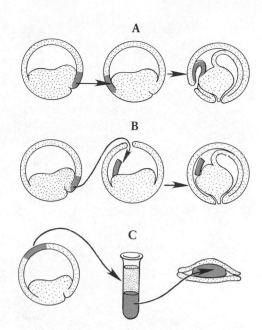

10–18   Three methods of exposing competent gastrula ectoderm to induction. A, transplantation of part of the dorsal lip onto the ventral, marginal surface of a second gastrula where it invaginates and forms a secondary archenteron; B, transplantation of part of the dorsal lip of the blastopore into the blastocoele through a slit in the animal hemisphere; C, inductor, such as centrifuged tissue homogenates, "sandwiched" between two pieces of presumptive ventral ectoderm.

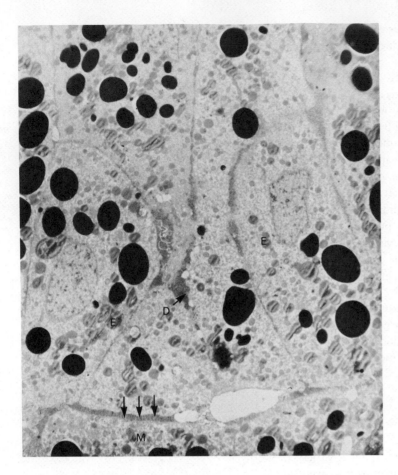

10–19 The ectoderm and chordamesoderm junction during neural induction in *Xenopus*. Aggregates of dark granules (D) are seen between the ectoderm (E) and chordamesoderm (M) layers. The arrows indicate the position of the chordamesodermal boundary. (From D. Tarin, 1972. J. Anat. 111, 1.)

(1969) and by Tarin (1972) report the presence of granules in the interzone between chordamesoderm and ectoderm during induction in *Xenopus* (Fig. 10–19). Many of these granules are sensitive to ribonuclease treatment, a property that aligns them to the active component of foreign inductors. (See studies of Yamada [1958] and Toivonen and Saxén [1968] below.) At present it is not known if the RNA-containing granules actually participate in the tissue interaction, whether they are transferred from one tissue to another, and what role the RNA plays in the inducing system.

Direct experimental evidence that the neural inductor is probably a diffusible molecule released from the chordamesoderm originated with classical studies by Niu and Twitty in 1953. They removed the dorsal lip of the blastopore from a salamander embryo and placed the tissue fragment in a small quantity of saline on the surface of a coverslip. The coverslip was then inverted over the hollow of a depression slide and sealed to prevent dessication. After 7 to 10 days, a fragment of competent ectoderm from the gastrula stage was added to the culture medium, now "conditioned" by the presence of dorsal lip tissue. Following a period of 24 hours, nerve and pigment cell types were detected in the medium (Fig. 10–20). If fragments of competent ectoderm were cultured in drops withdrawn from the original culture and containing no dorsal lip cells, nerve and pigment cells still differentiated from the ectodermal tissue. Competent ectoderm placed in Holtfreter's solution lacking dorsal lip tissue remained undifferentiated. If the chordamesoderm remained in the culture medium for 12 to 15 days, competent ectoderm incubated in drops of this conditioned medium differentiated into pigment, nerve, and precursor muscle cells. Niu and Twitty concluded that the chordamesoderm releases different substances into the medium. One appears early and induces neural tissue while the other appears later and induces mesodermal structures. Niu later found the conditioned medium to be rich in RNA and strongly suggested that this nucleic acid was the natural inducer.

During the last two decades, a number of studies have been conducted in an effort to analyze carefully the nature of inducing substances in gastrulating embryos and to determine if such substances actually pass from the chordamesoderm to the overlying ectoderm. Unfortunately, it has not been possible to obtain in sufficient quantities extracts of dorsal lip or primitive streak which will allow for detailed chemical analysis. However, a variety of adult tissues are known to display strong inductive capacities, imitating the action of the natural primary organizer. Extracts and pellets of these tissues have been made and the inducing power of the preparations subjected to various testing procedures. With few exceptions, each adult tissue is able to induce several kinds of structures. For example, Yamada and his colleagues in Japan use alcohol-treated guinea pig liver to induce primary archencephalic structures, such as brain vesicles and nose primordia. Guinea pig kidney following alcohol treatment is primarily a spinocaudal inductor; it stimulates the expression of spinal cord, notochord, and somites. Alcohol-treated guinea pig bone marrow induces almost exclusively the mesodermal structures found in the trunk of the embryo, these being notochord, somites, and kidney tubules. Tiedemann and his associates in Germany use an RNA-rich embryo extract, prepared from 9- to 11-day thick embryos, to induce structures of largely mesodermal origin.

The concept that neural induction may be due to the interaction of two chemically distinct inductive agents emerged from studies in which the inducing properties of adult tissues were experimentally

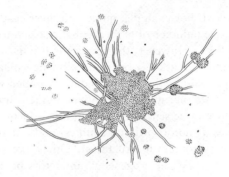

10–20 Chromatophores formed from gastrula ectoderm of *Triturus* after introduction into a 10-day-old culture conditioned by tissue presumptive to mesodermal structures of the tail and posterior part of the trunk. (After M. Niu and V. Twitty, 1953. Proc. Nat. Acad. Sci. U.S.A. 39, 985.)

altered. For example, guinea pig liver tissue continues to be an effective inductor of archencephalic structures even if heated to 70°C to 90°C. However, the spinocaudal inducing activity of guinea pig kidney is markedly reduced following similar heat treatment; yet, in some cases, the tissue induced archencephalic structures. This suggests that guinea pig kidney tissue contains two factors or substances, one sensitive to heat (and inducing such spinocaudal structures as notochord and somites) and one resistant to heat (and inducing forebrain structures). Other experiments employing these foreign (i.e., heterogeneous) inductors permit one to conclude that there are basically two responses during the induction process: *neuralization* and *mesodermalization*. Neuralization ultimately leads to the formation of cranial neural structures (forebrain, optic vesicles), whereas mesodermalization culminates in the expression of purely mesodermal structures (notochord, somites). Toivonen and Saxén proposed several years ago that two substances, extracted from a variety of tissues, were responsible for neuralization and mesodermalization: a *neuralizing agent* (thermostable and soluble in organic solvents such as petroleum ether) and a *mesodermalizing agent* (highly thermolabile and insoluble in organic solvents), respectively. The expression of mid- and postcranial structures, such as hindbrain and spinal cord, resulted from the combined action of the primary neuralizing and mesodermalizing agents.

Support for the "combined effect" hypothesis was obtained in elegant experiments by Toivonen and Saxén using pellets prepared from guinea pig tissues. Two pellets, one prepared from guinea pig liver (neuralizing action) and the other from guinea pig bone marrow (mesodermalizing action), were implanted simultaneously into the blastocoele of a young salamander gastrula (Fig. 10–21). The liver pellet alone induces only archencephalic structures. The bone marrow pellet alone induces only mesodermal structures. Together, however, the two pellets induce deuterencephalic and spinocaudal structures (hindbrain, inner ear vesicles, spinal cord) in the ectoderm, presumably because of the interaction of the diffusible, active components being released by the pellets.

Are the two proposed neuralizing and mesodermalizing agents two distinctly different substances or merely two different states of the same substance? Partial answers to these questions have been obtained from centrifuged fractions of heterogeneous tissues tested on isolated, competent ectoderm (Fig. 10–22). Generally, both ribonucleoprotein (PNP—pentose nucleoprotein) and protein fractions of these tissues have proved to be effective inductors. The active component of tissues inducing archencephalic and deuterencephalic structures appears to be a ribonucleoprotein (Fig. 10–22).

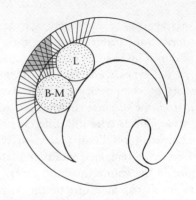

10–21 Simultaneous implantation of a neuralizing agent (L, liver) and a mesodermalizing agent (B–M, bone marrow) into the blastocoele of a salamander gastrula. Deuterencephalic and spinocaudal structures are induced where the effects of the two agents overlap. (From L. Saxén and S. Toivonen, 1962. Primary Embryonic Induction. Prentice-Hall, Englewood Cliffs.)

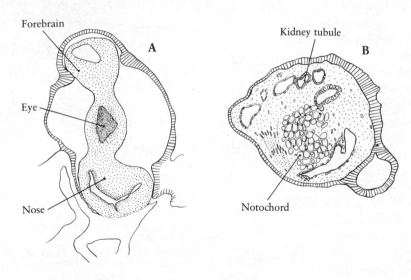

Forebrain

A

Eye

Nose

Kidney tubule

B

Notochord

10–22 A, nose, forebrain, and eye-type structures with pigment (archencephalic induction) induced by liver PNP in isolated *Triturus* ectoderm; B, notochord, somites, and kidney tubules are induced in isolated ectoderm by the non-nucleoprotein fraction of bone marrow. (After T. Yamada, 1958. Experientia 14, 81.)

Purification of the PNP by ultracentrifugation does not disturb its inducing capacity. Importantly, treatment of PNP fractions with ribonuclease does not reduce the original inducing capability of the preparation, thus suggesting that the nucleic acid moiety of the active agent is not the essential component of the inductor. However, archencephalic and deuterencephalic structures fail to develop if PNP fractions are treated with proteolytic enzymes such as pepsin. Indeed, there appears to be an enhancement of the differentiation of nonaxial structures in the presence of the treated fractions.

In short, the inductors of such axial structures as neural tube, notochord, and somites are proteins that may or may not be coupled with RNA. The mesodermalizing agent appears to be a protein that can be eluted from a chromatographic column at a pH of 7.0. The neuralizing agent appears to be ribonucleoprotein that can be eluted from a chromatographic column at a pH of 5.6. The presence of inducing activity in tissue ribonucleoprotein following ribonuclease treatment suggests that the nucleic acid component is not informationally essential in the inductive process. Recent studies by Niu conflict with this concusion. He claims that RNA extracted from calf testis (germ-cell RNA), when added to postnodal pieces of the definitive primitive streak of the chick, will induce a range of embryonic axial differentiations.

Assuming that the proteins of the neuralizing and medodermalizing agents are responsible for neural induction in the intact gastrulating embryo, where are they located and how are they organized to produce a combined action? The model of induction proposed by Toivonen and Saxén indicates that these substances are located in the chordamesodermal mantle or roof of the archenteron (Fig. 10–23). The regional differentiations along the axis of the embryo appear to be controlled by a balance between the neuralizing substance and the mesodermalizing substance, each of which is distributed in the form of a gradient. The dual gradient concept emerged from studies in which neural and predominantly mesodermal inductor cells were mixed semiquantitatively in various ratios and the cellular combinations then analyzed with respect to the types of neural and spinocaudal structures induced (Fig. 10–24). Forebrain was expressed when the combination consisted of only neural inductor cells. Progressive caudalization of neural structures was associated with a relative increase in the amount of the mesodermalizing inductor. Hence, the neuralizing agent is organized equally along the anteroposterior axis of the chordamesoderm with its highest concentration in the dorsal midline. It decines in concentration toward the lateral and ventral parts of the embryo. The mesodermalizing agent is absent from the extreme anterior region of the embryo. It begins in the presumptive hindbrain region of the embryo and progressively increases in concentration toward the tail.

The anterior end of the chordamesodermal layer (i.e., presumptive prechordal plate) produces only neuralizing agent and induces the ectoderm to form archencephalic structures. Slightly further in the posterior direction, the ectoderm is exposed to neuralizing agent and a small amount of mesodermalizing substance. This combination induces hindbrain and inner ear vesicles. As the relative amount of mesodermalizing to neuralizing substance increases in the anterior-to-posterior direction, trunk and tail structures are induced. The gradient of the neuralizing substance may also be responsible for the dorsal-to-ventral differentiations of such ectodermal derivatives as neural crest and sensory placodes (lens and nose primordia). Where the gradient of the neuralizing agent progressively diminishes, the ectoderm becomes epidermis. In the chordamesodermal mantle, the gradient of the mesodermalizing agent induces the differentiation of somites and lateral plates.

Nieuwkoop (1973) has put forth a slightly different hypothesis to explain the events of neural induction. He proposes that the ectoderm is initially determined to be a forebrain differentiation as a result of the activation of neural principles within its cells. A non-specific agent from the tip of the chordamesoderm induces this alteration in the overlying ectoderm as it slides forward during gastrulation. Subsequently, the activated ectoderm becomes transformed under the influence of a second agent released from the chordamesoderm. The differentiation of a given region of ectoderm is the result of a balance between the initial archencephalic tendency and the length of time that this layer has been exposed to the

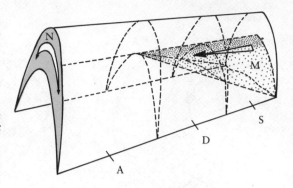

10–23 The two-gradient model of Saxén and Toivonen. The chordamesoderm contains both a neuralizing agent (N) and a mesodermalizing agent (M). The neuralizing agent is distributed in gradient fashion from dorsal to ventral. The mesodermalizing agent increases in concentration from the level of the future hindbrain to the tail of the embryo. A, D, S, levels of archencephalic, deuterencephalic, and spinocaudal inductions, respectively. (From L. Saxén and S. Toivonen, 1962. Primary Embryonic Induction. Prentice-Hall, Englewood Cliffs.)

10–24 Percentage of neural structures belonging to the central nervous system induced in experiments in which two types of foreign inductors were mixed in different ratios. (From L. Saxén and S. Toivonen, 1961. J. Embryol. Exp. Morphol. 9, 514.)

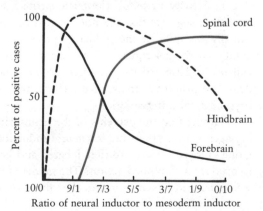

transforming agent. Since the posterior ectoderm is first to be influenced by the transforming agent, it is exposed for a longer period of time than the anterior ectoderm and therefore differentiates as trunk and spinal cord. The *activating* and *transforming agents* of Nieuwkoop are probably equivalent to the neuralizing and mesodermalizing agents, respectively, of Toivonen and Saxén. Both induction models are quite similar if one assumes that neuralizing and mesodermalizing agents are released at different rates or at different times from the chordamesodermal mantle.

That regionalization of the central nervous system is complex and cannot be due simply to a single inductive event has been experimentally shown by Saxén and his colleagues using the techniques of disaggregation and reaggregation (Fig. 10–25). Competent ectodermal cells from an amphibian gastrula were isolated and exposed to either guinea pig liver (culture A) or guinea pig bone marrow (culture B). Approximately 24 hours later, the inductors were removed from each culture, and the ectodermal cells disaggregated into single cell populations. When the suspensions were allowed to reaggregate, the cells in culture A formed forebrain and optic cups while those in culture B formed spinal cord, muscle blocks, kidney tubules, and notochord. However, if the two types of induced suspensions were mixed and cultured as a combined aggregate, hindbrain and inner ear vesicles were readily formed. It can be concluded that these structures were determined after the initial period of induction and before the regionalization of the central nervous system was stabilized. If presumptive forebrain cells from young amphibian neurulas are cultured in mixed aggregates of axial mesodermal cells, they can be "transformed" into hindbrain and spinal cord structures. Interestingly, a gradual increase in the ratio of axial mesodermal to forebrain cells results in the gradual caudalization of the central nervous system derivatives (Fig. 10–26).

These experiments strongly indicate that primary embryonic induction is a multistep process. During a short initial phase, the ectoderm of the embryo is probably determined in either a neural or mesodermal direction. Without further influence, cells determined in the neural direction will become forebrain structures. However, continued mesodermal influence alters their further morphogenetic pattern into caudal-neural structures. This secondary interaction, which affects the specificity of morphogenetic expression, operates in a quantitative fashion and acts to stabilize the initial determination.

It must be remembered that much of what we know concerning primary embryonic induction is based upon studies using heterogeneous (i.e., foreign) tissue inductors. Required is proof that inductor protein is present, located in the chordamesodermal mantle, and

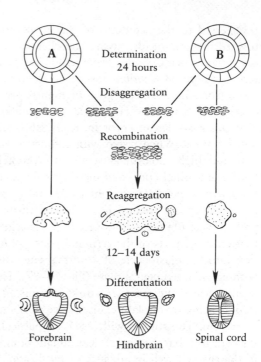

10–25 Experimental procedure demonstrating the differentiation of the central nervous system in cultures of competent ectoderm exposed to guinea pig liver (A) and bone marrow (B) utilizing the techniques of disaggregation and reaggregation. (From L. Saxén, S. Toivonen and T. Vainio, 1964. J. Embryol. Exp. Morphol. 12, 333.)

transferred to the ectoderm of the intact embryo. Some progress toward the goal of identifying and characterizing natural inductors is currently being made. From crude extracts prepared from different regions of *Xenopus* gastrulas, Deuchar has determined that those from the dorsal lip give the highest percentages of neural induction. Others have succeeded in separating whole extracts of *Xenopus* gastrulas into protein, RNA, RNA-protein, and DNA-protein fractions. When tested with competent ectoderm, certain protein and high molecular weight RNA-protein fractions induced hindbrain, spinal cord, and mesodermal structures. A protein fraction with a molecular weight of 25,000 to 30,000, isolated from chick embryonic tissues, has a mesodermalizing effect upon amphibian gastrula ectoderm. Recently, Malacinski (1974) has shown that crude extracts of the germinal vesicle of *Rana*, following injection into the blastocoele of a normal embryo, produce an embryo with an enlarged neural plate (Fig. 10–27). The substance or active agent, termed the *axial structure determinant* (ASD), is characterized as being thermolabile, insensitive to ribonuclease, but sensitive to trypsin. The studies with ASD are particularly exciting because they suggest that the neural determinant or inductor may be present in the egg cell well in advance of fertilization. Its association with the grey crescent or presumptive chordamesoderm is indicated by experiments in which UV-treated frog embryos can be corrected by the microinjection of crude extracts of germinal vesicle plasm. Ultraviolet irradiation normally alters the grey crescent and produces embryos with defective neural structures.

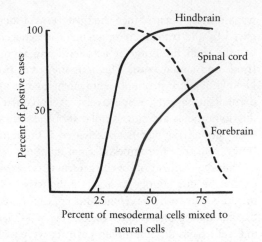

10–26 Percentage of neural derivatives (forebrain, hindbrain, and spinal cord) formed when cells of the axial mesoderm are mixed with neural cells of the forebrain region (neurulae). (From S. Toivonen and L. Saxén, 1968. Science 159, 539. Copyright 1968 by the American Association for the Advancement of Science.)

THE MODE OF ACTION OF THE INDUCTOR

There are two schools of thought, although not necessarily with an equal number of adherents, regarding the location of the substance(s) responsible for neural induction within the embryo. Since a wide spectrum of agents can induce competent ectoderm by sublethal cytolysis to form neural structures, there are those, particularly Waddington and his colleagues, who are inclined to believe that the inductor is resident within the cytoplasm of the reacting cells. According to them induction involves the unmasking, probably by some nonspecific signal (*indirect evocator*) of the inductor molecule (*direct evocator*) in the ectoderm. Activation of the direct evocator stimulates the transformation of the ectodermal cells into neural cells. Additional support for the views of Waddington on neural induction come from the phenomenon of *autoneuralization*. Competent ectoderm in salt solutions will form a neural tube in the

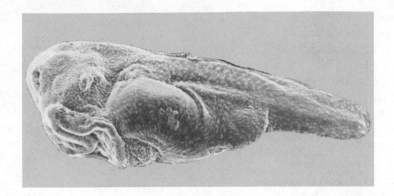

10–27 Microinjection of germinal vesicle plasm into the blastula of a frog embryo results in the development of an enlarged neural plate and a macrocephalic embryo. (From G. Malacinski, 1974. Cell Differ. 3, 31.)

absence of any inducer substance (i.e., self-neuralization). This suggests that all factors for neuralization are present in the responding ectoderm and simply await to be activated.

Chiefly from studies in vitro in which the induction process has been analyzed using selected filters interposed between interacting tissues, most investigators are of the opinion that primary embryonic induction is a case of the transmission of specific inductive stimuli across the ectodermal–chordamesodermal junction. Unfortunately, the characterization of the inductive substances has been limited, as previously pointed out, and concrete evidence for the passage of substances from the chordamesodermal mantle to the overlying ectoderm in the intact embryo is disappointing and still largely lacking. Experiments have been conducted in which competent ectoderm has been cultured with chordamesodermal tissue tagged with radioactive amino acids or fluorescently labeled proteins. Because label is detected in the ectoderm following induction, the results from such experiments are suggestive of a signal transfer between inducer tissue and the reacting ectoderm. However, there is still some question as to whether the labeled compounds were essential to the induction process. Also, it must be pointed out that induction does not always occur with the transfer of these labeled compounds.

Assuming that diffusible signals are involved in neural induction, how do they act upon the target ectocerm and what are the responses of the ectoderm. Some insight into these questions has been obtained by determining if synthetic mechanisms are stimulated into action during gastrulation and by establishing if these activities are essential to the process of neural differentiation. We now know on the basis of a variety of studies that the genes of the embryo, after being largely inactive through the period of cleavage and blastulation, begin to express themselves during gastrulation and subseqently assume greater control over the processes directing the development of the embryo. Evidence for the increased level of nuclear activity at gastrulation, manifested in the appearance of new proteins, enzymes, and nucleic acids, has been obtained, in part, from certain interspecific hybridization experiments.

A *true hybrid embryo* is formed by taking the egg of one species and fertilizing it, either naturally or artificially, with the spermatozoon of a second species (i.e., *Rana pipiens* ♀ X *Rana sylvatica* ♂). The extent to which these hybrid embryos will develop depends in great measure upon the phylogenetic distance between the two parents. Closely related species of the same genus are often able to produce hybrids capable of normal and complete development. In many interspecific hybrids of the genus *Rana,* however, the hybirds may develop through cleavage and blastulation, but become arrested at the gastrula stage. By contrast, viable hybrids between species of different genera, or even between genera of different families, have been produced in fishes.

The fertilized egg formed by a hybrid cross consists of maternal cytoplasm (the contribution by the spermatozoon of cytoplasm to the fertilized egg is negligible) and a nucleus, half of which is maternal and half of which is paternal in origin. The detection during development of gene products formed at the direction of the paternal chromosomes serves to mark that point in time when the genes of the embryo become active. The markers of this gene activity may be RNA, proteins, and individual enzymes or structural proteins.

In recent years, there has developed an increasing appreciation for the fact that enzymes, such as lactate dehydrogenase (LDH) and malate dehydrogenase (MDH), commonly exist in multiple molecular forms known as *isozymes*. A prominent feature of isozymes is that their distribution in adult tissues and organs is specific (i.e., the tissues and organs have characteristic distributions of activity of the multiple molecular forms). Additionally, variation in the number and properties of these molecular forms of an enzyme often exist between species of a given genus. For example, LDH is a tetramer that shows five forms of the enzyme in most vertebrate species. These five forms arise from the random combination of two distinct subunits (subunit A and subunit B). In the brook trout, the A subunit migrates more rapidly toward the anode in an electrical field (*electrophoresis*) than the A subunit of the lake trout. Since these subunits are distinguishable and represent products of gene loci, a comparison of LDH patterns during development of hybrids between the two parental species provides valuable information on the time of activation of the embryo's genes.

Interspecific hybridization studies of this type reveal that gastrulation is a period of major gene activity, expressed in the synthesis of a variety of new proteins and enzymes. As one might also suspect, there is positive evidence that the mRNA synthesized during gastrulation is quite different from that present in the cytoplasm of the egg or the cells of the blastula, thus indicating that genes previously inactive become active at this particular time of development. The observation that sequences of DNA are being transcribed for the first time at gastrulation was determined using an elegant technique known as DNA-RNA hybridization (Fig. 10–28). Likewise, supportive components in the chain of events leading to the formation of proteins, such as tRNA and rRNA, are known to be transcribed from nuclear genes at this time.

Since the activation of genes during gastrulation and the resulting synthesis of proteins are manifestations of the developing embryo, it is important to ask whether these activities are associated with the ectoderm and critical to the event of neural induction. A number of biochemical changes, apparently essential to neural differentiation, are detectable in the neural ectoderm immediately following induction. In *Triturus,* the neural plate contains several antigens not present in the ordinary epidermis. Using immunoelectrophoretic methods, Stanisstreet and Deuchar (1972) have shown that one of the earliest features of neural differentiation in *Xenopus* in response to induction by dorsal gastrula mesoderm is an increase in the concentration of three antigenic components when compared to ventral or noninduced ectoderm. Indeed, this particular biochemical change in the neural ectoderm is detected prior to any visible sign of the neural plate.

Neural induction, therefore, like any other mechanism that controls differentiative processes in embryonic cells, appears to act by initiating the synthesis of new proteins in the target cells. Is the presence of new protein in the neural ectoderm evidence of gene activity? Are these proteins essential for successful induction to occur? Partial answers to these questions are available based upon experiments in which inhibitors have been used to block key steps in the synthetic activities of the neural ectoderm.

If the dorsal lips of young *Triturus* gastrulas are cultured in either actinomycin D (transcriptional inhibitor) or puromycin (translational inhibitor) and then the treated tissue confronted with competent ectoderm, induction still occurs and the ectoderm responds by forming neural structures. This suggests that neither the transcription of mRNA nor the synthesis of proteins that may take place in the chordamesoderm at the time of gastrulation is essential for induction to occur. However, if the dorsal lip is explanted with the adjacent ectoderm and then treated with sufficient concentrations of actinomycin D to block synthesis of mRNA, the ectoderm will not differentiate into neural plate. Hence, for the reacting cells to move in the direction of neuralization, the formation of mRNA

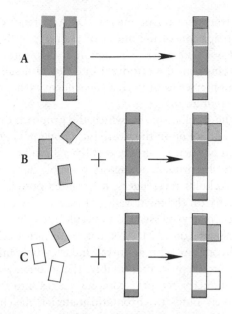

10–28 The purpose of DNA-RNA hybridization is to permit the investigator to determine whether mRNA synthesized at one stage of development (i.e., gastrulation) is the same as or different from mRNA formed at another stage of development (i.e., cleavage). Advantage is taken of the known binding specificity between whole sequences of bases of DNA and complementary bases of RNA. The principal steps in the technique are shown here with two transcriptive sites. A, double-stranded DNA is separated by heating into two single DNA strands; B, mRNA from the cleavage stage is added to one of the single DNA strands and hybridizes with the complementary section of the DNA; C, mRNA from the gastrula stage is then added and only those mRNAs that are different from the cleavage stage will attach to the DNA. The proportion of mRNA molecules that fail to hybridize gives an indication of the similarity in the mRNAs between the two stages.

by transcription of nuclear DNA is required. Without the active participation of the nuclei of the target cells, neural differentiation will not take place. The action of the neural inductor is not simply to transform the ectoderm into neural tissue, but rather to set into motion a series of nuclear-dependent events that will lead to neural differentiation.

The mechanism by which the proposed diffusible, chemical substances act upon the overlying ectoderm to stimulate a specific program of nuclear activity is still a subject of considerable speculation. Since the primary inductors resemble hormones in that they act as intercellular messengers, it has been postulated that they either act directly on the membranes of target cells, stimulating the release of a secondary messenger molecule (possibly adenosine 3',5' monophosphate or cAMP), or enter the target cells by simple diffusion and complex with an intracellular cytoplasmic-specific binding protein or receptor. Presumably, the secondary messenger molecule or the inductor-receptor complex passes into the nucleus where it selectively binds to chromatin material, thereby derepressing specific genes for transcription of mRNA. Unfortunately, there have been few studies to test the validity of these hypotheses. The cAMP secondary messenger hypothesis has recently been tested by Wahn and his associates (1975). They excised presumptive epidermis from the dorsal lip stage of several amphibian species and cultured the tissue fragments with various nucleotide compounds, including 3',5' monophosphate (dibutyryl cAMP). Although their results varied somewhat from one species of amphibian to another, in all cases several cell types characteristic of neural differentiation were recognizable in those cultures treated with dibutyryl cAMP. Their experiments do not prove per se that cAMP is the normal agent mediating the effects of the primary inductors. Further work is required to determine if, in fact, there is a rise in cAMP activity in presumptive neural plate cells during primary induction.

L. G. Barth and L. T. Barth, long interested in the problems of embryonic induction, have offered an hypothesis (1969) that attempts to associate local physiological factors, such as changes in ion concentrations, with consequent modification of gene activity leading to differentiation. They argue strongly that the actual process of induction is initiated by an alteration in cell membrane properties of the target ectoderm which, in turn, results in the release and redistribution of cations within the cells. Their hypothesis also holds that there are no net changes in total ion concentration, but only a change in the ratio of bound to free ions in the cells of the early gastrula. Their observations are based upon an extensive series of experiments in which it could be demonstrated that induction of nerve and pigment cells in the presumptive epidermis of the frog gastrula was dependent upon the concentration of the sodium ion in the culture medium. Nerve and pigment cells were induced at a sodium concentration of 88 millimolars; no inductions occurred at a lower concentration (44 mM). The dramatic increase in intracellular sodium during the period of induction would appear to promote neuralization. Whether free cations may regulate gene expression in the target cells of ectoderm by freeing segments of DNA from their histones is still very unclear. Sodium might compete with neighboring groups on DNA during induction, thereby resulting in a series of anabolic processes leading to the differentiation of neural tissue. Since the regulation of many metabolic processes and ionic concentrations is cAMP dependent, it is conceivable that the adenosine $3',5'$ monophosphate may play a role in the modification of the ratio of bound to free cations during induction.

Most of the investigators studying neural induction consider only the initial reactions of the target cells. Yet there is some evidence that communication between the target ectodermal cells may be an important aspect of the inductive process. Deuchar (1970) has shown that a minimum number of cells is necessary for neural differentiation in *Xenopus*. The success of neuralization appears to depend in this frog upon an adequate number of ectodermal cells. No neural differentiation was visible when less than 10 ectodermal cells from the neural plate region of late gastrulas were cultured with mesodermal cells. However, groups of fewer than 10 cells, when first cultured with dorsal lip and then seeded into a larger ectodermal mass, were able to stimulate the latter to form neural structures. The quality of the neural differentiation, therefore, possibly depends upon some second-stage interaction between the ectodermal cells.

REFERENCES

Barth, L. G. and L. T. Barth. 1969. The sodium dependence of embryonic induction. Dev. Biol. 20:236–262.

Deuchar, E. 1970. Neural induction and differentiation with minimal numbers of cells. Dev. Biol. 22:185–199.

Gallera, J., G. Nicolet, and M. Baumann. 1968. Induction neurale chez le oiseaux à travers un filtre millipore: Etude au microscope optique et électronique. J. Embryol. Exp. Morphol. 9:439–450.

Karfunkel, P. 1971. The role of microtubules and microfilaments in neurulation in *Xenopus laevis*. Dev. Biol. 25:30–56.

Karfunkel, P. 1972. The activity of microtubules and microfilaments in neurulation in the chick. J. Exp. Zool. 181:289–302.

Kelly, R. O. 1969. A electron microscopic study of chordamesoderm-neuroectoderm association in gastrulae of a toad, *Xenopus*. J. Exp. Zool. 172:153–179.

Malacinski, G. 1974. Biological properties of a presumptive morphogenetic determinant from the amphibian oocyte germinal vesicle nucleus. Cell Differ. 3:31–44.

Nieukoop, P. D. 1973. The "organization center" of the amphibian embryo: Its origin, spatial organization, and morphogenetic action. Adv. Morphog. 10:1–39.

Niu, M. and V. Twitty. 1953. The differentiation of gastrula ectoderm in medium conditioned by axial mesoderm. Proc. Nat. Acad. Sci. U.S.A. 39:985–989.

Portch, P. and A. Barson. 1974. Scanning electron microscopy of neurulation in the chick. J. Anat. 117:341–350.

Saxén, L., S. Toivonen, and T. Vainio. 1968. Initial stimulus and subsequent interactions in embryonic induction. J. Embryol. Exp. Morphol. 12:333–338.

Saxén, L. and S. Toivonen. 1962. Primary Embryonic Induction. London: Logos Press.

Schroeder, T. E. 1973. Cell constriction: Contractile role of microfilaments in division and development. Am. Zool. 13:949–960.

Spemann, H. 1938. Embryonic Development and Induction. New Haven, Conn.: Yale University Press.

Spemann, H. and H. Mangold. 1924. Über Induktion von Embryonalanlagen durch Implantation artfremder organisatoren. Wilhelm Roux' Arch. Entwicklungsmech. Org. 100:599–638.

Stanisstreet, M. and E. Deuchar. 1972. Appearance of antigenic material in gastrula ectoderm after neural induction. Cell Differ. 1:15–18.

Tarin, D. 1971. Scanning electron microscopical studies of the embryonic surface during gastrulation and neurulation in *Xenopus laevis*. J. Anat. 109:535–547.

Tarin, D. 1972. Ultrastructural features of neural induction in *Xenopus laevis*. J. Anat. 111:1–28.

Toivonen, S. and L. Saxén. 1968. Morphogenetic interaction of presumptive neural and mesoderm cells mixed in different ratios. Science 159:539–540.

Waddington, C. H. 1966. Principles of Development and Differentiation. New York: Macmillan.

Waddington, C. H. and G. A. Schmidt. 1933. Induction by heteroplastic grafts of the primitive streak of birds. Wilhelm Roux' Arch. Entwicklungsmech. Org. 128:522–563.

Wahn, H., L. Lightbody, T. Tchen, and J. Taylor. 1975. Induction of neural differentiation in cultures of amphibian undetermined presumptive epidermis by cyclic AMP derivatives. Science 188:366–368.

Yamada, T. 1958. Induction of specific differentiation by samples of proteins and nucleoproteins in the isolated ectoderm of *Triturus* gastrulae. Experientia 14:81–87.

11

Communication Between Nucleus and Cytoplasm—The Basis of Cellular Heterogeneity

The earliest stages in the life of the embryo are characterized by a certain amount of morphogenesis, manifest in the multiplication of cells and their organization into the blastula, and such intracellular events as membrane formation, mitotic spindle assembly, and the synthesis of proteins and nucleic acids. As we have seen in several animal groups, the various activities involved in the morphological and biochemical changes of the early embryo are not controlled directly by the genomes of its cells. Instead, they are controlled directly by constituents produced during oogenesis under maternal influence and stored in the cytoplasm. It is at the time of gastrulation that the embryo enters an extended period during which a vast array of new, specialized cell types appear and become rigidly ordered into tissues and organs. Hence, embryonic cells that are initially alike gradually come to acquire specialized functions.

The development and expression of specialized cell types and tissues is a central theme of embryogenesis. The process by which cells acquire distinctive morphology and function is known as *cell differentiation*. The differentiated cell is a unique functional phenotype, as reflected in its ability to synthesize tissue-specific proteins and assemble distinctive cytoplasmic organelles. The transition between the undifferentiated cell (or one without immediate specialized structure and function) and the differentiated cell is gradual, tends to occur at rather specific times during development, and generally requires the translation of a particular set of mRNAs. A major step toward the development of functionally different cells occurs in vertebrate embryos during gastrulation with the formation of ectoderm, mesoderm, and endoderm. Each of these broadly determined cell lines serves as a progenitor for cell populations that will undergo visible differentiation at selected stages of the postgastrular period.

The development of different cell types within a multicellular system is often dependent upon interactions with neighboring cell populations (i.e., induction phenomena). This communication may be effected either through contacts or specialized junctions between contiguous cells or by the movement of diffusible signal substances that pass through extracellular fluids. Ultimately, however, the acquisition of the unique properties associated with a differentiated cell is genotypic in origin and depends upon the control and regulation of pathways within the cell itself. In other words, the process of cell differentiation is promoted by the utilization of genetic information within the nucleus of the cell.

As previously pointed out, some 19th-century embryologists considered that differentiation could be accounted for on the basis of a parceling out of qualitatively diverse nuclear determinants to different cell nuclei. Specialization of cell type would then represent the temporal expression of a mosaic of partial cell genomes. Hence, each nucleus was viewed as possessing only those "genes" required to program the cell for a particular set of functional activities. We now know, largely on the basis of nuclear transfer experiments and spectrophotometric analyses of the DNA content within cells, that both undifferentiated and differentiated cells contain the same complete genome. The genome is biochemically and informationally equivalent to that present in the zygote nucleus. If the structural and functional characteristics of a cell are dependent upon its genome and if there is an equivalence of genomes between diverse cell types, then the proposition results that cell specialization involves the expression of selective portions of the genome. Since the relationship between the nucleotide sequence of DNA and the specificity of proteins found within a cell is now well established, different cell types must realize their characteristics as a result of the activity of different genes. Various types of evidence now lead us to believe that only a small fraction of the nucleotide sequence of DNA is transcribed in a differentiated cell. Most of the genetic information is regarded as being repressed or inhibited. An interesting question, therefore, is how large segments of the genome become progressively silenced as a cell passes from the undifferentiated to the differentiated state.

These two observations—that in any differentiated cell type only a small portion of the genes are transcribed at any given time and that most of the genome is repressed—form the basis of the *variable gene theory of differentiation*. Within the past 25 years, a variety of sources have contributed a rather substantial body of data to support this theory. How different genes are regulated to control the patterns of flow of genetic information within the cell is currently a question of major concern to developmental biologists. Theoretically, the regulation of gene activity can occur at any step between the transcription and the formation of a functional protein. Generally, however, the differentiated state of a cell is viewed as depending upon mechanisms controlling the selection of specific DNA sequences for transcription and translation.

MORPHOLOGICAL AND CYTOLOGICAL MANIFESTATIONS OF NUCLEOCYTOPLASMIC INTERACTIONS

The differentiation of any specific cell type requires a complex of interactions between nucleus and cytoplasm, most details of which are still imperfectly understood. The nucleus is obviously important in differentiation because it is the location of the genetic information that specifies the instructions for the synthesis of tissue-specific proteins. The cytoplasm has been shown to affect nuclear behavior, and during embryogenesis it assumes a primary role in determining the time and place for the expression of specific genes. The required interaction between nucleus and cytoplasm in establishing differences between cells has been demonstrated at the morphological, cytological, and molecular levels of biological organization.

One approach to exploring nucleocytoplasmic interactions has been by the techniques of grafting and nuclear transplantation. *Acetabularia* is a marine, unicellular green alga that has been extensively used for experimental studies on nucleocytoplasmic interactions. The mature cell is rather cylindrical and consists of the rhizoid, the stalk or stem (4–6 cm in length), and an apical cap (up to 1 cm in diameter) (Fig. 11–1 A). The nucleus of the cell resides in the basal portion or rhizoid. Various species of *Acetabularia* tend to show variations in the size and shape of the cap. In *A. crenulata,* the cap is lobate in shape with many fingerlike projections while the cap of *A. mediterranea* is smooth and circular (Fig. 11–1 A).

The large size of this single cell permits portions of the cytoplasm

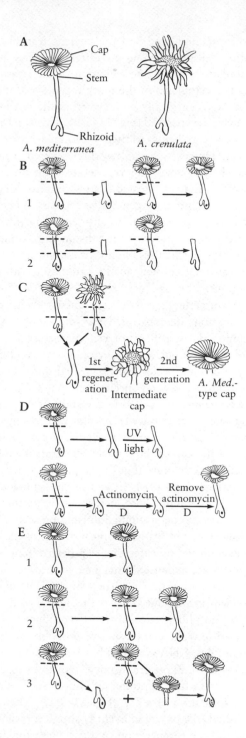

11–1 Nucleocytoplasmic interactions in the unicellular alga, *Acetabularia*. A, the structural organization of the cell in two species of *Acetabularia*. Note the differences in the shape of the cap between *A. mediterranea* and *A. crenulata;* B, a nucleated fragment from which the cap has been removed will repeatedly regenerate a new cap (1). A stem from which the cap has been removed will regenerate a new cap for only one generation (2); C, a uninucleate graft formed by an *A. mediterranea* rhizoid and a capless *A. crenulata* stem will regenerate a cap intermediate in characteristics between the two species. The cap of the second generation will have the characteristics of the species donating the nucleus; D, cap regeneration is sensitive to UV irradiation and actinomycin D; E, the nucleus divides when the cap reaches maximum size (1). If the cap is removed prior to reaching this size, the nucleus never divides (2). Grafting of a mature cap to a young rhizoid prematurely induces division of the nucleus (3).

to be manipulated and the nucleus transplanted or grafted to another cell of the same or different species. Such experimental manipulations allow an evaluation of the relative roles of the nucleus and/or cytoplasm in the morphogenesis of this cell. For example, if the cap is surgically removed from the rest of the cell, a new cap is quickly regenerated (Fig. 11–1 B). This can be successively repeated, a new cap being formed as long as there remains a nucleated stem. However, a capless stem severed from the rhizoid (i.e., an enucleated stem) can regenerate only once (Fig. 11–1 B). Additionally, if an enucleated stem is cut into three pieces, each fragment shows a different regenerative capacity. These observations indicate that cap regeneration, a light-dependent phenomenon, is under nuclear control and requires substances passing from the nucleus into the cytoplasm. Presumably, these substances are organized in an apical-basal gradient in the cytoplasm with the highest concentration near the cap.

Hammerling's classic experiments on interspecific nuclear transplantations demonstrated the importance of the nucleus in determining the specificity of cell characteristics. To establish the contributions of nucleus and cytoplasm in cap formation, an enucleated stem of one species can be grafted onto the nucleated fragment or rhizoid of a second species (Fig. 11–1 C). When the rhizoid of A. mediterranea is grafted to the stalk of A. crenulata from which the cap has been removed, the first cap to regenerate is an intergrade having features characteristic of the caps of both species (Fig. 11–1 C). If the cap of the interspecific graft is now severed, the regenerated cap resembles that of the parent which supplied the nucleated fragment (Fig. 11–1 C). Since the initial cap of an interspecific hybrid is intermediate in form, it is presumed that the cytoplasm contains cap-determining information stored from both species. The absence of cap features typical of one of the species after the initial regeneration indicates that cap-determining substances of the graft species are exhausted after one generation.

Information flowing from the nucleus appears to be responsible for cap formation. What is the nature of this nuclear information? The morphogenetic substances produced by the nucleus and released into the cytoplasm are probably in the form of stable RNA molecules. RNA synthesis has been shown to be essential in cap regeneration. Exposure of nucleated stalks to UV irradiation or treatment with transcriptional inhibitors such as actinomycin D prevent the formation of a cap (Fig. 11–1 D). The same nucleated rhizoid washed free of actinomycin D shows a resumption of RNA synthesis and the regeneration of a cap. Presumably, stable informational mRNAs produced by the nucleus are released into the stem where they are stored. Upon activation, these informational molecules are translated into proteins required for cap morphogenesis. Although these molecules are supplied by transcription of nuclear DNA, their expression is apparently regulated by control mechanisms in the cytoplasm.

Various processes in *Acetabularia* also demonstrate that activities within the cytoplasm strongly influence nuclear activity. Normally, the primary nucleus in this organism divides successively to produce numerous, small secondary nuclei when its cap reaches a maximum size. These secondary nuclei are carried by protoplasmic streaming into the cap where each forms a cyst. After a period of encystment, each secondary nucleus matures into a single gamete. If the cap of *Acetabularia* is excised prior to reaching its normal size, the divisions of the primary nucleus do not occur (Fig. 11–1 E). Division of this organelle to produce daughter nuclei will be delayed until a cap size of maximum dimensions has been produced. Conversely, division of the primary nucleus can be induced prematurely by grafting an enucleated fragment having a mature cap onto a young nucleated rhizoid without a cap (Fig. 11–1 E).

Evidence that variable gene activity can be correlated with cell type comes from a variety of studies in which alterations of the physiological activities of cells commence with visible changes in the gross organization of chromosomes. Since the late 1800s, it has been known that certain tissues of the Diptera, such as the salivary glands, Malpighian tubules, midgut, and rectum, possess highly visible, *giant* or *polytene chromosomes* (Fig. 11–2 A,B). The large size of each of these chromosomes reflects certain peculiarities in the growth of larval tissues, namely that the tissues grow by hypertrophy rather than by ordinary cell division. Consequently, the DNA replicates without chromosomal duplication. A mature, polytene chromosome contains up to 1024 strands of DNA. In various regions, portions of the chromosome are typically uncoiled and thrown into a series of lateral puffs and *Balbiani rings* (Fig. 11–2 B). Puffs have been the focus of considerable research over the past 30 to 40 years because their appearance on chromosomes coincides with changes in cellular functions.

Regions of a chromosome occupied by puffs appear to be sites of active gene expression. When giant chromosomes are exposed to radioactive precursors for RNA and protein syntheses, there is rapid incorporation of the label into the puffs. Also, puff regression is accompanied by a corresponding decrease in the uptake of labeled amino acid or uridine.

Patterns of puff formation and regression are particularly in evidence during *insect metamorphosis* when there are dramatic structural and physiological alterations in the activities of the insect's cells. Hemimetabolous insects, such as cockroaches and locusts,

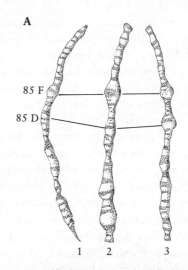

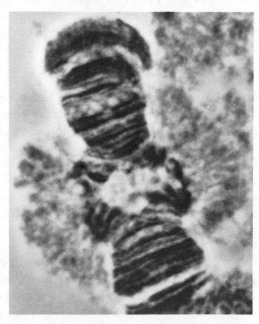

11–2 A, reconstructions of the puffing sequence in the proximal arm of chromosome III in *Drosophila*. The numbers refer to specific bands of this polytene chromosome (After M. Ashburner, 1967. Chromosoma 21, 398); B, a photograph of chromosome III in *Chironomus pallidivitatus* showing a large or giant puff (Balbiani ring). (From U. Grossback, 1973. Cold Spring Harbor Symp. Quant. Biol. 38, 619.)

pass through several larval stages or *molts* before they assume the adult form. In holometabolous insects, such as beetles, moths, and flies, the larva is transformed into a pupa stage before reaching adulthood. These major molts, from larval to pupal stages and from pupal to adult stages, are termed *metamorphoses*. Larval, pupal, and adult stages of the insect appear to require different sets of genetic instructions to form body parts.

Metamorphic events are controlled by neuroendocrine hormones derived from several major organs, including the brain (Fig. 11–3). A hormone synthesized by neurosecretory cells of the brain is released upon stimulation into the hemolymph or tissue fluid. With high titers of this hormone, the *prothoracic* or *ecdysial glands* of the thorax are, in turn, stimulated to release *ecdysone*. The brain hormone also causes the *corpora allata* to release *juvenile hormone*, an essential larval growth hormone.

Ecdysone and juvenile hormones interact in a complex way to determine the specific patterns of metamorphic change, particularly as they are recorded in the epidermis (Fig. 11–3). Ecdysone stimulates the epidermal cells of the integument to deposit or lay down a new cuticle and to release several hydrolytic enzymes charged with the destruction of the old cuticle. If the titer of juvenile hormone is high in the tissue fluids, the cuticle laid down will be larval in character. With a low concentration of juvenile hormone, the epidermis in the presence of ecdysone responds by forming a pupal instead of a larval cuticle. Hence, ecdysone and variable titers of juvenile hormone act in concert to control the temporal and phenotypic expression of the epidermis. The experimental manipulation of pieces of epidermis to alter the molting sequence provides additional support for this position. For example, a strip of pupal epidermis following transplantation into a young larva will secrete a larval cuticle when the larva molts.

The hormonally controlled events of insect metamorphosis are accompanied by patterns of puff expression and regression in various tissues, reflecting temporal changes in activity and inactivity of portions of the chromosomes. Generally, puffs are particularly evident just prior to molts and metamorphoses. Some 100 different puffs have been identified within tissues of insect larvae with most of these being common to all tissues. The tissues differ, however, in the time that the puffs form and disappear.

The dependence of puffing patterns upon the presence of both ecdysone and juvenile hormone has been shown by a number of investigators. U. Clever injected ecdysone into the last larval stage of *Chironomus tetans* and observed an immediate puff within 15 to 30 minutes on the first chromosome at a site designated as I–18–C (Fig. 11–4). This was closely followed by the appearance of a sec-

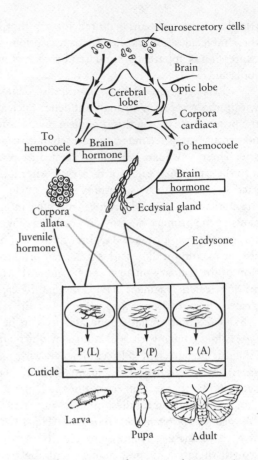

11–3 The sequence of metamorphic events in a typical holometabolous insect. Ecdysone and variable titers of juvenile hormone act in concert to control the temporal and phenotypic expression of the epidermis (i.e., type of cuticle). P(L), larval proteins; P(P), pupa proteins; P(A), adult proteins. (From G. Tombes, 1970. An Introduction to Invertebrate Endocrinology. Academic Press, New York.)

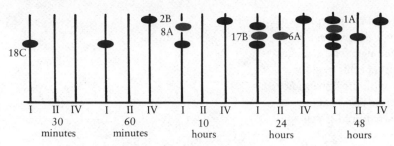

ond puff on chromosome number IV (Fig. 11–4; site IV–2–B). A second group of puffs is expressed between 6 and 48 hours after injection of the hormone (Fig. 11–4). One of these puffs (8A on chromosome I) appears and regresses within this interval of time. Ecdysone-stimulated puffs at sites I–18–C and IV–2–B can be blocked with actinomycin D. Larvae injected with puromycin or cycloheximide followed by treatment with ecdysone show normal puff formation on the first and fourth chromosomes, but later puffs fail to appear. These observations suggest that the activity of early puffs is essential for the sequential expression of later puffs. Presumably, proteins synthesized as a result of RNA synthesis at sites I–18–C and IV–2–B act as initiators of subsequent patterns of gene activity.

Juvenile hormone also affects puffing in the giant chromosomes of the salivary glands. When injected with juvenile hormone, *Chironomus* larvae often fail to metamorphose to the pupal stage. Some puffs affected by juvenile hormone are the same as those induced with ecdysone. Hence, ecdysone and juvenile hormone must act in synergistic rather than antagonistic fashion to determine the patterns of gene activity that underlie the physiological changes of metamorphic events.

The puffs of polytene chromosomes represent an "exaggerated" reflection of genes in action in selected tissues of metamorphosing insects. The basis of structural and functional change in tissues with nonpolytene chromosomes is presumably similar, with uncoiled sequences of DNA serving as templates for the synthesis of RNA. Proteins specified by these messenger transcripts may activate other genes or act to catalyze other processes required in differentiation.

CYTOPLASMIC CONTROL OF CELL TYPE AND NUCLEAR ACTIVITIES

Several examples from the development of both invertebrate and vertebrate embryos have been mentioned in previous chapters.

These examples suggest that the differentiation and the morphogenesis of early embryonic cells are achieved through the interaction of components initially resident within the fertilized egg. The segregation of cytoplasmic factors or determinants into specific regions of the dividing egg can be correlated subsequently with the appearance of particular cellular differentiations of the embryo. That an interaction between the nucleus and cytoplasm is required if cell specialization is to be realized is supported by several observations. First, alterations, either by extirpation or centrifugation, in the spatial arrangement of various cytoplasmic constituents of eggs produce embryos with predictable morphological and cellular defects. For example, removal of the anuclear polar lobe at the first or subsequent cleavage divisions in *Ilyanassa* produces embryos lacking mesodermal cells and other lobe-dependent structures. Extirpation of the grey crescent material of the fertilized egg blocks the appearance of neural cells and notochordal cells in frog embryos. Removal of the yellow cytoplasm of the egg of *Styela* disturbs mesodermal differentiation. Second, suppression of specific activities of the nucleus by the treatment of embryos with transcriptional inhibitors, such as actinomycin D, at specific times during development inhibits the subsequent expression of given cell types.

Although nuclear activity under the influence of these cytoplasmic localizations appears to be essential for the differentiation of early cell types, the demonstration of such an interaction experimentally requires an alteration in the activity of the nucleus by the cytoplasm around it. Efforts to determine if regions of the egg cytoplasm can exercise control over patterns of nuclear expression have been successful in some animal species. It has been considerably more difficult in the early embryo to associate the synthesis of particular proteins with the appearance of specific cells.

You will recall that removal of the first cleavage polar lobe in *Ilyanassa* produces a lobeless embryo that lacks such structures as the heart, intestine, eye, and foot. Muscle tissue, nerve ganglia, and stomach and pigment cells differentiate and are unaffected by this manipulation at the two-celled stage. Hence, lobeless embryos are characterized by an absence of certain cellular differentiations. Since removal of the polar lobe does not disturb any nuclear components of the cell, an experimental system is available to test the effects of the altered cytoplasmic environment upon various biosynthetic activities of the nucleus.

Both lobeless and normal embryos develop at about the same rate for the first several days and show few differences in their capacities to synthesize DNA and RNA. After three days of development, however, lobeless embryos generally incorporate less labeled amino acid into protein and less labeled uridine into total RNA when compared with normal, lobed embryos. As might be expected, the absence of certain differentiated tissues in lobeless embryos is reflected in a marked alteration of their total proteins. A number of investigators have shown that by about the fifth day of development there are significant differences between lobeless and lobed embryos in the patterns of proteins being synthesized. By this time, organogenesis has been initiated and many lobe-dependent structures have appeared in normal embryos.

On the basis of studies by Donohoo and Kafatos in particular, it is now certain that the polar lobe cytoplasm qualitatively affects the synthesis of proteins from very early development. They determined that the proteins synthesized in embryos cultured from isolated AB and CD blastomeres (two-celled stage) were clearly different, thus indicating a causal relationship between the presence of polar lobe cytoplasm and the expression of a unique set of proteins. Newrock and Raff (1975) subsequently showed that extirpation of the polar lobe disturbs patterns of protein synthesis long before the morphological effects of this manipulation were evident.

A key question regarding these studies can now be posed. Do the early cells of these developing embryos become different solely because of having received a different cytoplasm, or does the polar lobe cytoplasm influence cell specificity and protein synthesis by controlling the activities of the nuclei? Unfortunately, results of current research do not permit us to say with certainty whether the polar lobe cytoplasmic determinants act in some fashion on the structural genes of the nucleus. One possibility is that the polar lobe contains a qualitatively unique battery of maternal mRNAs. The presence of polysomes in the polar lobe and the known capacity of the polar lobe to synthesize proteins support the position that *Ilyanassa* embryos have maternal mRNA. The selection for translation of specific maternal mRNAs at specific times during development could account for the differences in protein synthesis patterns between lobed and lobeless embryos. However, an alternative hypothesis is that some of these proteins may act selectively to regulate gene activity and the production of embryonic mRNA. Newrock and Raff have demonstrated that when both lobeless and normal embryos are treated with actinomycin D and their newly synthesized proteins compared, highly significant differences are detected. Thus, the polar lobe could contain specific maternal mRNAs, some of which upon translation function to regulate transcriptional processes.

The primordial germ cells are examples of the expression of early embryonic cell types considered to be specified through the action of cytoplasmic factors localized in the egg cell. A particularly useful feature in following germ cell development is that the region of the

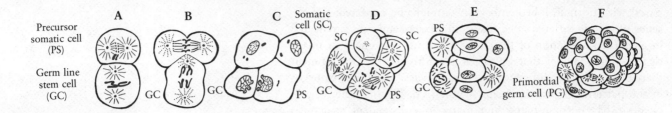

Precursor somatic cell (PS)

Germ line stem cell (GC)

A B C Somatic cell (SC) D E F

GC GC PS GC SC SC PS GC PS PS GC

Primordial germ cell (PG)

egg cytoplasm which participates in their formation is often marked by highly visible *polar granules*. Polar granules have been identified in eggs of a variety of animal species, including nematodes, insects, urochordates, fishes, and amphibians. Recent studies with amphibians suggest that these granules may contain the germinal determinants.

Before the turn of the century, Boveri observed that the eggs of *Ascaris* undergo unequal cleavages through the 32-celled stage. At each of these five divisions, one daughter blastomere retains a complete set of chromosomes while the other blastomere eliminates a large fraction of chromosomal material (Fig. 11–5). The blastomeres formed as the result of *chromosome diminution* will contribute to the somatic cells of the embryo and the adult organism. The single blastomere at the 32-celled stage retaining all chromosomes is the stem cell for all future germ cells. Manipulation of the germinal plasm by centrifugation or by the introduction of accessory nuclei into the egg yields additional insights into the differentiation of the germ cell lineage. If, for example, the fertilized egg is centrifuged just before cleavage so that each of the first two blastomeres receives germinal plasm, then after five divisions there will be 30 somatic cells and two germ-line stem cells (Fig. 11–6). The implication of this experiment is that the germinal plasm influences the resident nucleus of a blastomere to divide unequally. Also, if nuclei not normally found in the polar region of the egg cell are forced into this area, they become part of a population of blastomeres protected from chromosome diminution.

A special portion of the cytoplasm of the egg is also responsible for germ cell development in beetles. The egg of the beetle is typically oblong in shape and following fertilization undergoes an incomplete form of cleavage (Fig. 11–7). The zygote nucleus is initially located in the center of the cell (Fig. 11–7 A). Here it starts to divide, but without a corresponding division of the cytoplasm (Fig. 11–7 B). After several such nuclear divisions, the individual nuclei begin to migrate toward the periphery of the cell. The nuclei that arrive at one pole of the cell enter a special zone of cytoplasm with germinal determinants (Fig. 11–7 C,D). Only those nuclei that come under the influence of the germinal plasm will differentiate as

11–5 Chromosomal diminution and the determination of germ cells in *Ascaris*. A, the 2-celled stage with germlike stem cell (GC) and a presumptive somatic cell (PS); B, an advanced 2-celled stage in which chromatin is eliminated at the equator of the presumptive somatic cell; C, the 4-celled stage with eliminated chromatin on surface of two somatic cells; D, third cleavage division with second chromosome diminution in the precursor somatic cell; E, the 12-celled stage with third chromatin diminution; F, the 32-celled stage with the fourth chromatin diminution in progress. Note the single primordial germ cell. (From T. Boveri, 1925. The Cell in Development and Heredity by E. B. Wilson. The Macmillan Co., New York.)

11–6 Redistribution of the germ cell determinants by centrifugation of the *Ascaris* egg before cleavage typically produces two primordial germ cells (PG). Note chromatin diminution in the somatic cells (SC). A and B are two examples of such centrifuged eggs. (From M. Hogue, 1910. Wilhelm Roux' Arch. Entwicklungsmech. Org. 29, 109.)

A B

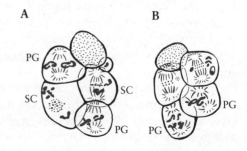

PG PG

SC SC

PG PG PG

germ-line stem cells. If the germinal plasm is destroyed by heat prior to the peripheral movement of the nuclei, no germ cells will form and the adult organism is sterile.

Strong support for the concept that there is communication between nucleus and cytoplasm during the differentiation of a cell comes from nuclear transfer studies with multicellular organisms, particularly by Gurdon and his colleagues on the Amphibia. Introduction of the nucleus of a given cell type into the cytoplasm of another cell type from which the nucleus has been removed permits an analysis of the effect of the foreign cytoplasmic environment upon the activities of the donor nucleus. The chief activity of the nucleus following fertilization is intense DNA synthesis; several experiments have shown that components in the egg cytoplasm control the synthesis of this gene product. A nucleus from the brain cell of an adult frog synthesizes RNA (mainly rRNA) but rarely produces DNA. When such a nucleus is isolated and injected into an artificially activated, enucleated frog's egg, the synthesis of RNA is observed to terminate and the nucleus engages in its own DNA synthesis (Fig. 11–8). The synthesis of RNA is not detected until the transfer embryo reaches a stage when this nucleic acid normally appears. If a nucleus from the same brain tissue is injected into a ripe, ovarian oocyte, whose primary activity is RNA but not DNA production, the nucleus responds by manufacturing only RNA (Fig. 11–8). Nuclei of mature red blood cells, which synthesize neither DNA or RNA, commence to produce both DNA and RNA following their transfer into the cytoplasm of a rapidly dividing cell population. One can conclude from these experiments that differentia-

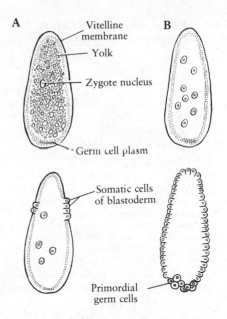

11–7 Determination of the germ cells in a typical beetle. A, recently fertilized egg; B, cleavage showing division of nuclei without corresponding division of cytoplasm; C, nuclei arriving at the periphery initiate blastoderm formation; D, nuclei which invade germ cell plasm become blastomeres differentiating as primordial germ cells. (After R. W. Hegner, 1911. Biol. Bull. 20, 237.)

11–8 Diagrammatic illustration of studies by Gurdon and others to show that a frog brain nucleus following transplantation into an enucleated, activated egg (which promotes DNA synthesis) or a young oocyte (which promotes RNA synthesis) produces a gene product dictated by the synthetic activity of the host cell.

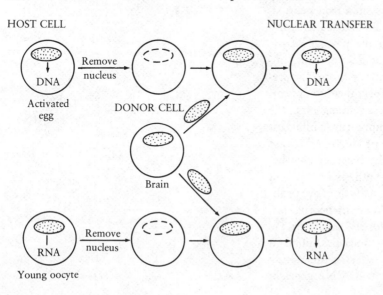

Table 11–1 Summary of nuclear transfer experiments in *Xenopus laevis* demonstrating an influence of living cytoplasm on nuclear activity[a]

	Synthetic activity of embryos[b]			
	DNA	nRNA	tRNA	rRNA
Neurula cell (donor nuclei)	−	++	++	++
Nuclear-transplant embryos				
Uncleaved egg (1 hour after transfer)	++	−−	−−	−−
Midblastula (7 hours after transfer)	+	++	−−	−−
Late blastula (9 hours after transfer)	+	++	++	−−
Neurula	−	++	++	++

[a] Single neurula nuclei were transplanted to enucleated eggs, which were labeled with uridine-^{3}H for 1 to 2 hours at various stages during their subsequent development. For details of experiments, see Gurdon and Woodland (1969).

[b] Symbols: −−, no detectable synthesis; −, ca. 10 percent of nuclei active; +, ca. 50 percent of nuclei active; ++, rapid synthesis in nearly all nuclei.

From J. B. Gurdon. 1969. Communication in Development. Ed. A. Lang. 28th Symposium of the Society of Developmental Biology. New York: Academic Press.

tion does not irreversibly alter the genome. In other words, the nuclear changes leading to a specific program of gene expression are at least potentially reversible.

Other experiments by Gurdon indicate that there is specificity in the cytoplasmic factors controlling the program of nuclear expression (Table 11–1). As pointed out previously, there is a predictable, temporal pattern of RNA synthesis in the developing eggs of most animal species. Nuclear, transfer, and ribosomal RNA molecules are sequentially synthesized in response to the activation of genes responsible for their formation. If the nucleus of a frog neurula, which actively produces RNA, is injected into an enucleated frog's egg, RNA synthesis ceases immediately. With the passage of the transplant embryo through the early stages of development, nuclear, transfer, and ribosomal RNA are sequentially formed at precisely those times when one would normally expect them to appear. Several conclusions can be drawn from these observations. First, the cytoplasm must contain a factor(s) which temporarily inhibits or shuts down the activity of genes specifying one product, in this case RNA. Second, the cytoplasmic factors must be heterogenous because the different genes responsible for the synthesis of different RNAs are selectively activated. These cytoplasmic factors are probably specific to each species. The injection of *Xenopus* neurula nuclei into enucleated eggs of the frog *Discoglossus* results in the expression of only some of the types of RNA molecules found in normal *Xenopus* eggs. The cytoplasm of *Discoglossus* apparently lacks certain cytoplasmic factors required to activate RNA genes in the donor nucleus.

A logical assumption is that an interaction between nucleus and cytoplasm is achieved by the passage of molecules from the cytoplasm into the nucleus. Unfortunately, efforts at isolating and identifying specific cytoplasmic components that can be demonstrated to alter nuclear activity have not been particularly successful. At least during early development, there is now ample evidence from studies with frogs and sea urchins that proteins synthesized in the cytoplasm do accumulate within nuclei. K. Arms (1968), for example, was particularly interested in the relationship between movements of cytoplasmic proteins and the onset of DNA synthesis in the amphibian fertilized egg. He introduced tritiated amino acids into the cytoplasm of a ripe oocyte. After approximately two hours when most of the amino acids were incorporated into protein, he injected brain nuclei and puromycin (a translational inhibitor blocking further protein synthesis) into the egg. Autoradiography of sectioned eggs fixed some one and a half hours later showed that the nucleus contained about twice as much of the labeled protein as did the cytoplasm. Since the egg cytoplasm represses RNA synthesis and induces DNA synthesis, a causal relationship is suggested between the entry of protein into the nucleus and the shift in the program of nuclear activity.

Some proteins known to be synthesized in the oocyte during maturation or in the cytoplasm of cells of the early embryo become localized in embryonic nuclei. Histone proteins are such an example. Active synthesis of histones has been known for some years to occur in early sea urchin embryos, an event that is temporally correlated with the high rate of DNA synthesis. Autoradiographic observations of sea urchin blastomeres have shown that a large proportion of the proteins synthesized in the cytoplasm accumulate in the nuclei and approximately half of these have been identified as histones. In *Xenopus* embryos, the rate of histone synthesis is not so directly correlated with the rate of DNA synthesis because of the large amount of histone mRNA and preformed histone stored in the egg during oogenesis. Additional experiments with actively dividing populations of cultured cells have shown that the influx of labeled cytoplasmic proteins is particularly pronounced during the S phase of the cell cycle, a time when histone synthesis is also high. It follows that histones may enter nuclei at this time in embryonic cell populations.

Deoxyribonucleic acid polymerase is another protein that has been demonstrated to shift from the cytoplasmic to the nuclear compartment of cleaving cells in both sea urchin and frog embryos. Substantial amounts of this protein accumulate in the cytoplasm of the egg during oogenesis. Investigators have long suspected that the quantity of DNA polymerase and/or its cyclic localization in the nucleus exercise control over the rate of DNA synthesis during development. More recently, Benbow and his colleagues have presented data suggesting that there is an additional cytoplasmic *control protein* or *initiation factor* controlling the synthesis of DNA. The nuclei of the liver cells of adult *Xenopus* produce very little DNA. When these nuclei were incubated in the cytoplasm of homogenates of oocytes, which possess all the necessary precursors—primed with deoxynucleoside triphosphates—for DNA production, there was little DNA synthesis under the influence of the endogenous liver DNA polymerase. By contrast, the same nuclei incubated in cytoplasmic homogenates of the fertilized egg actively supported the formation of DNA.

Although we know that cells of the early embryo differentiate, the precise role of elements of the cytoplasm and their influence in controlling nuclear activity in the differentiative process is not completely understood. Certainly, specific mRNAs and proteins preformed in the egg and subsequently parceled out to different cells can be associated with the appearance of early cell types in the embryo. The reality of cytoplasmic determinants in the egg and their capacity to affect protein synthesis cannot be questioned. A critical area for future research is how these determinants affect patterns of gene activity in the early embryo to account for the diverse types of cell lineages.

The importance of the heterogeneity of the cytoplasm in stimulating nuclear changes, which lead to specific cellular differentiations, is based largely upon studies with adult tissues or embryos at stages of organogenesis when functional tissues are forming. Some of these cases will be discussed in later chapters. It is becoming increasingly evident from such studies that various constituents of a cell (i.e., cyclic nucleotides, inorganic ions, and hormones), which are normally viewed as regulating the metabolic activities of cells, may also play critical roles in guiding cells through differentiation with their actions being mediated, in part, at the level of nuclear gene transcription. The presence simultaneously of these known initiators of differentiation within the same cell type provides the challenge of working out the precise pathways of interactions by which the nuclear activity is ultimately effected. For example, we have previously seen that ecdysone, a steroidlike hormone, when injected into insect larvae induces puff formation. Dibutyrl adenosine monophosphate (cAMP) also induces or represses puff formation in the larvae of *Drosophila* at different stages of development, thus suggesting that the gene expression induced in target cells under the influence of the hormone may, in fact, be regulated within the cell by the cyclic AMP acting as a *secondary messenger*.

Hormones are signals that activate a genomic program of dif-

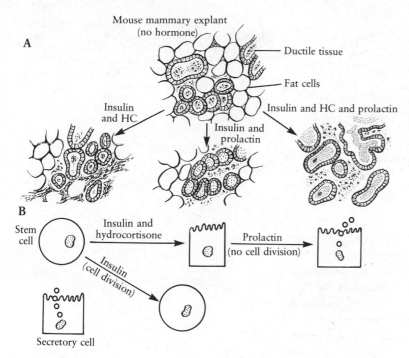

A Mouse mammary explant
(no hormone)

Ductile tissue

Fat cells

Insulin
and HC

Insulin and
prolactin

Insulin and HC and prolactin

B

Stem
cell

Insulin and
hydrocortisone

Prolactin
(no cell division)

Insulin
(cell division)

Secretory cell

11–9   The effect of hormones on the differentiation of alveoli in the mammary gland of the mouse. A, appearance of sections of mammary gland explant after exposure to selected combinations of hormones; B, scheme to show the interactions of hormones in the differentiation of gland tissue. Only the presence of all three hormones will lead to a functional secretory epithelium. HC, hydrocortisone. (From R. Turkington, 1968. Current Topics in Developmental Biology. Λ. Moscona and Λ. Monroy, eds. Vol. 3. Academic Press, New York.)

ferentiation in target cells some distance from the site of their production. *Erythropoietin,* whose level in the blood is controlled by the level of oxygen tension, stimulates the formation of the erythrocyte and the synthesis of hemoglobin in the bone marrow of mammals (Chapter 18). In reptiles and birds, the liver is modified into an organ that produces the bulk of egg-specific yolk proteins (plasma lipovitellin and plasma phosvitin) under elevated levels of or prolonged exposure to estrogen. It has been shown that the synthesis of these proteins requires DNA-dependent RNA synthesis with the mRNAs specific to lipovitellin and phosvitin being formed rapidly under the influence of elevated levels of estrogenic substances.

Several hormones act in concert to bring about the functional differentiation of the alveolar cells of the mammary gland. The alveolar cells synthesize and secrete milk proteins, the principle one of which is *casein*. Normally, the alveolar sacs do not arise until the last half of pregnancy. At this time, there is a rapid proliferation and differentiation of the alveolar epithelium from a primordial milk duct system in response to the presence of three hormones (*insulin, hydrocortisone,* and *prolactin*). When mammary gland tissue from young mice is cultured with these three hormones, alveolar cells will differentiate and produce secretory material (Fig. 11–9 A). By withholding one or several of these hormones from the

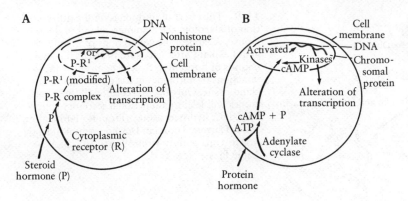

A

DNA
Nonhistone protein
or
P-R¹
Cell membrane
P-R¹ (modified)
P-R complex
Alteration of transcription
P
Cytoplasmic receptor (R)
Steroid hormone (P)

B

Cell membrane
Activated
DNA
Kinases
Chromosomal protein
cAMP
Alteration of transcription
cAMP + P
ATP
Adenylate cyclase
Protein hormone

11–10   Diagrams showing proposed pathways by which steroid (A) and protein (B) hormones act on target cells. (A, from G. Stein, T. Spelsburg, and L. Kleinsmith, 1974. Science 183, 817. Copyright 1974 by the American Association for the Advancement of Science.)

organ culture, the precise role that each hormone plays in the development of the alveolar epithelium can be determined (Fig. 11–9 A,B). Insulin appears to stimulate DNA synthesis and the proliferation of mammary gland cells, but it has no effect upon overt alveolar cell differentiation. However, unless it is present and stimulates cell division, further development under the influences of hydrocortisone and prolactin will not take place. Hydrocortisone must be present at some time when insulin acts upon the presumptive alveolar cells in order for prolactin to elicit synthetic activity and the production of casein in these cells. Only prolactin is capable of inducing the formation of the functional milk proteins associated with the differentiated cell type. Since cell division is apparently required in this system for the expression of a new cell type, it is likely that the genome is programmed during this step to activate the transcription of genes coding for milk proteins.

Cells that respond to hormones do so by at least two different mechanisms. For steroid hormones, such as estrogen, progesterone, hydrocortisone, and androgens, each hormone is postulated to complex or bind with a specific *receptor protein* (cytosol) in the cytoplasm of the target cell (Fig. 11–10 A). After undergoing some modification, the receptor protein transports the hormone through a specialized nuclear membrane where the receptor-hormone complex binds to the chromatin. The movement of the hormone-receptor complex has been demonstrated by adding labeled hormone, such as progesterone, to the cytosol fraction of a target organ, such as chick oviduct. When the hormone-receptor complex is incubated with nuclei isolated from the oviduct, an uptake of the label by the nuclei is consistently observed. Little uptake of the hormone is noted if nuclei are incubated in the hormone alone.

Protein hormones effect their actions on target cells by a totally different mechanism (Fig. 11–10 B). Molecules of the hormone attach to special receptor sites on the cell surface, an event that results in the release of membrane-bound adenylate cyclase into the cytoplasm. Adenylate cyclase then catalyzes the conversion of ATP into cAMP ($3',5'$ adenosine-monophosphate) and pyrophosphate. The cyclic nucleotide is proposed to activate certain protein enzymes (*kinases*) within the nucleus, which subsequently mediate the phosphorylation of chromosomal proteins. The uptake of phosphate by chromatin protein (see below) is an early event that is often observed after hormonal stimulation of target cells and preceding extensive gene activation. Prolactin appears to act on the alveolar epithelial cells of the mammary gland in this fashion. Indeed, the function of hydrocortisone in the mammary gland system described above may well be to stimulate the synthesis of prolactin receptor sites on surface membranes of newly formed gland cells.

NUCLEAR PROTEINS AND THE MECHANISM OF GENE REGULATION

The process of gene transcription is vitally important during development because information encoded in the nuclear DNA is utilized in the synthesis of complementary RNA molecules which, in turn, act as templates specifying the cytoplasmic proteins of differentiated cells. Different cell types are characterized by a unique spectrum of proteins. Presumably, these different proteins are specified by different regions of the genome. Depending upon the requirement of the cell, therefore, specific regulatory molecules must be present at the level of the nucleus to activate and inactivate particular regions of the genome. A central question in any genetic model of differentiation is how regulatory molecules act on cells with identical genomes to initiate and maintain different regimens of protein synthesis. Unfortunately, the mechanism(s) by which genes are selected and regulated in cells of higher organisms is still largely unknown. Considerably more information is available on gene control systems in viruses and bacteria. In *Escherichia coli,* for example, a specific repressor protein has been isolated and shown to regulate transcription by binding to a specific site on the bacterial DNA. Small molecules such as lactose, in turn, control the binding affinity of the repressor protein by inducing alterations in its conformational organization.

As pointed out in previous sections, changes in gene expression are correlated with the uptake by the nucleus of cytoplasmic proteins, cyclic nucleotides, and hormone-receptor complexes. These apparently bind to the chromatin material once within the nucleus. Chromatin consists of DNA, large amounts of histone and nonhistone proteins, and small amounts of RNA. Although much remains to be determined regarding the functional roles played by these various chromatin components, there is increasing evidence that changes in the expression of a cell's genetic information are controlled at least in part by the nuclear proteins. In other words, the molecules responsible for specific gene regulation are to be found among the chromosomal proteins. Historically, the proposed regulatory proteins have been divided into two classes: (1) the histones, and (2) the nonhistones or nuclear acidic proteins.

Histones comprise about 70 percent of the nuclear proteins of adult nuclei and are best defined as proteins with a positive charge and rich in such basic amino acids as arginine and lysine. Initially, because of their known preference to bind tenaciously to DNA and demonstrated function to inhibit the ability of DNA to serve as a template for RNA synthesis, it was thought that histones were specific repressors of gene transcription. An attractive hypothesis was that histones might function in the differentiation of cell types during embryogenesis by progressively silencing selected DNA sequences. Although new histone proteins do appear during some critical stages of sea urchin and amphibian development, there are really very few developmental changes that can be correlated with variations in the appearance of basic proteins. Also, since histones exhibit remarkable uniformity among tissues and cells (crude histone preparations can only be fractionated into five major classes), they apparently lack sufficient specificity to recognize and influence the activity of specific genes. The absence of sufficient heterogeneity among histones suggests that these proteins probably act as regulatory molecules of gene transcription in some nonspecific way.

As early as the 1940s, Stedman and Stedman proposed that the nonhistone chromosomal proteins were potential regulators of specific gene activity. Acid nuclear proteins constitute approximately 30 percent of the nuclear proteins, are frequently rich in aspartic and glutamic acids, and—like histones—are synthesized in the cytoplasm of the cell. In contrast to histones, the nonhistone proteins display tremendous structural and functional differences in different cell types. At least some of the proteins are probably involved in the specific activation of genes during the differentiation and specialization of cells. Unfortunately, although some information is available on acid nuclear protein changes during development, the proposed role of these proteins as regulatory molecules is largely based upon studies with fully differentiated tissues and not on early embryos. The most direct evidence that nonhistones play a role in tissue-specific transcription comes from *chromatin reconstitution experiments* in which the activity of DNA of a given cell type, which is measured by the synthesis of a specific RNA, is evaluated in the presence of histones or nonhistones from another cell type (Fig.

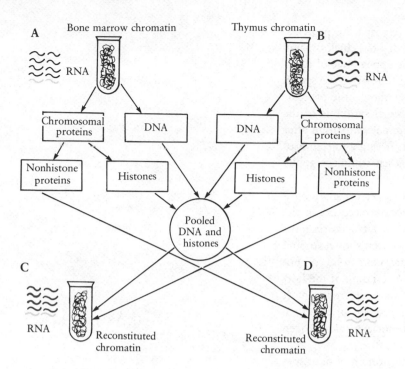

A   Bone marrow chromatin

Chromosomal proteins

DNA

Nonhistone proteins

Histones

RNA

B   Thymus chromatin

DNA

Chromosomal proteins

Histones

Nonhistone proteins

RNA

Pooled DNA and histones

C

RNA

Reconstituted chromatin

D

Reconstituted chromatin

RNA

11–11 The technique of chromatin reconstitution permits an analysis of the role of nonhistone proteins in tissue-specific transcription. This figure illustrates experiments conducted by R. Gilmour and J. Paul using rabbit thymus and rabbit bone marrow chromatin. Chromatin from bone marrow and thymus can be dissociated into DNA, histones, and nonhistones (A, B). When DNA and histones from both tissues are pooled and combined with nonhistone proteins from thymus, the reconstituted chromatin synthesizes RNA characteristic of thymus (C). When DNA and histones from both tissues are pooled and combined with nonhistone proteins from bone marrow, the reconstituted chromatin synthesizes RNA, which behaves like bone marrow RNA (D). (From G. Stein, T. Spelsburg, and L. Kleinsmith, 1974. Science 183, 817. Copyright 1974 by the American Association for the Advancement of Science.)

11–11). In famous experiments by Gilmour and Paul at the Institute for Cancer Research in Glasgow, rabbit thymus and rabbit bone marrow cells were dissociated into DNA, histone, and nonhistone fractions (Fig. 11–11). When all of these components of the thymus were reconstituted, the RNA that formed behaved just like normally synthesized thymus RNA. When DNA and histones from thymus and bone marrow were pooled together and the chromatin fully reconstituted with the addition of thymus nonhistone proteins, the RNA synthesized had all of the characteristics of thymus RNA. This occurred even though DNA and histones were available from the bone marrow. When the same types of DNA and histones were recombined with nonhistones from bone marrow, the RNA synthesized from the combined chromatin behaved like bone marrow RNA. From these observations, it can be concluded that the specificity of gene transcription is regulated by the tissue-specific nonhistone chromosomal proteins.

The specification of gene function as a property of nonhistone proteins has also been demonstrated, using the chromatin reconstitution technique, in cells stimulated to differentiate under the influence of hormones. The epithelial layer of the oviduct of the recently hatched chick is immature and shows little evidence of specialized cell types. Under the influence of the sex steroids estrogen and progesterone, however, the oviduct epithelium becomes differentiated into cells that synthesize and secrete very specific proteins. For example, continuous treatment of the five-day-old chick oviduct with estrogen will, after 96 hours, result in the appearance of tubular glands in the epithelial tissue. After an additional two days with hormone treatment, the cells of these glands synthesize the proteins *ovalbumin* and *lysozyme*. Goblet cells, the sites of synthesis of the eggwhite protein *avidin,* differentiate in the luminal epithelium after nine days of exposure of oviduct to estrogen. A single injection of progesterone into the estrogenized chick will then stimulate goblet cells to manufacture avidin.

The lining of the oviduct is one of several target organs for estrogen; its epithelial cells possess estrogen-specific receptors in the cytoplasm which bind the hormone. The oviduct estrogen-receptor complex is not only taken up by nuclei, but has been shown to bind with chromatin isolated from the oviduct. If the nonhistone component is selectively extracted from oviduct DNA, binding of the hormone-receptor complex to the chromatin is markedly reduced. It would appear, therefore, that the acid nuclear proteins of the chromatin material are the target site within the nucleus for estrogen and probably other hormones.

Does binding of estrogen to the nonhistone protein initiate specific gene transcription? The answer to this question is probably affirmative. Following the entrance of the estrogen-receptor complex into oviduct nuclei, there is rapid synthesis of actinomycin D sensitive RNA molecules. Several types of experiments clearly indicate that the new kinds of RNA include specific messenger molecules for ovalbumin. If RNA is extracted from oviduct tissue stimulated by estrogen and is then added to a cell-free protein synthesizing system, the presence of ovalbumin can subsequently be detected. By contrast, no ovalbumin is formed if the extracted RNA is obtained from nontreated chick oviduct tissue. Indeed, the mRNA specifying pure ovalbumin has now been isolated and used in vitro with *reverse transcriptase* to construct strands of DNA. Since the mRNA acts as a template upon which complementary DNA molecules are formed, the DNA strands are essentially genes coding for ovalbumin. With these DNA strands, it has been possible using DNA-RNA hybridization techniques to determine how much ovalbumin-specific RNA is made in estrogen-treated oviducts and nontreated oviducts. Hormonally stimulated oviduct tissue is about eight times more active in synthesizing specific ovalbumin messenger molecules. Again, the nonhistone component of chromatin appears to specify ovalbumin synthesis. Nonhistones extracted from the chromatin of estrogen-stimulated oviduct, when reconstituted with DNA and histones obtained from nonstimulated oviduct, will give a transcriptive

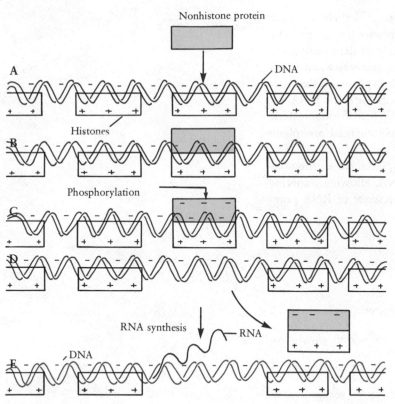

Nonhistone protein

A

DNA

Histones

B

Phosphorylation

C

D

RNA synthesis

RNA

DNA

E

11–12 A model showing regulation of gene activity by nonhistone protein. A, a nonhistone protein recognizes a specific site on DNA that is repressed by histone protein; B, the nonhistone protein binds to the site; C, the nonhistone protein undergoes phosphorylation and becomes negative; D, the nonhistone-histone complex is displaced from the negatively charged DNA, leaving a segment of the DNA available for the transcription of RNA (E). (From G. Stein, J. Stein, and L. Kleinsmith, 1975. Sci. Am. 232, 47.)

capacity for this protein equivalent to that of normally stimulated oviduct chromatin.

The action of progesterone on estrogen-treated oviduct is rapid and specific with avidin being detected within 12 hours. Qualitative changes in the RNA content of the cells shortly after hormonal stimulation suggests that a portion of the RNA molecules are specific for avidin.

Assuming that nonhistone chromosomal proteins play an essential role in regulating the transcription of individual genes during the differentiation of cell types, how is the control exercised? Although several models have been proposed to account for the molecular mechanism by which this regulation is effected, the histone-displacement model as set forth by Stein and his colleagues, is consistent with a number of observations regarding the behavior of both histone and nonhistone proteins. Histones bind vigorously to DNA and apparently they function to silence large blocks of genes. Therefore, synthesis of specific proteins in response to initiators of differentiation would require the removal of histones from selected DNA sites.

A striking property of the nonhistone proteins is their extensive phosphorylation or capacity to rapidly incorporate phosphate. The uptake of radioactive phosphate is particularly evident during the synthetic or S phase of the cell cycle, a time interval when genes also appear to be more actively transcribed. It is proposed that specific nonhistone proteins complex with specific sites of DNA repressed by histone protein (Fig. 11–12 A). When the nonhistone protein becomes phosphorylated, its negatively charged phosphate groups are repelled by the negatively charged DNA (Fig. 11–12 B,C). Consequently, there follows displacement of the nonhistone-histone protein complex from the DNA, allowing a specific region to be transcribed into RNA in the presence of RNA polymerase (Fig. 11–12 D,E).

REFERENCES

Arms, K. 1968. Cytonucleoproteins in cleaving eggs of *Xenopus laevis*. J. Embryol. Exp. Morphol. 20:367–374.

Asburner, M. 1967. Patterns of puffing activity in the salivary gland chromosomes of *Drosophila*. Chromosoma 21:398–428.

Britten, R. and E. Davidson. 1969. Gene regulation for higher cells: A theory. Science 165:349–357.

Clever, U. 1964. Actinomycin and puromycin: Effects on sequential gene activation by ecdysone. Science 146:794–795.

Clever, U. 1966. Gene activity patterns and cellular differentiation. Am. Zool. 6:33–41.

Donohoo, P. and F. Kafatos. 1973. Differences in proteins synthesized by the progeny of the first two blastomeres of *Ilyanassa*, a "mosaic" embryo. Dev. Biol. 32:224–229.

Grossbach, U. 1973. Chromosome puffs and gene expression in polytene cells. Cold Spring Harbor Symp. Quant. Biol. 38:619–627.

Gurdon, J. 1968. Changes in somatic cell nuclei inserted into growing and maturing amphibian oocytes. J. Embryol. Exp. Morphol. 20:401–414.

Gurdon, J. and H. Woodland. 1968. The cytoplasmic control of nuclear activity in animal development. Biol. Rev. Cambridge Philos. Soc. 43:233–267.

Gurdon, J. and H. Woodland. 1969. The influence of the cytoplasm on the nucleus during cell differentiation, with special reference to RNA synthesis during amphibian cleavage. Proc. Roy. Soc. Lond. Serv. B. 173:99–111.

Hammerling, J. 1963. Nucleocytoplasmic interactions in *Acetabularia* and other cells. Ann. Rev. Plant Physiol. 14:65–92.

Hegner, R. 1911. Experiments with chrysomelid beetles. III. The effects of killing parts of the eggs of *Lepitinotersa decemlineata*. Biol. Bull. (Woods Hole, Mass.) 20:237–251.

McMahon, D. 1974. Chemical messengers in development: A hypothesis. Science 185:1012–1021.

O'Malley, B. and A. Means. 1976. The mechanism of steroid hormone regulation of transcription of specific eukaryotic genes. Progr. Nucleic Acid Res. Mol. Biol. 19:403–419.

Newrock, K. and R. Raff. 1975. Polar lobe specific regulation of translation in embryos of *Ilyanassa obsoleta*. Dev. Biol. 42:242–261.

Stein, G., J. Stein, and L. Kleinsmith. 1975. Chromosomal proteins and gene regulation. Sci. Am. 232:47–57.

Stein, G., J. Stein, L. Kleinsmith, W. Park, R. Jansing, and J. Thomson. 1976. Nonhistone chromosomal proteins and histone gene transcription. Progr. Nucleic Acid Res. Mol. Biol. 19:421–445.

Subtelny, S. 1974. Nucleocytoplasmic interactions in development of amphibian hybrids. Int. Rev. Cytol. 39:35–88.

Tsai, S., S. Harris, M. Tsai, and B. O'Malley. 1976. Effects of estrogen on gene expression in chick oviduct. J. Biol. Chem. 251:4713–4721.

Turkington, R. 1968. Hormone-dependent differentiation of mammary gland *in vitro*. Current Topics in Developmental Biology, Vol. 3, pp. 199–218. Eds., A. A. Moscona and A. Monroy. New York: Academic Press.

12

Early Human Development, Embryonic Membranes, and Placentation

EARLY HUMAN DEVELOPMENT

Because of the obvious difficulties in obtaining material, the study of the early development of the human presents many gaps in the series of embryos available for observation. Nevertheless, by comparison of the available human material with other mammalian, particularly primate, species, the early development of the human ovum can be seen to differ little from that in other primate species. The timing, although necessarily based on assumed times of fertilization, in comparison with other species and studies of in vitro development, is probably quite accurate within the limits of biological variability.

Development Through the First Week: Cleavage and Blastocyst Formation

Four examples of in vivo cleaving human ova have been described—2, 12, 58, and 107 cells. The two-cell embryo (Fig. 12–1), removed from the uterine tube, shows two blastomeres of about equal size surrounded by an incomplete zona pellucida inside of which a polar body is visible. The egg's diameter is 179 μ. On the basis of the time of coitus and the estimated time of ovulation (based on uterine histology), this two-cell embryo is considered to be about 36 to 40 hours postfertilization.

A 12-cell stage with a diameter of 173 μ was also recovered from the uterine tube, but unfortunately this specimen was lost during its examination and no photographs are available. At this stage, the blastomeres differed in size. There was one large central blastomere with a diameter approximately double that of the average of the other 11 blastomeres. Presumably the large blastomere was embryonic in potential—destined to form embryonic structures—and the smaller ones were *trophoblastic* cells—destined to form extraembryonic membranes. This embryo was estimated to be about 72 hours in age.

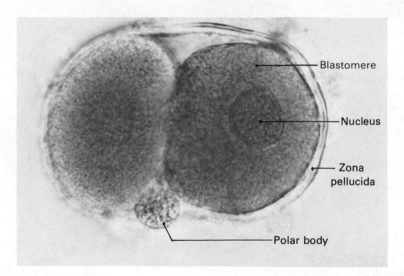

Blastomere

Nucleus

Zona pellucida

Polar body

12–1 Two-celled human embryo, about 36–40 hours postfertilization. (Courtesy of the Carnegie Institution of Washington, Department of Embryology, Davis Division.)

12–2 A, 58-cell human embryo, about 96 hours. Formation of the inner cell mass and blastocoele; B, 107-celled human embryo, about four and a half days. Unilaminar blastocyst with inner cell mass at the embryonal pole. (Courtesy of the Carnegie Institution of Washington, Department of Embryology, Davis Division.)

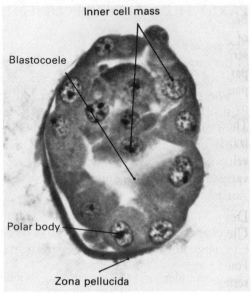

Inner cell mass

Blastocoele

Polar body

Zona pellucida

A

The 58-cell embryo (Fig. 12–2 A), still surrounded by its zona pellucida, shows a continuing divergence in cell specialization with 5 large *formative* (embryonic) cells and 53 small trophoblastic cells. The formative cells are more central in position and represent the beginning of the development of the *inner cell mass* or *germ disc* which will locate at one pole of the embryo, the embryonal pole. Coalescing intercellular spaces represent the beginning of the formation of the segmentation cavity or the blastocoele. The age of this embryo, which was found free in the uterine cavity, was approximately 96 hours.

The 107-cell embryo (Fig. 12–2 B) consists of 8 formative cells and 99 trophoblastic cells. The larger more vacuolated formative cells make up an excentrically located inner cell mass at the embryonal pole of what may now be termed the *blastocyst*. The trophoblast cells are flattened and elongated and form a complete covering for the blastocyst. The zona pellucida has disappeared. This embryo, also found free in the uterine cavity was estimated to be four and one half days old.

Implantation

Implantation is the process by which the developing mammalian egg penetrates the outer layers of the uterine wall and, by means of its expanding trophoblast cells, begins to establish a relationship with the maternal tissues which will result in the formation of the placenta. Development of the placenta is a necessary and crucial

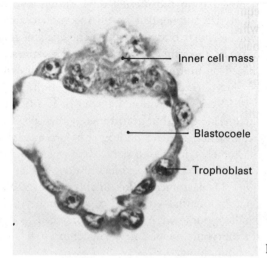

Inner cell mass

Blastocoele

Trophoblast

B

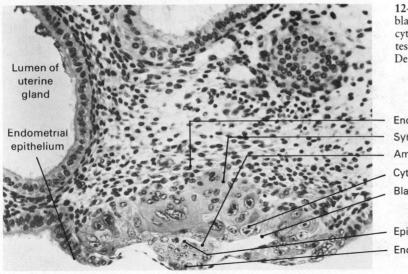

12–3 Seven-day-old human embryo. Bilaminar blastocyst, partially collapsed. Differentiation of cytotrophoblast and syncytiotrophoblast. (Courtesy of the Carnegie Institution of Washington, Department of Embryology, Davis Division.)

Lumen of uterine gland

Endometrial epithelium

Endometrial stroma
Syncytiotrophoblast
Amniotic cavity
Cytotrophoblast
Blastocoele

Epiblast
Endoderm

step since it is this organ—partly of maternal and partly of fetal origin—which must function in providing the nutritive, excretory, and respiratory needs of the developing fetus until parturition. The intimacy of contact between fetal and maternal tissues varies in different species and will be considered in a separate section on comparative placentation. Implantation and placentation are the functions of extraembryonic trophoblast cells, not a part of the development of the embryo proper, which is formed from the inner cell mass. However, it is an integral part of development and does concern the growth of tissue derived from the fertilized egg; thus, we will consider the early stages of implantation in conjunction with the progressive stages of embryonic development rather than describing them separately.

The youngest human embryo in the process of implantation (Fig. 12–3) is judged to be seven to seven and one half days of age. The embryonic pole of the blastocyst has eroded the uterine epithelium and is starting to penetrate into the endometrium. The blastocyst, in this section, has collapsed so that the abembryonal trophoblast lies up against the under surface of the germ disc, partially obscuring the blastocoele—probably not a normal occurrence. The trophoblast wall varies from a thin mesothelial or membranous structure at the abembryonal region to a thick proliferating mass of cells at the embryonal pole. The trophoblast in the embryonal region, which is actively invading the maternal tissues, can be separated into an inner cellular layer that lines the segmentation cavity, the *cytotrophoblast,* and an outer syncytial mass, the *syncytiotrophoblast.* The embryonic disc at this time shows the beginning of the develop-

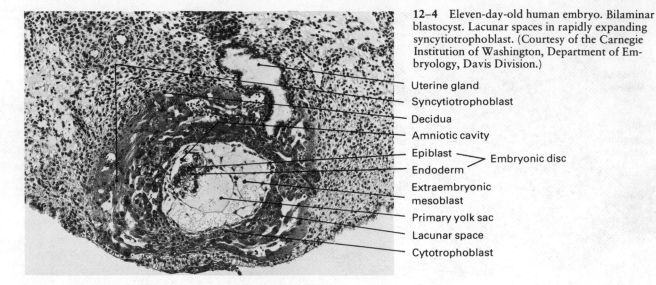

12–4 Eleven-day-old human embryo. Bilaminar blastocyst. Lacunar spaces in rapidly expanding syncytiotrophoblast. (Courtesy of the Carnegie Institution of Washington, Department of Embryology, Davis Division.)

Uterine gland
Syncytiotrophoblast
Decidua
Amniotic cavity
Epiblast
Endoderm
Embryonic disc
Extraembryonic mesoblast
Primary yolk sac
Lacunar space
Cytotrophoblast

ment of a bilaminar form. It consists of a layer of columnar cells, the ectoderm (or epiblast, since the cells in this layer will also contribute to the formation of the mesoderm), beneath which is a layer of irregularly arranged polyhedral cells, the endoderm, adjoining the blastocoele. Clefts may be seen between the epiblast and the overlying trophoblast. These represent the beginning of the formation of the amnionic cavity, which will result from the coalescence of these clefts. The precocious formation of the amnion by cavitation or delamination should be compared with its formation by the growth and folding of sheets of cells as described for the chick and the pig in a later section of this chapter.

Development Through the Second Week

The eleven-day embryo (Fig. 12–4) is almost completely embedded within the uterine tissues and the uterine epithelium has closed in over it. The continuation of the invasive process is seen in the marked expansion of the trophoblast cells. The cytotrophoblast cells still appear as a single layer around the blastocoele and are easily distinguished from the rapidly expanding syncytiotrophoblast cells. The increase in the number of nuclei in the latter layer is not due to division of the syncytiotrophoblast nuclei themselves, but to cell divisions taking place in the cytotrophoblast. Spaces or lacunae have developed as the result of the coalescence of cavities appearing in the syncytiotrophoblast and this stage of trophoblast development is termed the *lacunar* or *previllous* stage. The uterine endomentrium in contact with the fetal syncytiotrophoblast is un-

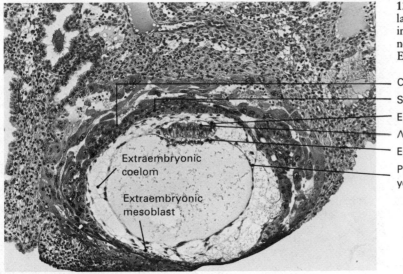

12–5 Twelve-day-old human embryo. Late bilaminar blastocyst. Intercommunicating spaces in the syncytiotrophoblast. (Courtesy of the Carnegie Institution of Washington, Department of Embryology, Davis Division.)

Cytotrophoblast
Syncytiotrophoblast
Epiblast
Amniotic cavity
Endoderm
Primary
yolk sac

dergoing a decidual reaction forming the *decidua* with its characteristic larger pale cells containing glycogen and lipid droplets in the cytoplasm. The term decidua is indicative of the fact that this part of the uterine lining will be cast off at parturition as the so-called afterbirth. Glandular enlargement and vascular congestion are apparent in the uterine tissue. The embryo proper has also undergone significant change. A continued differentiation of epiblast and endoderm is apparent. The amniotic cavity has developed further and cells apparently differentiated from the overlying cytotrophoblast have formed its roof, giving rise to a complete membrane, the amnion. A thin layer of cells attached to the embryonic endoderm forms a second cavity within the blastocoele. This layer of cells, variously termed *Heuser's membrane, exocoelomic membrane,* or *primary yolk-sac membrane* is considered to be formed from extraembryonic mesothelial cells of the cytotrophoblast, since no embryonic mesoderm has as yet developed. The blastocoele may now be called the *exocoelomic cavity* and the blastocyst is now considered to be in its bilaminar stage.

At 12 days (Fig. 12–5) the trophoblast has expanded still further and the syncytiotrophoblast shows an intercommunicating system of lacunar spaces. Maternal blood and engulfed endometrial cells in the lacunar spaces present evidence of the active erosion of uterine tissue by the fetal trophoblast. The cytotrophoblast shows areas where it has started to extend into the syncytiotrophoblast, the beginning of the formation of the *chorionic villi.* The embryo is still in a bilaminar stage. Some cells from the borders of the endoderm

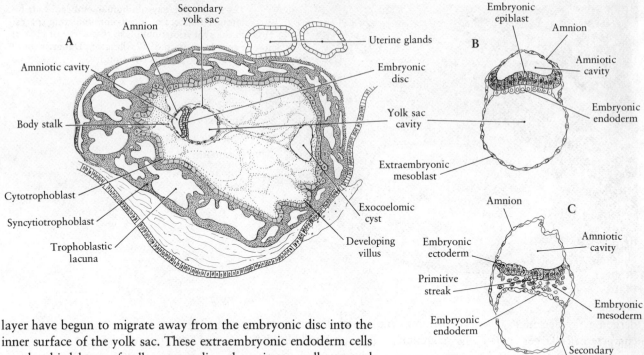

12–6   A, drawing of a 13-day-old human embryo. Trilaminar blastocyst. Amnion, chorion, and yolk sac developed. Body stalk present; B, cross section through the middle of the embryonic disc; C, section through the caudal end of the embryonic disc. Embryonic mesoderm differentiating from the early primitive streak.

layer have begun to migrate away from the embryonic disc into the inner surface of the yolk sac. These extraembryonic endoderm cells are the third layer of cells surrounding the primary yolk sac and thus represent the beginning of a trilaminar blastocyst. We thus have a bilaminar embryo but an early trilaminar blastocyst. A space has appeared between the primary yolk sac and the cytotrophoblast, and this space is occupied by a loose network of stellate-shaped cells representing a further contribution of the trophoblast to the extraembryonic mesoderm.

Figure 12–6 A represents a section through a 13-day embryo. The abembryonal region of the blastocyst is completely enclosed by the uterine endometrium and the trophoblast is beginning to show proliferative changes in this region also. Local proliferation of cytotrophoblast cells surrounded by syncytiotrophoblast, representing *primary stem villi,* are more apparent than in the previously described embryo. The continued proliferation of cells from the endodermal layer of the embryonic disc has now completely lined a cavity much smaller than the primary yolk-sac cavity. These endodermal cells are covered by mesoblast and together they make up the *secondary* or *definitive yolk sac.* Apparently, large portions of the primary yolk sac are pinched off in the process of forming the smaller definitive yolk sac. Exocoelomic cysts found in what is now the extraembryonic coelom are considered to be these pinched off remnants of the primary yolk sac. The extraembryonic coelom thus splits the extraembryonic mesoderm into two layers. One, the outer layer of the yolk sac and the other, the inner of the cyto-

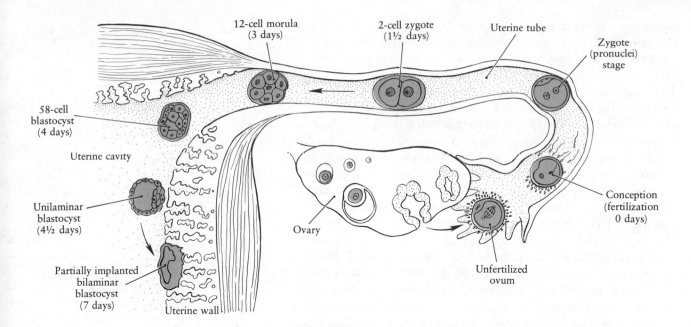

Figure labels:
- 12-cell morula (3 days)
- 2-cell zygote (1½ days)
- Uterine tube
- Zygote (pronuclei) stage
- 58-cell blastocyst (4 days)
- Uterine cavity
- Unilaminar blastocyst (4½ days)
- Ovary
- Conception (fertilization 0 days)
- Partially implanted bilaminar blastocyst (7 days)
- Uterine wall
- Unfertilized ovum

trophoblast—which may now be called the chorion. The mesoderm also forms the outer layer of the amnion.

The embryo is still in the form of a flat bilaminar disc. At the caudal end of this disc, a band of mesoderm stretches across the extraembryonic coelom connecting the embryo and the amnion to the cytotrophoblast. This is the *body stalk.* At the cranial end of the embryonic disc an area of columnar endoderm cells forms the prechordal plate, the future site of the mouth. A cross section through the middle of the embryonic disc (Fig. 12–6 B) shows the typical pseudostratified columnar ectoderm, the loosely connected cuboidal endoderm, and the amnionic and yolk-sac cavities. A cross section near the caudal end of the embryo (Fig. 12–6 C) shows the beginning of the formation of a third layer, the embryonic mesoderm, between the ectoderm and the endoderm. This is occurring in the region of the forming primitive streak.

Figure 12–7 is a diagrammatic review of the development of the human embryo during the first two weeks showing the stages described, their estimated age, and their position within the female reproductive tract.

12–7   Composite of the first two weeks of human development showing the age of the embryo and its general location within the female reproductive tract. (After R. F. Gasser, 1975. Atlas of Human Embryos. Harper & Row, Publishers.

EMBRYONIC MEMBRANES

Fishes and amphibians, collectively called *anamniotes,* deposit large numbers of eggs that develop rapidly to an independent free-swimming stage in an aquatic environment. Because of the rapid development and the acquatic environment these eggs do not require complex auxillary membranes to assist them in respiration, excretion, and nutrition during their embryonic stages. However, the eggs of the anamniotes may form protective coverings such as the chorion of the fishes and the jelly membranes of the amphibians. In addition, fishes also develp a membrane, which is termed a yolk sac. It overgrows and surrounds the yolk and, when vascularized, makes the yolk available to the embryo. The yolk sac is formed by the growth of the edges of the blastoderm (as described in Chapter 8), which consists of ectoderm, mesoderm, and periblast. It does not have any endoderm and therefore is not homologous to the yolk sac of higher forms, although it does serve the same function.

In reptiles and birds that lay their eggs on land, development takes place within a system in which the embryo is largely closed off from the outside environment by the egg shell. This closed (*cleidoic*) system necessitates the development of structures whose sole function is to protect the embryo and provide for its nutritive, excretory, and respiratory needs. These structures are called extraembryonic membranes. They function only during development; they do not form any part of the embryo itself. Four membranes are developed in reptiles and birds, the *serosa* (*chorion*), *amnion*, *yolk sac*, and *allantois*. The first two develop from somatopleure; the last two, from splanchnopleure.

In the mammal, development takes place in the uterus but the same embryonic membranes are formed, although their function may be different. The placenta, which is partly of embryonic and partly of maternal origin, is the major extraembryonic membrane in mammals.

The Yolk Sac

In the chick, the splanchnopleure and somatopleure extend out in all directions over the yolk beyond the region in which the body of the embryo is forming. Where these layers lie beyond the limits of the embryo proper, they are termed extraembryonic. At first, there is no definite boundary between the extrembryonic and the embryonic splanchnopleure and somatopleure, which form continuous sheets. However, as the embryo takes shape, a series of folds appear all around it and grow downward to undercut it and separate it from the underlying yolk. These folds, which then define the limits of the embryonic body, are known as the *body folds*. The first to appear is the *head fold* (Fig. 12–8). During the second day of incubation it becomes continuous with the *lateral body folds* developing along both sides of the embryo (Fig. 12–9). During the third

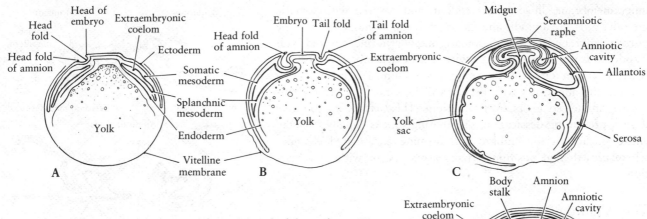

12–8 Schematic diagrams of sagittal sections of the chick showing the formation of the head and tail folds and the extraembryonic membranes. A, 24 hours; B, 72 hours; C, 5 days; D, 9 days. (From B. Patten and B. M. Carlson, 1974. Foundations of Embryology. McGraw-Hill Book Company.)

day a *tail fold* begins to undercut the caudal end of the embryo (Fig. 12–8 B). The net result is a progressive separation of the embryo from the yolk, establishing the shape of the body and indicating the boundary between the embryonic and extraembryonic structures.

When the head and tail folds have undercut the embryo, the embryonic gut may be divided into three regions: a closed foregut in the head fold, a closed hindgut in the tail fold, and an open midgut between them, whose floor is the yolk. The extraembryonic splanchnopleure of the yolk sac is continuous with the splanchnopleure that forms the lining of the gut of the embryo. The extraembryonic splanchnopleure gradually grows over the surface of the yolk in all directions and encloses it in a covering membrane, the yolk sac. As the body folds continue to undercut the embryo, the fore and hindguts becomes progressively longer and the midgut becomes progressively shorter. The connection between the splanchnopleure of the yolk sac and the midgut thus becomes restricted to a narrow band of tissue termed the *yolk stalk* (Fig. 12–8 D). The mesoderm of the yolk sac forms a highly vascular network that establishes connection with the circulatory system of the embryo by way of the vitelline blood vessels. By 40 hours of incubation, blood is circulating through the vascular network of the yolk sac. Vascularized projections of the yolk sac penetrate into the yolk and aid in its breakdown and absorption.

The Amnion and Serosa

The amnion and serosa arise together as the *seroamniotic folds,* upwardly directed folds of the somatopleure just outside of the body folds (Figs. 12–8, 12–9). The head, tail, and lateral seroamniotic folds meet and fuse dorsally at the *seroamniotic raphe* and completely enclose the embryo. When the somatopleure fuses, the embryo is now covered by two double-layered membranes. The inner membrane, lined with ectoderm and covered with somatic mesoderm, is the amnion and its cavity is the amniotic cavity. The outer membrane, lined with somatic mesoderm and covered with ectoderm, is the serosa and its cavity is the extraembryonic coelom, which is continuous with the embryonic coelom. Following its formation, the amniotic cavity becomes filled with fluid and the embryo is immersed in its own aquarium. This acts as a protective device, preventing dessication, distributing shocks equally over the entire surface of the embryo and forming an isolated chamber where growth and positional changes may occur without restriction.

The Allantois

The last of the four embryonic membranes to develop appears late in the third day of incubation. The allantois differs from other membranes in that it develops as an extension of a part of the embryo itself, specifically as an evagination of the splanchnopleure of the hindgut (Figs. 12–8, 12–10). During the fourth day, this evagination is carried out into the extrembryonic coelom between the amnion and the serosa, where it continues to grow until it entirely fills up this space (Fig. 12–8 C,D). The allantoic sac remains attached to the hindgut by the allantoic stalk, which is traversed by the allantoic blood vessels going to and from the embryo. The yolk stalk and the allantoic stalk lie along side of each other in the body stalk.

The splanchnic mesoderm of the allantoic diverticulum becomes closely associated with the somatic mesoderm of the serosa. When the former becomes vascularized, a rich vascular network is formed just beneath the entire surface of the egg shell. This network provides the mechanism for the exchange of respiratory gases between the outside air and the fetal red cells. The combined serosa and allantois thus function in this respect as the embryonic lung. The similarity of this condition in the chick to the chorioallantoic placenta of the mammal will be apparent when we consider the latter.

In addition to its respiratory responsibility, the allantois also has an excretory function, serving as a large reservoir for the storage of wastes. During the early stages of development, urea is the main breakdown product of protein metabolism in the chick embryo. This compound, however, is soluble in water so that large amounts of water would be necessary to keep the urea below toxic levels if it were to continue to be formed throughout development. The breakdown product of protein during the later stages of development, however, is uric acid. This compound is relative insoluble in water

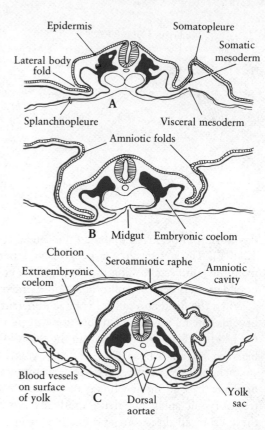

12–9 Cross sections through the early chick embryo showing the relationship of the body folds to the seroamniotic folds during the formation of the serosa and the amnion.

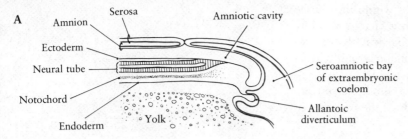

A

Amnion
Serosa
Amniotic cavity
Ectoderm
Neural tube
Notochord
Endoderm
Yolk
Seroamniotic bay of extraembryonic coelom
Allantoic diverticulum

12–10 Diagrams of sagittal sections through the caudal end of the chick embryo showing the formation of the allantois and its relationship to the extraembryonic coelom and the serosa. A, 72 hours; B, 3½ days; C, 4½ days. (From B. Patten and B. M. Carlson, 1974. Foundations of Embryology. McGraw-Hill Book Company.)

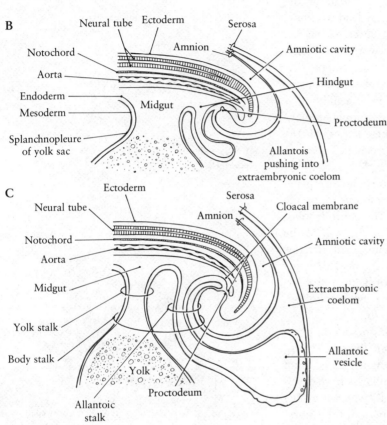

B

Neural tube   Ectoderm
Serosa
Notochord
Amnion
Amniotic cavity
Aorta
Hindgut
Endoderm
Mesoderm
Midgut
Splanchnopleure of yolk sac
Proctodeum
Allantois pushing into extraembryonic coelom

C

Ectoderm
Neural tube
Serosa
Cloacal membrane
Amnion
Notochord
Amniotic cavity
Aorta
Midgut
Extraembryonic coelom
Yolk stalk
Body stalk
Yolk
Allantoic vesicle
Proctodeum
Allantoic stalk

so that large quantities can be stored as crystalline material in the allantoic sac without ill effects to the embryo.

PLACENTATION

In describing the first two weeks of development we have seen how the blastocyst loses its zona pellucida, attaches to the uterine wall, and then rapidly becomes completely embedded within the uterine endometrium. The early period of implantation is characterized by the rapid proliferation of the trophoblast cells, particularly the syncytial layer, which actively erode the uterine endometrium and its glands and blood vessels to establish lacunar spaces lined with syncytiotrophoblast and filled with maternal blood. Blood moves into the lacunar spaces from the open ruptured ends of the branches of the uterine spiral arteries.

The normal implantation site is in the posterior wall of the uterus. Implantation in other areas of the uterus may lead to abnormal development, particularly if it occurs near the cervix. When implantation occurs outside of the uterus, this known as an *ectopic pregnancy*. Less than 2 percent of all pregnancies are ectopic, the large percentage of these occurring in the uterine tube. Tubal pregnancy usually results in rupture of the tube and severe hemmorhaging during the second month of pregnancy. Less commonly, implantation may occur in the ovary or in the mesenteries of the abdominal cavity. Rarely does any extrauterine pregnancy come to full term.

Early in the third week of development the cytotrophoblast penetrates into the bases of the syncytiotrophoblast columns lining the lacunae and forms primary villi (Fig. 12–11 A). The entire trophoblast is proliferating rapidly to keep pace with the growth of the blastocyst. However, mitotic activity in the trophoblast still remains restricted to the cytotrophoblast, which supplies the nuclei for the expansion of the syncytiotrophoblast as well as for its own proliferation into the syncytiotrophoblast columns. The cytotrophoblast cells in the developing villi are called *Langhans cells*.

Shortly after the formation of the primary villi, mesoderm penetrates them and converts them into *secondary villi* (Fig. 12–11 B). The mesoderm is probably of extraembryonic origin derived from the trophoblast. By the end of the third week, capillaries have developed in situ in the mesodermal cores of the villi, which are now termed *tertiary villi* (Fig. 12–11 B). During this period, the embryonic circulatory system is becoming established; early in the fourth week communication between the embryonic umbilical arteries and veins and the vessels of the chorion, by way of channels in the body stalk, provides a pathway of circulation of blood between the fetus and the placenta. The vessels that are found in the body stalk develop from the allantoic mesoderm (Fig. 12–12). Although the allantois itself is rudimentary, its splanchnic mesodermal component forms these important vessels. Because both the chorion and the allantois contribute to the formation of the placenta, it is called a *chorioallantoic* placenta. When the heart begins to beat during the fifth week, the placenta now functions to supply the embryo's

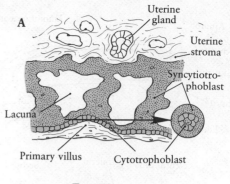

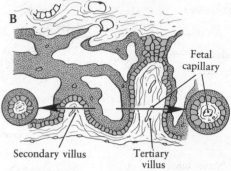

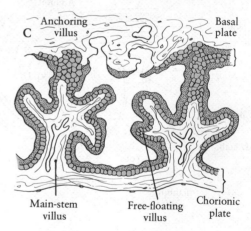

12–11 Development of chorionic villi. A, primary villus; B, secondary villus with mesodermal core and tertiary villus with fetal capillary; C, anchoring villi connecting chorionic and basal plates of the placenta.

needs, which have been taken care of prior to this time by diffusion only.

A further development of the placenta is marked by the proliferation of the cytotrophoblast at the tips of the villi into the overlying syncytiotrophoblast until it reaches the maternal endometrium (Fig. 12–11 C). Cytotrophoblast cells from adjacent villi make interconnections and form a thin cytotrophoblast shell, which marks the line of contact between the fetal and the maternal parts in the placenta. This development starts at the embryonal pole but soon occurs over the entire circumference of the placenta. Cytotrophoblast and syncytiotrophoblast in contact with the maternal decidua form the *basal plate* of the placenta. The fetal area from which the villi develop is termed the *chorionic plate*. Between the basal plate and the chorionic plate, the coalesced lacunae form the *intervillous space*. This space is still lined with syncytiotrophoblast. The villi crossing the intervillous space and attaching to the basal plate are called *anchoring villi* (Fig. 12–11 C).

As the placenta continues to develop, the villi branch extensively and each main stem forms branches that end freely in the intervillous space as well as branches that acquire secondary connections to the basal plate and thus increase the number of the anchoring villi. Each main stem villus thus resembles the root system of a bush. There are estimated to be from 60 to 200 stem villi in the mature placenta, and their branches form a dense network of villi filling in the intervillous space.

The amount of tissue separating the fetal capillaries from the intervillous space—mesenchyme, cytotrophoblast, and syncytiotrophoblast in that order—becomes progressively reduced throughout gestation, accompanied by a great increase in the number and a considerable reduction in the cross-sectional diameter of the individual villi. The capillaries increase in size and move from a central to a peripheral position directly under the trophoblast. After the first trimester the cytotrophoblast, which at first forms a complete layer in each villus, partially disappears, while the syncytiotrophoblast thins out considerably. Although at term the capillaries may often appear to bulge into the intervillous space covered only by an attenuated layer of syncytiotrophoblast, the Langhans cells never completely disappear from the villi, despite the fact that they are difficult to find in histological sections.

We may list a number of changes that occur during the development of the placenta that apparently increase the efficiency of placental transport: (1) the ratio of the surface to volume of the villi increases, (2) the thickness of the syncytiotrophoblast decreases and the cytotrophoblast becomes discontinuous, (3) the amount of villous connective tissue decreases relative to the amount of tropho-

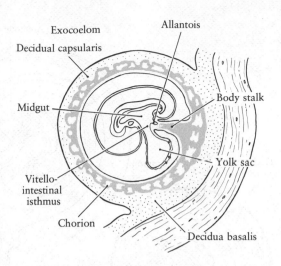

12–12 Embryo and its membranes at about the end of the first month. The allantois is rudimentary but the allantoic mesoderm has formed the body stalk blood vessels.

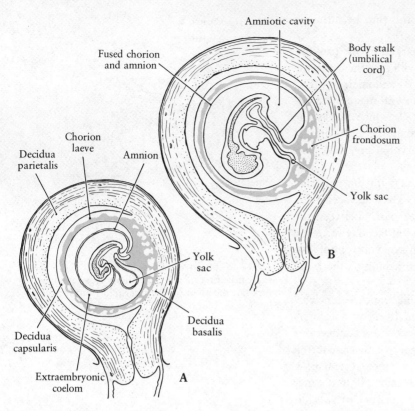

Amniotic cavity

Fused chorion
and amnion

Body stalk
(umbilical
cord)

Chorion
frondosum

Chorion
laeve

Decidua
parietalis

Amnion

Yolk sac

Yolk
sac

Decidua
basalis

Decidua
capsularis

Extraembryonic
coelom

A

B

12–13   A, the uterus, the fetus, and its membranes at about the middle of the second month.
Note remnant of the yolk sac; B, about the middle of the third month.

blast, and (4) the number of villous capillaries increase and move
closer to the surface of the villous. These changes increase the absorptive surface and reduce the amount of tissue between the maternal and the fetal systems and thus should increase the efficiency of
transport, especially for those substances that pass through the placenta by simple diffusion.

During their early development, the villi cover the entire circumference of the chorion (Fig. 12–12). During the second month, however, they become restricted to a disc-shaped region centered about
the embryonal pole. This area is termed the *chorion frondosum*
(leafy chorion). The remainder of the villi atrophy and form the
chorion laeve (smooth chorion) (Fig. 12–13).

At the margin of the disc-shaped chorion frondosum, the
chorionic plate and the basal plate fuse and this part of the placenta
is made up of several layers of cytotrophoblast cells enclosing occasional degenerating villi. The chorion laeve is lined internally with
avascular chorionic mesoderm associated with the extraembryonic
coelom. By the end of the third month the expansion of the amnion
obliterates the extraembryonic coelom and brings together the avas-

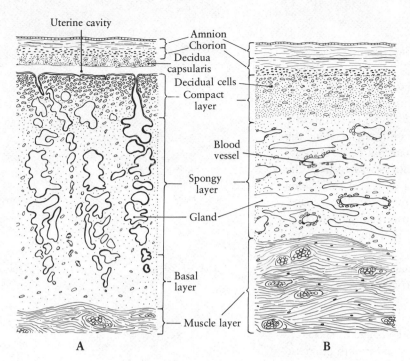

Uterine cavity

Amnion
Chorion
Decidua
capsularis
Decidual cells
Compact
layer

Blood
vessel

Spongy
layer

Gland

Basal
layer

Muscle layer

A   B

12–14 Relation of the decidua capsularis to the decidua parietalis. A, at three months, before fusion; B, at six months, after fusion and obliteration of the uterine cavity. (From L. B. Arey, 1974. Developmental Anatomy. W. B. Saunders & Company, Philadelphia.)

cular mesoderm of the amnion with that of the chorion. What is termed an *amniochorion* is thus formed (Fig. 12–13 B).

Changes in the fetal chorion are also associated with changes in the surrounding maternal tissues. On the basis of its position in relation to the embryo, the maternal decidua is divided into three areas, a *decidua basalis* over the embryonal pole and the chorion frondosum, a *decidua capsularis* over the abembryonal pole between the blastocyst and its chorion laeve and the uterine cavity, and a *decidua parietalis,* all of the remainder of the uterine decidual tissue (Fig. 12–13). Before the differentiation of the chorion frondosum and the chorion laeve, the decidua basalis and the decidua capsularis are similar in structure. As the functional villi become restricted to the embryonal region of the chorion and the embryo and its membranes increase in size, the decidua capsularis becomes stretched and begins to degenerate. Continued expansion brings the decidua capsularis into contact with the decidua parietalis of the opposite wall of the uterus. By the end of the first trimester, the uterine cavity has been obliterated and the epithelial layers of the opposing decidua capsularis and decidua parietalis have fused and degenerated and the remaining endometriums of these two parts of the uterus are no longer distinguishable (Fig. 12–14).

Placental Circulation

We have described the intervillous space as the region of the disc-shaped placenta between the chorionic and basal plates occupied by the syncytial-covered chorionic villi bathed by maternal blood. In fact, this space is partially subdivided into compartments formed by the growth of a number of septa, the *decidual septa,* projecting from the basal plate into the intervillous space but not reaching the chorionic plate. These septa with a core of maternal tissue are covered by the syncytiotrophoblast. If the placenta is viewed from the maternal side, some 15 to 20 slightly bulging domes of *cotyledons* mark this partial compartmentalization of the intervillous space. Each compartment or cotyledon contains its own stem and anchoring villi and villous network. Despite the fact that there is continuous communication between compartments in the region of the chorionic plate, the circulation of the maternal blood is concerned mainly with what takes place in each of the cotyledenary areas.

Maternal Circulation

Maternal blood reaches the placenta through the coiled or spiral arteries of the uterine endometrium. From the second month on, these arteries open directly into the intervillous space often at the apices of projections. In the intervillous space, the maternal blood is of course outside of the maternal capillaries and in contact with the syncytiotrophoblast. Within this space there are no anatomical channels to conduct the blood around the villi and back to the maternal veins. The blood entering the intervillous space from the open ends of the spiral arteries is propelled by the maternal blood pressure toward the chorionic plate, since the maternal pressure is much higher than that in the intervillous space. In this space, the blood runs into the irregular projections of the septa and the network of villi that slow it down, reduce its pressure, and spread it throughout the intervillous space. The blood is pushed along by the inflow of additional blood and eventually moves out of the space at the basal plate into the open ends of the endometrial veins. The amount of blood flowing through the placenta increases about tenfold during the last two trimesters of pregnancy owing to an increase in the diameter of the spiral arteries and dilation of their openings into the intervillous space.

Fetal Circulation

Fetal blood reaches the chorionic plate by way of the umbilical arteries passing from the fetus through the body stalk and from here into the capillaries of the villi. Its return to the fetus is through the umbilical veins of the body stalk. It was at one time proposed that the fetal blood within the villous capillaries flowed parallel but in the opposite direction from the maternal blood. Although this relationship of countercurrent flow would provide the greatest potential for exchange, the arrangement of the fetal villi precludes the existence of such a system in the human. Fetal blood flows from artery to vein through the capillaries of a single villous. Single villi are tiny compared to the intervillous space and are oriented in all varieties of directions. Maternal blood in its movement through the intervillous space passes many villi in which the capillary blood flow may be oriented differently in each villous. This type of arrangement of blood flow has been termed *multivillous flow* (Fig. 12–15).

Comparative Placentation

Membranes Involved

As noted previously, the human placenta in which the allantois, specifically the allantoic mesoderm, contributes to the vascularization of the chorion is an example of a chorioallantoic placenta. This type of placenta predominates in all mammals above the marsupials. The most primitive mammals, the monotremes, which include the fascinating Australian duck-billed platypus, are egg layers and of course do not develop a placenta. Most marsupials evidence a specialized type of prenatal development in that their young are born at very immature stages after going through a short gestation period. Since, during development the yolk sac is the first embryonic membrane to form, in these species with such short gestation periods it is the only membrane that has time to develop. As it appears, it assumes a relationship with the chorion to form what is called a *yolk-sac placenta,* or what may be better termed a *choriovitelline placenta.* In most other mammals—man is an exception—a portion of the yolk sac fuses with the chorion and its splanchnic mesoderm vascularizes a temporary choriovitelline placenta. This however, disappears when the exocoelom extends into the area and imposes itself between the yolk sac and the chorion. In some species (e.g., rabbits, mice, bats) a part of the choriovitelline placenta may persist and supplement the chorioallantoic placenta.

Placental Shape

The region of the chorion that becomes vascularized and persists in the mature placenta shows considerable variation and provides a method of classification based on the distribution pattern of the functional villi. Thus, man and most other primates with a cup-shaped region of functional villi have what is called a *discoid placenta.* Bats and rodents also have discoid placentas. *Diffuse placentas,* in which the villi cover the entire surface of the chorion, are

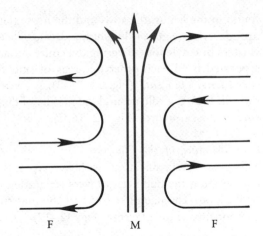

F   M   F

12–15 Schematic diagram of the relation of fetal (F) to maternal (M) blood flow in the human placenta.

found in the lemur, the sow, and the horse (Fig. 12–16 A). In most artiodactyles (e.g., cattle, sheep, deer), villi appear as prominent clusters of cotyledons covering the entire surface of the placenta but separated from each other by areas of smooth chorion forming a *cotyledenary placenta* (Fig. 12–16 B). A *zonary placenta,* in which the villi form a girdle around the middle of the chorion is characteristic of the carnivores (Fig. 12–16 C).

Fine Structure of the Placenta

This basis of classification, with five types, is based essentially on enumerating the number of layers separating the maternal and the fetal blood. The names reflect first the maternal and then the fetal components of the placenta (Fig. 12–17).

1. In the *epithelialchorial* type, found in the sow and the horse, the fetal villi of the chorioallantoic placenta rest against the intact uterine epithelium. Extensions of the villi may fit into depressions in the epithelium of the uterus.

2. Cattle and most ruminants have a *syndesmochorial*-type placenta, where uterine erosion occurs but is kept to a minimum. The chorionic villi penetrate through the uterine epithelium into the connective tissue.

3. A further step in the elimination of the amount of tissue between fetus and mother is seen in the *endothelialchorial* placenta, where the invading trophoblast lies up against the endothelium of the maternal capillaries. Carnivores have this type of placenta.

4. In man and most primates, we have seen that the endothelium of the maternal vessels is broken down and the fetal villi are found in the intervillous space bathed in maternal blood released from the open ends of the maternal vessels. The chorionic villi still retain all of their tissue—trophoblast plus connective tissue and capillary endothelium—and hence this type of placenta is termed *hemochorial*. There are two types of hemochorial placentas. One is that found in man and most higher primates with a single communicating intervillous space containing the villous network—a *villous* type. In the second type, *labyrinthine,* the trophoblastic columns are fused and the maternal blood flows in delimited channels. This type is characteristic of some insectivores, rodents, and bats.

5. The closest approach to an intermingling of fetal and maternal blood is found in the *hemoendothelial* type of placenta. Here, in some areas of the mature placentas of some rodents, the trophoblast and the connective tissue overlying the fetal capillaries disappear and only the fetal capillary endothelium separates the two systems.

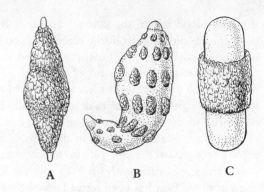

12–16   Types of placentas based on the gross distribution of villi. A, diffuse (sow); B, cotyledonary (cow); C, zonary (dog).

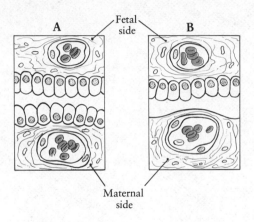
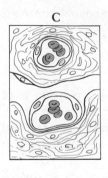
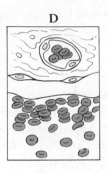
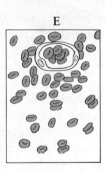

A — Fetal side

Maternal side

While the above five classifications appear rather straightforward and apparently present an easily understood picture of progressive thinning of the layers between maternal and fetal blood systems, a number of reservations must be mentioned.

1. The placenta changes with age. As we have seen from the description of the development of the human placenta, the amount of tissue between the fetal and maternal systems diminishes progressively.

2. The placenta is not uniform throughout, and considerable variation in the kind and amount of intervening tissue exists in different regions in any single placenta.

3. The classification places emphasis on the placental barrier and in so doing may suggest that the less the barrier the greater the efficiency of placental transport. While this may be true for some compounds that pass through by simple diffusion, it neglects the physiological function of the placenta during transport.

In addition, more recent electron microscope studies reveal that the classification may not be quite so clear-cut or accurate as heretofore suggested. The syndesmochorial placenta of the sheep and the goat is more like an epithelialchorial type, since remnants of the epithelium persist in some parts of the placenta. The term *vasochorial* has been suggested for some of the endothelialchorial placentas, since some connective tissue is probably necessary to support the maternal capillaries. This connective tissue may be fetal trophoblast connective tissue rather than maternal. In the endothelialchorial placenta of the cat and dog, however, maternal connective tissue persists, and these placentas should then be classified as syndesmochorial. Again, the hemoendothelial placenta

12–17 Schematic drawing of placental classification on the basis of the tissue between the maternal and fetal blood. A, epithelialchorial; B, syndesmochorial; C, endothelialchorial; D, hemochorial; E, hemoendothelial.

is really hemochorial since at least one layer of trophoblast persists throughout gestation.

Placental Transfer

Exchange between fetus and mother through the placenta is of course essential for normal intrauterine development. In this capacity the all important placenta serves as a substitute for the fetal lung, kidney, and gastrointestinal tract. We have already seen that it also serves as an endocrine organ.

We often speak of the "placental barrier." This places an emphasis on the placenta as an organ that restricts exchange between fetus and mother. While the placenta does act as a barrier in many instances, this terminology fails to focus attention on the real function of the placenta, which is to provide a mechanism for fetal-maternal exchange.

Substances pass through the placental membrane by four mechanisms: simple diffusion, facilitated diffusion, active transport, and pinocytosis. These mechanisms are not unique to the placenta but are mechanisms that occur and have been studied in other epithelial membranes such as those of the intestine and the kidney.

Simple Diffusion

Diffusion—movement of molecules from a region of higher to a region of lower concentration—is responsible for the placental transfer of many important compounds including the respiratory gases, oxygen and carbon dioxide. In the transfer of respiratory gases, the placenta approaches the efficiency of the lung. Although the thickness of the interposed tissues plays a role in transfer by diffusion, other factors are also important. These include molecular size, concentration gradient, rate of uterine and fetal blood flow, and the amount of the substance metabolized by the placenta during transfer. Generally, the amount of oxygen reaching the fetus is dependent largely on the rate of blood flow, and fetal hypoxia is usually the result of factors that diminish either the fetal or the maternal blood flow.

Facilitated Diffusion

Some substances cross the placenta in response to concentration gradients but do so at a rate more rapid than that which would result from the laws of simple diffusion. Glucose, the primary source of energy for fetal metabolism, is one such substance. In facilitated diffusion, compounds combine with a carrier molecule in a process that requires no endogenous energy source supply from the placenta. The carrier-substrate complex then crosses the placental membrane with the concentration gradient faster than that which the substrate alone would accomplish in what may be called a "rapid downhill transfer" system.

Active Transport

This type of transfer requires the presence in the placenta of an active energy-requiring transport system by means of which a compound may be transported across the membrane against a gradient. In terms of a carrier system, this means an energy-consuming chemical alteration of the carrier substance in order to effect a transport in an "uphill" direction. Some amino acids and divalent ions are transported by this method.

Pinocytosis

This involves the surrounding and engulfing of the compound to be transported by the plasma membrane of the cell and its transfer intact by what appears as a vacuole in the cytoplasm. Large molecules such as gamma globulins and lipoproteins may use this system.

Transfer of Some Specific Types of Compounds

Electrolytes: Electrolytes cross the placenta in significant quantities. Most univalent ions, such as Na^+, K^+, and Cl^-, appear to cross by simple diffusion. On the other hand, the divalent ions, such as Fe^{++}, Ca^{++}, P^{++}, and Zn^{++}, are present in higher concentrations in the fetal than in the maternal system, a distribution reflecting an active transfer system.

Proteins: The fetus synthesizes most of its proteins from amino acids transferred across the placenta. There is a net transfer from mother to fetus and a higher concentration of amino acids in the fetal than in the maternal blood, suggesting an active transfer system. Additional evidence supporting transplacental movement by means of an active transport system is: (1) the placenta shows a stereospecificity (the L-isomers usually being transported more rapidly than the D-isomers); (2) the different amino acids compete for transfer; and (3) the rate of transfer diminishes in the presence of energy-uncoupling inhibitors. Nitrogenous end products of amino acid and protein metabolisms, such as urea and creatinine, however, occur in equal concentrations in fetal and maternal blood, indicating their transfer by simple diffusion.

Many high molecular weight polypeptides cross the placenta slowly or not at all. This is true of the pancreatic hormone, insulin, and the pituitary trophic hormones, ACTH and TSH. Maternal serum proteins apparently cross the placenta intact. Gamma globulins cross in large quantities. However, only small amounts of alpha and beta globulins cross. The serum proteins are probably transferred by pinocytotis.

Carbohydrates: Pentoses and hexoses cross at the same rate and proportional to the concentration gradient—indicating simple diffusion. High molecular weight carbohydrates, such as inulin and some dextrons, do not cross, but those with molecular weights less than about 650 cross readily. Fructose and other sugars with similar molecular weights cross more slowly than glucose.

Vitamins: The water soluble vitamins, riboflavin, ascorbic acid, thiamin, and B_{12}, are present in the fetal blood in concentrations higher than in the maternal, while the reverse is true for the fat soluble vitamins. Due to the lipid nature of membranes this is unexpected. One reason for the higher concentration of water soluble vitamins in the fetal blood may be their conversion by the fetus to an impermeable product—possibly by binding to a protein.

Lipids: Acetate and many free fatty acids cross rapidly but cholesterol passes only slowly and phospholipids not at all. The immobility of the latter two lipids is probably due to their metabolism in the placenta, phospholipids being hydrolyzed to phosphate and cholesterol being used in steroid synthesis.

Drugs: Birth defects occur with alarming frequency. Although some have been shown to have a genetic basis, the cause for many others remains unknown. The thalidamide incident of the early 1960s focused attention on the fact that drugs taken during pregnancy may have damaging effects on the fetus. The fact that this tranquilizer produced an easily recognizable bizarre effect, *phocomelia,* in almost 100 percent of the cases when taken between days 34 and 45 of pregnancy was striking evidence that drugs may be teratogenic. If thalidamide had produced a more common defect—such as cleft lip—in a smaller percentage of cases, its effect may well have gone unnoticed. This implies that teratogenic drugs or chemicals are probably the unknown cause of many birth defects simply because the defects are not specific nor readily directly related to particular drugs. If this is true of a large number of drugs, both prescribed and self-administered, despite our lack of knowledge of specific effects, it leads to the sensible proposal that any drug, unless indicated on serious medical grounds, should be avoided during pregnancy. This injunction can be made despite the fact that: for most agents the defects are not specifically known; they may be varied and inconsistent; they may occur in only rather sensitive individuals in low incidence; and they do not universally follow drug administration. Despite the uncertainty about drugs, they are taken in large quantities, often by pregnant women. In one recent study in England involving 1369 pregnant women, it was reported that 97 percent were taking some form of a prescribed drug and 65 percent some form of a self-administered drug. These included analgesics, antihistamines, vitamins, diuretics, tranquilizers, antibiotics, laxatives, cough medicines, and appetite suppressors.

It is beyond the province of this book to attempt to document the evidence implicating specific compounds in the production of fetal defects. Much of the evidence is as yet inconclusive and controversial. Our knowledge of drug effects on the human fetus is necessarily slim and often circumstantial. Nevertheless, clinicians and researchers are rightly concerned about the effects of indiscriminate use of drugs during pregnancy.

Disease organisms: Fortunately, the placenta presents a true barrier to most disease organisms. Although viruses may cross the placenta, only two viral infectious agents, rubella and cytomegalovirus, have been shown to act on the fetus in the production of congenital defects.

Of these two, rubella has been thoroughly studied since it was first recognized in the early 1940s. At first it was considered effective only during the first trimester when it was shown to produce cataracts, heart lesions, hearing defects, microcephaly, and mental retardation in order of decreasing frequency. Although the defects are most frequent when infections occur in the first month, the incidence may still reach 6 percent for infections during the third, fourth, and fifth months.

Cytomegaloviruses, so named because of the characteristic enlargement of the cells containing the virus, are also able to cross the placenta. Congenital defects produced include microcephaly, microphthalmia, blindness, hepatomegaly, and sometimes encephalitis.

Other viruses may cross the placenta but they do not lead to developmental anomalies. These include the agents of polio, smallpox, vaccinia, and mumps, which may produce chronic infections in the fetus.

A number of nonviral organisms are also known to result in fetal infection. This is evidenced as a pathological expression of the disease in the fetus and the newborn rather than as any developmental defect. One such infection is syphilis, which is incurred by the fetus following transmission from the mother through the placenta. The fetus has little resistance to the spirochetes that live and multiply rapidly and are found in practically all of the fetal tissues in numbers far greater than in the adult. Approximately 25 percent of the infected fetuses die before term and a high percentage are born prematurely.

Erythroblastosis fetalis: Despite the fact that the tissues of the mother and the fetus, which are immunologically incompatible, develop side by side without tissue destruction—possibly due to some trophoblastic barrier intervening between the two—there is one situation in which the barrier is shown to be defective. This involves cases in which the blood cell antigens of the fetus and the mother are different. Most studied and publicized is Rh incompatibility where an Rh-positive fetus is carried by an Rh-negative mother. Rh-negative individuals are double recessives. Thus, the fetus, if both parents are Rh negative, presents no problem. However, the fetus of an Rh-negative mother and an Rh-positive father could be either Rh positive or negative depending on well-known genetic laws and probabilities. If the fetus is Rh positive, and red blood cells get through the placenta into the maternal circulation, they will trigger an immune response from the Rh-negative maternal system which will produce antibodies against the foreign antigen. These antibodies, gamma globulins, will pass through the placenta and into the fetal circulation; the resulting antigen-antibody reaction will destroy fetal red cells, lead to anemia and jaundice and cause liver and spleen enlargement. Because of the extensive red cell destruction, this disease is also called hemolytic disease of the fetus. Since there is no connection between maternal and fetal circulatory systems, fetal red cells must reach the maternal circulation through some defect in the placenta. Placental transfer of red cells is now well documented; in a recent study, fetal red cells were found to be present in 71 percent of all pregnant women. However, the numbers present were small and in most cases the amount of fetal blood which crosses the placental barrier is usually less than that necessary to initiate a primary maternal response.

There are factors, other than the number of fetal red cells, which affect the maternal antibody response. One is the suppression of the maternal response by the elevated levels of steroids present during pregnancy. Also, if the fetal cells are incompatible with the mother's ABO blood group antigens, their survival time in the maternal system is limited and may not be long enough to initiate an immune response. New techniques for prediction, prevention, diagnosis, and treatment have significantly decreased the serious consequences of Rh incompatibility. Even prior to the introduction of these measures only 1 in 20 to 26 Rh-incompatible matings resulted in involvement of the fetus.

Passive Immunity
The adult acquires immunity over a period of time, responding to the challenges of invading organisms by establishing specific defense mechanisms mediated in a large part through serum antibodies. The fetus is not only to a large extent effectively—but not completely—isolated from these challenges but also is not capable of

responding to them by synthesizing any significant amounts of antibodies. Thus, at birth, the fetus is projected into a potentially hostile environment filled with microbial challengers, at a time when it has not had the opportunity to develop its defense against these challengers. Fortunately, the fetus is provided with a defense mechanism that it in a sense has borrowed from its mother by means of the passage of maternal antibodies across the placental membrane. In this instance, the introduction of maternal antibodies into the fetal circulation is not undesirable, as in the case of Rh antibodies, but is instead of definite advantage to the fetus. Almost any infection that the mother has contracted—measles, mumps, whooping cough, influenza—will cause her to develop antibodies against these disease organisms which, after they cross the placenta, provide the newborn with a built-in defense mechanism. This passive immunity lasts for several months of postnatal life, during which time the infant progressively acquires its own immunity in response to the challenges offered to it.

Fetal-Maternal Immunological Reactions

Grafts or transplants that are genetically alien to a host are quickly rejected. Yet the fetus is genetically distinct from the mother and despite the fact that the fetal placental unit is in intimate contact with the immunocompetent maternal tissues, it is not rejected. It has been suggested that the uterus is an immunologically privileged site. However, the occurrence of ectopic pregnancies in such places as the uterine tube or the ovary, where the fetus is not rejected either, does not support this. In fact, the decidual reaction of the uterus appears to resist the invasive tendencies of the fetus, and this invasiveness is much more apparent in ectopic sites. A balance must be achieved between the aggressive invasive activities of the fetal trophoblast and the tendencies of the maternal organism to rid itself of a foreign graft. Such a mechanism probably resides at the site of contact between the fetal trophoblast and the maternal decidua. In fact, it has been suggested that there is actually no significant contact between maternal and fetal tissues. This may be due to the fact that the trophoblast surrounds itself with an extracellular acid mucopolysaccharide deposit or fibrinoid, which effectively isolates it from the maternal tissues. This anatomical barrier erected by the fetus acts to prevent the passage of fetal antigens into the maternal system where they would trigger an antibody reaction. It has also been proposed that human chorionic gonadotrophin (HCG) may play a role in this process by inhibiting the response of the maternal lymphocytes to fetal antigens.

ANALYSIS OF EARLY
MAMMALIAN DEVELOPMENT

With relatively few exceptions, it was not until the 1960s that experiments on the early stages of the mammalian embryo were reported in the literature. The main reason for this was that early attempts at culturing and manipulating mammalian embryos outside of the maternal environment met with limited success. An additional factor involved the low rate of egg production and the difficulty of obtaining embryos. This has left unanswered or speculative the question of regulative versus determinative development as the causal basis of the establishment of developmental patterns in mammalian systems. Gradients in the distribution of cytoplasmic components have been described in the mouse egg, and they may have a causal relationship to early differentiation, thus classifying the mammalian egg as determinative. Other investigations of the development of one of the two-cell or four-cell blastomeres also supported the idea that the direction of development of the early blastomeres was dictated by the character of the inherited cytoplasm.

However, the refinement of in vitro culture techniques and the development of better manipulative procedures have produced a greater amount of experimentation under controlled conditions and have modified and contradicted earlier conclusions. The more recent experiments have contributed the general concepts that the mammalian egg is indeed regulative, that the early blastomeres are totipotent probably to the eight-cell stage and that the basis of determination of which blastomeres will form the inner cell mass and which will form trophoblast is the position they assume in the morula stage rather than differential distribution of cytoplasmic determinants.

Development of Individual Blastomeres

A number of studies have shown that single blastomeres of the two- or four-cell mouse or rabbit embryo are capable of regulation in culture to form normal blastocysts composed of inner cell mass and trophoblast. Blastocysts from one-half or one-quarter embryos have been transferred to foster mothers and brought to term, and the offspring were normal and fertile. In the rabbit, when seven blastomeres of the eight-cell embryo were destroyed and removed, a single blastomere remaining within its own zona pellucida and reimplanted into a foster mother survived to term in 11 percent of the operations performed. Since the surviving blastomere is chosen at random, this experiment does not prove that each and every one of the eight blastomeres is capable of this performance. In fact, since the percentage of blastomeres that survive to term decreases from the four-cell to the eight-cell stage, it might even suggest the opposite. However, a greater susceptibility to damage and a greater difficulty in manipulating embryos with larger numbers of blastomeres could also account for the result.

Attempts have been made to follow the development of all of the blastomeres of the four- or eight-cell mouse embryo. Since this necessarily involves culture of naked (zona pellucida removed) eggs and since naked blastomeres cannot be transferred to foster mothers, development can be followed only to the blastocyst stage. In these experiments there was no indication of isolated blastomeres from any one embryo developing complementary structures—as one would expect if segregation of cytoplasmic factors into individual blastomeres was responsible for differentiation. In fact, it was demonstrated that every cell in the embryo up to the eight-cell stage has the potentiality of developing into a trophoblast. In addition, about one third of the single blastomeres developed from four-cell embryos and 11 percent of the single blastomeres developed from the eight-cell embryo formed more or less normal blastocysts with an inner cell mass covered by a trophoblast.

Disaggregation and the Development of Chimeras

Regulative activity may also be demonstrated by disaggregation studies in which zona-free eggs are disaggregated and pooled and then groups of cells from the pooled mass are removed and cultured. Complete disassociation of embryos from the eight-cell to the early blastocyst stage is followed by reaggregation and development to morphologically normal blastocysts in 90 percent of the cases of pooled cells of the same developmental age and 77 percent of the cases of pooled cells from eggs of different developmental ages (4-cell and 16-cell; 4-cell and 32-cell). Pooling of embryos results in a varied mixture of blastomeres, and it is unlikely that blastomeres in the reaggregate take up positions corresponding to any original polarity. Thus, any spatial or gradient-forming relationships between the original blastomeres are completely destroyed. It is apparent that any polarity present in the uncleaved egg and the early embryo is unnecessary for differentiation up to the blastocyst stage.

Regulative development can also be demonstrated through the formation of chimeras by fusing the cells from two or more embryos. Again, extensive rearrangement of the blastomeres will result. The development of a high percentage of normal blastocysts (Fig. 12–18) under conditions in which migration and rearrangement or sorting out of fused cells to reestablish a particular pattern

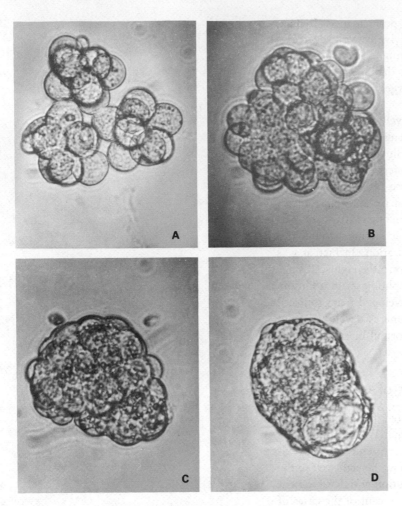

12–18 In vitro aggregation of three eight-celled mouse embryos. A, at 1 hour after fusion, a few blastomeres from each embryo are in contact; B, at 8 hours, a single compact embryo is beginning to form; C, at 19 hours, a morula three times larger than normal; D, at 25 hours, a small blastocoele has formed. (From M. S. Stern and I. B. Wilson, 1972. J. Embryol. Exp. Morphol. 25, 247.)

or location of specific blastomeres is impossible, also supports the conclusion that cytoplasmic segregation is not responsible for early differentiation. It is not even necessary to fuse embryos of the same age. A good percentage of eight-cell embryos fused with late morulas or early blastocysts can regulate for these chronological differences as well as develop into morphologically normal, but giant, blastocysts (Fig. 12–19).

Differentiation of the Trophoblast and the Inner Cell Mass

By three and a half days of development, the fully expanded blastocyst is made up of two distinct populations of cells, the inner cell mass and the trophectoderm, committed to different directions of

A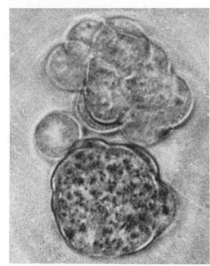

B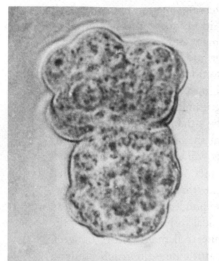

C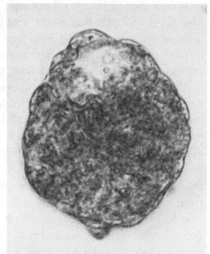

development. On the basis of their experiments on culturing isolated blastomeres from early mouse embryos, Tarkowski and Wroblewska (1967) proposed that the factor that determines which of the two routes of development any blastomere takes depends upon its position in the developing embryo. Those cells that remain on the outside develop into trophectoderm. Those cells that occupy the interior form the inner cell mass by virtue of their isolation from influences of the external environment. The initially totipotent cells of the early cleavage stages, as they develop into the morula, recognize their position as either "outside" or "inside" and develop trophectoderm or inner cell mass accordingly. A variety of experiments have since been reported to support this hypothesis.

At the fully expanded blastocyst stage, both of these types of cells are fully committed to divergent pathways of development. Trophectoderm cells may be dissected free and cultured or transplanted, and under no condition will they form anything but trophectoderm. Conversely, isolated inner cell masses never develop any trophectoderm. The trophectoderm of a blastocyst may be lysed away, leaving only inner cell mass tissue, by reacting the blastocyst with antispecific antisera (immunosurgery). When this inner cell mass free of trophectoderm is cultured in vitro, it forms only a compact cell mass with no trophectoderm evident.

Although the three-and-a-half-day blastocyst is committed to two divergent pathways of development, we still have to find out at what point in development this commitment occurs. At the eight-cell stage the blastomeres, which are at first spherical in shape and loosely arranged, compact into a single columnar layer in which the

D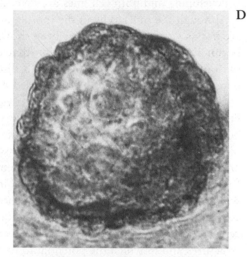

12–19   Fusion of developing mouse eggs of different ages. A, an eight-celled egg joined with a morula; B, A after 4 hours in culture; C, A after 21 hours in culture. Cavitation is apparently starting in the older partner; D, blastocyst developed from A after 45 hours in culture. (From C. L. Markert and R. M. Peters, 1978. Science 202, 56. Copyright 1978 by the American Association for the Advancement of Science.)

cells now show a structural polarity, having inner and outer ends. It was suggested that this might result in an unequal distribution of cellular contents in which inner cell mass and trophectoderm "materials" may be segregated in the inner and outer regions of the cell. However, cell marking experiments do not support this contention.

As soon as cells become positioned in the interior, their potencies can be tested by isolating them using immunosurgery. We have already seen that at three and a half days the inner cell mass cannot form any trophectoderm. However, at the morula stage, inner cells differentiate into miniature blastocysts, which show typical trophectoderm as well as inner cell mass. In fact, inner cell masses isolated from cavitating blastocysts only some three to four hours away from the three-and-a-half-day fully expanded blastocyst stage can also form normal blastocysts with typical trophectoderm. Thus, the commitment to trophectoderm or inner cell mass occurs between three and three and a half days, just at the time the trophectoderm is developing and both cell lines are determined at the same time.

Although the inner cells in the morula and developing blastocyst are not as yet determined, it has been shown that they have already begun to differentiate in a direction that distinguishes them from the outer cells. The inner cells have a distinct pattern of alkaline phosphatase activity and a higher labeled thymidine uptake as early as the morula stage. In the early blastocyst they show evidence of fluid accumulation and will not phagocytose melanin granules— both properties that distinguish them from the outer potential trophectoderm cells. Of the five groups of tissue-specific proteins that are present in the embryonic cells of the mature blastocyst, one is found in the 16-cell stage and two more in the morula. This stepwise divergent differentiation finally reaches a point when the inner cell mass is determined to follow a path of development in which its cells are destined to form only embryonic and some extraembryonic structures and in which the potential to form trophectoderm is lost. The two cell lines are distinct.

Differentiation Within the Trophectoderm

By day four and a half the trophoblast shows regional differences. The mural cells—those cells not lying above the inner cell mass— stop dividing and form primary giant cells. The polar cells continue to divide. They form the ectoplacental cone above the inner cell mass. As the ectoplacental cone increases in thickness, secondary giant cells appear in the region furthest away from the underlying inner cell mass. The regional differentiation of the trophoblast has been ascribed to inductive influences from the inner cell mass. Trophoblast cells lose the capacity to divide and become giant cells unless they are exposed to influences from the inner cell mass. Secondary giant cells are formed in the ectoplacental cone by progeny of the dividing polar cells, which are pushed to peripheral regions where they are no longer influenced by the inner cell mass. The nature of the inductive influence is not known.

Regulation Within the Inner Cell Mass

We may now return to the inner cell mass cells. Their fate is to form the egg cylinder that will form the embryo proper, the amnion, the yolk sac, and part of the chorioallantoic placenta. However, regulation within these prospective fates is still possible. A number of experiments demonstrate that the cells of the inner cell mass are not committed to specific developmental pathways but that a high potentiality for regulation within the system is still present.

1. When part of the inner cell mass is removed, a normal offspring may result.

2. Whole blastocysts, when cut in half, will develop into fetuses that are morphologically normal.

3. An inner cell mass from a three-and-a-half-day blastocyst may be transplanted to a host three-and-a-half-day blastocyst where it will aggregate with the host inner cell mass and produce a normal chimeric offspring.

4. When a single, marked inner-cell mass cell is injected into a host blastocyst, the progeny of this cell are widely distributed when the resulting 11-½- to 17-½-day embryos are examined. Donor cells have been found in the embryo proper and in its membranes and in derivatives of all three germ layers.

Further Development of the Inner Cell Mass

As the inner cell mass develops from three and a half to four and a half days, a monolayer of cells appears on its blastocoelic surface, which may be distinguished from the other cells of the inner cell mass on the basis of their morphology, the formation of tight junctions, and the presence of cytoplasm rich in rough endoplasmic reticulum. This layer is the *primitive endoderm,* which will contribute to the formation of the yolk sac and the placenta. The remaining inner cell mass, the *primitive ectoderm,* will form all of the fetal germ layer material.

The prospective fates of the primitive endoderm and primitive ectoderm are different but are their potencies also restricted? They are. Culturing primitive endoderm yields only primitive endoderm

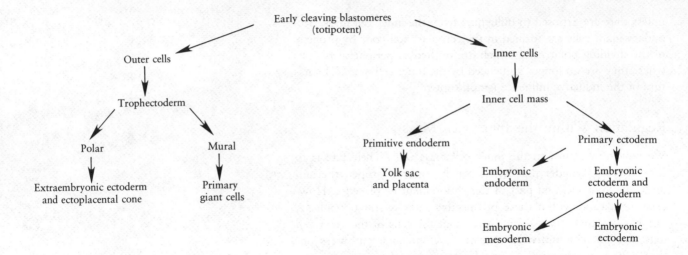

and indicates that it is at four and a half days committed to only a single developmental direction. Conversely, the primitive ectoderm cells will form only embryonic ectoderm, endoderm, and mesoderm and cannot form primitive endoderm. However, within the framework of these potentialities, the primitive ectoderm is not as yet determined to develop in any specific direction. Up to the primitive streak stage, the ectoderm can still form both endoderm and mesoderm. At the time the embryonic endoderm develops—in the primitive streak stage—the ectoderm then loses its capability to form more endoderm. Later, when the mesoderm develops, it also loses its capability to form more mesoderm. There is a progressive restriction of developmental potencies.

Apparently, at the time certain cells in the inner cell mass become committed to some specific line of development, the remaining cells lose the capability of forming any more cells of this line. When the trophectoderm cells appear, the inner cell mass loses its potential to form more trophectoderm; and when the primitive endoderm differentiates, the inner cell mass then loses its potential to form more primitive endoderm; and so on down the line. Each step means the formation of a determined cell line and the restriction of potency in the as yet undetermined cells to form any more cells of the determined line. A scheme of development of the mouse embryo is diagrammed in Figure 12–20, showing in both the inner cell mass and the trophectoderm the same type of progressive restriction of developmental potencies.

It is questionable if all the conclusions drawn from the analysis of differentiation in one mammal can be applied to all of the others. However, there appears to be no question that the mammalian egg may be considered to be a regulative system in which neither polar-

12–20 Schematic diagram of the progressive steps in the development of the mouse embryo. (After R. L. Gardner, 1975. The Developmental Biology of Reproduction, C. L. Markert and J. Papacandantinau, eds. Academic Press, New York.)

ity nor the differential distribution of cytoplasmic factors are important for future development. The inner-outer determination of inner cell mass and trophoblast differentiation and the regulative properties of the inner cell mass cells appear to be general mammalian characteristics. However, the inductive influence of the inner cell mass on the differentiation of the polar trophoblast has not been completely substantiated in all the species studied.

REFERENCES

Bartels, H., W. Moll, and J. Metcalfe. 1962. Physiology of gas exchange in the human placenta. Am. J. Obstet. Gynecol. 84:1714–1730.

Dalcq, A. M. 1957. Introduction to General Embryology, pp. 103–108. London: Oxford University Press.

Gardner, R. L. 1975. Analysis of determination and differentiation in the early mammalian embryo using intra- and interspecific chimeras. In: The Developmental Biology of Reproduction, pp. 207–236. Eds., C. L. Markert and J. Papaconstantinau. New York: Academic Press.

Johnson, M. H., A. H. Handyside, and P. R. Braude. 1977. Control mechanisms in early mammalian development. In: Development in Mammals. Ed., M. H. Johnson, New York: North-Holland.

Mintz, B. 1964. Synthetic processes and early development in the mammalian egg. J. Exp. Zool. 157:85–100.

Moore, N. W., C. E. Adams, and L. E. A. Rowan. 1968. Developmental potential of single blastomeres of the rabbit egg. J. Reprod. Fertil. 17:527–537.

Nelson, M. M. and J. O. Forar. 1971. Association between drugs administered during pregnancy and congenital abnormalities of the fetus. Br. Med. J. 1:523–527.

Ramsey, E. M. 1973. Placental vasculature and circulation. In: Handbook of Physiology, Endocrinology II, Part 2. Ed., R. O. Greep. Baltimore: Williams and Wilkins.

Rasmussen, D. M. 1968. Syphilis and the fetus. In: Intra-Uterine Development. Ed., A. C. Barnes. Philadelphia: Lea and Febiger.

Rossant, J. 1977. Cell commitment in early rodent development. In: Development in Mammals. Ed., M. H. Johnson. New York: North-Holland.

Seeds, A. E. 1968. Placental transfer. In: Intra-Uterine Development. Ed., A. C. Barnes. Philadelphia: Lea and Febiger.

Seidel, F. 1960. Die Entwicklungsfähigkeiten isolierter Furchungszellen aus dem Ei des Kaninchens, Oryctolagus cuniculus. Wilhelm Roux' Arch. Entwicklungomech. Org. 152:44–130.

Sever, J. L. 1971. Viral infections and malformations. Fed. Proc., Fed. Am. Soc. Exp. Biol. 30:114–117.

Stern, M. S. 1972. Experimental studies on the organization of the pre-implantation mouse embryo. II. Reaggregation of disaggregated embryos. J. Embryol. Exp. Morphol. 28:255–261.

Stern, M. S. and I. B. Wilson. 1972. Experimental studies on the organization of the pre-implantation mouse embryo. I. Fusion of asynchronously dividing eggs. J. Embryol. Exp. Morphol. 28:247–254.

Tarkowski, A. K. 1959. Experiments on the development of isolated blastomeres of mouse eggs. Nature (London) 184:1286–1287.

Tarkowski, A. K. and J. Wroblewska. 1967. Development of blastomeres of mouse eggs isolated at the 4- and 8-cell stage. J. Embryol. Exp. Morphol. 18:155–180.

Wynn, R. M. 1973. Fine structure of the placenta. In: Handbook of Physiology, Endocrinology II, Part 2. Ed., R. O. Greep. Baltimore: Williams and Wilkins.

13

Principles of Morphogenesis

By the end of gastrulation, each germ layer, occupying a different topographical position in the embryo, is broadly committed to develop into specific tissue and organ primordia. In both amniote and anamniote embryos, the basic body plan at this time is that of a tube within a tube. The inner, endodermal tube is separated from the outer or ectodermal tube by coelomic tubes of mesoderm. The free surface of each tube is initially organized as a sheet of cells or an *epithelium*. An epithelium is a monolayer of cells whose tight-knit cohesiveness is maintained by specialized intercellular junctions and extracellular materials. An important property of embryonic epithelia is the capacity for their individual cells to change shape. Alterations in the shapes of individual cells are translated and integrated into morphogenetic movements involving many cells. Transformation of epithelia in multicellular animal embryos by modifications in the shape of cells is an important instrument in the establishment of definite form in many organs.

Organogenesis can be considered to occur during that period of time when organs and organ systems become fashioned from germ layer organ rudiments. Most organs develop from rudiments that consist of an epithelial tissue and a mesenchymal tissue. Analysis of organ development shows that the processes of morphogenesis and cytodifferentiation must occur if tissues and organs are to acquire their proper structural and functional features. The importance of these two events is readily apparent in most cases of organ development. For example, it would be futile for the embryo to differentiate cells capable of producing bile (liver) or secretory enzymes (pancreas) without the development of a network of small ductules and ducts (morphogenesis) to carry the products to the small intestine.

The precise relationships between the differentiation of the functional cell types of an organ and the development of that organ's morphology (i.e., shape, form) are still imperfectly understood. Since the synthesis of specific molecules within a differentiating cell is dependent upon its gene activity, it is natural to ask whether the genes controlling macromolecular synthesis and the genes controlling morphogenesis are functionally coupled or independently regulated. Based primarily on studies using embryonic pancreas, thyroid gland, and glands of the oviduct, it appears that specific steps in the development of the morphology of an organ can be temporally correlated with the differentiation of its unique cell types. For example, Rutter and his colleagues (1968) have examined the relationships between cytodifferentiation and morphogenesis in the development of the mouse pancreas. The dorsal pancreas in the mouse arises as a hollow diverticulum from the endoderm; this epithelial rudiment pushes into the investing mesodermal tissue (Chapter 15). Subsequently, fingerlike groups of cells develop from the epithelial outpocketing that branch to form a labyrinth of ductules and ducts. Special cell clusters termed acini arise at the terminal ends of the ductules. These differentiate as exocrine cells and will produce the digestive enzymes of the pancreatic juice. Using sensitive biochemical assays for the detection of pancreatic proteins, Rutter was able to identify, although at very low levels, the first pancreatic proteins at about the time that the initial form of the gland was taking shape. Increased levels of the enzymes were subsequently detected several days later when ducts, ductules, and acini were clearly formed. Hence, the morphogenetic phase of an organ can be correlated with levels of differentiation of its cell types.

Of the morphogenetic and cytodifferentiative phases that characterize organ development, it is fair to state that the bulk of work has centered on how individual cells acquire their special structural and chemical properties. Less well understood are the processes that account for the morphogenetic phase of organ formation. The processes involved in this phase of organ development include localized cell division, cell movements, localized cell death, and alterations in the extracellular matrix.

MORPHOGENESIS OF EMBRYONIC EPITHELIA BY CHANGES IN CELL SHAPE

Most of the internal organs of the vertebrate organism, such as lungs, pancreas, salivary glands, and so on, originate from primordia consisting of two dissimilar cell populations. One population of cells is epithelial in its organization. These cells line tubes, ducts, cavities, and so forth and differentiate into specific functional components of organs. The other population of cells, generally of mesodermal origin, is less regularly or uniformly organized and will contribute to the connective and supportive functions of organs.

The form and shape associated with many internal organs relate to the localized transformation of the epithelial component of primary organ rudiments. Commonly, the initial phase in the formation of an organ is expressed as a thickening in an embryonic

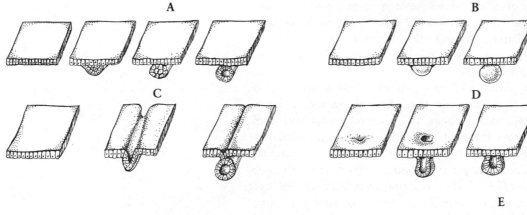

A

B

C

D

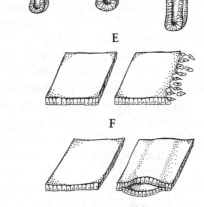

E

F

epithelial layer, as in the case of the neural tube. Paired (lens placodes) or multiple (hair follicles) organs initially appear as two or many thickenings, respectively, within the same embryonic layer. As described in Chapter 10. the neural plate of *Triturus* forms as a result of a middorsal thickening in the outer, epithelial layer of ectoderm. Tall, columnar-shaped cells characterize the neural plate and stretch from its internal to external surfaces. Rather than being due to localized differences in rates of cellular mitoses, the neural plate thickening can be correlated with the elongation of individual cells in the middorsal region of the embryo. Thickenings representing the early primordia of the lenses and inner ears arise as the result of a rearrangement of cells within an epithelial layer. Although each cell of the thickening changes shape drastically, it does not shift in position relative to its neighbors.

Thickenings within an epithelial layer may be directed outward or inward. Often, the thickening may secondarily lose its connection with the epithelial layer and remain solid (thyroid gland) or acquire an internal cavity (Fig. 13–1A). For example, in hagfishes and bony fishes the neural plate arises as a longitudinal thickening in the ectoderm. It subsequently separates itself from the epidermis. Internally, a rearrangement of cells leads to the construction of a central cavity (neurocoele) within the longitudinal thickening. The lenses of frogs and bony fishes also form in similar fashion (Fig. 13–1B). A localized, thickened group of ectodermal cells separates from the adjacent epidermis and slips beneath the surface as a solid mass. Here, an internal reorganization of cells leads to the formation of a hollow body or lens vesicle.

The folding of an epithelial sheet, either by invagination or by evagination, is perhaps the most common method in the formation of organs. Recall that the invagination of the primitive gut in echinoderms and cephalochordates, as well as the initial indentation of the endoderm in amphibian gastrulas, is essentially the infolding of

13–1 A diagram showing various types of transformations in an embryonic epithelium that may occur during the formation of an organ. A, development of a tube from a solid, longitudinal thickening of the epithelium; B, development of a vesicle from a localized thickening of the epithelium; C, a longitudinal groove in an epithelium giving rise to a hollow tube; D, a localized pit may give rise to a vesicle or to a tubule continuous with the epithelial surface; E, disaggregation of an epithelium to produce mesenchymelike cells; F, splitting of an epithelial layer into two layers (i.e., coelom formation). (From B. I. Balinsky, 1975. An Introduction to Embryology. W. B. Saunders Company, Philadelphia.)

an epithelial layer of cells. The reverse of invagination—evagination—is utilized in constructing diverticula from the germ layer tubes formed by gastrulation. The gut tube, for example, evaginates to form the visceral pouches, the laryngotracheal groove, and the pancreatic and liver primordia.

Two types of epithelial foldings can be identified in organ formation (Fig. 13–1C,D). If the infolding of the epithelial sheet is linear, there results a longitudinal groove (i.e., a neural groove with complete separation from the epithelial layer produces a closed tube [i.e., a neural tube]) (Fig. 13–1C). If the separation is incomplete, then the tube remains connected to the epithelial layer by an opening (i.e., a trachea). The infolding of a portion of the epithelial layer may be quite localized, producing a depression or pocketlike structure (Fig. 13–1D). Separation of these pocketlike formations yields epithelia-lined, hollow vesicles. The eye lenses and the inner ear vesicles of amniote embryos are fashioned in this way.

The foldings of an epithelial sheet are manifestations of cells that actively undergo morphogenetic movements. Movements are accomplished by the coordination of changes in the shapes of individual cells within the sheet which are translated into changes in the form of a population of cells. Two types of cell shape are recognized during the morphogenesis of epithelia. First, individual cells may elongate, as in the early formation of such organs as the neural plate, lens, thyroid gland, and pancreas. Second, individual cells may narrow or constrict at either their apical or basal ends. Recall that apical constriction produces wedge-shaped cells and converts a flattened, thickened surface into a curved surface (i.e., the basis of an infolding) (Chapter 10).

While the changes in the shapes of cells during morphogenesis of epithelia appear to be rather complicated, available evidence now indicates that only a few cellular forces are involved and that these are used again and again. The forces responsible for the morphogenetic movements of epithelia are within their constituent cells and generally held to be due to the coordinate activities of two kinds of organelles: microtubules and microfilaments. As pointed out in Chapter 10, microtubules, long, cylindrical, unbranched structures, generate changes in cell shape by virtue of their orientation and distribution within epithelial cells. Microtubules are almost always observed to be oriented parallel to the long axis of lengthening cells (i.e., lens placode and neural plate formation). Also, various inhibitors (e.g., colchicine, colcemid) cause disruption of the microtubules, which results in the disappearance of cell asymmetry. The elongation of cells is clearly dependent upon intact microtubules.

It is still unclear as to how microtubules function in the elongation of cells in epithelia. Several hypotheses have been put forth (Chapter 10). Microtubules might "push" the elongating ends of a cell by the polymerization of additional subunits at its poles. Force against the apical and basal ends of a lengthening cell may be generated by the active sliding of an apical set of microtubules against a basal set of microtubules, thereby decreasing overlap. Other investigators have suggested that the microtubules may function as rigid tracts along which the flow of cytoplasm is directed from the apical to the basal end of the cell. All three of these hypotheses account for the lengthening of a cell.

Microfilaments are generally held to be responsible for changing the shape of epithelial cells through their contractile activity. Microfilaments can be temporally and spatially correlated with localized constriction of epithelial cells (i.e., neural plate cells). Experiments with cytochalasin B, which disrupts the integrity of microfilaments in some cell types, suggest a correlation between the presence of these organelles and the apical constriction of epithelial cells. Bundles of microfilaments are considered essential in the formation of such organs as the neural tube, the lens vesicle, and the pancreatic diverticulum. It might seem rather surprising that nonmuscle embryonic, epithelial cells have contractile properties. Yet, numerous biochemical studies have shown actin and myosin to be present in many varieties of nonmuscle cell types. There is compelling evidence that actin, considered to be the major protein of microfilaments, extracted from nonmuscle cell types behaves physiologically and biochemically like the actin of skeletal muscle. Although there is the suspicion that morphogenetic movements of epithelia are mediated by musclelike proteins, there needs to be a careful assessment of the properties of these "motility proteins" and their exact form of distribution within filaments of nonmuscle cells.

INDIVIDUAL CELLS AND THEIR MOVEMENTS

Although the spreading, folding, and branching of cohesive sheets of cells are instrumental in rearranging cells and thereby giving shape to an organ, individual cells or clusters of cells are an important source of materials for organ formation. Mesenchymal cells, primordial germ cells, and neural crest cells migrate, often over considerable distances from their point of origin, to accumulate at specific sites in the embryo where they will aggregate to give rise to organ rudiments or disperse and participate in organ construction. Generally these cells migrate as individual units, crawling over a substratum that may be the basal lamina underlying an epithelium or the extracellular matrix between epithelia. Properties of embryonic substrata are important in determining when cells begin to move, where cells move, and when cells stop moving.

Both mesenchyme and neural crest cells are examples of individual cell types produced by the breaking up or disaggregation of epithelial tissues (Figs. 13–1E; 13–2). Neural crest cells arise dorsally from the epithelial cells at the lateral edges of the neural plate. They detach from the ectodermal epithelium during neurulation and become organized above the neural tube as an axial ribbon of tightly clustered cells. Subsequently, the neural crest cells disaggregate in an anteroposterior sequence and give rise to migratory cells that move away from the neural tube in two discrete streams (Fig. 13–2). A dorsal stream moves laterally and glides beneath the overlying ectoderm. A second stream of cells migrates laterally and ventrally to a position medial to the somites. Pigment cells of the dermis, nerve cells of the spinal ganglia, ganglia of the sympathetic and parasympathetic divisions of the nervous system, and the cartilages of the embryonic pharynx are derivatives of neural crest cell populations.

Since neural crest cells follow different pathways during cellular migration, invade and aggregate in specific regions of the embryo, and differentiate into such varied cell types, they have been used as an experimental model system in the investigation of several questions regarding morphogenetic movements of individual cells in the embryo. Do individual cells migrate to specific sites because of their intrinsic genetic properties, or do they utilize preformed, directional pathways provided by other tissues or the extracellular matrix? Why do cells stop at a specific site in the embryo? Are they directed to a specific target because of the special properties of that site?

Where the movements of individual cells can be demonstrated to be oriented and directed rather than random, as is the case with neural crest cells, it appears that the properties of the extracellular environment or matrix mediate and guide the cells to their specific destinations. The neural crest cells appear to recognize and selectively to make adhesive contacts with the extracellular substratum. The cells cease movement at specific places in the embryo when their tendency to adhere to each other is stronger than the adhesion between them and the extracellular matrix. Consequently, the cessation of movements of cells results in dense masses or aggregates of cells. P. Weiss coined the term *contact guidance* to refer to the orientation given by the substratum to cells during their migratory activities. It needs to be emphasized, however, that contact guidance is a concept that has emerged from studies utilizing cell culture techniques. Its application to an understanding of morphogenetic

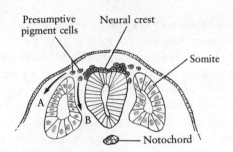

13–2 Diagram of a cross section through an early vertebrate embryo showing the two alternative pathways for the migration of neural crest cells. One (A) dorsolateral stream leads to the formation of epidermal pigment cells. The other (B) stream leads to the formation of posterior root ganglia, autonomic nervous system ganglia, and cells of the medulla of the adrenal gland.

movements in the embryo must currently be considered with reservation.

Mesenchyme cells are individual, stellate-shaped cells that migrate away from mesodermal epithelia and aggregate at specific target sites in the embryo. Here, they differentiate as rudiments of organs (e.g., cartilage and bone cells of the skeletal system) or as connective tissues for the support of the epithelial components of organs. The movement of individual mesenchyme cells between their site of origin and their final destination has been studied in remarkable detail in the sea urchin using cinemicrography (Chapter 8). Prior to the onset of gastrulation, the primary mesenchyme cells of the vegetal plate begin locomotory activity by pulsating and forming hemispherical protrusions called blebs. Following their separation from neighboring cells as well as from each other, presumably because of a decrease in cell-to-cell adhesiveness, the mesenchyme cells round up and move into the blastocoele. Each cell sends out long, thin dendritic pseudopodia or filopodia whose tips probe the inner surface of the blastocoele wall. When an adhesive contact with the blastocoele wall is made (i.e., at the junction between ectodermal cells), the filopodium contacts and thus pulls the cell along. The movement of these primary mesenchyme cells along the inner surface of the ectoderm appears to be rather like an inchworm, accomplished by the filopodia alternately making and breaking contacts with the cellular substratum.

The migratory behavior of mesenchyme cells in the intact vertebrate embryo has not been studied to any great extent. One organ that has received some attention is the eye of the chick. On the fourth day of chick embryonic development, mesenchyme cells migrate as individuals into an area between the cornea and the lens. Following their rearrangement into an epithelial sheet, these cells will differentiate into endothelial tissue (e.g., blood vessels) along the anterior chamber of the eye. The presumptive endothelial cells, although somewhat flattened, appear to move into the eye region by the extension of numerous filopodia. On the sixth day of embryonic development, mesenchymelike cells termed fibroblasts (here of neural crest origin) also migrate into the region beneath the cornea. Bard and Hay (1975) have observed that these fibroblasts have spindle-shaped bodies and extend numerous branched filopodia during their migratory activities. It appears that their locomotion is accomplished by the flow of cytoplasm from the cell body into certain filopodia and not into others. A particularly interesting observation is that these fibroblasts, when isolated and cultured in vitro on a glass substratum, behave like typical fibroblasts. Ordinary fibroblasts are the predominant cell type in connective tissues; they differentiate from mesenchyme cells. When observed in culture under phase microscopy, fibroblasts glide across the glass surface without filopodia formation or internal cytoplasmic flow. During movement, the fibroblast is in contact with the substratum only at its leading edge (i.e., the direction of movement) and its trailing edge. The leading edge of the cell is drawn out into a broad, thin, fanlike membrane known as a *lamellipodium*. Locomotion depends on the advance of the lamellipodium over the substratum. Localized protrusions or *ruffles* along the margin of the lamellipodium undulate and intermittently make and break contacts with the surface over which the cell moves. The cell typically moves in the direction from which a major lamellipodium extends from its surface. As the leading edge of this lamella advances, the cell becomes elongate in that direction because its trailing edge remains adherent to the substratum for a time.

Differences in the migratory behavior of the chick-eye fibroblast cells, when observed in situ and in vitro, point out the importance of the substratum and its influence upon cell form. When these same cells were cultured on a collagen gel, they assumed a spindle shape, formed filopodia, and behaved the same way as in vivo. This lends support to the suggestion that a collagen gel may very well simulate the embryonic environment in which the cells normally move.

Contact and adhesion with a substratum are important features in the morphogenetic movements of individual cells whether in vitro or in vivo. As in the case of the folding of epithelial sheets, the locomotion of cell types is invariably accompanied by changes in cell form. A variety of special surface modifications appear to serve as locomotory "organs" and effect the movement of a cell from one place to another place. These structures include filopodia, lamellipodia, and blebs or lobopodia (Chapter 8). Since these structures appear to move the cell by pulling it along, one might suspect that the basis of cell form changes is contractile and effected by the same intracellular organelles previously identified in the filopodia of primary mesenchyme cells, in the lobopodia of *Fundulus* deep cells, and in the lamellipodia of fibroblast cells. The availability of antibodies to actin and other major cytoplasmic structural proteins has enabled investigators to use indirect immunofluorescence to follow the distribution of these molecules under conditions of individual cell movement. Using this technique with a variety of fibroblast cells, Lazarides has demonstrated the presence of actin filaments in the membrane ruffles of lamellipodia. The actin filament pattern observed with immunofluorescence corresponds to the microfilament pattern observed with electron microscopy. Also, microtubules have been seen to extend from the main part of the fibroblast into the main body of a lamellipodium, thus indicating that they are probably the structural supporting elements of this type of membrane extension. The conclusion is warranted, therefore, that individual cells move by contractility that is effected through a complex intracellular system of filaments.

THE EXTRACELLULAR MATRIX

Within recent years, there has been an increased awareness of the importance of the extracellular environment or matrix (ECM) in both the morphogenetic and cytodiffereniative phases of organ formation. Virtually every organ of the adult organism arises as the result of interactions between an epithelial tissue and a mesenchymal tissue.. A complex network of macromolecules is found in the extracellular matrix between these two tissues. These materials of the extracellular environment exert a controlling influence over such processes as cell migration and short-range inductive interactions between groups of cells. Also, this medium acts as a vehicle through which a variety of chemical messages, such as nucleic acids, proteins, and ions, pass and function to alter the activities of neighboring cells.

The extracellular matrix or interface between epithelial and mesenchymal tissues undergoing morphogenesis is fluid-filled, colloid-like, and fibrous. Typically, the matrix is organized into a distinct basement membrane or basal lamina beneath the epithelium and a series of associated fibrous materials. *Collagens* and *glycosaminoglycans* (GAGS) are the chief molecular constituents of the extracellular matrix. Collagen, a high molecular weight structural protein, is fashioned into fibers that vary in dimensions of both length and thickness. The abundance of fibrillar collagen frequently varies among specific sites within an organ. For example, in the early branching lung, it is abundant around the trachea but thinner around the lung buds. Glycosaminoglycans are polysaccharides of high molecular weight which are composed chiefly of amino sugars. They are found at the interface between embryonic epithelia and mesenchymal tissues, frequently being linked to proteins to form *glycoproteins* (i.e., proteoglycans). Combinations of collagen and proteoglycans produce an array of fibrous complexes over epithelial surfaces during embryogenesis.

The extracellular, fibrous scaffolding serves as an important substratum over which individual cells, such as mesenchyme and neural crest cells, move. Where the cell movement is nonrandom, the orientation and directionality of cell migration to a target site appear to be provided by the specific arrangement of the fibrillar matrix.

A

3 days

B

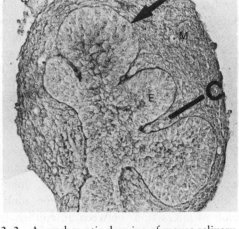

13–3 A, a schematic drawing of mouse salivary gland epithelial morphogenesis. The in vivo development of the gland takes about three days from the time of the initial appearance of the rudiment (After B. Spooner, 1973. Am. Zool. 13, 1007); B, photograph of a 13.5-day-old submandibular salivary gland of the mouse showing glycosaminoglycans on epithelial surface (dark line at base of arrow). Note the interlobular clefts (c). E, epithelium; M, mesenchyme. (From M. Bernfield, R. Cohn, and S. Banerjee, 1973. Am. Zool. 13, 1067.)

Indeed, glycosaminoglycans, particularly hyaluronic acid, are suspected of initiating, controlling, and stopping the movements of mesenchyme cells. Karp and Solursh (1974) have observed that there is a marked increase in the synthesis of GAGS at the beginning of echinoderm gastrulation when the primary mesenchyme cells emerge from the vegetal plate. The movement of neural crest-derived fibroblasts into the region beneath the cornea of the chick is preceded by a sudden burst in the synthesis of hyaluronic acid. Just as hyaluronic acid may be an important extracellular factor facilitating migration, a reduction in its concentration could cause migratory movement to cease. Cessation of the movements of corneal fibroblast cells is accompanied by a decline in the formation of hyaluronic acid and an increase in hyaluronidase activity beneath the corneal epithelium. Observations such as these are particularly provocative because they suggest that the migratory activities of cells, and hence the stability of tissue configurations of organs, may be controlled by localized fluctuations in the composition of the extracellular environment.

The extracellular matrix of collagen and GAGS has also been implicated in controlling the branching morphology of many tubular type organs, such as the salivary glands, lungs, and kidneys. Branching involves the epithelial component and is repetitive, continuing until the complex, definitive shape of the organ is achieved. Generally, the particular pattern of branching is characteristic for any given organ. Since the morphogenesis of the salivary gland has received considerable attention, let us examine it in some detail.

Each salivary gland arises as a small epithelial bud in the oral cavity, which pushes into the underlying mesodermal mesenchyme (Fig. 13–3). The early primordium consists of a bulbous distal tip that joins the oral cavity by a stalk or primary duct. Subsequently, the epithelium undergoes substantial growth and repetitive branching. Branching is initiated by an invagination that deepens into a distinct cleft at the bulbous tip of the primordium, thereby separat-

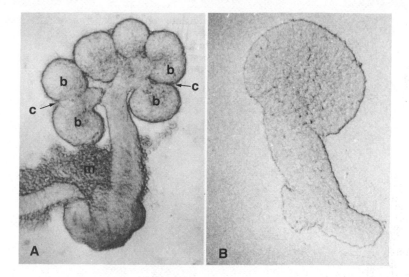

13–4 A, photomicrograph of living salivary gland epithelium after removal of the surrounding mesoderm (m). Note the clefts (c) and branches (b); B, photomicrograph of salivary gland epithelium that has been treated with cytochalasin B. Note the absence of clefts. (From B. Spooner, 1973. Am. Zool. 13, 1007.)

ing it into two lobes. A cleft then appears in the tip of each lobe, and the level of branching is increased. The dual processes of growth, supported by mitosis, and cleft formation establish the branching pattern of the salivary gland. The process of cleft formation is accompanied by a change in cell shape (i.e., cells become wedge-shaped). This alteration in cell shape during epithelial branching is presumably due to contraction of a system of filaments. Treatment of cultured salivary glands with cytochalasin B stops cleft formation and blocks further branching of the epithelial component (Fig. 13–4). Studies by Spooner with the electron microscope have shown bundles of microfilaments concentrated in basal ends of epithelial cells or in the outer surface of each distal branch. Although microtubules are also present in the epithelial cells, they are not required for salivary cleft formation. Treatment of cultured salivary glands with colchicine or colcemid stunts their growth but does not interfere with the clefts present in the epithelium.

The importance of salivary gland mesoderm in epithelial tube morphogenesis has been demonstrated in several types of experiments by Spooner (Fig. 13–5). If the salivary epithelium is enzymatically isolated from the underlying mesoderm and then grown in culture, it rounds up and fails to branch (Fig. 13–5 A). When the epithelial primordium is combined in organ culture with salivary mesoderm on one side and lung mesoderm on the other side (Fig. 13–5 B), branching morphogenesis occurs only in the portion of the epithelium associated with the salivary mesoderm. Although the epithelium does not branch where it is in contact with the lung mesoderm, a basal lamina and deposited GAGS can be identified at

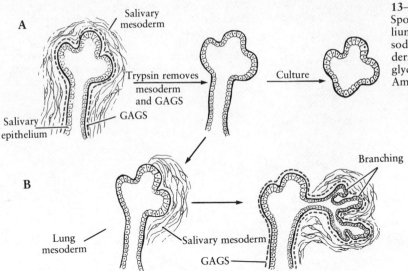

A

Salivary mesoderm

Salivary epithelium

Trypsin removes mesoderm and GAGS

GAGS

Culture

B

Lung mesoderm

Salivary mesoderm

GAGS

Branching

13–5 Schematic illustration of experiments by Spooner showing that isolated salivary epithelium fails to branch when divested of its own mesoderm (A) or associated with a foreign mesoderm such as lung mesoderm (B). GAGS, glycosaminoglycans. (After B. Spooner, 1973. Am. Zool. 13, 1007.)

the interface between the two tissues. Also, microfilaments are identified in the epithelial cells associated with the lung mesoderm, suggesting that salivary mesodern is not specifically required for the continued presence of these organelles. However, salivary mesoderm is absolutely required for epithelial morphogenesis. It induces a very specific pattern of branching in the epithelium by controlling microfilament activity.

Extracellular materials between the salivary epithelium and the salivary mesoderm appear to mediate the interaction between these two tissues. The precise roles of the collagen fibrils and the GAGS in controlling growth and cleft formation in the salivary epithelium remain to be fully determined. However, studies by Bernfield and others (1973) have given some insight into this problem.

Both collagen and glycosaminoglycans can be detected between the epithelial rudiment and the mesenchyme cells during branching. Early experiments using labeled precursors of collagen showed that this protein is synthesized by the mesenchyme and subsequently deposited in the basal lamina of the salivary epithelium. Treatment of salivary epithelia undergoing morphogenesis with collagenase, an enzyme which digests away the collagen protein, stops the branching process. Although it appears that collagen is crucial to branching, Bernfield subsequently discovered that the collagenase he used was contaminated with traces of enzyme, which also digested away certain polysaccharides. The role of collagen in salivary gland formation is, therefore, still a mystery. It is speculated that the collagen fibrils somehow stabilize the older formed clefts.

With other kinds of enzymatic treatments, it is possible to remove selectively specific GAG components from the extracellular matrix to determine which are important in tubule development (Fig. 13–6). When GAGS are removed from the basal surface of the epithelial rudiment by trypsinization, branching morphogenesis ceases; morphogenesis resumes if the epithelium is combined with salivary mesenchyme and new GAG components synthesized (Fig. 13–6 B). Bernfield and his co-investigators have also treated epithelial rudiments with a low concentration of pure collagenase (which does not remove GAGS) and then exposed them to trypsin, hyaluronidase, or chondroitinase. All of these treatments disrupt the basal lamina and prevent branching of the salivary epithelium. The subsequent addition of an investing layer of mesenchyme restores branching of the epithelium (Fig. 13–6 C-E). Bernfield has concluded that the morphogenetically critical GAGS are chondroitin, hyaluronic acid, and chondroitin sulfates. They are probably major constituents of the basal lamina whose structural integrity is needed for branching.

What is the mode of action of these GAG molecules in controlling epithelial morphogenesis? A hypothetical model constructed by Bernfield and his colleagues from their studies explaining the relationship between the extracellular materials and branching is shown in Figure 13–7. A continuous basal lamina containing newly synthesized GAGS lies beneath the basal side of an epithelial bud or primary lobule (Fig. 13–7 A). On either side of such an epithelial bud, GAGS accumulate at a very low rate, but well-defined bundles of collagen fibers are visible. All cells of the epithelium contain apical (inner) and basal (outer) microfilaments. Contraction of the basal microfilaments at the tip of the bud produces a localized group of wedge-shaped cells, thereby generating an infolding or cleft (Fig. 13–7 B). As the cleft deepens, the primary bud is converted into two branches or secondary lobules. Collagen fibers, whose precursors are synthesized, in part, from the adjacent mesenchyme, are drawn into the cleft where they act to stabilize the branched morphology. Continued cleft formation is due to contraction of the microfilaments and a high level of mitotic activity in the cells of the secondary lobules (Fig. 13–7 C). The entire sequence is repeated as each new cleft is formed. The disappearance of GAGS from the clefts is an essential step in the branching process, and it may be related to the release of hydrolytic enzymes from the salivary mesenchyme cells.

The relationship between the contraction of microfilaments and the GAGS of the basal lamina during branching morphogenesis is very speculative. Calcium ions are considered to have a regulatory role in the contractile systems of both muscle and nonmuscle cells.

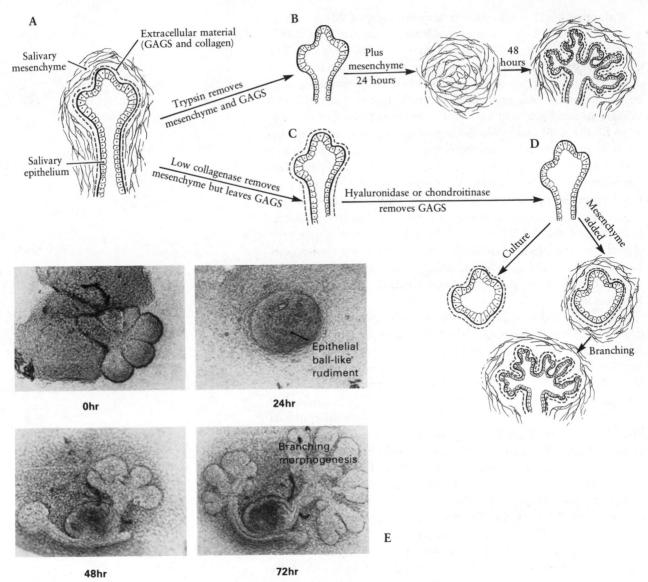

13–6 The role of extracellular materials in the branching morphogenesis of salivary epithelium. A, isolated gland rudiment consists of an epithelial bud surrounded by mesenchyme; B, trypsin treatment of rudiment removes the mesenchyme and the glycosaminoglycans (GAGS). The epithelial bud initially rounds up, but it will resume branching some 48 hours after being reassociated with salivary mesenchyme; C, low concentrations of collagenase remove the mesenchyme but leave the layer of GAGS intact. Without the addition of mesenchyme, the epithelium treated in this way loses its branching pattern; D, if C is followed by treatment with hyaluronidase or chondroitinase, all GAGS are removed and the epithelium rounds up unless combined with salivary mesenchyme; E, photograph of trypsin-isolated living salivary epithelium showing its response to contact with fresh mesenchyme (0 hr) after 24, 48, and 72 hours. GAGS are re-synthesized but there is no branching without the mesenchyme. (From M. Bernfield, R. Cohn, and S. Banerjee, 1973. Am. Zool. 13, 1067.)

Papaverine, a drug that blocks smooth muscle contraction by interfering with the flow of calcium ions, inhibits the morphogenesis of salivary glands in organ culture. It is postulated, therefore, that GAGS, which can bind calcium ions, control the morphogenetic events at the tips of branching epithelial tubules by regulating the availability of this cation.

THE LIMB: AN INTERACTION BETWEEN AN EPITHELIAL SHEET AND MESODERM

During the past several decades of analyzing the development of organs, it has become evident that many organs during their formation require complex inductive interactions between an epithelial tissue, generally of ectodermal or endodermal origin, and a mesenchymal tissue. An exchange of signals between these two types of tissues takes place in such varied organs as the salivary glands, lungs, lenses, liver, pancreas, skin, and limbs. The vertebrate limbs have received particular attention from investigators because their development exhibits all of the basic phenomena associated with organ formation: morphogenesis, histodifferentiation, cytodifferentiation, sequential inductions, gene control, and self-regulation. Also, the primordia of the limbs are rather large, at least in avian embryos, and special techniques permit their manipulation for the purposes of examining the interrelationships between these various processes. We will examine the development of the paired limbs in some detail here and not return to them again.

The Limb Field and Limb Bud

The initial signs of paired limb development in vertebrates are internal and visible in the lateral plate mesoderm on either side of the embryo (Fig. 13–8). The upper edge of the somatic layer of the lateral plate mesoderm thickens. Gradually, many of these cells lose their association with the mesodermal epithelium and migrate laterally beneath the overlying ectoderm. In the case of amphibian embryos, the limb mesenchyme proliferates locally and consequently produces two pairs of discrete, disclike masses (*limb discs*) at sites representing the future pectoral and pelvic appendages. By contrast, the length of the lateral plate mesoderm thickens on either side of the amniote embryo and its mesenchyme cells accumulate beneath the ectoderm as a distinct horizontal ridge (*Wolffian ridge*). Enlargement of each ridge in the pectoral and pelvic positions, coupled with the gradual disappearance of the intermedi-

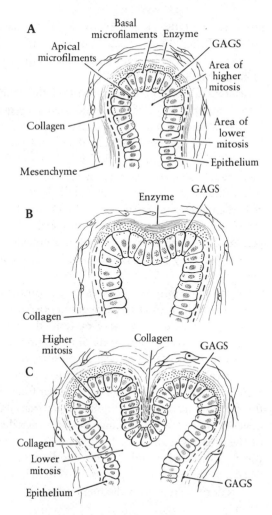

13–7 Schematic model according to Bernfield and colleagues depicting the relationships between extracellular material and cleft formation in a branching organ. A, the tip of an epithelial bud is a major site of GAG synthesis. Newly synthesized GAGS accumulate in the basal lamina region but turn over rapidly, perhaps due to "remodeling" by hydrolytic enzymes; B, early cleft formation is due to the contraction of microfilaments in the epithelial cells at the tip of the bud. Collagen fibers begin to form at the top of the cleft because of the regional synthesis of tropocollagen by mesenchymal cells; C, deepening of the cleft and the formation of secondary buds or lobules. The branch points are now stabilized by bundles of collagen. The tips of the secondary lobules show the bulk of newly synthesized GAGS. These are the sites for the next clefts. (From M. Bernfield, R. Cohn, and S. Banerjee, 1973. Am. Zool. 13, 1067.)

ate portion of the ridge, results in the formation of the definitive *limb buds* (Fig. 13–9). Each limb bud, therefore, consists of a central core of condensed mesenchyme surrounded by an overlying cap of ectoderm (Fig. 13–10).

Briefly, subsequent development of the limb bud is as follows. Rapid multiplication of the mesodermal cells quickly transforms the limb bud into an elevated mass projecting from the ventrolateral body wall of the embryo. The distal end of the limb primordium becomes flattened and considerably broader than its proximal end (i.e., paddle-shaped). The paddle-shaped part of the limb rudiment will differentiate as either the hand or the foot. The mesodermal cells then aggregate regionally to block out discrete masses that represent the precursors for the various skeletal components of the appendage. Cell proliferation, cell movements, and cell death (see below) play key roles in the definition of the final contours of the limb.

Of the two embryonic tissues that contribute to the construction of the limb, the mesoderm appears to possess the property of "limbness" and is determined very early in development or well in advance of any visible sign of the limb rudiment. This can be demonstrated by excising a fragment of presumptive limb mesoderm from the lateral plate and transplanting it beneath the flank ectoderm. When the mesodermal fragment is taken from embryos shortly after the stage of neural tube formation, its transplatation results in the development of a supernumerary limb. Ectoderm from any region of the embryo at this stage appears fully competent to contribute to the formation of a limb. If the ectoderm of the limb region is excised and the presumptive limb mesoderm is then covered by a piece of ectoderm taken from the head or trunk, a normal limb bud will form.

As in the case of other organs, such as the lens and the inner ear, the area of tissues capable of giving rise to the limb bud (i.e., prospective limb bud potential) is larger than that area normally contributing to the rudiment of this organ. For example, extirpation of the area normally giving rise to the limb disc in an early stage salamander embryo is followed after a short delay by the appearance of a limb. Presumably, ectodermal and mesodermal cells adjacent to the site of the extirpated tissues move in and reconstitute the limb disc. If the extirpation is enlarged to include both the presumptive limb bud as well as the surrounding cells, no limb will subsequently develop. This larger region, which represents the whole prospective limb bud potential, is referred to as the *limb field*.

The term *primary field* is often employed to describe the general region in an embryo from which a particular organ will develop. Just as in the case of the egg, which can be separated mechanically

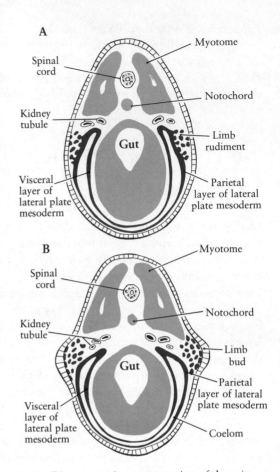

13–8 Diagrammatic representation of the origin of the limb mesenchyme from the lateral plate mesoderm (A) and its association with the ectoderm to form the limb bud (B) in a typical vertebrate embryo.

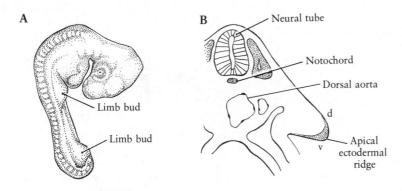

13–9 A, the limb buds appear as prominent swellings on the body wall of the chick embryo (stage 21); B, cross section through the wing bud of a stage 19 chick embryo. Note the differences in the thickness of the wing bud ectoderm between dorsal (d), ventral (v), and lateral surfaces.

into two parts with each part capable of forming a miniaturized whole, a primary organ field can be split into two halves and each half will develop into a complete organ. Up until the limb bud stage in amniote embryos, the limb rudiment can be divided into two halves and each half, following transplantation to an appropriate site, will develop into a whole limb. Cells within a field, therefore, appear to recognize their position within the whole. If the field is disrupted either by the removal or addition of cells, there is the property of regulation by the constituent cells such that a normal organ still forms. Another basic property of a primary field is the gradual and progressive determination of its parts. Initially, the parts of a primary field are totipotent and each can form the entire organ. As the potency of a part becomes restricted to its prospective significance, it can then only form a part of the whole organ. Successive determinations subdivide the primary organ field into secondary fields, tertiary fields, and so on until all parts of an organ are fully fixed with respect to their fate.

The Roles of Ectoderm and Mesoderm in Limb Differentiation

During the early growth of the limb bud in amniotes, a sharply defined epidermal thickening appears distally along the edge of the flattened bud (Fig. 13–10). The constituent cells of this *apical extodermal ridge* (AER) originate from the in situ proliferation of the ectoderm as well as from ectodermal cells migrating distally over the dorsal and ventral surfaces of the limb bud. The cells of the ridge are organized as a pseudostratified, columnar epithelium, an organization in distinct contrast to the cuboidal shape of the adjacent, nonapical ridge cells. Ridge cells contain numerous pinocytotic vesicles and oriented microtubules. Observations with the scanning electron microscope now indicate that apical ridges are characteristic of amphibian and mammalian limb rudiments.

13–10 A photograph of the apical ectodermal ridge (AER) at the apex of the left wing bud in a chick embryo. (From J. Saunders, 1948. J. Exp. Zool. 108, 363.)

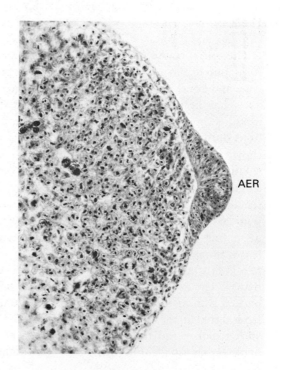

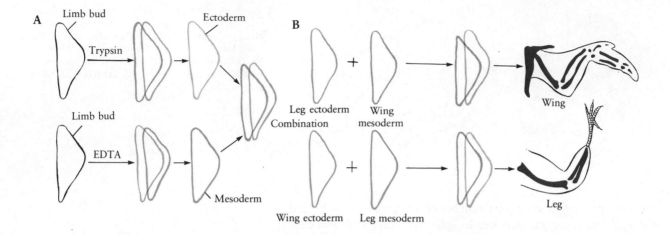

The AER appears to be induced by the underlying mesenchymal component of the limb bud. When the prospective limb mesoderm from chick embryos (stages 12 to 17) is isolated and transplanted beneath flank epidermis, it will induce cells of the latter to form an AER and subsequently a supernumerary limb bud. Mesoderm transplanted before stage 12 fails to initiate the development of an AER. It has been suggested by some investigators that an association with the somites at the level of the limb bud may be required for the acquisition of inductive properties by the limb mesoderm. Flank ectoderm loses its ability to respond to the limb inductive stimulus and form an AER by about stage 17.

The role(s) of the AER and the limb bud mesoderm in the transformation of the limb primordium into an organ with muscle, cartilage, and bone, arranged in particular configurations about definite axes, has been the subject of considerable study. A particularly useful technique in examining the processes and cellular interactions during limb morphogenesis was developed by Zwilling and is shown in Figure 13–11 A. By treating chick limb buds with a trypsin solution, he was able to separate intact the outer ectodermal layer from the inner mesenchymal mass. Since the mesoderm cells do not remain viable after trypsinization, other limb buds were treated with an EDTA solution. Ethylenediaminetetraacetic acid acts by disrupting the epithelial integrity of the ectodermal cells, but it leaves the mesoderm intact and in a healthy state. An in vitro system is thus made available to test the importance of the two limb tissues. The isolated ecoderm can be rolled into a sleeve and then packed with mesodermal tissues obtained from different sources or from different age embryos. The tissues of the composite limb bud stick together and the bud itself can then be implanted onto the flank or chorioallantoic membrane of another embryo. For ex-

13–11 The importance of the mesoderm in limb morphogenesis. A, diagram to show the procedure developed by Zwilling for the separation of intact ectoderm and mesoderm from either wing bud or leg bud. The mesoderm is then stuffed into the jacket of ectoderm and the recombinant graft placed on the flank or chorioallantoic membrane of a host embryo; B, wing-bud mesoderm surrounded by leg-bud ectoderm grows out as a wing. Leg-bud mesoderm surrounded by wing-bud ectoderm grows out as a leg structure.

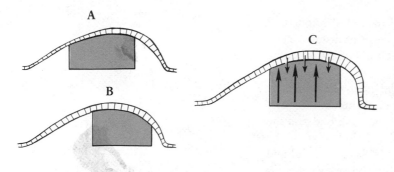

13–14 Distribution of the mesodermal maintenance factor in wing-bud mesoderm according to
Zwilling (A) and Saunders (B). C, the Zwilling-
Saunders model of limb development proposes
that the mesodermal maintenance factor (large
arrows) acts on the apical ectodermal ridge and
the apical ectodermal ridge (small arrows) exerts
an influence on the mesoderm by controlling its
outgrowth activity. (From R. Amprino, 1965.
Organogenesis. R. H. DeHaan and H. Ursprung,
eds. Holt, Rinehart and Winston, New York.)

through the mutant mesoderm to maintain the AER of the graft.
The ability of the MF to sustain the AER diminishes with age.

In the normal chick limb, the position of the AER becomes asym-
metric as the bud elongates. Gradually, the AER along the anterior
margin of the bud degenerates because the mesoderm in this region
no longer produces MF. Hence, according to the Saunders-Zwilling
model of limb morphogenesis, the MF is present in a limited portion of the mesoderm (largely postaxially), distributed asymmet-
rically, and transmissible in a proximodistal direction (Fig. 13–14).
The distribution of MF along the anteroposterior axis of the bud
appears to be the condition that ultimately determines the craniocaudal length of the apical ridge, the thickness of the ridge, and
probably the number and arrangement of developing limb elements.
Early studies by Saunders and others (1962) in which the tip of an
early wing bud was rotated through 180 degrees led to the production of duplicated distal wing parts with reversed symmetry anteriorly. In the normal wing, the anteroposterior sequence of the
digits is II, III, and IV. The sequence produced in the rotated wing
tip was IV, III, II, II, III, and IV. The conclusion from these experiments was that MF from the postaxial mesoderm maintained
the AER preaxially which, in turn, elicited the outgrowth and differentiation of postaxial structures in the preaxial mesoderm.

Other experiments with polydactylous mutant chicken strains
suggest that the anterior or preaxial portion of the limb mesoderm
does not normally produce MF. Extra preaxial digits are characteristic of polydactylous mutants. If ectoderm isolated from the limb
bud of a normal strain is combined with the limb mesoderm of a
polydactylous strain, the preaxial section of the apical ridge increases in thickness and induces supernumerary preaxial digits. It is
assumed that the production of MF is extended to the preaxial portion of the limb mesoderm in polydactylous forms.

The various portions of the overlaying apical ectodermal ridge
respond to MF by promoting the outgrowth of specific regions of
the subadjacent mesoderm. Figure 13–15 shows the consequences

of removing the cranial or the caudal half of the apical ectodermal ridge of a wing bud. Outgrowth and development of distal skeletal structures are apparent only in the bud mesoderm that is covered by the remaining part of the ridge.

The specification of skeletal parts along the anteroposterior axis of the wing also appears to be related to a special zone of mesodermal cells located at the posterior junction of the wing bud and the body wall. This small region of mesodermal cells is known as the *zone of polarizing activity* (ZPA). When the ZPA is transected and grafted to other sites such as the distal tip of the wing bud, there is subsequent outgrowth of a supernumerary wing tip. In most cases the posterior side of the duplicated wing tip faced the graft site. Hence, the ZPA has both an inductive capacity in causing outgrowth and polarizing activity in determining the anteroposterior sequence of wing parts. The relationship between the ZPA and the MF is still very unclear. Some investigators have proposed that the ZPA induces the production of the MF in neighboring mesodermal cells. A complication regarding the ZPA is that it may play no role in normal limb morphogenesis. Fallon and Crosby (1975) have demonstrated that extirpation of the ZPA between stages 15 and 24 does not interfere with limb development.

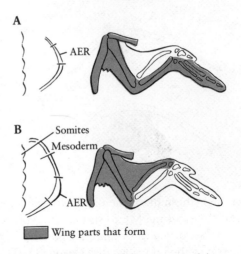

Wing parts that form

13–15 Consequences of the removal of the cranial (A) or the caudal (B) half of the apical ectodermal ridge on the development of the wing bud. (From J. Saunders, 1948. J. Exp. Zool. 108, 363.)

Determination of the Limb Axes

The growth and differentiation of the limb skeleton normally proceed in an ordered, proximodistal sequence. In amniote embryos, the limb girdles, which develop from the same mass of mesoderm as the limb skeletal parts, differentiate at the same time as the *stylopodium* (femur, humerus). Successively the *zeugopodium* (radius and ulna of forelimb, tibia and fibula of hindlimb) and *autopodium* (manus of forelimb, pes of hindlimb) are laid down. Each skeletal element is intially blocked out in mesoderm, which subsequently becomes converted to cartilage. The muscles that will attach to the skeleton of the limb originate from mesenchyme cells of the myotomes.

It is apparent that the organization of the various components of the normally developed limb is complex and asymmetrical. Ross Harrison (1921) in a classical study analyzed the origin of the axial polarity of the embryo by transplanting limb primordia. Using the salamander, rudiments of the limb were excised at different stages following neurulation, rotated or inverted in such a way that one or several of its axes were altered with respect to the axial polarity of the host embryo, and transplanted (Fig. 13–16). For example, transplantation of the left limb primordium shortly after neurulation can be accomplished by moving the transplant over the back and onto the right flank. Such a transplant reverses the dorsoventral axis with respect to the host, but the anteroposterior axes of host and graft coincide (Fig. 13–16 A). The graft transplanted in this manner develops normally with the limb growing caudally (Fig. 13–16 B). If, however, the same graft is rotated 180° on the right flank such that the anteroposterior axis is reversed with respect to the host (Fig. 13–16 C), the limb grows forward instead of caudad and subsequently shows the posterior digits placed anteriorly (Fig. 13–16 E). Hence, the anteroposterior axis is determined and irreversibly fixed at the time of the transplantation. The dorsal and ventral surfaces were undisturbed in these two experiments (i.e., the dorsal part of the limb rudiment differentiated ventral structures). Transplantation of a right forelimb primordium to the right flank after rotation of 180° produces a similar limb (Fig. 13–16 D). When the limb disc area was excised from an embryo whose tail rudiment was beginning to elongate and transplanted as in Figure 13–16 A, the dorsoventral axis was observed to by fully determined at this time. Such a graft showed no disturbances in the development of the proximodistal axis. The proximodistal axis is determined at about the time that the limb bud becomes visible morphologically.

The sequential determination of the axes of the limb has also been demonstrated by grafting experiments in the chick. The anteroposterior axis is the first to be determined (five somite stage). Subsequently, the dorsoventral and proximodistal axises become fixed to establish the complete axial relationships of the adult limb.

A summary of the events of the development of the limb as interpreted by most investigators is presented in Figure 13–17. Initially, there is a morphogenetic phase during which major limb form arises as a consequence of the interaction between limb mesoderm and ectoderm. The properties of these two tissues are distinctive, not shared by cells of other tissues, and must involve a characteristic set of genes. "Limbness" is a morphogenetic property that is transitory, terminating at about the time that cells enter into an active phase of cytodifferentiation. Cytodifferentiation is characterized by a marked augmentation of the synthesis of chondroitin sulfate, the chief GAG of cartilage. The specific program of cytodifferentiation by the mesoderm cells is probably a consequence of their position within the limb.

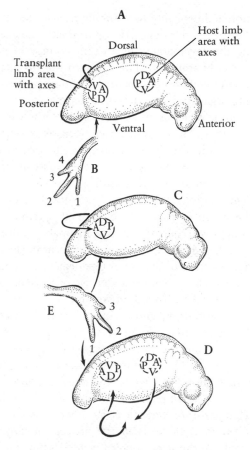

13–16 Specification of the axes of the amphibian limb. A, transplantation of a left limb primordium with inversion of the dorsoventral axis; B, the normal limb resulting from this operation; C, transplantation of a left limb primordium to the right flank with inversion of the anteroposterior axis; D, transplantation of a right forelimb primordium to the right flank after rotation of 180 degrees; E, the limb resulting from the operations in C and D grows forward, indicating that the anteroposterior axis is irreversibly fixed. A, anterior; D, dorsal; P, posterior; V, ventral. (After F. Swett, 1937. Q. Rev. Biol. 12, 322.)

CELL DEATH: A MORPHOGENETIC AGENT

One can conclude from the previous sections of this chapter that many factors interact to account for the morphogenesis of tissues and organs in multicellular animal embryos. A process that is common and probably necessary in many cases of organ development is that of cellular degeneration or death. The destruction of cells during the development of an embryo may be massive and quite dramatic. Examples include the removal of many larval tissues at the time of metamorphosis in amphibians and insects (e.g., tadpole tail, intersegmental muscles of pupating insects). More typically, cell death is regional in character where it is employed in the definition of pattern of an organ. Cell necrosis is often observed to precede changes in the shape of an epithelial organ, such as during the invagination of the optic cup (eye) and the olfactory pit (nose). The separation of the lens rudiment from the ectoderm requires cell degeneration. The removal of unwanted or superfluous cells after the union of parts, the closure of openings, and the formation of lumens is frequently effected through cell death.

Although cell death is a prominent occurrence in several embryonic systems of the vertebrate organism, it has been analyzed most extensively as a morphogenetic process in the development of the limb. Figure 13–18 illustrates the areas of necrosis in the superficial mesoderm of the chick wing as detected by supravital straining with Nile blue sulfate. Most of the cell deaths between stages 21 and 23 occur along the anterior edge of the wing bud and the adjacent body wall. This degeneration assists in shaping the contours of the future shoulder region. By stage 24, cells begin to die in large numbers at the posterior margin of the wing bud and the body wall. This *posterior necrotic zone* (PNZ), which contains approximately 1500 to 2000 cells in the process of degeneration at one time, results in the separation of materials that form the distal part of the scapula from those that contribute to the elbow region and the posterior portion of the upper arm. The PNZ appears to be unique to the chick wing bud. Its cells are quickly phagocytized by macrophages. At later stages, there is a distinct correlation between the topographical distribution of cell deaths and the emergence of the definition of the manus or hand with its three major digits.

A comparison between the leg primordia of the chick and the duck clearly shows the relationship between the distribution of necrotic areas and the modeling of the appendage (Fig. 13–19). In the chick, massive destruction of cells in the interdigital zones brings about the separation of the individual hindlimb digits. In the duck, areas of necrosis are limited to the peripheral regions between the digits. Most of the epidermis remains intact to contribute to the webbing of the foot.

Evidence from transplantation experiments by Saunders and his collaborators indicates that the death of the cells of the necrotic zone appears to be set by stage 17. If the PNZ is excised between stages 17 and 22 and then transplanted to a suitable environment,

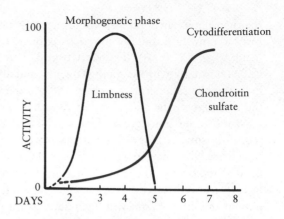

13–17   Relationships of the relative activities of the morphogenetic and cytodifferentiative phases in the development of the chick limb. Note that chondroitin sulfate, the major constituent of cartilage cells, is initially synthesized during the morphogenetic phase. (From E. Zwilling, 1968. The Emergence of Order in Developing Systems. M. Locke, ed. 27th Symposium of the Society for Developmental Biology. Academic Press, New York.)

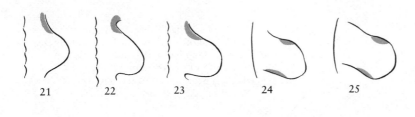

21 22 23 24 25

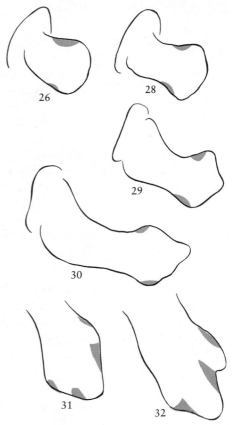

26 28
29
30
31 32

such as the somite region of the host embryo, the cells of the graft die on schedule or at stage 24. Control grafts, prepared from the dorsal side of wing mesoderm, when transplanted into the somite area remain healthy. Also, cells that migrate into and replace the excised PNZ do not undergo cell death. These experiments allow the conclusion that the degeneration of PNZ cells can be attributed to an intrinsic "death clock."

Although the death clock is set by stage 17 in the wing bud, other grafting experiments show that the death program can be reversed prior to stage 22. If the PNZ of stage 21 embryos is removed and grafted to the dorsal mesoderm of the wing bud, there is no triggering of the death clock and the PNZ cells remain alive. After stage 22, however, transplants of the PNZ unequivocally demonstrate that its cells are irreversibly directed toward massive necrosis at stage 24. Additional in vitro experiments on the ability of the dorsal wing mesoderm to prevent scheduled PNZ necrosis suggest that this portion of the wing produces a diffusible substance that in some way sustains the PNZ cells. Presumably, the mesodermal cells of the PNZ in the intact embryo lose the ability to synthesize this substance and die.

A similar area of necrosis, termed the *opaque patch,* is also clearly important to the patterning of the forearm. This region of cell death appears in the wing between stages 24 and 25 and effectively separates the condensations of mesoderm that will give rise to the radius and ulnar bones. In contrast to the cells of the PNZ, cells of the opaque patch show distinct signs of death, such as condensed chromatin and vacuolated cytoplasm, prior to being phagocytized. All cells of the central mesoderm of the forearm actively produce chondroitin sulfate until stage 24. At this time, however, the opaque cells suddenly cease synthesizing chondroitin sulfate and change their programming from presumptive cartilage cells to cells endowed with a death clock.

It has not been possible to detect in the PNZ cells prior to stage 24 morphological changes that would overtly indicate the operation of the death clock. However, alterations in the synthesis of particular macromolecules have been identified in PNZ cells before stage 24 and the onset of phagocytosis. If chick embryos between stages 19 and 23 are injected with tritiated thymidine, the PNZ cells at

13–18 The wing bud in late paddle stages and stages of contour formation to show regions of massive necrosis in the superficial mesoderm. (From J. Saunders, M. Gasseling, and L. Saunders, 1962. Dev. Biol. 5, 147.)

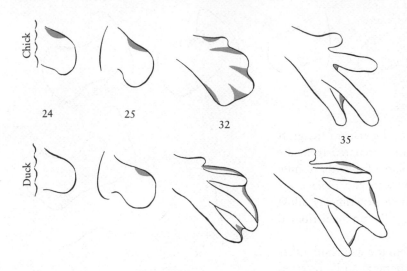

13–19 Patterns of necrosis at different stages in the leg primordia of the chick and the duck. (From J. Saunders and J. Fallon, 1966. Major Problems in Developmental Biology. M. Locke, ed. 25th Symposium of the Society for Developmental Biology. Academic Press, New York.)

stage 22 (when they are irreversibly committed to death) show a marked reduction in thymidine incorporation and hence in DNA synthesis. Shortly after the depression in the rate of DNA synthesis, neighboring cells begin to engulf PNZ cells. Substantially fewer labeled amino acids are incorporated into protein in the PNZ after stage 22. Since these changes in patterns of DNA and protein synthesis occur after the commitment of PNZ cells to death, they are symptomatic of death rather than determinants of cell death differentiation.

Patterns of cell death in the chick limb probably involve inductive interactions between the central mesoderm and the overlying epidermis. When the mesoderm of a duck leg is isolated and covered by a strip of epidermis from the wing of a chick, the recombinant limb graft grows and displays a pattern of necrosis similar to that of the duck (i.e., the limb is webbed). The reciprocal recombinant limb graft, or mesoderm of a chicken leg covered by wing epidermis of the duck, shows a pattern of interdigital necrosis that is similar to that of the chick (Fig. 13–20 A,B). Hence, specificity of patterns of necrosis in the limbs appears to be established in the mesoderm. By some unknown mechanism, the mesoderm is able to elicit localized patterns of cell death in the epidermis.

Obligatory cellular necrosis is also required in the remodeling and differentiation of portions of the digestive tract in a number of vertebrates, including amphibians, birds, and mammals. In the chick embryo, for example, the esophagus characteristically becomes occluded anteriorly at approximately five days of incubation. A period of intense epithelial proliferation then follows for the next several days. The degeneration of epithelial cells in this part of the gut is initiated at about eight days of incubation. Numerous inter-

cellular vesicles appear between the moribund epithelial cells and through coalescence produce a new, definitive esophageal lumen. As in other systems showing necrosis (e.g., developing limbs, chick oviduct), biochemical data indicate that there is a marked increase in acid hydrolase activity, particularly of acid phosphatase and β-glucuronidase, during the remodeling process. The increases in the specific activities of these hydrolytic enzymes between days 7 and 12 link them temporally with cell death and remodeling. Failure of the epithelial cells to degenerate results in the formation of a highly vesiculated and partially obstructed lumen, a condition present in homozygous crooked neck dwarf mutant chick embryos. The mechanism controlling the death of these gut cells remains to be determined. There is the possibility that the hydrolytic enzymes are released intracellularly from a lysosomal system to effect degeneration.

A dramatic example of cell death in insects is the degeneration of the intersegmental muscles in the silkmoth (*Antheraea*) following ecdysis from the pupa to the adult stage. Within 48 hours of the emergence of the pupa from the old cuticle, these muscles have degenerated. They appear to provide the motive force for ecdysis itself. Presumably, their contraction drives hamolymph or tissue fluid into the thorax of the pupa and thus assists in the rupture of the cuticular encasement. After ecdysis into the adult stage, these same muscles propel hemolymph into the wings in order to expand them. Developmentally, therefore, it is imperative that these muscles remain functional until the moth has emerged from the pupa stage.

Since hormonal balance is critical in insect metamorphosis (Chapter 11), the role of the endocrine system in setting the death clock for the intersegmental muscle breakdown has been examined by Lockshin and Williams in a series of studies. They found that three weeks before ecdysis the combination of a high level of ecdysone and a low level of juvenile hormone acted as a potentiator for the degeneration of the muscle cells after the emergence of the moth. If juvenile hormone was experimentally injected into the thorax of the pupa at this time, metamorphosis into the adult form was blocked and the breakdown of the intersegmental muscles prevented.

Ecdysone by itself does not appear to initiate directly the actual degeneration process in the muscles. Additional experimental studies by Lockshin and Williams have shown that the stimulus that triggers the differentiated death mechansim is neural in nature. There is observed a marked cessation of motor impulses to the intersegmental muscles shortly after ecdysis. The absence of a neuromuscular transmitter substance in some way then causes lysosomal-

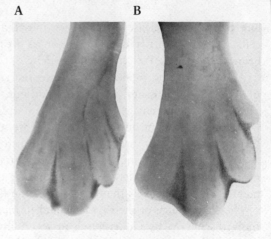

13–20   Patterns of necrosis revealed between the digits by Nile blue staining. A, chimeric limb bud grown as a flank graft composed of a core of mesoderm from chick leg bud and a jacket of ectoderm from the wing of a duck embryo; B, foot of a control chick embryo. Note the extent of necrosis in A is considerably less than in B. (From J. Saunders and J. Fallon, 1966. Major Problems in Developmental Biology. M. Locke, ed. 25th Symposium of the Society for Developmental Biology. Academic Press, New York.)

like particles to release cytolytic enzymes that destroy the muscle cells. Cessation of nervous stimulation as a cause of cell death has been observed in other embryonic systems.

As in insects, hormones play an essential role in the destruction of specific larval tissues, such as tail and gut, during the metamorphosis of amphibians. Amphibian metamorphosis is an important postembryonic event during which there are spectacular changes in larval structures in preparation for transformation to a lung-breathing, terrestrial animal. Almost every tissue and organ system of the larval frog undergoes alterations. A dramatic part of the metamorphic process is the regression of the tail.

The significance of the thyroid gland in metamorphosis was initially discovered by Gudernatsch in 1912. By feeding mammalian thyroid gland tissue to tadpoles, it was shown that the tadpoles exhibited precocious metamorphosis. Conversely, the elimination of iodine (an elemental constituent of *thyroxine*) or of thyroxine by thyroidectomy prevents metamorphosis from taking place. Regression of the tail depends upon stimulation by thyroxine. Morphologically, experimental data indicates that the thyroid hormone acts upon the tail tissues and induces their lysis. Histolysis of tail tissues always begins at the tip and proceeds toward the base of the tail. A typical pattern of destruction includes thickening of the epidermis, migration of pigment cells, and involution of notochord, neural tube, and muscle cells. Tissues undergoing regression have high activity levels of such hydrolytic enzymes as cathepsin, acid phosphatase, and collagenase. Visible tail resorption is accomplished by phagocytic digestion.

How does thyroxine act at the level of the cell to stimulate cell destruction? The process of tail resorption has been studied on the biochemical level using amputated larval tails cultured in an artificial medium. When such tails are exposed to low concentrations of triiodothyronine (a thyroid hormone related to thyroxine), they undergo resorption at a rate comparable to that observed in control larvae. The effect of the hormone can be completely eliminated by adding actinomycin D (to inhibit RNA synthesis) or cycloheximide or puromycin (to inhibit protein synthesis) to cultures of hormone-stimulated tails. This indicates that mRNA synthesis and protein synthesis are required for cell death and tail regression. It would appear that the thyroid hormone in the tail turns on a specific genetic program of transcription and translation, the result of which is the production of destructive hydrolytic enzymes.

A particularly fascinating feature of the hormonal control of amphibian metamorphosis is that thyroxine elicits a wide range of responses in different larval tissues. Depending upon the target tissue, some of these alterations are constructive while others are de-

structive. Some tissue cells die while other tissue cells proliferate. For example, the same thyroid hormone accelerates the destruction of larval blood cells and stimulates the proliferation of blood cells characteristic of the adult frog. A major and largely unresolved problem is: What properties of the thyroid hormone or of the target cells are responsible for these different responses? An attractive hypothesis is that the response of a given tissue at a given time may relate to the presence of mature thyroxin-binding receptors on its cell surfaces.

CELL SORTING AND
ORGAN CONSTRUCTION

Embryogenesis in vertebrates proceeds through a complicated series of cellular interactions in which cells of organ rudiments sort out and associate into specific multicellular groupings that give rise to tissues and organs. In the cases of some organs, such as the gonads, heart, and adrenal cortex, cells that contribute to their organization must migrate considerable distances to their final destinations before they reassociate to establish various tissue and organ primordia. Organs are not haphazard collections of cells and tissues. Rather, each organ has a distinctive, characteristic form, a precisely ordered arrangement of cells, and specific relationships to other organs. Topographic stability of cells and tissues lies at the basis of the integrity of organs. The performance of normal function could not proceed without it.

It is now a generally held view that molecular events occurring at the cell surface are of considerable importance in controlling cell movements and in determining cell associations within an organ. Of very specific significance in the construction of tissues and organs are the processes of cell recognition and selective cell adhesion. We have previously seen in Chapter 10 that there is specificity of cell adhesion in multicellular organisms. Several decades ago, Holtfreter dissociated the germ layers of early amphibian embryos and then observed that the resulting single cells were in many cases able to reaggregate to form a tissue of remarkable likeness to the one from which they came. Cells of the same type have a way of recognizing each other, and they prefer to interact with cells of their own kind. If two different types of embryonic cells are dissociated and then intermingled in the same suspension, the resulting aggregate incorporates both types of cells. However, in the course of the further development of such heterotypic aggregates, the diverse cell types sort out according to kind and form distinct, histogenetically uniform groupings. Since the early 1950s, the dissociation-reaggregation technique has made possible an analysis of the behavior of embryonic cells in vitro as it relates to the organization of tissues in organ construction. The method assumes that the interactions observed between particular cell types in vitro are similar to those taking place during in vivo organogenesis.

The ability of cells to recognize each other, and hence to sort out and segregate into distinct, cellular fabrics, appears early in vertebrate development. Recognition is displayed at gastrulation when tissue fragments from the different germ layers are combined in vitro (Chapter 10). Each germ layer possesses its own adhesive properties and germ-layer specificity. During the course of further development, different populations of cells within the same germ layer acquire characteristic recognition specificities. Hence, cell populations of the same germ layer sort out from one another.

The capacity of different populations of cells from the same germ layer to recognize each other and sort out is apparent during the early morphogenetic phase of organ formation. Zwilling (1968) has shown, for example, that nonlimb mesodermal cells cannot participate with limb bud mesodermal cells to construct an integrated, chimeric organ. He dissociated mesodermal cells from chick leg bud (stages 18 and 19) and mesodermal cells from chick somites (stages 13 to 15), mixed them randomly, and placed the resulting pellet of cells into a jacket of limb bud ectoderm. The ectoderm-mesoderm "assembly" was then grafted onto the dorsal wing bud of an appropriate host embryo. Within a period of 18 to 20 hours there was unequivocal evidence that the mesodermal cells were sorted out. Typically, the somitic cells usually moved to a central position within the graft, while the limb mesodermal cells occupied a more peripheral position. Similar observations were made on grafts formed by combining limb mesodermal cells with flank mesodermal cells isolated from chick embryos between stages 14 and 18. Despite the fact that somitic mesoderm and limbbud mesodermal cells have the capacity to differentiate into the same cell types (i.e., cartilage and bone cells), they segregated on the basis of their rudiment of origin within the mesodermal germ layer.

The cells of the embryo appear to pass through different recognition states, which probably explain their morphogenetic properties at different stages of organogenesis. For example, suppose the chondrocytes from limb cartilages (derivatives of the limb mesoderm) and the chondrocytes of the vertebral cartilages (derivatives of the somitic mesoderm) are digested from their matrices (eight-day-chick embryo) and then randomly mixed within limb bud ectoderm. Several days after transplantation, the resultant limb graft shows internally a single, chimeric mass of differentiated cartilage (i.e., limb and vertebral chondrocytes did not segregate but remained ran-

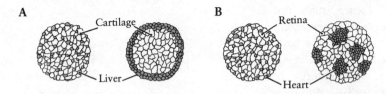

13–21 Two types of sorting out patterns as observed in mixtures of embryonic cells. A, liver and cartilage cells; B, heart and retinal cells.

domized). The intrinsic surface properties that probably cause these cells to segregate from each other during the morphogenetic phase of limb development are apparently no longer present. This suggests that when the morphogenetic phase of an organ is over and the cytodifferentiation of specialized cell types is under way, the surface properties of cells likewise become altered to permit them to associate into highly organized cellular fabrics.

Sorting out studies in mixed aggregates using tissues from older chick embryos have provided most of what is known about the mechanism by which individual cells of organs are held together in their specific groupings and ordered arrays. A variety of cell combinations have been used, including retina and heart cells, cartilage and heart cells, and heart and liver cells. Figure 13–21 illustrates two types of sorting out patterns that are commonly exhibited by a mixture of embryonic cells. When dissociated, four-day limb bud chondrogenic cells are randomly mixed with five-day liver cells, the cultured heterotypic aggregate within several days shows the formation of a discrete outer liver tissue completely enveloping the inner, chondrogenic tissue. A different pattern of segregation is observed when heart cells of five-day old embryos are mixed with retinal cells of seven-day old embryos. Following the mixing of the two types of embryonic cells, the heart cells withdraw from the surface of the aggregate. Gradually, the heart cells organize as a series of clusters throughout the larger, continuous association of retinal cells. The number of coherent masses of heart tissue is dependent upon the proportion of heart cells in the original cell aggregate.

Analysis of the behavior of many types of embryonic cells in heterotypic aggregates has led to the conclusion that tissues demonstrate a distinct hierarchy of segregation. Liver cells always occupy an outside position in cultures with heart cells, while heart cells are always superficial to cartilage cells. Predictably, and as described above, dissociated liver cells sort out and envelope cartilage cells. Some investigators have questioned this concept of the hierarchy of tissues based on segregation patterns, maintaining that sorting out in mixed cell cultures is probably due to artifacts related to the preparation of the cells rather than to any specific differences in recognition. Since cells for mixed culture studies are commonly dissociated with trypsin, it is conceivable that different cell types may be unequally sensitive to the enzymatic treatment. Hence, might not patterns of sorting out simply reflect these differences in sensitivity to the enzyme? A partial answer to this question has come from studies by Steinberg in which nonenzymatically prepared tissue fragments were brought together in culture. The patterns of segregation of these tissue fragments, including inside-outside relationships, were observed to be very similar to those in suspensions of mixed cells produced by enzymatic dissociation. It would appear, therefore, that patterns of sorting out do reflect intrinsic differences between cells in their surface adhesive properties.

Although there are no precise definitions of such terms as specificity, selectivity or preference, and adhesion, these have long been used in describing the morphogenetic behavior of embryonic cells during development. The absence of uniform definitions of these terms has undoubtedly impeded progress on our understanding of how cells move and assemble in the construction of an organ. However, most models explain the segregation of cells and the formation of tissues during organogenesis on the basis of the capacity of cells to discriminate from one another (recognition specificity) and to selectively form stable bonds between each other (cell adhesion). There is specificity in both the recognition process and in the adhesive process. Specificity of a given cell type is a property of its cell surface and presumably reflects specific patterns of macromolecular organization which are determined by a specific set of genes. Several hypotheses to account for the sorting behavior of embryonic cells in culture have been proposed (Chapter 8). Moscona has proposed that sorting out is largely based on qualitative differences in adhesive sites between cell types. The formation of such sites within a cell type may depend upon the incorporation of specific sugars into cell surface glycoproteins. Alternatively, Steinberg's hypothesis proposes that the adhesive sites between cells are quite similar; differences in adhesive properties between cells are reflected in the number and/or distribution of adhesive sites over the cell surface. The differential adhesion hypothesis of Steinberg appears to best account for the spectrum of cellular activities that take place during the sorting process.

The normal architecture of an organ requires that cells of a specific function be organized into a given tissue and that these tissues be arranged in a very specific way. Cell sorting plays a central role in the construction of homogeneous tissues and in their arrangement into specified patterns. Since cell movements also assist in the formation of normal tissue arrangements, analysis of the mechanisms controlling cell movement during cell sorting may provide additional insight into mechanisms governing cell movements during organ formation.

REFERENCES

Amprino, R. 1965. Aspects of limb morphogenesis in the chicken. In: Organogenesis. Eds., R. DeHaan and H. Ursprung. New York: Holt, Rinehart and Winston.

Bard, J. and E. Hay. 1975. The behavior of fibroblasts from the developing avian cornea. Morphology and movement *in situ* and *in vitro*. J. Cell Biol. 67:400–418.

Bernfield, M., R. Cohn, and S. Banerjee. 1973. Glycosaminoglycans and epithelial organ formation. Am. Zool. 13:1067–1083.

Fallon, J. and G. Crosby. 1975. Normal development of the chick wing following removal of the polarizing zone. J. Exp. Zool. 193:449–455.

Harrison, R. G. 1921. On relations of symmetry in transplanted limbs. J. Exp. Zool. 32:1–136.

Karp, G. and M. Solursh. 1974. Acid mucopolysaccharide metabolism, the cell surface, and primary mesenchyme cell activity in the sea urchin embryo. Dev. Biol. 41:110–123.

Lockshin, R. A. 1971. Programmed cell death. Nature of the nervous signal controlling breakdown of intersegmental muscles. J. Insect Physiol. 17:149–158.

Lockshin, R. A. and C. M. Williams. 1965. Programmed cell death. III. Neural control of the breakdown of intersegmental muscles of silkmoths. J. Insect Physiol. 11:601–610.

Moscona A. A. 1974. Surface specificities and embryonic cells: Lectin receptors, cell recognition, and specific cell ligands. In: The Cell Surface in Development. Ed., A. A. Moscona. New York: John Wiley & Sons.

Rubin, L. and J. Saunders. 1972. Ectodermal-mesodermal interactions in the growth of limb buds in the chick embryo: Constancy and temporal limits of ectodermal induction. Dev. Biol. 28:94–112.

Rutter, W., J. Kemp, W. Bradshaw, W. Clark, R. Ronzio, and T. Saunders. 1968. Regulation of specific protein synthesis in cytodifferentiation. J. Cell Physiol. 72:1–18.

Saunders, J. 1948. The proximo-distal sequence of origin of the parts of the chick wing and the role of the ectoderm. J. Exp. Zool. 108:363–403.

Saunders, J. 1966. Death in embryonic systems. Science 154:604–612.

Saunders, J. and J. Fallon. 1966. Cell death in morphogenesis. In: Major Problems in Developmental Biology, pp. 289–314. Ed., M. Locke. New York: Academic Press.

Saunders, J. and C. Reuss. 1974. Inductive and axial properties of prospective wing bud mesoderm in the chick embryo. Dev. Biol. 38:41–50.

Saunders, J., M. Gasseling, and L. Saunders. 1962. Cellular death in morphogenesis of the avian wing. Dev. Biol. 5:147–178.

Spooner, B. 1973. Microfilaments, cell shape changes, and morphogenesis of salivary epithelium. Am Zool. 13:1007–1022.

Tarin, D. and A. Sturdee. 1971. Early limb development in *Xenopus laevis*. J. Embryol. Exp. Morphol. 26:169–179.

Trinkaus, J. 1976. On the mechanism of metazoan cell movements. In: The Cell Surface in Animal Embryogenesis and Development, Vol. 1., pp. 227–329. Eds., G. Poste and G. Nicolson. New York: North-Holland.

Zwilling, E. 1961. Limb morphogenesis. Adv. Morphog. 1:301–330.

Zwilling, E. 1968. Morphogenetic phases in development. In: The Emergence of Order in Developing Systems, pp. 184–207. Ed., M. Locke. New York: Academie Press.

Zwilling, E. 1974. Effects of contact between mutant (wingless) limb buds and those of genetically normal chick embryos: Confirmation of a hypothesis. Dev. Biol. 39:37–48.

14

Development of the Face,
Palate, Oral Cavity,
and Pharynx

The ventrolateral aspect of the head of the early embryo shows a number of barlike processes separated from each other by a series of grooves. The ridges are the *visceral arches* and the grooves are the *visceral furrows* (Fig. 14–1). Four well-defined arches are seen at the end of the first month (Fig. 14–1 A). The fifth arch always remains rudimentary. A lateral view of a slightly older embryo shows the formation of the *mandibular* and *maxillary processes* from the first arch (Fig. 14–1 B).

THE FACE

At the beginning of the second month when the pharyngeal membrane ruptures to establish connection between the ectodermal stomodeum and the endodermal foregut, the lateral boundaries of the stomodeum are formed by the mandibular and the maxillary processes (Fig. 14–2 A,B). In a frontal view of the face at this time most of the structures that will contribute to the formation of the face are distinguishable (Fig. 14–2 A,B). The lower jaw, the caudal boundary of the stomodeum, is formed by the mandibular processes whose origin from a pair of lateral primordia is evident in this figure. The maxillary processes, which form a large part of the upper jaw, are present only as small rudiments at this time. The maxillary and mandibular processes, both derivatives of the first visceral arch, merge with each other at the lateral boundary of the stomodeum. The transverse diameter of the stomodeum is considerably greater than that of the definitive oral opening. Present also are a pair of nasal placodes that represent the beginning of the development of the nose. Between them is the unpaired *frontonasal prominence*. During the next two weeks (Fig. 14–2 B–D) the maxillary processes become more prominent and the olfactory placodes invaginate to form the *olfactory pits*. The rim of each olfactory pit is deficient where it communicates with the oral cavity, and the olfactory pit might well be termed the olfactory groove at this time. *Lateral nasal*

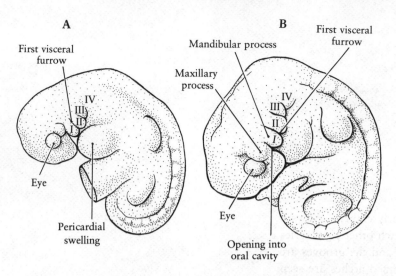

A

First visceral furrow

IV
III
II
I

Eye

Pericardial swelling

B

Mandibular process

Maxillary process

First visceral furrow

IV
III
II
I

Eye

Opening into oral cavity

14–1 External appearance of the visceral arch system. A, 4.2 mm (week 5); B, 6.3 mm (week 6). (From E. Blechschmidt, 1961. The Stages of Human Development before Birth. W. B. Saunders Company, Philadelphia.)

processes and *medial nasal processes* form the lateral and medial ridges of each olfactory pit.

The outline of the face emerges as the structures named above continue to grow (Fig. 14–2 E,F). A deepening of the nasal pits and the stomodeum is brought about by the forward growth of the mesodermal structures surrounding these orifices. The olfactory pits approach each other in the midline gradually squeezing out the frontonasal prominence. The maxillary processes grow medially and fuse with an extension of the medial nasal process. The junction of the maxillary processes and the median nasal processes forms the *philtrum* of the adult lip. Fusion of these processes closes the externally observed connection between the olfactory grooves and the oral cavity and converts the olfactory grooves into blind passageways whose external openings are the nostrils (*external nares*). The median nasal processes fuse to form the *median nasal septum* separating the two nasal cavities. The external nares thus are brought closer together from their original lateral positions. A transverse furrow develops between the nasal region of the frontonasal prominence and the frontal region of the skull, setting off the nose as a separate structure.

The developing eyes and ears are also seen in a frontal view of the face during the second month (Fig. 14–2 D,E). A groove extends between the maxillary process and the lateral nasal process from the corner of the eye. This is the *nasolacrimal furrow*. It marks the beginning of the formation of the nasolacrimal canal, which connects the orbital and nasal cavities in the adult. The first visceral furrow between the first and second visceral arches marks the position of the future external auditory meatus. Contributions from the areas of the first and second arches surrounding the first visceral furrow will form the external ear.

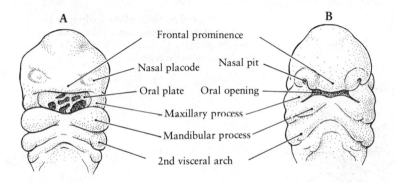

A

- Frontal prominence
- Nasal placode   Nasal pit
- Oral plate   Oral opening
- Maxillary process
- Mandibular process
- 2nd visceral arch

B

14–2   Development of the human face as seen from the frontal aspect. A, four weeks; B, five weeks; C, five and a half weeks; D, six weeks; E, seven weeks; F, eight weeks.

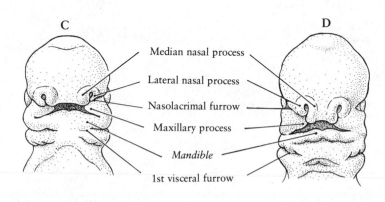

C

- Median nasal process
- Lateral nasal process
- Nasolacrimal furrow
- Maxillary process
- *Mandible*
- 1st visceral furrow

D

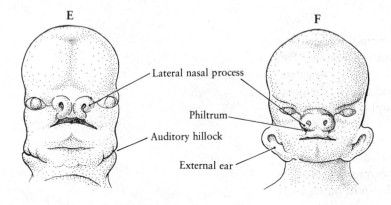

E

- Lateral nasal process
- Philtrum
- Auditory hillock
- External ear

F

These external modifications occur during the second month and are followed by the development of the underlying bony structures of the jaws. The most medial part of the upper jaw forms from an extension inward of the fused median nasal processes and is homologous to the premaxillary process and bone of lower forms. It bears the incisor teeth. The remainder of the upper jaw, carrying all of the other upper teeth, develops from the maxillary portions of the first

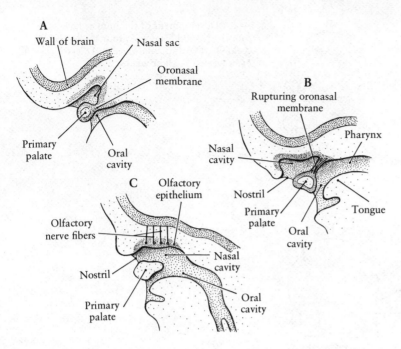

A
Wall of brain
Nasal sac
Oronasal membrane
Primary palate
Oral cavity

B
Rupturing oronasal membrane
Pharynx
Nasal cavity
Nostril
Primary palate
Oral cavity
Tongue

C
Olfactory epithelium
Olfactory nerve fibers
Nostril
Primary palate
Nasal cavity
Oral cavity

14–3 Sagittal sections of the early human embryo showing the formation of the nasal cavities and the primary choanae. A, five weeks; B, six weeks; C, seven weeks.

arch, while the tooth bearing portions of the lower jaw are formed from the mandibular division.

THE PALATE

The deep end of each olfactory pit is separated from the underlying oral cavity by an epithelial plate, the *oronasal membrane* (Fig. 14–3 A) and thus at first each olfactory pit ends blindly. When the oronasal membrane perforates late in the second month, the nasal cavity now opens into the anterior part of the oral cavity by way of a pair of foramina, the *primitive choanae* (Fig. 14–3 B,C). The most anterior part of the nasal cavity is separated from the oral cavity by the *median palatine process (primary palate)*, which is the inner extension of the fused median nasal processes mentioned above as being homologous to the premaxillary bone. The short passageway from the anterior nares to the primitive choanae is extended during the third month by the formation of a much larger roof over the oral cavity, the *secondary palate*. Only a small anterior part of the definitive palate is formed by the median palatine process. The major part of the palate is formed by the medial growth of a pair of *lateral palatine processes*, shelflike outgrowths of the maxillary processes (Fig. 14–4). When they fuse in the midline, they roof over the oral cavity and extend the posterior openings of the nasal cavities back to the region of the pharynx (Fig. 14–4 F, H). The respiratory

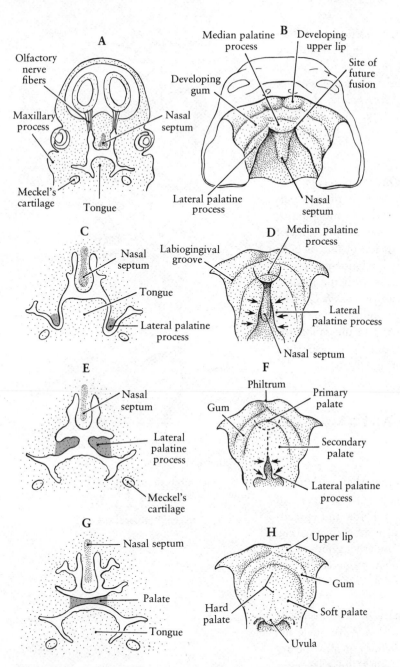

14-4 Drawings of frontal sections (A, C, E, and G) and of the roof of the oral cavity (B, D, F, and H) illustrating the development of the palate from week 6 to week 12.

A

Olfactory nerve fibers

Maxillary process

Nasal septum

Meckel's cartilage

Tongue

B

Median palatine process

Developing upper lip

Developing gum

Site of future fusion

Lateral palatine process

Nasal septum

C

Nasal septum

Tongue

Lateral palatine process

D

Median palatine process

Labiogingival groove

Lateral palatine process

Nasal septum

E

Nasal septum

Lateral palatine process

Meckel's cartilage

F

Philtrum

Gum

Primary palate

Secondary palate

Lateral palatine process

G

Nasal septum

Palate

Tongue

H

Upper lip

Gum

Hard palate

Soft palate

Uvula

and alimentary passageways thus establish separate external entrances but open in common posteriorly into the pharynx. The two nasal cavities are completely separated from each other by the *nasal septum,* which fuses with the palate (Fig. 14–4, C,E,G). The nasal septum differentiates from the medial mass of the cartilaginous model of the ethmoid bone. The lower portion of the septum that joins the palate remains cartilaginous. The upper portion ossifies to form the perpendicular plate of the ethmoid bone, thus completing the nasal septum. The anterior part of the palate ossifies to form the *hard palate.* The most posterior part, posterior to the nasal septum, however, contains no bone and becomes the *soft palate,* its most posterior portion forming the triangular *uvula* (Fig. 14–4 H).

Cleft Palate and Cleft Lip

Failure of fusion of any part of the palatine processes results in a gap in the roof of the mouth, known as *cleft palate.* In the soft palate, the gap is commonly in the midline. However, in the anterior part of the hard palate, the cleft is located on one or both sides of the midline, resulting from the failure of the fusion of one or both of the lateral palatine processes with the medial palatine process.

Failure of the fusion of the maxillary process with the median nasal process results in a common anomaly known as *cleft lip.* The gap in the lip is at one side of the midline at the philtrum. The name "harelip" is thus somewhat of a misnomer since in the rabbit the gap is in the midline. A cleft lip may occur on one or on both sides and may be continuous posteriorly with a cleft palate.

THE ORAL CAVITY AND THE PHARYNX

The Teeth

A sagittal section through the primitive jaws shows that up until the sixth week they are solid masses. At this time a thickened plate of epithelium, the *labial lamina,* appears in the midline and spreads outwardly in a semicircle in both directions around each jaw (Fig. 14–5 A). As the labial lamina sinks into the underlying mesoderm the central cells disappear and a groove, the *labial groove* is formed (Fig. 14–5 B). The labial groove becomes the *vestibule* separating the lips from the gums (Fig. 14–5 C).

Projecting inwardly from each labial lamina is a second semicircular shelf of tissue, the *dental lamina* (Fig. 14–5 A,B). Since the dental lamina is an ingrowth of the oral epithelium, it must be appreciated that it contains the rapidly proliferating cellular layers of normal surface epithelia. Through the mitotic activity of these cells, the dental lamina increase rapidly in size. During the third month, specialized regions, the *enamel organs,* develop (Fig. 14–5 B,C). They form as cup-shaped structures that sink into the mesoderm but remain connected to the gum epithelium by way of the dental lamina, now a constricted cord of cells. Five of these struc-

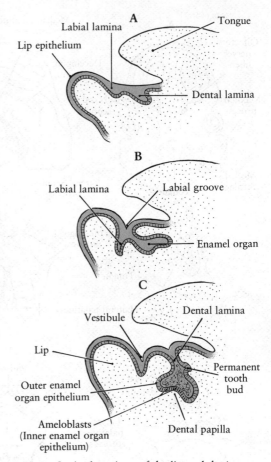

14–5 Sagittal sections of the lip and the jaw showing the separation of the lip and the gum by the labial groove and the early development of a tooth. A, 7 weeks; B, 8 weeks; C, 11 weeks.

tures develop on each side in both the upper and the lower jaws. They will form the deciduous or milk teeth. On its mesenchymal side each enamel organ becomes indented by a core of mesoderm, the *dental papilla* (Figs. 14–5 C; 14–6). Both the enamel organ and the dental papilla are surrounded by a connective tissue sheath, the *dental sac*. The entire structure is known as the *tooth germ* or *tooth bud*.

The enamel organ consists of an inner concave group of columnar cells, the *inner enamel organ epithelium,* which is continuous with an outer convex layer of cuboidal cells, the *outer enamel organ epithelium.* Between these two epithelia, the ectodermal matrix forms a stellate reticulum that contans large amounts of intercellular fluid rich in mucopolysaccharides, morphologically resembling embryonic mucous connective tissue (Fig. 14–6; 14–7 A). The indented inner epithelium gives rise to the *enamel* of the tooth. Its cells are termed *ameloblasts.* The cells of the enclosed dental papilla closest to the ameloblast layer differentiate into a *dentine*-forming layer of cells called *odontoblasts* (Fig. 14–7 B). The remainder of the mesodermal core of the dental papilla differentiates into the *pulp* of the tooth. The pulp consists of a framework of reticular tissue binding together the blood vessels, lymphatics, and nerves of the tooth. Enamel and dentine are formed simultaneously by continued secretions from the ameloblasts and odontoblasts, the oldest enamel and dentine being in apposition in the center of the developing tooth. Enamel, dentine, and bone have similar characteristics consisting of an organic framework in which are deposited inorganic salts. Bone contains approximately 33 percent organic material, dentine somewhat less, and enamel only about 5 percent. The root of the tooth begins to form after the crown is almost completed and has not yet completed development even at the time the tooth erupts.

The dental sac has an important function. As the tooth erupts, both the dental sac and the enamel organ are sloughed off in the part that has erupted. However, the dental sac that surrounds the root differentiates into an organ closely applied to the dentine of the tooth on one side and the bony alveolar socket of the jaw on the other. Both of these layers of periosteal tissue together constitute the *periodontal* membrane. The cells of the dental sac closest to the dentine differentiate into *cementoblasts.* The cementoblasts secrete a substance, *cementum,* histologically and chemically similar to bone, around the root of the tooth. The remaining cells of the dental sac form fibers that hold the tooth in place by embedding themselves in both the dentine of the tooth and the bone of the alveolar socket (Fig. 14–8).

Each deciduous tooth will eventually be replaced by a permanent tooth. The permanent teeth develop from lingual extensions of the

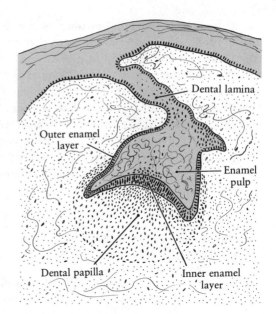

14–6 Developing human tooth at three months.

14–7 Developing human incisor at seven months. A, sagittal section; B, detail of rectangle in A.

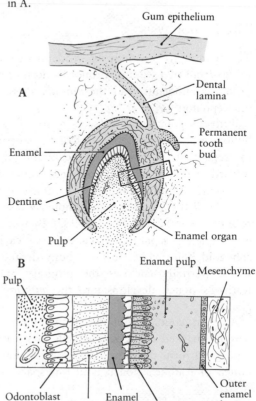

dental lamina in the same manner as the deciduous teeth (Figs. 14–7; 14–8). Those permanent teeth that have no deciduous precursors, the molars, develop from backward growing extensions of the ends of the semicircular dental lamina of each jaw. The permanent teeth grow slowly at first, but gradually their growth exerts a pressure on the deciduous teeth. This pressure, along with a partial absorption of their roots, results in the milk teeth being shed.

The order in which the deciduous teeth erupt is generally from the midline laterally. However, their replacement does not follow this pattern. The approximate times of eruption of the deciduous and permanent teeth are as follows:

Deciduous teeth		Permanent teeth	
central incisors	6–8 months		7 years
lateral incisors	7–10 months		8 years
canines	14–20 months		12 years
1st molars	12–16 months	1st bicuspids	11 years
2nd molars	20–30 months	2nd bicuspids	11 years
		1st molars	6 years
		2nd molars	12 years
		3rd molars	17–25 years (often later— or never)

The Hypophysis

The hypophysis is entirely an ectodermal derivative. However, it develops from two separate primordia, *Rathke's pouch,* an outgrowth of the stomodeum, and the *infundibulum,* an outgrowth of the diencephalon.

Rathke's pouch may be seen in the 4.2 millimeter embryo as a hollow evagination of the roof of the stomodeum just in front of the region of the pharyngeal membrane (Fig. 14–9 A), extending toward the floor of the overlying brain. When Rathke's pouch meets the infundibulum, its oral attachment becomes constricted (Fig. 14–9 B,C), and it then completely loses its connection to the roof of the oral cavity (Fig. 14–9 D). By week 12 the buccal anlagen is completely separated from the oral cavity by the developing sphenoid bone which forms a bony depression, the *sella turcica,* which partially encloses the pituitary anlagen (Fig. 14–9 E). Rathke's pouch develops into the *anterior lobe* of the pituitary gland.

After its contact with the infundibulum, the anterior lobe undergoes marked changes. The cells of its anterior wall proliferate rapidly to form the *pars distalis.* In so doing they impose on the lumen of Rathke's pouch until this space is reduced to a narrow

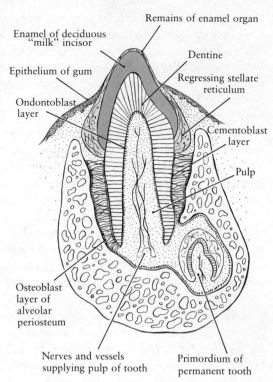

14–8 Drawing of an erupting tooth showing its relation to its bony alveolar socket in the jar.

cleft, the *residual lumen*. The wall of Rathke's pouch in contact with the infundibulum forms the *pars intermedia* of the anterior lobe. This part of the pituitary may be well-defined in the fetus and the infant but, in the adult, it merges with the *pars nervosa* of the *posterior lobe* and becomes obscure. Paired lateral extensions of the pars distalis grow out, fuse, and form a collar around the infundibular stalk. This is the *pars tuberalis*.

The pars distalis becomes highly vascularized and its cells become arranged in interlaced columns forming a network around the blood vessels. Most of the blood vessels are branches of the internal carotid artery. During the third month of development, there is evidence of cell specialization when secretory granules appear in a number of cells, indicating their differentiation into cells that are destined to synthesize specific pituitary hormones. These functional fetal pituitary cells may secrete trophic hormones that are necessary for the complete development and function of the thyroid and adrenal glands. However, the majority of the cells of the pars distalis remain chromophobic during fetal life and do not show accumulations of the characteristic acidophilic and basophilic granules found in the adult gland.

The infundibulum forms the posterior lobe of the pituitary. Its distal end enlarges to become the pars nervosa, which remains connected to the hypothalamus by way of the mostly solid *infundibular stalk* (Fig. 14–9 E). The cells of the pars nervosa differentiate into cells known as *pituicytes,* which are modified neuroglia cells. Nerve cells are not found in the pars nervosa, but many nerve fibers grow into this area from nuclei in the hypothalamus. These are the neurosecretory fibers whose function was described in Chapter 5.

DERIVATIVES OF THE VISCERAL ARCH SYSTEM

A section through the pharyngeal region at the end of the first month (Fig. 14–10 A) shows that behind the oral cavity the pharynx has flattened and broadened and developed a series of endodermal diverticula, *pharyngeal pouches,* growing laterally toward the corresponding ectodermal visceral furrows. In fishes the pharyngeal pouches and the visceral furrows break through and join to form *visceral clefts*. These visceral clefts are also termed gill slits since the visceral (branchial) arches bear respiratory structures, the gills. The gill slits provide exit for the respiratory water, which enters through the mouth. In amniotes, visceral clefts usually do not develop and, if they do, are only temporary and never serve any respiratory function. Thus, it is quite incorrect to say that the amniote embryo—

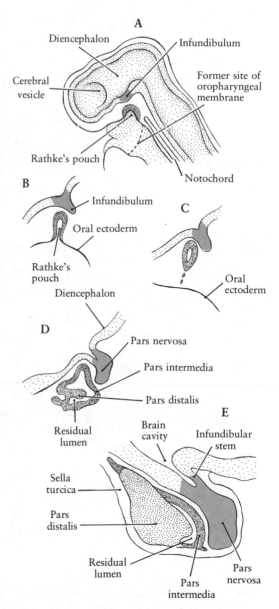

14–9   Diagrams of sagittal sections illustrating the development of the hypophysis. A, end of the first month showing the dual origin of the gland from the roof of the oral cavity (Rathke's pouch) and the floor of the diencephalon (infundibulum); B, C, meeting and fusion of two primordia during month 2; D, 8 weeks; E, 11 weeks.

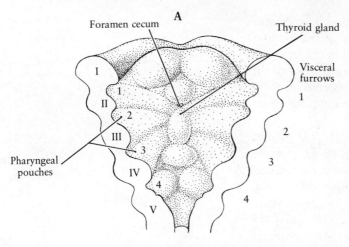

A

Foramen cecum

Thyroid gland

Visceral
furrows

I

1

II

2

III

3

IV

4

V

Pharyngeal
pouches

1

2

3

4

14–10 Diagrams of three stages in the differentiation of the visceral arch system. A, about four weeks; B, formation of the cervical sinus (week six); C, differentiation of the pouches (week six).

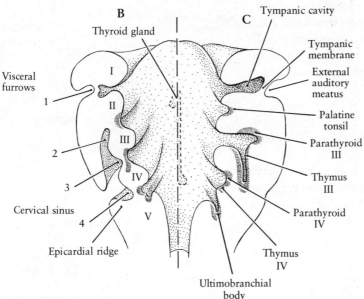

B

C

Thyroid gland

Tympanic cavity

Tympanic
membrane

External
auditory
meatus

Visceral
furrows

I

II

III

IV

V

1

2

3

4

Palatine
tonsil

Parathyroid
III

Thymus
III

Parathyroid
IV

Cervical sinus

Epicardial ridge

Thymus
IV

Ultimobranchial
body

despite the fact that it develops in an aquatic environment—is ever a fish (or even fishlike). Although the visceral arch system in the amniotes gives up its respiratory function, the furrows, arches, and pouches develop into a wide variety of other specialized structures.

Visceral Furrows

The first visceral furrow forms the external auditory meatus. It is the only visceral furrow that forms an adult structure, the rest forming indistinguishable parts of the neck contour.

Visceral Arches

At the end of week six, the second arch grows over the more caudal ones, sinking them into a depression known as the *cervical sinus* (Fig. 14–10 B). When the second arch fuses with the epipericardial ridge, the cervical sinus is cut off from the surface and is eventually obliterated (Fig. 14–10 C). The caudal growth of the second arch may be likened to the same event in the bony fishes, which forms the flaplike operculum over the posterior gill arches. Thus, after a short existence of only about two weeks, any resemblance to the gill-bearing branchial arch system of the teleosts is lost.

Each visceral arch has three components: (1) an artery, (2) a nerve, and (3) mesenchyme—which will form cartilage, bone, and muscle.

The visceral arches at one time or another provide a pathway for the paired aortic arches from the aortic sac to the dorsal aorta, although many of these connections are only transitory. The transformation of the aortic arches into the adult pattern will be described in the chapter on the circulatory system.

The motor fibers of cranial nerves V, VII, and IX supply the muscles derived from visceral arches one, two, and three, respectively. The Xth nerve supplies muscles derived from the remaining arches. This one-to-one relationship between the muscles derived from specific arches and their motor innervation does not hold true for their sensory supply. This is particularly true for the exteroceptors, almost all of which are supplied by the trigeminal (Vth) cranial nerve. However, there does seem to be a relationship between visceral arch origin and sensory nerve supply to visceral structures (mucous membranes, taste buds).

The differentiation of the mandibular and the maxillary processes into the jaws has already been described. In addition, the first and second arches also form the middle ear ossicles as will be described in the section on the ear. The second arch mesenchyme also forms the lesser cornu and the upper part of the body of the hyoid bone. The third arch forms the remainder of the hyoid bone—the greater cornu and the lower half of the body. The fourth and fifth arches form the laryngeal cartilages (Fig. 14–11).

The first arch mesoderm forms the muscles of mastication and also the anterior belly of the digastric, the mylohyoid, and the tensor tympani. The muscles of facial expression are all derived from the second arch mesoderm, which also forms the posterior belly of the digastric, the stylohyoid, and the stapedius. The third arch mesoderm forms the more cranial pharyngeal muscles, and the fourth and fifth arches form the lower pharyngeal and the laryngeal muscles.

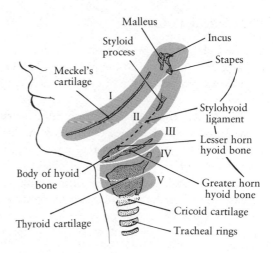

14–11 Diagram of the contributions of the five visceral arches to the skeletal system.

Pharyngeal Pouches

The first pharyngeal pouch forms the tympanic cavity of the middle ear and its connection to the pharynx, the Eustachian tube. Again, their development will be discussed more completely in the section on the ear.

The dorsal and most of the ventral portions of the second pharyngeal pouch becomes obliterated by the proliferation of the endoderm. However, a small recess persists, the *tonsillar fossa,* the primordium of the *palatine tonsil* (Fig. 14–10). It is invaded by mesenchyme and at about the fifth month begins to develop aggregations of lymphatic material. Similar aggregations of lymphatic tissue (but not of second pouch origin) occur in the *lingual tonsil* and the dorsal wall of the nasopharynx to form the *pharyngeal tonsil (adenoids).*

In the third pouch, communication to the pharynx becomes constricted during the third month. The lateral end of the pouch, however, continues to expand and forms a large pouchlike region with dorsal and ventral sacculations (Fig. 14–10 B,C). The dorsal sacculations give rise to parts of the *parathyroid glands,* and the ventral sacculations form the major portion of the *thymus gland* (Fig. 14–10 C). In the 13 millimeter embryo, during week six, the constricted connection to the pharynx is lost and the developing thymic and parathyroid tissues become free from any pharyngeal attachments. The third pouch now shows an accelerated rate of growth, particularly in the region that will form the thymus (Fig. 14–12). This region pushes caudally and its lumen is gradually eliminated (Fig. 14–12 D). During the early caudal movement of the thymic rudiment, the parathyroid remains attached to it and is pulled caudally past the position of the part of the fourth pouch, which is also developing a part of the parathyroid gland. This explains the definitive position of parathyroid III caudal to that of parathyroid IV.

At about the 20 millimeter stage, toward the end of month two, the rudiments of the thymus and the parathyroid of pouch three separate. The thymic rudiment continues its caudal migration and its caudal end extends into the thoracic cavity where it meets and fuses with its counterpart of the other side. The cranial end remains in the cervical region and some cords persist up to or higher than the level of the thyroid gland.

Each fourth pharyngeal pouch develops a parathyroid rudiment, parathyroid IV, from its dorsal portion, in the same manner as the third (Fig. 14–10). The pair from the fourth pouch does not become associated with the caudally growing thymus and thus retains its position and ends up at the level of the cranial end of the thyroid, becoming the *superior parathyroid* of the adult. Both pairs of

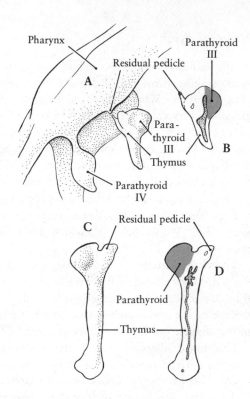

14–12 Later development of the parathyroid and thymus. A, parathyroid III and thymus III separated from the pharynx; B, section through A; C, D, caudal elongation of the thymus and the beginning of the obliteration of its cavity. (From G. L. Weller, 1932.)

parathyroids become embedded in the thyroid tissue (Fig. 14–13).

The fate of the ventral region of the fourth pouch is in some doubt. A small portion may contribute to the thymus gland. A pair of large *ultimobranchial bodies* is found in this region in the sixth week (Fig. 14–10). The ultimobranchial bodies have variously been considered as a part of the fourth pouch or as rudimentary fifth pouches. The ultimobranchial bodies lose their connection with the pharynx and become embedded in the thyroid gland as it grows caudally. The ultimate fate of the tissue of these bodies has been considered to be: (1) nothing, (2) thyroid tissue, or (3) special tissue in the thyroid gland, parafollicular cells, responsible for the secretion of thyrocalcitonin.

The Floor of the Oral Cavity

The Thyroid Gland in Man

The thyroid gland develops in close association with the pharyngeal pouches. It is recognizable in early somite embryos as a thickening in the floor of the pharynx between the first and second pouches just caudad of the region that will form the tuberculum impar of the tongue (Fig. 14–14 A). In man, at 16–17 days, the thickening forms a ventral outpocketing that becomes closely associated with the underlying endothelium of the developing heart. The evagination develops into a flask-shaped vesicle attached to its origin by a narrow neck, the *thyroglossal duct* (Figs. 14–14 E; 14–15 A,B). The vesicle quickly becomes bilobed. The lumen of the thyroglossal duct soon becomes occluded and early in the second month the stalk breaks up and the bilobed terminal portion loses its connection to the pharynx (Figs. 14–14 C; 14–15 C). The lumen of the vesicle also disappears at this time, and the gland becomes a solid mass of expanding tissue.

As the heart moves caudally, the thyroid gland moves along with it, and by the end of the seventh week it becomes located in its adult position in the anterior lower neck region where it lies ventral to the developing larynx as a bilobed U-shaped structure, its two lobes connected by a narrow *isthmus* (Fig. 14–15 D). Subsequent morphological development involves a progressive increase in size.

The histological and biochemical differentiation of the thyroid gland has been studied in a number of mammals, including man. In man, there are three histological stages: (1) a precolloid stage (from 47–72 days), (2) a beginning colloid stage (from 73–80 days), and (3) a stage of follicular growth (from 80 days to birth). Colloid appears in canaliculi between the developing follicles. The canaliculi open into a central clover-shaped colloid space that is surrounded by the developing follicles.

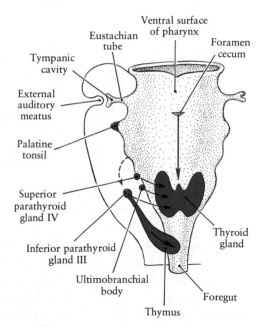

14–13 Diagram of the caudal migration of the thyroid, thymus, parathyroids, and ultimobranchial bodies.

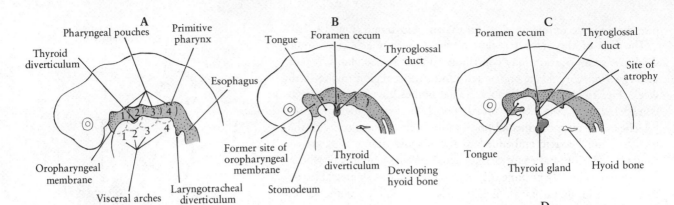

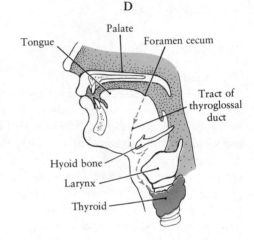

14-14 Diagrams of sagittal sections of the head showing successive stages in the development of the thyroid gland at four, five, and six weeks (A, B, and C); D, adult head showing path of the thyroid gland to its position anterior to the larynx.

There are some species differences in the time of the development of an iodine-concentrating mechanism and in the sequence of the synthesis of the active thyroid hormone, thyroxin (triiodothyronine, T_4). In the mouse, organic binding of iodine and formation of colloid occur on days 15–16, a day before the appearance of follicles and the production of T_4. In most subprimate mammals there is a stepwise development of synthetic activity that begins with the ability to trap iodine, next develops the mechanism to synthesize iodotyrosine, and then develops the mechanism to couple iodotyrosine to form iodothyronine—the same steps that take place during the synthesis of the hormone in the adult gland. However, in man and in the monkey, the ability to concentrate iodine and the mechanism for synthesizing T_4 appear at the same time—about day 74 in man—when the follicles are forming lumens and the colloid is present centrally in the cloverleaf pattern.

The Thyroid Gland in the Chick

The development of the thyroid gland in the chick embryo follows the same morphological pattern described above. It can be divided into five stages: (1) primordium formation, (2) vesicle formation, (3) stalk formation and detachment, (4) bilateral division, and (5) mesenchyme invasion. Up until 48 hours of incubation (stage 12), the floor of the pharynx consists of a single layer of loosely connected cuboidal cells all having the same appearance. At stage 12, the thyroid primordium is first seen when a small group of cells between the second pair of arches develops differences that distinguish them from the surrounding cells. They become more tightly packed, the cell surface open to the pharynx becomes scalloped, large characteristically staining droplets appear in the apical cytoplasm, and an indication of a fibrillar band stretching across several cells appears in the apical cytoplasm.

Shortly thereafter, the lateral walls of the primordium become elevated and a shallow depression is formed. At this time, the density of the apical fibrous band increases, particularly in the region of maximum bending. This is in agreement with the suggested involvement of microfilaments in a purse-string-like action associated with tissue folding as has been described in the development of the neural folds. EM photographs of the cup-shaped thyroid primordium show these microfilaments as a band around the entire rim of the vesicle.

In the next two days, as the thyroid gland moves away from the floor of the pharynx, a short thyroid stalk develops whose lumen soon becomes occluded. As it elongates, it also narrows and at about four and one half days (stage 24) breaks up. At this time, the primordium is bilobed, but the connection between the lobes becomes increasingly stretched. By day five (stage 26), the lobes separate.

The thyroid primodium, which is closely associated with the ventral aorta during its early development, moves caudally along with the caudal movement of the heart to assume its definitive position in the lower neck region about day six and one half (stage 29). Here it becomes encapsulated by mesenchyme, which also invades the gland to form the thyroid lobules. Follicle formation begins at the time the gland reaches its adult position.

In the chick, T_4 can be detected chromatographically at stage 12, the time the thyroid primordium can first be distinguished morphologically. This appearance of an organ-specific product at the time the organ can first be distinguished morphologically has been reported so far in only one other organ, the pancreas, where insulin can be detected in the early primordium.

T_4 accumulation in the cells of the developing glands does not show a steady increase with time, but shows at first a rapid logarithmic increase to about day four and one half (stage 24), a plateau until about day six and one half (stage 29), and then a second slower rise to a second plateau at day 12, which level is maintained until hatching (Fig. 14–16 A). The number of cells per gland follows almost the same pattern, rising to a plateau between days five and six and one half and then steadily increasing until hatching (Fig. 14–16 B). It should be noted that plateaus in T_4 accumulation and cell number occur at a time of complex morphogenetic activity—formation of a bilobed structure, detachment of the lobes, and mesenchymal invasion. The second rise in T_4 accumulation and cell number is correlated with the formation of the thyroid follicles. It has been suggested that the cessation of cell division during an important morphogenetic (or biochemical) phase of differentiation may be important to the later development of the thyroid gland.

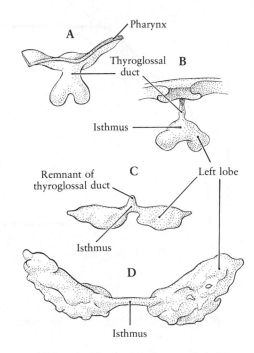

14–15 Development of the human thyroid gland. A, formation of bilobed rudiment showing its connection to the pharynx by the hollow thyroglossal duct; B, thyroglossal duct elongates as gland grows caudally; C, connection to the pharynx is lost and the two lobes are connected by an isthmus; D, large right and left lobes connected by a thin isthmus.

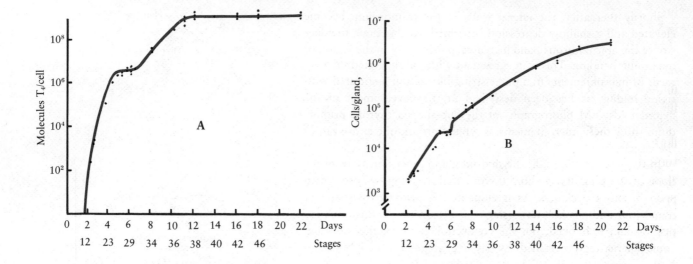

This stage has been compared to the "protodifferentiation" period described in the development of the pancreas.

The Tongue

The tongue is derived from the floor of the oral cavity and the pharynx. At the end of the first month of development, in the 6 millimeter embryo, the visceral arches are well defined and the ventral ends of the pharyngeal grooves and the arches between them extend toward the midline (Fig. 14–17 A). Between and caudal to the first arches is a small median elevation, the *tuberculum impar.* From it and the adjacent mandibular region the anterior two thirds of the tongue, the body, will be formed. The posterior third of the tongue, the root, will be formed by the union of the second visceral arches and also will receive some contributions from the third and fourth arches. The *foramen caecum* is an important landmark located just posterior to the tuberculum impar. It marks the point of origin of the thyroid evagination and also separates the body from the root of the tongue.

The major part of the body of the tongue arises from paired *lateral lingual swellings* of the first arch (Fig. 14–17 B,C). The lateral lingual swellings increase rapidly in size and unite with the tuberculum impar, which itself lags in development, is obscured by the lingual swellings, and contributes little of significance to the definitive organ. The fusion of the lingual swellings is indicated on the dorsum of the tongue as the *medium sulcus* (Fig. 14–17 C,D) and appears internally as the *septum* of the tongue. The foramen caecum persists as a small depression on the dorsal surface of the tongue at the apex of a V-shaped sulcus, the *sulcus limitans.* Just

14–16 A, changes in the amount of thyroid hormone per cell during the development of the chick; B, changes in the number of cells per thyroid gland during the development of the chick. (From W. G. Shain, S. R. Helfer, and V. G. Fonte, 1972. Dev. Biol. 28, 202.)

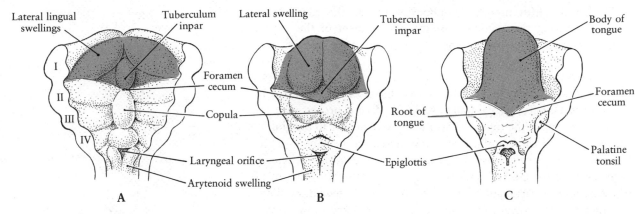

Lateral lingual swellings — Tuberculum inpar — Lateral swelling — Tuberculum impar — Body of tongue

Foramen cecum — Copula — Root of tongue — Foramen cecum

Laryngeal orifice — Arytenoid swelling — Epiglottis — Palatine tonsil

A   B   C

anterior to the sulcus limitans are located the large circumvallate papillae.

The formation of the root of the tongue is somewhat more complicated. Between and uniting the second and third visceral arches, posterior to the tuberculum impar, is a swelling known as the *copula* (Fig. 14–17 B). The root of the tongue is formed by the copula and from the ventral parts of the second, third, and fourth arches. In its development, the material of the third arch migrates anteriorly and encroaches on the territory of the second, and a large part of the sensory innervation to the root of the tongue is by way of cranial nerve IX, the nerve of the third visceral arch. The vagus nerve, the nerve of the fourth arch, also supplies the root of the tongue, indicating the contribution of fourth arch material.

The main sensory supply to the body of the tongue is by way of branches of cranial nerves V and VII, nerves of the first and second arches, respectively. However, a small part of the tongue anterior to the sulcus limitans is supplied by the glossopharyngeal nerve indicating some third arch contribution to the body.

The tissue beneath the epithelial membrane of the tongue consists mainly of skeletal muscle and connective tissue. The connective tissue is formed from the mesoderm of the visceral arches. However, the mesoderm of the visceral arches probably does not form the tongue muscles. Both on the basis of comparative anatomy and the fact that the hypoglossal nerve supplies the tongue muscles, it appears that this tissue is derived from more caudally located somatic muscle of the occipital myotomes.

The oral surface of the tongue develops specialized gustatory receptors, the taste buds. In addition to the circumvallate papillae already mentioned, foliate papillae appear during the third month, and fungiform and filliform papillae appear still later. All types develop as elevations of the surface epithelium.

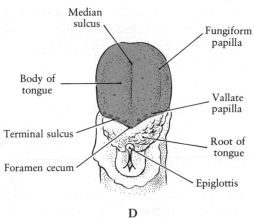

Median sulcus — Fungiform papilla — Body of tongue — Vallate papilla — Terminal sulcus — Root of tongue — Foramen cecum — Epiglottis

D

14–17   Development of the human tongue seen from above. A, five weeks; B, six weeks; C, five months; D, adult.

During the fifth month, lymphocytes invade the root of the tongue marking the beginning of the development of the lingual tonsil. Its crypts, however, do not develop until after birth.

The Epiglottis

The slit-shaped opening into the larynx, the *glottis,* is apparent in the fifth week between the fourth and fifth visceral arches just caudad of the root of the tongue (Fig. 14–17 A). Anterior to the glottis, between it and the copula, a swelling marks the beginning of the formation of the *epiglottis* and a pair of *arytenoid swellings,* one on either side of the glottis, mark the beginning of the development of these laryngeal cartilages (Fig. 14–17 A). The arytenoid swellings migrate rostrally toward the epiglottis and in so doing form a transverse component on the upper end of the glottis so that the opening now becomes T-shaped (Fig. 14–17 D). Later, the upper part of the opening becomes more ovoid, although a deep interarytenoid notch persists in the sagittal plane.

Salivary Glands

The epithelium of the oral cavity gives rise to a number of solid evaginations that will develop into the salivary glands. The *submandibular gland* develops during the third month as an outgrowth from the floor of the oral cavity between the tongue and the gum. The *parotid gland* appears somewhat later as an outgrowth from the cheek immediately posterior to the angle of the jaw and the primordium of the *sublingual gland* develops lateral to it. The openings of the ducts of the salivary glands in the adult are somewhat more anterior than the point of the original evagination owing to the closure of the posterior parts of the gutterlike grooves from which they are derived. The original solid epithelial outgrowths undergo repeated branching and by the sixth month the numerous branches become completely canalized.

REFERENCES

Burnet, F. M. 1962. The thymus gland. Sci. Am. 207:50–57.

Fisher, D. A. and J. H. Dussault. 1976. Development of the mammalian thyroid gland. Handbook of Physiology, Section 7, Vol. 3, pp. 21–38. Eds., R.O. Greep and E. B. Astwood. Baltimore: Williams and Wilkins.

Shain, W. G., S. R. Hilfer, and V. G. Fonte. 1972. Early organogenesis of the embryonic chick thyroid. Dev. Biol. 28:202–218.

Weller, G. L. 1932. Development of the thyroid, parathyroid and thymus glands in man. Contr. Embryol. Carnegie Inst. 24:93–139.

15

The Digestive Tube
and Associated Glands

THE DIGESTIVE TUBE

The Pharynx

The *pharynx* is connected cranially with the oral and the nasal cavities and caudally with the *larynx* and the *esophagus*. Following the development of the nasal cavities and the palate, the pharynx may be divided into three areas. The *oropharynx* communicates with the oral cavity from which it is marked off by an indistinct fold of mucous membrane, the *palatoglossal fold* (anterior pillar of the fauces). A second fold of mucous membrane connects the palate to the floor of the pharynx, the *palatopharyngeal fold* (posterior pillar of the fauces). The palatine tonsil develops between these two sheets of mucous membrane. The *nasopharynx* is the portion of the pharynx that communicates with the nasal cavities by way of the posterior nares. The Eustachian tubes open into the lateral walls of the nasopharynx. The *laryngopharynx,* the most caudal part of the pharynx, communicates posteriorly with the esophagus and, by the way of the glottis, with the larynx.

The Esophagus, Stomach, and Intestine

The alimentary tract caudal to the pharynx differentiates into the esophagus, *stomach,* and the *small* and *large intestine,* and the *rectum.* The alimentary tract shows a basic similarity of development throughout its length, and differences exist only in the degree and extent of changes in size, shape, and position and in the production of a number of specialized glandular outgrowths. The basic histological differentiation of the tract will be described after a consideration of the gross morphological changes.

The esophagus is the portion of the foregut into which the pharynx opens. At first only a very short connection between the pharynx and the stomach, the esophagus increases rapidly in length with the development of the lungs and the caudal shift in position of the heart and the stomach (Fig. 15–1). It remains, however, as a relatively straight, unspecialized connection between the pharynx

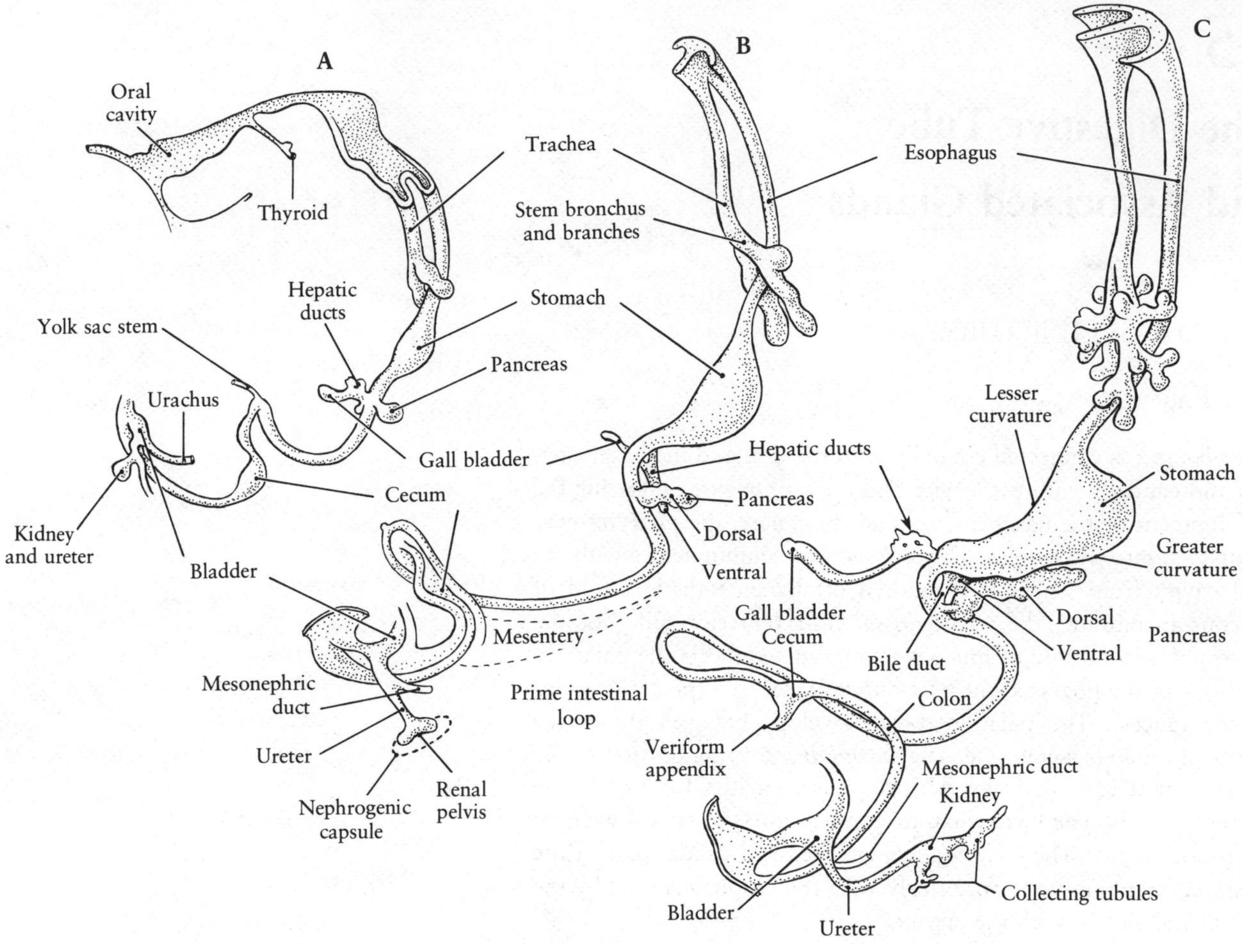

A
Oral cavity
Thyroid
Hepatic ducts
Yolk sac stem
Urachus
Kidney and ureter
Bladder
Gall bladder
Cecum
Mesonephric duct
Ureter
Nephrogenic capsule
Renal pelvis
Prime intestinal loop
Mesentery
Trachea
Stem bronchus and branches
Stomach
Pancreas
B
Hepatic ducts
Pancreas
Dorsal
Ventral
Gall bladder
Cecum
Veriform appendix
Bladder
Ureter
C
Esophagus
Lesser curvature
Stomach
Greater curvature
Dorsal
Ventral
Pancreas
Bile duct
Colon
Mesonephric duct
Kidney
Collecting tubules

15–1 Drawings of reconstructions of three stages in the development of the digestive tube in man. A, 7–8 mm, 31–32 days; B, 8–11 mm, 32–34 days; C, 11–13 mm, 34–35 days. (From G. L. Streeter, 1948. Carnegie Contributions to Embryology 32, 211.)

and the stomach. It is the most constricted part of the alimentary tract.

The stomach is the caudal continuation of the esophagus. It shows a fusiform dilation as early as the end of the first month, which forecasts its future expansion about a week later (Fig. 15–1 A). Continued growth develops a greatly enlarged organ that already shows the adult configuration with a cranial *lesser curvature,* a caudal *greater curvature,* and a bulge near the esophageal junction, the *fundus* (Fig. 15–1 B,C). Dorsal and ventral mesenteries (mesogastria) are attached to the greater and lesser curvatures, respectively, indicating that during this stage of development the stomach goes through a 90° rotation to the right.

The intestine is the portion of the digestive tube between the stomach and the cloaca. The major portion of both the small and the large intestine develops from the roof of the open midgut be-

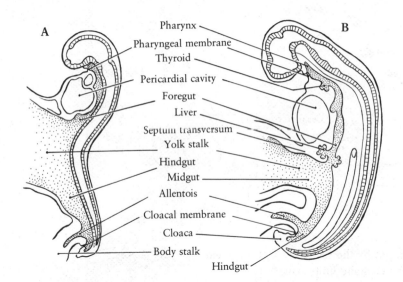

A

- Pharynx
- Pharyngeal membrane
- Thyroid
- Pericardial cavity
- Foregut
- Liver
- Septum transversum
- Yolk stalk
- Hindgut
- Midgut
- Allentois
- Cloacal membrane
- Cloaca
- Body stalk

B

Hindgut

15–2 Sagittal sections of early human embryos showing the digestive tract. A, 2.5 mm, 18 somites; B, 2.5 mm, 25 somites.

tween the anterior and the posterior intestinal portals. The midgut is at first in open and broad communication with the yolk sac, and the entire tract lies in the sagittal plane of the body (Fig. 15–2). As the body folds develop and undercut the embryo, the connection between the embryonic and extraembryonic structures is by way of the body stalk. At the end of the first month, the embryonic intestine, which has begun to increase rapidly in length, begins to herniate into the body stalk and its original broad connection to the yolk sac is marked by the point of attachment of the yolk stalk (vitelline duct) at the end of the hairpin-shaped herniation (Fig. 15–3 A). This small diverticulum may be used as a landmark in respect to which the midgut may be divided into cephalic (proximal) and caudal (distal) limbs. The cephalic limb will form the caudal part of the *duodenum,* the *jejunum* and the greater part of the *ileum.* The caudal limb will form the caudal part of the ileum, the *cecum,* the *ascending colon,* and about half of the *transverse colon.* The cranial part of the duodenum develops from the foregut. The caudal part of the colon and the rectum develop from the hindgut. The cecum marks the point of transition from the small to the large intestine. It appears early in the second month as a dilation caudal to the point of attachment of the yolk stalk (Fig. 15–1 A,B).

The positional relationship between the small and large intestine in the adult may readily be understood by a consideration of the rotation of the herniated midgut and the sequence of its return into the embryonic abdominal cavity as diagrammed in Figure 15–3. The midgut moves into the extraembryonic coelom owing to a lack

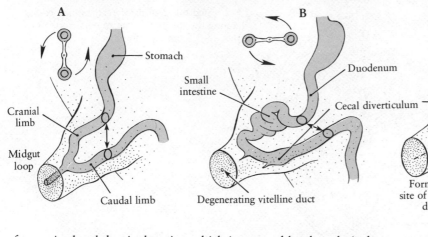

A

Stomach

Cranial
limb

Midgut
loop

Caudal limb

B

Small
intestine

Duodenum

Cecal diverticulum

Degenerating vitelline duct

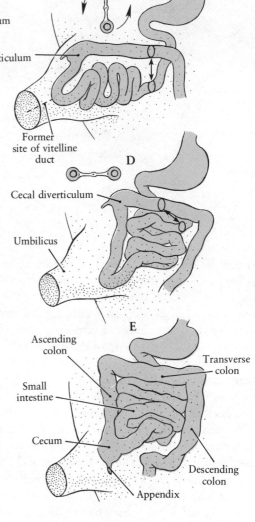

C

Former
site of vitelline
duct

D

Cecal diverticulum

Umbilicus

E

Ascending
colon

Transverse
colon

Small
intestine

Cecum

Descending
colon

Appendix

of space in the abdominal cavity, which is usurped by the relatively massive embryonic liver and mesonephros. The cephalic limb now elongates rapidly and is thrown into coils. The caudal limb does not coil and shows little change except the development of the cecum (Fig. 15–3 B).

The entire midgut, within the body stalk, starts a counterclockwise rotation around the superior mesenteric artery (a branch of the dorsal aorta that will supply all of the midgut derivatives). About 90° of the entire rotation is completed while the midgut is herniated (Fig. 15–3 B).

As about the tenth week, the relative size of the liver and the mesonephros decreases and the abdominal cavity expands and the herniated midgut begins to return to the abdominal cavity (Fig. 15–3 C). As it does so, the rotation continues and eventually goes through about 270° (Fig. 15–3 D). The small intestine, the cephalic limb of the midgut, moves out of the body stalk first and, in so doing, pushes the caudal part of the large intestine (hindgut) to the left of the body cavity. The jejunum is the first part to return, and its cranial coils come to be located on the left side, the more caudal folds of the jejunum and the ileum gradually filling up the remainder of the cavity. The caudal limb of the midgut is then withdrawn, the cecal region being the last part to leave the body stalk to occupy a position just below the liver in the upper right quadrant of the abdominal cavity (Fig. 15–3 D). The large intestine then occupies the left and cranial parts of the abdominal cavity, and the much coiled small intestine occupies the central part. Further changes involve a descent of the cecal region so that the small intestine becomes completely enclosed in the C-shaped large intestine, the latter consisting of ascending, transverse, and descending portions (Fig. 15–3 E).

15–3 Diagrams of the herniation of the midgut into the yolk stalk and its subsequent rotation and return to the abdominal cavity. A, about five weeks. Midgut beginning to herniate; B, beginning of rotation of the gut while it is in the yolk stalk; C, continued rotation as the gut begins to return into the abdominal cavity; D, midgut completely within the abdominal cavity after rotation of 270 degrees; E, final positional changes completed as the cecum descends into the lower right quadrant. The insets, which indicate the rotation of the intestine, represent cross sections through the cranial and caudal limbs at the levels indicated by the circles and arrows in the diagrams. (After K. L. Moore, 1977. The Developing Human. W. B. Saunders Company, Philadelphia.)

The cecum continues to mark the transition between the small and the large intestine. As the cecum increases in size, the original end-to-end connection between these two areas is changed, and the small intestine enters the large intestine at a right angle (Fig. 15–4). The cecum then appears as a pouch below this *ileocolic junction*. The growth of the distal end of the cecum lags behind the other parts of the organ from the third month on, resulting in the formation of a small conical projection at the caudal end. This is the *appendix*. It is highly variable in both shape and position.

Histology of the Alimentary Tract

The characteristic histological structure of the adult alimentary tract is that of an epithelial lined tube surrounded by layers of muscle and connective tissue. The lining of the tract and the glands developed from it are the only parts derived from embryonic endoderm. The connective tissue and muscle are the products of the splanchnic mesoderm that becomes associated with the endodermal lining. The general pattern consists of four layers: (1) mucosa, (2) submucosa, (3) muscularis, and (4) serosa—named in order from the inside to the outside (Fig. 15–5).

The mucosa consists of the epithelial lining plus a thin layer of connective tissue and in some areas a thin layer of muscle. The epithelium shows some variation throughout the tract and, although it is generally simple columnar, in the esophagus it is stratified squamous. In the stomach and the intestine, it forms characteristic glands with various kinds of secretory and absorptive cells that begin to function at different times of development in different regions of the tract. Proteolytic enzymes and digestive ferments of the small intestine have been detected during the fourth month; and although some enzymes such as amylase may not be present until birth, it is apparent that the alimentary tract is ready to commence functional activitiy well in advance of the time it will be called on to do so.

For the first few months of development, the tract is usually devoid of solid material. After this time, an increasing amount of material begins to accumulate in the lumen. Swallowed amniotic fluid contributes sloughed epithelial cells and lanugo hairs. The tract itself adds more epithelial cells, mucus, and bile secretions. The contents of the neonatal gut are called *meconium* and, owing to their long retention in combination with bile secretions, they are greenish in color. The green color of the stool quickly changes during the first few days after birth to the normal yellowish color.

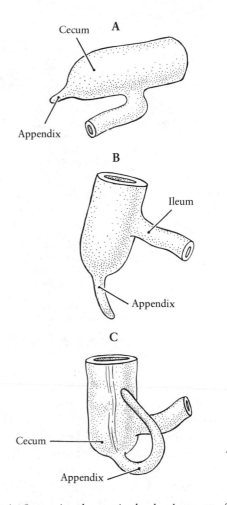

15–4 Successive changes in the development of the caecum, the appendix and the small intestine. A, about 7 weeks; B, about 12 weeks; C, at birth.

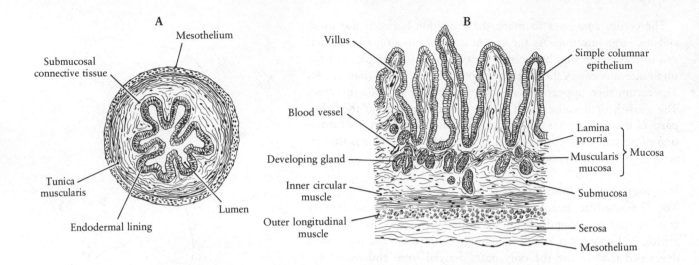

A

Mesothelium
Submucosal connective tissue
Tunica muscularis
Endodermal lining
Lumen

B

Villus
Simple columnar epithelium
Blood vessel
Developing gland
Inner circular muscle
Outer longitudinal muscle
Lamina prorria
Muscularis mucosa
} Mucosa
Submucosa
Serosa
Mesothelium

15–5   Two stages in the histogenesis of the intestine. A, month 2; B, month 5.

ASSOCIATED GLANDS

The Liver and the Gall Bladder

The liver is the most precocious of the glandular derivatives of the alimentary tract. It is first indicated in the third week as a thickening of the endodermal lining of the ventral wall of the foregut in the region of the anterior intestinal portal (Fig. 15–2 A). This is the region of the tract that will become the duodenum. The thickening soon gives rise to an outgrowth, the *hepatic diverticulum,* which grows into the septum transversum (Fig. 15–2 B). The septum transversum is a mesodermal partition lying between the pericardial cavity and the yolk stalk. It will form the major part of the diaphragm separating the pericardial and abdominal cavities (Chapter 17). The rapidly proliferating cells divide into two components, a more cranial, larger, *pars hepatica,* which will form the liver tissue and its duct system, and a more caudal, smaller, *pars cystica,* which will form the gall bladder and the cystic duct (Fig. 15–6 A, B).

The pars hepatica develops a maze of anastomosing cords of epithelial cells that continue to proliferate as they invade the septum transversum. The cords break up the vitelline and umbilical veins transforming these vessels into hepatic sinusoids. This results in an intermingling of hepatic cords and sinusoidal channels. The sinusoids form a network interspersed between the veins bringing blood to the liver (the vitelline and umbilical veins—the paired vitelline veins later differentiating into the single hepatic portal vein) and the veins draining the liver (the hepatic veins). The parenchyma of the liver develops from the hepatic cords, forming what are actually

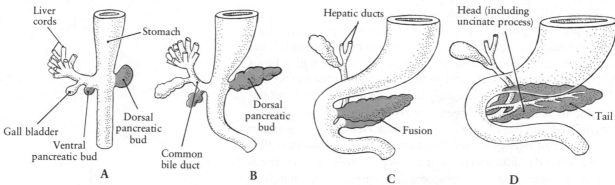

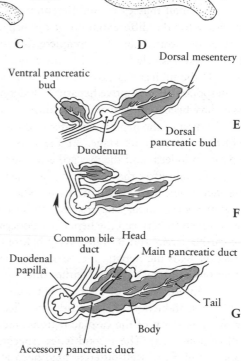

anastomosing sheets of epithelium, each consisting of a single layer of cuboidal cells. Bile canaliculi develop between the hepatic cords. They connect to intrahepatic bile ducts. These, in turn, connect to the larger hepatic ducts that drain into the common bile duct (Fig. 15–6 B).

The mesoderm of the septum transversum differentiates into the connective tissue, the hematopoietic tissue, and the Kupffer cells of the liver. Blood cells are differentiated in the second to the seventh month, but at birth the hematopoietic activity of the liver has stopped. The blood-forming function of the embryonic (fetal) liver is largely responsible for the rapid increase in the size of this organ, which in the third month makes up about 10 percent of the total weight of the fetus.

The gall bladder begins its development at the distal end of the pars cystica as a solid cylindrically shaped group of cells, connected to the common bile duct by a stem, the cystic duct (Fig. 15–6). The gall bladder grows ventrally but does not invade the tissue of the septum transversum.

Owing to the rotation of the duodenum, the opening of the common bile duct into the duodenum shifts from an anterior to a posterior position (Fig. 15–6, C,D). Consequently, the common bile duct will be found running posterior to the duodenum.

15–6 A–D, diagrams of successive stages in the development of the liver, the gall bladder and the pancreas from the fifth to seventh weeks; E–G, cross sections of B, C, and D at the levels indicated. (After K. L. Moore, 1977. The Developing Human. W. B. Saunders Company, Philadelphia.)

Epithelial-Mesenchymal Interaction in the
Development of the Chick Liver

The localization of the liver-forming areas of the chick embryo have been well documented by the work of Rudnick and Rawles. Early in development, hepatic and cardiac potencies are closely associated in the region just anterior to the primitive streak. Later, in the 10- to 15-somite stage, the hepatic region covers a large part of the blastoderm on either side of the somites, the bilateral areas merging anteriorly in the floor of the foregut and the cardiac fold. The presumptive liver tissue, which is located in the region of the anterior intestinal portal, represents presumptive hepatic endoderm and the remainder represents presumptive hepatic mesoderm. What is the relationship between the presumptive endoderm, which forms the proliferating epithelial cords of the liver, and the mesoderm into which the cords grow? If the early hepatic bud from which the underlying mesenchyme has been removed is cultured in vitro or transplanted into the coelom of a host chick embryo, it degenerates or forms small masses of undifferentiated cells. Mesoderm is thus necessary for the differentiation of the hepatic cells. In fact, it has been demonstrated that for complete differentiation the endoderm must be successively subjected to the action of two mesodermal tissues: (1) the midventral cardiac mesoderm and (2) the lateral hepatic mesoderm. Presumptive hepatic endoderm from which the mesoderm has been removed will not differentiate even when grafted into the area of the hepatic mesoderm, if the operation is performed before the five-somite stage. At the five- to six-somite stage, the hepatic endoderm and the precardiac mesoderm meet in the cardiac fold, and only after the endoderm has been exposed to the cardiac mesoderm will it form hepatic tissue when transplanted to the hepatic mesoderm area. The first step in liver differentiation, then, is the interaction between the hepatic endoderm and the mesoderm of the cardiac area; and it is necessary before the second step, the interaction with the hepatic mesoderm, can exert its effect. Both interactions must take place. Neither one, by itself, will result in the normal differentiation of the hepatic tissue.

The first induction is apparently specific. It can only be exerted by the mesoderm of the cardiac region, and only hepatic endoderm will respond to it. The second is less specific, since the hepatic endoderm will form well-differentiated hepatic cords when associated with mesenteric or metanephric mesoderm. Although these cords appear normal, the cells are unable to synthesize glycogen. However, if they are now put into association with hepatic mesoderm, they will begin to synthesize it. Apparently the inductive action of the foreign mesoderm is an incomplete one, and the secondary induction itself may be considered to consist of two steps: (1) the formation of hepatic epithelial cords—histological differentiation— and (2) the onset of specific metabolic activitiy—functional differentiation. Only hepatic mesoderm can bring about the latter.

Neither the mode of action nor the chemical nature of the liver-inducing substances is known. However, there is little doubt that they differ chemically from the inducing substances playing roles in the differentiation of other organs such as the lung, the limb, and the kidney.

The Pancreas

The pancreas is the second largest gland in the body. It has a dual function and consists of an exocrine portion that synthesizes digestive enzymes, which pass by way of a duct system into the duodenum and an endocrine portion that synthesizes insulin and glucagon, two hormones essential to the regulation of carbohydrate metabolism.

The Morphological Development of the Pancreas

The pancreas develops from the duodenal epithelium in the region of the liver as a pair of evaginations, one dorsal and one ventral, which later fuse with each other. The dorsal pancreas arises from the dorsal wall of the duodenum opposite and slightly cranial to the liver diverticulum and pushes into the dorsal mesentery. The ventral pancreas arises from the ventral region of the duodenum in the angle of the hepatic diverticulum, but as the hepatic diverticulum grows, the ventral pancreas establishes connection with it and opens into the common bile duct (Fig. 15–6 A). When the duodenum rotates to the right, the ventral pancreatic diverticulum is carried into the dorsal mesentery lying below and behind the dorsal pancreas and separated from it by the part of the left vitelline vein that will contribute to the formation of the hepatic portal vein. The two pancreatic primordia fuse (Fig. 15–6, C,D). The ventral pancreas contributes the tissue that will form the lower portion of the head; and the dorsal pancreas forms the remainder of the head, the tail, and the body of the adult pancreas. When the two primordia fuse, their duct systems also become interconnected. Then, the proximal part of the dorsal duct degenerates, and the pancreas empties into the persistent ventral pancreatic duct, a tributary of the common bile duct. Within the pancreatic tissue, the duct of the dorsal pancreas persists and drains the tail and the body of the organ. Although in man the ventral duct (duct of Wirsung) persists as the only definitive opening into the duodenum, in other species—the pig and the cow—only the dorsal duct (duct of Santorini) persists. In the horse and the dog, both ducts persist.

The Exocrine Pancreas in the Rodent

The development of the pancreas in the mouse and the rat has been thoroughly studied, and some interesting facts on the biochemical and ultrastructural aspects of development have been described. In these rodents the pancreas also develops from a dorsal and a ventral diverticulum that later fuse. The dorsal pancreas appears first, in the 20-somite embryo about the middle of the gestation period (9½ days in the mouse, 11 days in the rat). It original broad connection to the gut soon narrows, and the pancreas develops as a ramified system of tubules whose lumens form a connecting network throughout the pancreatic tissue. Each tubule consists of a single layer of polarized cuboidal cells whose apical ends are joined together by junctional complexes. Microvilli project into the narrow lumen. The basal end of the cells is covered by a common basal lamina continuous with that of the gut. Early in its formation, mesodermal cells accumulate around the pancreatic diverticulum. This contact with the mesoderm or with some factor passing from the mesoderm to the pancreatic cells is necessary for further differentiation. The tubules grow rapidly for several days and acinar, duct, and endocrine tissues develop from the epithelium.

The biochemical and cytological differentiation of the exocrine pancreas. The pancreas goes through a number of stages in its differentiation. If cells of the nine-day mouse embryo from the region of the gut where the pancreatic diverticulum will form are grown in vitro, they will develop pancreatic tissue and enzymes, provided mesoderm is also present. Before this time, they will not. Thus, even before the pancreatic diverticulum forms, some of the endoderm cells of the gut have acquired the capability of forming pancreatic tissue. At this time there is no morphological, cytological, or biochemical difference between these cells and any other cells of the gut.

When the pancreatic diverticulum first develops, its cells pass through what has been termed a *primary transition phase* when small amounts of the characteristic digestive enzymes can be detected in the cells (Fig. 15–7 A). After the primary transition, the cells enter a *protodifferentiation* state in which a constant low level of enzymes is present, cell division is rapid, and no cytodifferentiation has occurred. The protodifferentiation state lasts for three to four days. The low level of enzyme is probably not due to the fact that a few of the pancreatic cells have differentiated completely to a point at which they are synthesizing the adult level of enzyme. Rather it is due to all of the acinar cells of the pancreatic diverticulum synthesizing enzymes at a constant low level.

A *secondary transition* then occurs in which the rate of enzyme synthesis increases, and there is a dramatic increase by 1000 times or more of the concentration within the cells. Cytochemical changes now appear during this transition phase. First, there is an increase in the amount of rough endoplasmic reticulum, the site of enzyme synthesis, and this increase is followed by the appearance of zymogen granules in which the enzymes are stored. After the secondary transition, the acinar cells are considered to be fully differentiated.

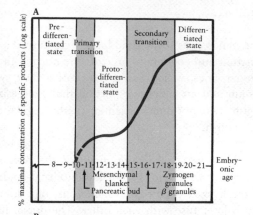

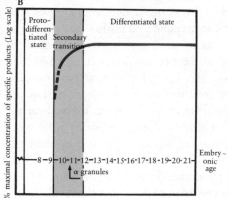

15–7 Model of the differentiation of the epithelial cells of the pancreas. A, exocrine cells and insulin-secreting cells. Concentrations of specific cell products rise from an undetectable level to a detectable low level during the primary transition phase as the pancreatic diverticulum forms and becomes associated with the mesoderm. Products remain at a constant low level in the protodifferentiated state and then rise to high levels during the secondary transition phase, which leads to the differentiated stage. The appearance of characteristic granules occurs in the secondary transition stage; B, glucogon secretion. Levels of glucogon rise rapidly during the primary transition stage of the cells diagrammed in A. Primary transition and protodifferentiated stages have not been identified. (From R. Pictel and W. J. Rutter, 1972. Handbook of Physiology, Section 7, Vol. 1. R. Greep and E. B. Astwood, eds. The American Physiological Society, Bethesda.)

The mesodermal factor. The need for a *mesodermal factor* (MF) to induce the differentiation of pancreatic tissue has been mentioned. MF is neither tissue nor species specific. Kidney or salivary gland mesoderm as well as mesoderm from the chick embryo will all support differentiation of the epithelial cells of the pancreas.

If pancreatic epithelium and mesoderm are cultured on opposite surfaces of a porous filter, the mesoderm can still produce its effect. Although the amount of differentiation is affected by the thickness of the filter and the size of the pores, contact between the two tissues is probably not necessary, as has been demonstrated in a number of other mesenchymal–epithelial-reacting systems. The mesodermal factor has been extracted and partially purified. It is trypsinsensitive and therefore proteinaceous. Its activity is also destroyed by sodium periodate, indicating it has a carbohydrate moiety.

At the time the cells of the gut first develop the capability of forming pancreatic derivatives, mesoderm must be present to achieve this result. However, late in the protodifferentiation state, about a half a day before the secondary transition, the inductive process has been completed and MF is no longer needed. The inductive influence of the mesoderm thus takes place over a relatively short span of three to four days. What is happening during the time the mesoderm is necessary? The major event is the rapid increase in DNA synthesis and cell division. This is apparently necessary for differentiation, since inhibition of DNA synthesis results in a failure of differentiation. Inhibition of mRNA synthesis during the protodifferentiation state also results in a failure of differentiation. It may then be concluded that new mRNA is being synthesized at this time as a preliminary to enzyme synthesis, and this RNA synthesis in turn depends upon DNA synthesis. When cell division ceases, differentiation takes place. This is easily demonstrated since cell division shows a gradient of activity toward the end of the protodifferentiation state, with the peripheral cells continuing to divide after the central cells have stopped. It is in the nondividing central cells that zymogen granules first appear. Also, inhibitors of DNA synthesis no longer have any effect on the differentiation of the central cells but still inhibit differentiation in the peripheral cells. Thus, a loss of proliferative activity appears to be associated with the attainment of the secondary transition stage leading to the final differentiation state.

The mechanism by which MF exerts its influence is speculative. There is good evidence that it acts at the cell surface. If MF is covalently bound to large insoluble beads of Sepharose (a derivative of agar) that are then placed among a culture of pancreatic epithelial cells, the cells attach to the beads, become oriented, synthesize

DNA, and divide. It has been proposed that MF promotes close contacts between cells. In the absence of MF, epithial cells in culture tend to spread out in a loose arrangement; something that does not happen if MF is present. Changes in membrane permeability and cell shape may also be produced and, in turn, stimulate cell division.

The Endocrine Pancreas in the Rodent

The epithelium of the developing pancreatic tubules consists of a single layer of cuboidal cells whose apical ends are closely connected by junctional complexes. The orientation of the mitotic spindle and the resulting cleavage plane are apparently instrumental in maintaining this single-layered configuration. The spindles are oriented parallel to the cell surface, and the cleavage planes thus develop perpendicular to the lumen. The cleavage furrow first appears at the basal region of the cell and moves apically. Each daughter cell remains firmly attached by its junctional complex to its neighbor cell and, in turn, the daughter cells develop apical junctional complexes between themselves before the cleavage plane is completed.

At the time of the early formation of the pancreatic diverticulum, the endocrine cells, which can be distinguished histologically from the exocrine cells, may be present in small numbers as a part of the single-layered tubule epithelium linked to the exocrine cells. Later formation of endocrine cells probably takes place by an orientation of the mitotic spindle perpendicular to the apical surface; the cell division then results in the formation of one apical daughter cell still linked to its neighbors and another separated from its neighbors and "escaped" from the single-layered epithelium—although still retained within the exocrine complex beneath the basal lamina (Fig. 15–8 A). There is a marked increase in the number of endocrine cells during the protodifferentiation period. Since it has been demonstrated that there is very little DNA synthesis or cell division among the endocrine islet cells, this increase must be the result of a continued supply from the dividing exocrine cells. Islet cells accumulate in small groups but still beneath the basal lamina (Fig. 15–8 B). Some of these groups may join to form larger outpocketings of islet cells. The islets later separate completely from the exocrine complex by the fusion of the basal lamina at the point of the outpocketing (Fig. 15–8 C). Capillaries invade the islets and the endocrine secretions of the islet cells are removed by way of this vascular supply.

Biochemical and cytological differentiation of the endocrine pancreas. The biochemical and cytological differentiation of the insulin-secreting B cells of the islets follows the same pattern just described

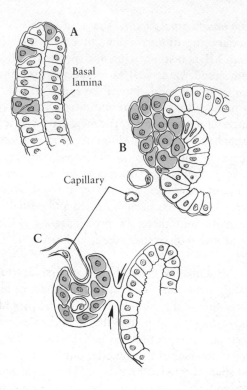

15–8 Histogenesis of the islet tissue. A, islet cells develop and some become located between the cells lining the lumen and the basal lamina. B, islet cells increase in number and form small clusters; C, islet cells become completely separated from exocrine cells by pinching off (at arrows) of the basal lamina at the point of outpocketing. Islets are penetrated by capillaries. (From R. Pictel and W. J. Rutter, 1972. Handbook of Physiology, Section 7, Vol. 1, R. Greep and E. B. Astwood, eds. The American Physiological Society, Bethesda.)

for the exocrine pancreas (Fig. 15–7 A). Following a preliminary initiating event leading to a primary transition phase, the synthesis of insulin takes place in the early pancreatic diverticulum and continues at low levels during the protodifferentiation state unaccompanied by any cytodifferentiation. Increasing quantities of insulin are synthesized during the secondary transition phase, and this event is accompanied by cytodifferentiation ending in the appearance of beta granules and the attainment of the differentiated state. The A cells, which synthesize glucagon, present a different picture. At the time of the formation of the pancreatic diverticulum during the primary transition phase, glucagon is already present at high concentrations—some 1000-fold higher than insulin (Fig. 15–7 B). This is correlated with the presence of A cells containing alpha granules. Glucagon levels and cytodifferentiation of the A cells reach the completely differentiated state while the exocrine pancreas and the insulin-secreting islet cells are still in the protodifferentiation state. The lack of a method for assaying low levels of glucagon does not at present allow an answer to the question of whether or not A cells also pass through a primary transition and a protodifferentiation state. If they do, this would occur before the formation of any morphologically or histologically recognizable pancreatic tissue.

REFERENCES

Pistil, R. and W. J. Rutter. 1972. Development of the embryonic endocrine pancreas. In: Handbook of Physiology, Section 7, Endocrinology, I. Eds., R. Greep and E. B. Astwood. Am. Physiol. Soc. Baltimore: Williams & Wilkins.

Rawles, M. E. 1936. A study of the localization of organ-forming areas in the chick blastoderm of the head-process stage. J. Exp. Zool. 72:271–315.

Rudnick, D. and M. E. Rawles. 1937. Differentiation of the gut in chorio-allantoic grafts from chick blastoderms. Physiol. Zool. 10:381–395.

Shephard, T. H. 1965. The thyroid. In: Organogenesis. Eds., R. L. DeHann and H. Ursprung. New York: Holt, Rinehart and Winston.

Streeter, G. L. 1942, 1945, 1948, 1949, 1951. Developmental horizons in human embryos. Contr. Embryol. Carnegie Inst. 30:211–245; 31:29–64; 32:133–203; 33:149–167; 34:165–196.

16

The Respiratory System

The tissues of the embryo, as well as those of the adult organism, require energy to carry out their various activities. The bulk of this energy is derived from a series of complex chemical reactions within the cell that involve the utilization of oxygen (*internal respiration*). An end product of pathways designed to capture this energy (in the form of ATP) is carbon dioxide, a gas that is either modified or eliminated directly from the internal environment of the organism.

For survival, both embryos and adult organisms have developed specialized systems for the supply of oxygen to and the elimination of carbon dioxide from their cells and tissues. The organs exchanging gases with the external environment (*external respiration*) in adult vertebrates are chiefly *internal gills* (fishes) and *lungs* (tetrapods). Both gills and lungs represent specialized structural derivatives of the embryonic pharynx. Other sites where external respiration may occur include the integument (amphibians), oral cavity (amphibians), and cloaca (reptiles).

The supply of oxygen and the elimination of carbon dioxide in most young developing embryos takes place by simple diffusion and exchange with the external environment. However, the energy requirements in rapidly growing embryos are such that specialized organs must be developed to promote these vital functions. In the placental mammal, the fetal and maternal tissues of the placenta serve as the site where carbon dioxide produced by the embryo diffuses into the maternal blood, and oxygen carried by the maternal circulation diffuses into the embryonic circulation. In reptiles and birds, the allantois with its extensive system of blood vessels acts as a respiratory organ. The allantois continues to function in this capacity until the embryo hatches from the eggshell and begins to breathe the surrounding air. The frog tadpole utilizes the moist skin and a series of pharyngeal gills.

Both gills and lungs are laid down during embryogenesis. To anyone who has dissected and examined these organs of respiration, the morphology of gills and lungs appears to be complex and quite different. In several respects, however, the structural differences between gills and lungs are superficial and primarily relate to the "conducting portion" of the respiratory organ. The basic requirement of any respiratory organ is a surface area across which gaseous exchange between the blood vascular system and the oxygen-

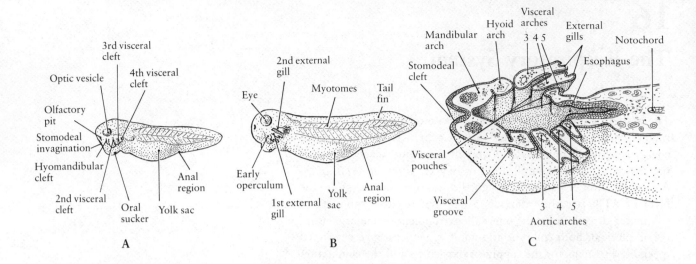

A

B

C

containing medium can take place. The efficiency of the exchange is enhanced if the surface area is large enough to permit sufficient flow and a diffusion distance short enough to allow rapid movement of molecules. Large surface areas are achieved by folding or branching of the respiratory surface. Short diffusion distances are created by making the cells of the blood-air (or blood-water) barrier thin. Whether the organ of respiration is a gill or a lung, therefore, the physical principles governing gaseous exchange dictate a common structural design at the site of external respiration.

16–1 Development of gills in the frog tadpole. A, the gill area in a 6 mm tadpole; B, external gills in a 9 mm tadpole; C, a reconstruction of a frog tadpole to show the topographical relationships between internal and external gills. (From R. Rugh, 1977. A Guide to Vertebrate Development. Burgess Publishing Company, Minneapolis.)

THE BRANCHIAL OR GILL RESPIRATORY ORGAN

Recall that the pharyngeal region of the embryonic foregut consists in all vertebrates of a series of laterally directed *pharyngeal* or *visceral pouches*. Ectodermal folds opposite to the visceral pouches push inward, thus producing a series of *visceral grooves* on the surface of the embryo. Temporarily, a *pharyngeal membrane* is formed by the lateral endodermal wall of the visceral pouch and the adjacent inner wall of the ectodermal groove. A *gill cleft* is formed when the pharyngeal membrane ruptures or becomes perforated, thus affording an open channel between the cavity of the pharynx and the external environment.

Most aquatic vertebrates use *gill lamellae* or *gill filaments* as sites of gaseous exchange (i.e., adult sharks and teleost fishes; larval frogs) (Fig. 16–1). These structures arise as the result of the covering epithelium of the visceral pouches being thrown into a complex labyrinth of primary and secondary foldings. Although the number of pouches participating in gill lamellae or filament formation varies among vertebrate species, the gills formed in this fashion are of the *internal type* since they are specializations of the inner or endodermal germ layer. Typically, gill lamellae are anchored onto the anterior and posterior surfaces of the *gill septum,* the latter being a flattened, lateral extension of the gill arch. The gills on each surface of the gill arch constitute a *demibranch,* while the two surfaces on either side of a gill arch form a complete gill or *holobranch.* Internal changes in the gill arches stimulate the vascularization of the lamellae or filaments. A large blood vessel beneath the pharynx (i.e., the ventral aorta) supplies a *branchial artery* to each gill arch. With the formation of the gill lamellae or filaments, each branchial artery eventually becomes divided into an *afferent branchial artery* and an *efferent branchial artery.* An extensive capillary network with a large surface area join together the afferent and efferent vessels. The afferent artery carries blood from the ventral aorta to the thin-walled capillaries; the efferent artery returns blood from the gills toward the dorsal aorta.

True *external gills* are primarily an embryonic or larval respiratory organ and occur in such forms as lungfishes, frogs, and salamanders. However, in some adult amphibians that continue a completely aquatic existence, such as the mudpuppy (*Necturus*), external gills are retained as the major organ of respiration. External gills are formed during the larval stage in all amphibians and, in the case of frogs, they are replaced by gills of the internal type. Gills of the external type originate as fleshy outgrowths from the dorsal ends of the visceral arches, particularly from the third, fourth, and fifth visceral arches. From these conicallike structures, finger-shaped projections or gill filaments extend outward. As in the case of internal gills, the vasculature of the external gill filaments is supplied by the branchial arteries of the visceral arches. External respiration is achieved by the movement of the external gill filaments in the surrounding medium.

THE LUNGS

Lungs or homologous structures are present in most major classes of vertebrates, from bony fishes, to amphibians, to mammals. Without exception, the lungs arise from a ventral pharyngeal diverticulum that appears relatively early in embryonic life. Both pharyngeal endoderm and pharyngeal mesoderm will participate in the construction of the postpharyngeal parts of the respiratory system, including the lungs proper.

Among vertebrates, the lungs show a range in the complexity of their structural organization. In the amphibians, particularly the salamanders, the lungs are a pair of simple, smooth-lined sacs that develop as expansions at the distal ends of an initially single respiratory primordium. By contrast, the lungs in mammals consist of many lobules composed in turn of a complicated system of branching tubes that terminate in thin-walled sacs or alveoli. The association of special air-storage compartments or *air sacs* with the air passageways distinguishes the lungs of birds from those of amphibians and mammals. Despite these dissimilarities, the lung in all vertebrate species basically develops in similar fashion, but to different stages of complexity. The degree of complexity can be directly correlated with the extent of internal subdivision and compartmentalization.

The Mammal—Human

The primordium of the postpharyngeal components of the respiratory system—the larynx, the trachea, the primary bronchi, and lungs—initially appears in the form of a midventral trough or furrow in the endoderm of the pharynx. Seen in the human embryo at approximately four weeks of development, this *laryngotracheal ridge* (or *tracheobronchiolar ridge*) is bluntly rounded and has an extensive communication with the ventrocaudal part of the pharynx (Fig. 16–2 A). Beginning posteriorly at the junction of the laryngotracheal ridge and the future esophagus, a pair of lateral grooves, one on either side, pinch inward and produce a pair of lateral folds (Fig. 16–2 B). The paired folds grow toward each other and fuse to form a temporary *tracheoesophageal septum*. As the lateral grooves deepen and gradually extend in the cranial direction, the septum is split, thereby separating a *laryngotracheal* (or *tracheobronchial*) *tube* from the rest of the gut tract except at the level of the future glottis or *laryngeal aditus* (approximately at the level of the fourth pair of visceral arches) (Fig. 16–2 C,D). The laryngotracheal tube elongates in the caudal direction, ventral to and approximately parallel to the esophagus. While this is occurring, the distal end of the tube enlarges and divides to form a pair of rounded swellings known as *lung buds*. These are probably better termed *primary bronchial buds* since each is a rudiment for the major branch to each future lung. By approximately the four-millimeter stage, the components of the future respiratory system are morphologically represented by the laryngeal region, the tubular trachea, and the paired primary bronchial buds (Fig. 16–2 D).

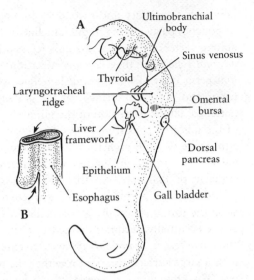

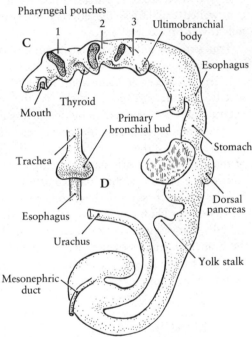

16–2   A, outline drawing of the gut endoderm to show the laryngotracheal primordium in a 3 mm human embryo; B, a lateral view of the laryngotracheal primordium at the same stage to show the lateral furrows as they pinch in between the future esophagus and trachea; C, outline drawing of the gut endoderm to show the respiratory primordium in a 4 mm embryo; D, ventral view of the respiratory primordium in a 4 mm embryo. (A, C, from G. Streeter, 1945. Carnegie Contributions to Embryology 31, 27.)

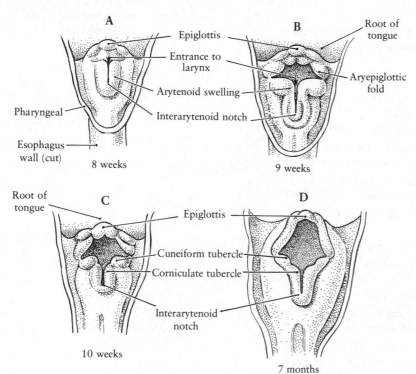

The Larynx

The larynx is a complicated organ of elastic and muscular tissues, supported by several cartilages, whose foundations are laid down very early in development (Fig. 16–3). It develops primarily around the site of the evagination of the primary respiratory primordium.

The slit that opens from the floor of the pharynx into the trachea is the laryngeal aditus or laryngeal orifice. Located between the bases of the third and fourth visceral arches, it is a narrow, longitudinal slit bounded cranially by a rounded pronounced thickening of the floor of the pharynx known as the *hypobranchial eminence.* The hypobranchial eminence will gradually become modified in shape, assume the form of a transverse flap, and give rise to the *epiglottis* (Fig. 16–3 A). The epiglottis will become muscular and act to protect against the entrance of foreign objects into the larynx and respiratory passageways during swallowing.

Concurrently, two additional thickenings, the *arytenoid swellings,* form on either side just caudal to the laryngeal aditus (Fig. 16–3 A). They arise as thickenings of mesodermal tissues originating from the fourth and fifth pairs of visceral arches. Each arytenoid swelling then thickens and lengthens toward the hypobranchial eminence. The two ridges of the tissue formed in this fashion, the *aryepiglottic folds,* convert the laryngeal aditus into a T-shaped orifice (Fig. 16–3 B).

For a short period of time (between 7 and 10 weeks of development), the entrance into the larynx ends blindly because the epithelial lining of the upper part of the larynx becomes fused together. The epithelial union then breaks down, and the lumen of this part of the respiratory system recanalizes, leaving an enlarged, oval laryngeal orifice and a pair of lateral recesses termed the *laryngeal ventricles.* Anteroposterior folds of the respiratory epithelium along the cranial and caudal walls of each laryngeal ventricle form the *vestibular folds* (false vocal cords) and the *vocal cords* (true vocal cords), respectively.

As with the rest of the postpharyngeal parts of the respiratory system, the inner or endodermal layer differentiates as the epithelial lining of the larynx. Dense mesenchyme from the fourth and fifth pairs of visceral arches supports the epithelium. The skeletal tissue of the larynx, chiefly in the form of several *laryngeal cartilages,* develops during the seventh week as the localized arytenoid swellings. Shortly thereafter, the primordia of the elastic cartilage plates, the *cuneiform* and *corniculate tubercles,* are clearly visible along the margins of the lumen of the larynx (Fig. 16–3 C,D). Later in fetal life the epiglottis becomes reinforced with a plate of cartilage. The *laryngeal muscles* originate from the same mesenchymal masses that form the laryngeal cartilages and hence are innervated by branches of the vagus nerve. The definitive topography of the larynx is assumed during the last third of gestation (Fig. 16–3 D).

The Trachea, Primary Bronchi, and Lungs

Following its separation from the foregut, the tracheal portion of the respiratory primordium grows rapidly and carries the primary bronchial buds caudally until they reach their definitive position in the thorax (Fig. 16–4). A cross section through the lung region at this time shows that each primary bronchial bud consists of an innermost epithelial layer surrounded by vascularized mesenchyme (Fig. 16–5). Initially, the primary bronchial buds tend to be symmetrically arranged (Fig. 16–6 A). Quickly, however, the lung buds become noticeably different in size and orientation. The right primary bronchial bud becomes larger in appearance and tends to be less sharply directed to the side (Fig. 16–6 B). This particular pattern of the primary bronchial tubes readily explains why foreign objects, postnatally, more frequently enter the right main bronchus than the left main bronchus. During the fifth week, each endodermal lung bud gives rise in *monopodial* fashion to a lateral diverticulum or bud; subsequently, the right lung bud gives origin on its craniodor-

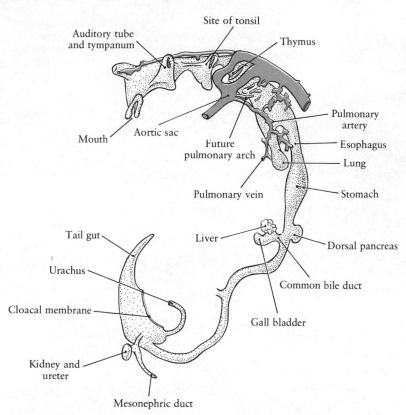

16–4 Outline drawing of the gut to show the caudal growth of the respiratory primordium in the 5.7 mm human embryo. (From G. Streeter, 1945. Carnegie Contributions to Embryology 31, 27.)

sal side to a second monopodial diverticulum (Fig. 16–6 C). By about the beginning of the second month, the right lung bud has differentiated into an undivided, proximal *right primary* or *main bronchus* and distally three *stem bronchi;* the left lung bud has differentiated into an undivided proximal *left primary* or *main bronchus* and distally two stem bronchi. Each stem bronchus is destined to branch and rebranch and, with the surrounding pulmonary mesenchyme, will give origin to the definitive *pulmonary lobes* that characterize adult lung organization. Hence, the right lung typically has three lobes (upper, middle, and lower) and the left lung two lobes (upper and lower).

The early branching of the primary bronchial buds tends to be monopodial. That is, a branch or diverticulum is formed on one side while the main branch continues to grow beyond the point of branching without any significant change in direction. The subsequent branching pattern of the stem bronchi tends to be *dichotomous* with a given branch being bifurcated into two symmetrically placed branches (Fig. 16–6 E). By these processes a large and arboreous system of tubes forms, which is termed the early bronchial or *respiratory tree.* With enlargement of the bronchial tree, the *pulmonary mesenchyme* surrounding the stem bronchi and their de-

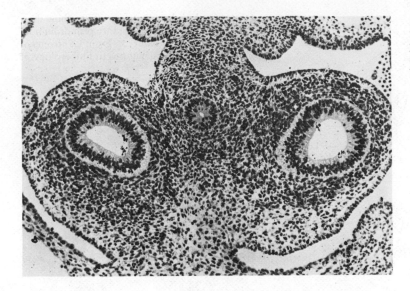

16–5 A photomicrograph of a cross section through the 6.7 mm human embryo showing the paired primary bronchi and the esophagus. (From G. Streeter, 1945. Carnegie Contributions to Embryology 31, 27.)

scendant tubes becomes furrowed, thereby yielding the principal lobes of the lung (Fig. 16–6 F). By the seventh week, ten bronchi of the third order of branching have appeared in the right lung and eight for the left lung. Each of these bronchial tubes supplies the remaining branches for the clinically important *bronchopulmonary segments* or lobules. These lobules are separated from each other by connective tissue partitions derived from mesenchyme.

It is now generally recognized that human lung development can be subdivided into four periods. Up until approximately 16 weeks (*pseudoglandular period*), the lung resembles an exocrine gland and consists of a complex of branching bronchial tubes that will constitute the air-conducting portion of the organ. The passageways formed include the *primary bronchi, secondary bronchi, segmental bronchi, terminal bronchi, bronchioles,* and *terminal bronchioles.* The epithelial lining of these tubes is cuboidal.

Between 16 and 24 weeks (*canalicular period*), the functionally important respiratory portion of the lung becomes delineated with the appearance of new, tubular branches, the *respiratory bronchioles.* Each respiratory bronchiole terminates in two or three thin-walled dilations termed *terminal sacs* or *primitive alveoli.* Also, there is observed an increase in the size of the lumens of the bronchi and bronchioles.

From six months until birth, the terminal ends of the respiratory bronchioles rapidly subdivide into an array of thin-walled, primitive alveolar ducts and primitive alveoli (*terminal sac period*). The immature alveoli are lined by a continuous vascularized epithelium that becomes progressively attentuated during this time. There is

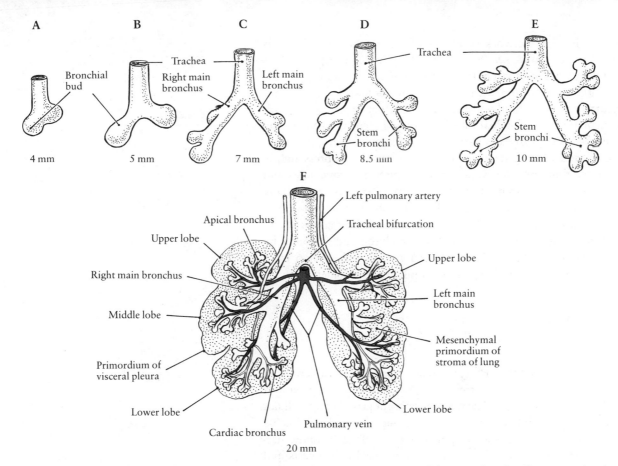

A Bronchial bud 4 mm

B Trachea Right main bronchus 5 mm

C Trachea Left main bronchus 7 mm

D Trachea Stem bronchi 8.5 mm

E Trachea Stem bronchi 10 mm

F

Left pulmonary artery

Apical bronchus

Tracheal bifurcation

Upper lobe

Upper lobe

Right main bronchus

Left main bronchus

Middle lobe

Mesenchymal primordium of stroma of lung

Primordium of visceral pleura

Lower lobe

Lower lobe

Cardiac bronchus

Pulmonary vein

20 mm

16–6 Diagrams showing the progressive development of the major bronchi of human lungs (ventral views). (After L. Arey, 1965. Developmental Anatomy. W. B. Saunders Company, Philadelphia.)

sufficient respiratory surface in the fetus at this time for gaseous exchange, represented by the terminal sac epithelium, to permit survival in case of premature birth.

Current information tends to indicate that definitive alveolar ducts and mature alveoli probably do not form until very late in fetal life and after birth (*alveolar period*). Alveolar ducts and alveoli arise as the result of the extreme attentuation of prenatal terminal sacs into narrow ducts and sacs lined by a simple squamous epithelium.

Increase in the size of the lung after birth is largely attributable to additional branching of the fetal respiratory tree. New respiratory bronchioles and alveoli are produced postnatally for six or seven generations of branchings. Also, postnatal enlargement of the lung results from an increase in the length and diameter of all respiratory bronchioles and their associated passageways.

Development of an adequate pulmonary vasculature is critical to the proper functioning of the lung at birth. Vascularization of the embryonic lung is initially evident at the time of primary bronchial bud formation (Figs. 16–4; 16–5). Each bronchial bud becomes invested with a fine network or plexus of capillarylike blood vessels arising from the *aortic sac* (See Chapter 18). Subsequently, branches descending from the sixth pair of aortic arches, the rudiments of the *pulmonary arteries,* join with the lung bud capillaries. The pulmonary artery to each lung will branch and rebranch, tending to follow the pattern of bronchial tube branching. Extensive proliferation of pulmonary capillaries is particularly noticeable during the canalicular period of lung development. These capillaries press tightly against the thin epithelial walls of the respiratory bronchioles and terminal sacs. With attentuation of the terminal sacs, the underlying capillaries bulge into the lumens of the alveoli. The air-blood barrier, therefore, is formed by two adjacent and tightly apposed epithelial membranes, one contributed by the alveoli and the other by the pulmonary capillaries. The pulmonary veins will develop from pulmonary mesenchyme lying between pulmonary lobules.

GENERAL MECHANISMS OF LUNG DEVELOPMENT

The dual origin of the lung—pulmonary epithelial endoderm and pulmonary mesenchyme—permits an analysis of the contributions made by each embryonic layer to the morphogenesis and cellular structure of the adult organ. As pointed out above, the epithelial component of the mammalian lung branches into a complex network of bronchial tubes. The pulmonary mesenchyme invests and condenses around the bronchial tubules as the respiratory tree takes form and shape.

Since early studies by Rudnick (1933), the fetal lung has always been considered to be capable of self-development or self-differentiation. That is, the primordium of the lung when removed and cultured under proper experimental conditions will develop to form an organ with a remarkable likeness to the lung in vivo. The lung explant can differentiate most of the cellular elements found in the adult lung. Also, many of the patterns of chemical change within differentiating cells are faithfully repeated in the lung explant. Since the lung is a self-developing entity, its epithelial and mesenchymal components can be manipulated in culture to determine their role in lung morphogenesis and the relationship between morphogenesis and the differentiation of various cell types.

Presumably, the laryngotracheal ridge appears during embryogenesis in response to some initiating induction in the foregut. However, the nature and the source of the inducing stimulus remain unknown. In the laryngotracheal area there are several chemical changes (such as increases in glycogen, alkaline phosphatase, and

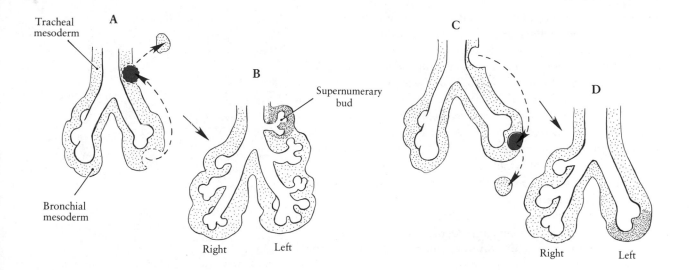

Tracheal
mesoderm

A

B

Supernumerary
bud

C

D

Bronchial
mesoderm

Right   Left

Right   Left

ribonucleoprotein) that accompany the formation of the early lung primordium, but their significance, if any, to the induction process has not been elucidated.

Concrete evidence that the epithelial and mesenchymal layers of the pulmonary primordium interact in an inductive relationship and that they are indispensable for lung morphogenesis and cytodifferentiation come from organ culture studies utilizing the more advanced fetal lung. Much attention has been given to the dependence of pulmonary epithelial branching upon the presence of the surrounding mesenchyme. Rudnick first demonstrated that branching of the bronchial tree fails to occur if the pulmonary epithelium is deprived of its investing mesenchyme. Also removal of the mesenchyme during the epithelial branching will immediately interrupt the latter process. Other investigators have also shown that epithelial morphogenesis is dependent upon underlying mesenchyme by grafting a piece of *bronchial mesoderm* next to the tracheal endoderm (Fig. 16–7 A). After approximately six hours in culture, a supernumerary bud appears in the explant at the original grafting site (Fig. 16–7 B). The extra bronchial bud is then observed to grow and branch profusely in a pattern reminiscent to that seen in vivo. Note that the left primary lung bud in the absence of investing pulmonary mesenchyme fails to subdivide. If *tracheal mesoderm* is excised and grafted to the base of one of the primary lung buds (Fig. 16–7 C), the lung bud with the investment of tracheal mesoderm fails to branch (Fig. 16–7 D). Hence, the pulmonary mesenchyme appears to exhibit very different capacities to stimulate epithelial budding in the developing lung. The proximal, older, or more mature tracheal mesoderm prevents or inhibits epithelial budding and

16–7   Grafting a piece of bronchial mesoderm next to the tracheal endoderm (A) will induce a supernumerary lung bud (B). A lung bud with an adjacent graft of tracheal mesoderm (C) fails to subdivide (D).

thus accounts for the undivided nature of the structural trachea. The distal, younger mesenchyme stimulates the epithelial budding to form the respiratory tree. Electron microscopic studies by Wessells (1970) have shown that the tracheal mesoderm is structurally different from the bronchial mesoderm. Cells of the former are highly ordered and form a tight investment around the tracheal endoderm. A layer of highly oriented collagen fibers is situated along the tracheal endoderm. At the tip of active bronchial buds, these same collagen fibers are randomly oriented (Fig. 16–8). Such an arrangement of fibers along the trachea could conceivably effect an inhibiting action by preventing the passage of an inducing stimulus from the pulmonary mesenchyme.

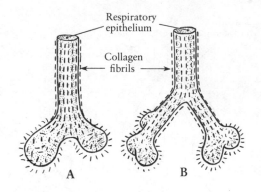

16–8   A diagram after studies by Wessells and others showing the distribution of collagen along the tracheobronchial epithelium of a mammalian embryo at two successive steps in lung morphogenesis. Note that branching occurs where there is a random arrangement of collagen fibrils.

How specific is the pulmonary mesenchyme in inducing epithelial budding? A variety of foreign mesoderms, such as those excised from gut or salivary gland, will elicit formation of the laryngotracheal or primary lung bud primordium. However, the branching of the primary lung buds is always dependent upon an appropriate interaction with bronchial mesoderm. Although the first step in lung formation occurs in the presence of what we might term *nonspecific mesoderm,* the shape and form of the respiratory tree require a very specific or *homologous mesoderm.*

Whether the morphogenetic factors controlling the species-specific pattern of branching are initially resident in the bronchial mesenchyme or bronchial epithelium is still a major unresolved question. For example, during normal chick lung morphogenesis, monopodial branching leads to a system of tubes and expanded air sacs. By contrast, mouse lung epithelium is more active and exhibits both dichotomous and monopodial branching in constructing a complex system of bronchial tubes. Taderera (1967) has observed that the in vitro combination of mouse lung epithelium and chick lung mesenchyme (a *chimeric explant*) initially exhibits a bronchial branching pattern characteristic of intact mouse lung explants. However, after some time, a few of the terminal branches appeared distinctively chicklike. This suggests that the mesoderm may play an important role in determining branching pattern. Unfortunately, the reciprocal chimeric explant (chick lung epithelium and mouse lung mesenchyme) failed to exhibit any branching.

The placement of a Millipore filter (25 μ thick; 0.45 μ pore size) between pulmonary epithelium and pulmonary mesenchyme does not disturb lung induction as measured by epithelial branching. This indicates that direct cell contact is not required between the interacting tissues in order for induction to occur. In this respect, the lung induction system is very similar to a number of other inductive systems studied, such as salivary gland, kidney, and skin (see Chapter 23). The mesenchyme, however, remains simple in organization and shows only a few histologic cell types with the transfilter technique. Normally, in the complete absence of pulmonary epithelium, the pulmonary mesenchyme fails to differentiate any of the characteristic connective tissue and smooth muscle cell types, thus showing that the mesenchyme and epithelium are reciprocally dependent upon each other for their differentiation. The failure of the pulmonary mesenchyme to differentiate smooth muscle, for example, across the filter may mean that either contact between the interacting tissues is necessary or that inductively active materials are impeded by the filter due to molecular size or lowered mobility.

The key to understanding the lung epithelial-mesenchymal interaction undoubtedly lies in analysis of the activities at the interface between the two tissues. Studies using electron microscopy, histochemistry, and biochemistry have revealed that collagen and glycosaminoglycans are major constituents of substances at the junction between the epithelium and the mesenchyme (Chapter 13). The source of these materials and their role(s) in induction and morphogenesis of lungs are areas of current investigation. It is known that the normal branched epithelial morphology is lost following treatment with collagenase. This clearly suggests that materials of the extracellular matrix are essential for stabilization of epithelial morphology. The division of an epithelial bud into two branches is probably dependent upon a sequence of events. An actively dividing bud shows a high rate of mitosis at its tip. Additionally, its epithelial cells are observed to synthesize and secrete glycosaminoglycans into the extracellular space. In contrast to nondividing portions of the respiratory epithelium, there is a rapid turnover of the newly synthesized glycosaminoglycans at the tip of a dividing epithelial bud. It has been proposed that the glycosaminoglycan turnover is induced by hydrolytic enzymes released from the pulmonary mesenchyme. The tip region is thus maintained in an unstable state. Stabilization of the branching of the pulmonary epithelium is probably accompanied by reduced turnover in extracellular glycosaminoglycans and by modification of the nature of the extracellular substances.

Finally, all current evidence tends to indicate that the differentiation of the cell types of the lung and the expression of shape and form of the lung are coupled events in the development of this organ. Permanent structural and chemical changes in both epithelial and mesenchymal layers occur in wavelike fashion from proximal to distal (i.e., from trachea to alveoli). The mesenchyme differentiates into cartilage, connective tissue (particularly elastic tissue), and smooth muscle. The differentiation of these various cell types tend to lag slightly behind the differentiation of the epithelium.

RESPIRATORY MOVEMENTS

As long as the fetus remains in the aquatic uterine environment, respiratory exchange occurs in the placenta and the lung does not perform any respiratory function. Nevertheless, it has been known for many years that the fetus may show contractions of the thoracic musculature and diaphragm which resemble normal respiratory movements. The majority of investigators report that the respiratory movements of the fetus are irregular and not constant, thus casting serious doubt on the view that respiratory movements in the newborn are merely a resumption of the normal physiological, intrauterine movements that had been interrupted by the birth process.

Fetal respiratory movements can be elicited in human embryos from the third month onward. Although opinions are divided, a generally accepted view is that respiratory movements occur only when the fetus fails to receive an adequate supply of oxygen by way of the placental circulation. It is known, for example, that in experimental animals artificially induced *anoxia* of the fetus stimulates vigorous respiratory movements. The amount of amniotic fluid that finds its way into the lungs is normally not of any consequence. Experimentally, the presence of amniotic fluid in the lungs has been demonstrated by the detection of labeled amniotic fluid (produced by injecting ink or thorotrast, a radio-opaque substance, into the amniotic cavity) in the trachea and bronchi. During late fetal life, there appears to be a state of respiratory movement inhibition. Near birth when the placenta becomes increasingly less efficient as a center of respiratory exchange and when some anoxia probably exists, there are surprisingly few respiratory movements. The neuromusculature architecture for initiating and controlling these movements is fully functional at this time.

Most of the spaces within the fetal lung are filled with fluid derived from the lung itself, the glands of the trachea, and the amniotic cavity. Aeration of the lungs, therefore, is due to the rapid replacement of fluid by air and not due to the simple inflation of a collapsed, empty lung. The fluid from the lungs is eliminated by several routes. Most of it enters the networks of pulmonary capillaries and lymphatic vessels which surround the pulmonary alveoli. Some fluid is also probably cleared from the lungs through the mouth and nose as the result of pressure exerted on the pleural cavities during the birth process.

The newborn animal apparently expands the soggy lungs by increasing the size of the pleural cavities. The original expansion must overcome the cohesion of the wet adhesive walls of the air passageways as well as the pressure exerted by the fluid of the pleural cavities. This is a remarkable feat when one considers that the muscular system at birth is weak and incompletely developed. It is not surprising that for as long as 10 days after birth portions of the lungs are likely to remain uninflated (*atelectasis*).

ABNORMALITIES OF THE RESPIRATORY SYSTEM

As one might expect, there are departures from the normal pattern of size and shape of various parts of the respiratory system (i.e., larynx, bronchial tubes), but these generally have little serious effect upon the individual. Occasionally, an entire lung or lung lobe may be absent (*agenesis*).

A serious congenital anomaly that is detected in approximately 1:3000 to 1:4000 births is *tracheoesophageal fistula*. The fistula is commonly visible at the level of the seventh cervical or first thoracic vertebra and appears as an opening between the trachea and esophagus below the level of the larynx (Fig. 16–9 A). Typically, the opening between the trachea and esophagus is large with the upper part of the esophagus terminating as a blind tube (*esophageal atresia*; Fig. 16–9 B). The difficulties for the nursing infant are self-evident. Milk is regurgitated from the atretic esophagus and, if passed into the lungs, may result in pneumonia. The fistula arises during the fourth week when the laryngotracheal primordium is separating from the esophagus. Presumably, the laryngotracheal primordium grows caudally more rapidly than the digestive tube, a process that disturbs the normal activity of the paired lateral grooves. The result is a posterior connection between esophagus and trachea, typically in the vicinity of the paired primary bronchi (Fig. 16–9 C). If the rate of tracheal elongation is excessive, the lower portion of the esophagus is drawn out into a narrow muscular ridge and the upper portion of the esophagus into a distended blind sac (Fig. 16–9 D). For many infants, the fistula can be surgically ligated and an anastomosis effected between the upper and lower esophageal components.

Bronchiestasis is a congenital anomaly of the bronchial tubes, particularly the terminal bronchi. It is manifest in irregular saccular enlargements or evaginations from the bronchi. Postnatally, they are subject to chronic infection because they fail to drain properly. Prenatally, some of these sacs may become completely blocked to form fluid-filled *bronchial cysts*.

Hyaline membrane disease is a serious affliction of the respiratory system that is caused by a lack of *surfactant*, a detergentlike substance that is normally produced by alveolar cells and acts to reduce

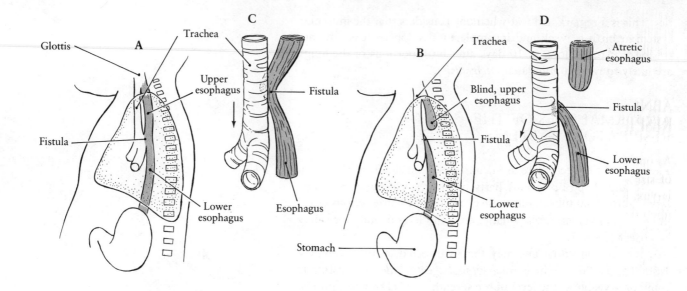

surface tension forces within the alveoli. Alveoli tend to collapse without surfactant. Some investigators support the hypothesis that disturbances in the development of the pulmonary vasculature, resulting in anoxia, affect the capacity of alveolar cells to produce surfactant. Obstetric techniques (*amniocentesis*) now make it possible to measure the levels of fetal surfactant.

16–9   A and B are sketches illustrating conditions encountered in two cases of tracheoesophageal fistula (After C. Haight, 1944. Ann. Surg. 120, 623); C and D illustrate the suggested mechanical basis for the origin of the fistula in A and B, respectively. The rate of tracheal elongation is excessive (arrows) and determines the severity of the fistula syndrome (After P. Gruenwald, 1940. Anat. Rec. 78, 293.)

REFERENCES

Corliss, C. E. 1976. Patten's Human Embryology, pp. 296–306. New York: McGraw-Hill.

Hamilton, W. J. and H. W. Mossman. 1972. Human Embryology, 4th ed., pp. 291–376. Baltimore: Williams and Wilkins.

Rudnick, D. 1933. Development capacities of the chick lung in chorioallantoic grafts. J. Exp. Zool. 66:125–154.

Sorokin, S. 1965. Recent work on developing lungs. In: Organogenesis, pp. 467–491. Eds., R. L. DeHaan and H. Ursprung. New York: Holt, Rinehart and Winston.

Spooner, B. and N. Wessells. 1970. Mammalian lung development: Interactions in primordium formation and bronchial morphogenesis. J. Exp. Zool. 175:445–454.

Streeter, G. L. 1945. Developmental horizons in human embryos. Description of age group XIII, embryos about 4 or 5 millimeters long, and age group XIV, period of indentation of the lens vesicle. Carnegie Contrib. Embryol. 31:27–63.

Streeter, G. L. 1948. Developmental horizons in human embryos. Description of age groups XV, XVI, XVII and XVIII, being the third issue of a survey of the Carnegie Collection. Carnegie Contrib. Embryol. 32:133–203.

Taderera, J. V. 1967. Control of lung differentiation *in vitro*. Dev. Biol. 16:489–512.

Wessells, N. 1970. Mammalian lung development: Interactions in formation and morphogenesis of tracheal buds. J. Exp. Zool. 175:455–466.

Wessells, N. and J. Cohen. 1968. Effects of collagenase on developing epithelial *in vitro:* Lung, ureteric bud, and pancreas. Dev. Biol. 18:294–309.

17

The Coelom and Mesenteries

Coelomic cavities are fluid-filled spaces that come to surround the various viscera of the vertebrate body during the course of development. These include the *pericardial cavity* around the heart, the *pleural cavities* surrounding the lungs, and the *peritoneal cavity* in which lie the stomach, intestines, pancreas, and other organs. Only the pericardial cavity and the peritoneal cavity are common to all vertebrates. Lungs present in such forms as amphibians, reptiles, and birds are located in the peritoneal cavity, which is more appropriately termed the *pleuroperitoneal cavity.*

The coelomic cavities of the mammal (pericardial, paired pleural, peritoneal) arise through the subdivision of the early *intraembryonic coelom* by the following partitions or membranes: the unpaired *transverse septum,* which effects an initial separation between pericardial and peritoneal cavities; the paired *pleuropericardial folds,* which fuse with the transverse septum and separate pericardial from pleural cavities, and the paired *pleuroperitoneal* folds, which also join with the transverse septum and complete the separation of each pleural cavity from the peritoneal cavity. These various membranes unite to contribute to the formation of the *diaphragm,* a muscular partition between pleural and abdominal cavities found only in mammals.

THE INTRAEMBRYONIC COELOM

The early intraembryonic coelom in all vertebrates originates on either side of the body as the result of the confluence of small isolated spaces that appear in the lateral plate mesoderm (Fig. 17–1). At the embryonic disc stage in the mammal, these cavities extend forward on either side to fuse anteriorly in the region of the future heart mesoderm (*cardiogenic mesoderm*) (Fig. 17–2). The cranial portion of the horseshoe-shaped intraembryonic coelom represents the primordium of the pericardial cavity. The right and left limbs represent the presumptive pleural cavities, as each will subsequently receive a developing lung bud, and the presumptive peritoneal cavity. Note that at approximately the level of the first pair of somites the intraembryonic coelom is continuous on either side with the *extraembryonic coelom.* As the body of the embryo is progressively

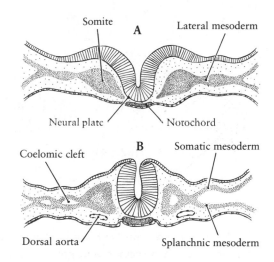

17–1   Origin of the vertebrate coelom by confluence of spaces in the lateral plate mesoderm. A, human embryo, two-somite stage; B, human embryo, seven-somite stage.

17–2   A diagrammatic reconstruction of a young human embryo (2.5 mm stage) to show the relationships between the intraembryonic coelom, the extraembryonic coelom, and the mesoderm. The arrow indicates the site of union between intraembryonic and extraembryonic coeloms. (From W. Hamilton and H. Mossman, 1972. Human Embryology. Macmillan Press, London.)

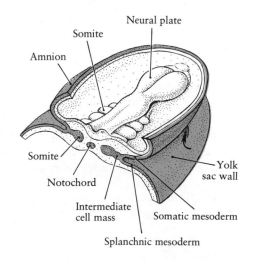

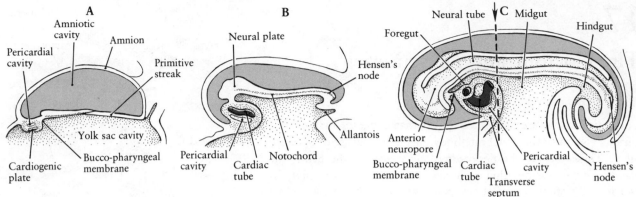

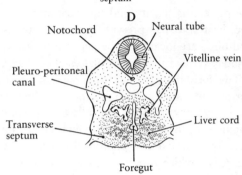

17–3 A series of schematic drawings in sagittal view (A–C) to show the formation of the pericardial cavity and the transverse septum in the human embryo. A, presomite embryo illustrating the anterior position of the pericardial cavity; B, formation of the head fold and the beginning of the rotation of the heart and pericardial cavity in a 7-somite human embryo; C, formation of the transverse septum in a 14-somite stage embryo; D, a cross section in the plane indicated in C (arrow) to show position and relationships of the transverse septum.

folded off from the extraembryonic membranes, the extraembryonic and intraembryonic portions of the coelom are thereby separated from each other. It is only the intraembryonic coelom that is partitioned to accommodate the embryonic viscera.

The intraembryonic coelom divides the lateral plate mesoderm into a *somatic (parietal) layer,* continuous with the extraembryonic mesoderm of the amnion, and a *visceral (splanchnic) layer* continuous with the extraembryonic mesoderm of the yolk sac (Figs. 17–1; 17–2). The somatic mesoderm and the embryonic ectoderm form the body wall or *somatopleure* and the visceral mesoderm and the endoderm form the gut wall or *splanchnopleure.*

THE PERICARDIAL CAVITY

The presumptive pericardial cavity is initially located anterior to the level of the neural plate (Fig. 17–3). With the formation of the head fold, the heart primordium, in the form of a pair of developing *endothelial tubes,* and the coelomic space in which it resides are bent ventrally and caudally beneath the foregut (Fig. 17–3 A,B). As a consequence of this reversal of position of the presumptive pericardial cavity, the original cranial wall of this chamber now becomes its definitive caudal wall. The mass of mesoderm, representing fused somatic and splanchnic layers of mesoderm, which occupies the space between the gut, yolk stalk and ventral body wall constitutes the *transverse septum* (Fig. 17–3 C,D). However, caudally, the dorsolateral corners of the pericardial cavity are still connected to the remaining portion of the intraembryonic coelom by somewhat restricted passageways now termed the *pericardioperitoneal canals* (Figs. 17–3; 17–4; 17–5). Hence, the transverse septum never extends all the way to the dorsal body wall.

The transverse septum represents the initial step in diaphragm formation and clearly foreshadows the division of the intraembryonic coelom into thoracic and abdominal regions. Only the cranial portion of the original transverse septum will continue in its role as a partition. The rapidly growing liver primordium penetrates the more caudal part of the septum and, as the liver increases in size and withdraws, this portion of the partition is drawn out as part of the ventral mesentery. Since both heart and liver abut against the transverse septum, the stems of all major embryonic and extraembryonic veins pass through the transverse septum.

THE PLEURAL CAVITIES

Dorsal to the transverse septum, the region of the pericardial cavity is continuous with the pericardioperitoneal canals (Fig. 17–4). Beginning at about four weeks of human development, each endodermal lung bud with its surrounding mass of pulmonary mesenchyme pushes into the pericardioperitoneal canal. The splanchnic mesoderm forms a covering for the lung primordium. At this time, the pericardioperitoneal canals are better termed the pleural cavities. The communication between the pericardial cavity and the pleural cavity on either side is the *pericardiopleural opening;* each pleural cavity communicates with the peritoneal cavity by the *pleuroperitoneal opening* (Figs. 17–4; 17–5 A). The pleural cavities are initially very narrow and slitlike, but they soon become greatly enlarged to accommodate the expanding respiratory tree.

The separation of the pericardial cavity from each pleural cavity is effected by the closure of the pericardiopleural opening through the development of the *pleuropericardial membrane.* The steps in this closure process can be traced in Figure 17–5 A–D. In the dorsal margin of the transverse septum, the *common cardinal vein* or *duct of Cuvier* passes transversely and medially to enter the sinus venosus (Fig. 17–5 B). Laterally, each vein tends to course in a crescentic-shaped ridge of somatic mesoderm termed the *pulmonary ridge* as it passes from the lateral body wall to the transverse septum. As the heart descends caudally, the common cardinal vein is forced to pass obliquely and ventromedially to enter the sinus venosus. This shift in the course of the common cardinal vein causes the pulmonary ridge to be drawn out into a curtainlike partition, the *pleuropericardial membrane* (Figs. 17–5 C–D; 17–6 A,B). By about the sixth week of development, the free edge of the pleuropericardial membrane fuses with the median mass of esophageal mesen-

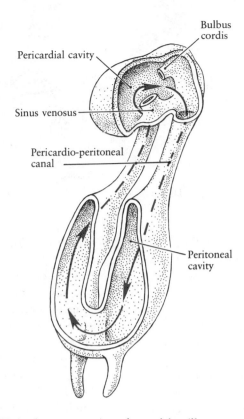

17–4 A reconstruction of a model to illustrate the continuity (arrows) between pericardial cavity, pericardioperitoneal canals, and the peritoneal cavity in a late somite human embryo. (From W. Hamilton and H. Mossman, 1972. Human Embryology. Macmillan Press, London.)

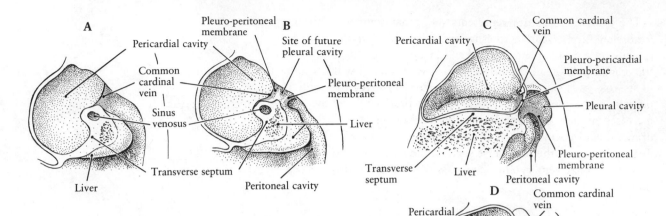

chyme (the *primitive mediastinum*) to close off the pleuropericardial opening (Fig. 17–6 C).

Closure of the pleuroperitoneal openings to separate the pleural cavities from the peritoneal cavity occurs during the seventh week of development when the lungs show extensive growth and lateral expansion. On either side, a pleuroperitoneal membrane arises in the dorsolateral aspect of the caudalmost part of the pleuroperitoneal canal as a crescentic-shaped fold of mesoderm extending between the cephalic portion of the kidney (*mesonephros*) and the transverse septum (Figs. 17–5 B; 17–6 A). The membranes extend medially and somewhat caudally, leaving a rapidly diminishing angle between the dorsal body wall and the esophageal mesentery (Figs. 17–5 C; 17–6 B). Fusion of their free edges with the esophageal mesentery and the transverse septum closes the communication between the pleural and peritoneal cavities (Figs. 17–5 D; 17–6 C).

Increasing size of the lung is accompanied by extension and enlargement of the pleural cavity, an event that takes place at the expense of the loose mesenchymal tissue of the lateral body wall (Fig. 17–6 C,D). Mesenchyme is added to the pleuropericardial and the pleuroperitoneal membranes as the lungs expand, particularly in the lateral and ventral directions, and separates the body wall tissue. Gradually, the lungs and the pleuropericardial membranes come to lie on either side of the heart in their typical adult relationships (Fig. 17–6 D). The original cardiac surface of each pleuropericardial membrane now constitutes the lateral wall of the pericardial cavity. The partition separating heart from lung represents the original pleuropericardial membrane plus mesenchymal additions captured from the body wall. The fibrous partition formed in this fashion encloses the heart like a sac and is termed the *pericardium* (Fig. 17–6 D).

17–5 Drawings showing partitioning of the human intraembryonic coelom. A, various regions of the coelom (right-side view) before partitioning; B, a 5 mm embryo, cut longitudinally near the midline, showing origin of the pleuropericardial and pleuroperitoneal membranes; C, complete separation of the pericardial cavity from the right pleural cavity by the right pleuropericardial membrane in a 13 mm embryo; D, complete separation of the peritoneal cavity from the right pleural cavity by the right pleuroperitoneal membrane in a 15 mm embryo.

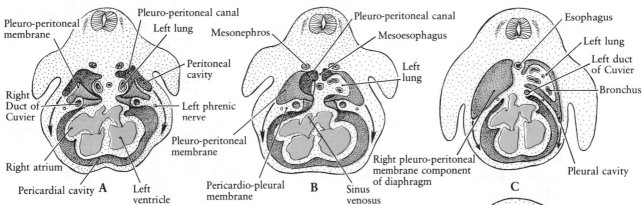

Pleuro-peritoneal membrane · Pleuro-peritoneal canal · Left lung · Right Duct of Cuvier · Left phrenic nerve · Right atrium · Pleuro-peritoneal membrane · Pericardial cavity **A** · Left ventricle · Peritoneal cavity

Mesonephros · Pleuro-peritoneal canal · Mesoesophagus · Left lung · Pericardio-pleural membrane **B** · Sinus venosus · Pleuro-peritoneal membrane

Esophagus · Left lung · Left duct of Cuvier · Bronchus · Right pleuro-peritoneal membrane component of diaphragm · Pleural cavity **C**

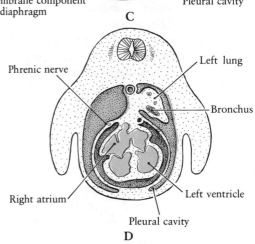

Phrenic nerve · Left lung · Bronchus · Right atrium · Left ventricle · Pleural cavity **D**

17–6 A series of schematic cross sections through human embryos to show the roles of the pleuropericardial and pleuroperitoneal membranes in the partitioning of the intraembryonic coelom. The lung has been removed from the right side. The arrows indicate extension of the pleural cavities in the body wall. A, 5 mm stage; B, 9 mm stage; C, 22 mm stage; D, approximately 25 mm. (A–C, from W. Hamilton and H. Mossman, 1972. Human Embryology. Macmillan Press, London.)

THE DIAPHRAGM

The complete separation of the pleural cavities from the peritoneal cavity is effected by a composite partition known as the diaphragm. Its origin is complex, but its chief components have been referred to above and include the following: (1) an anterior, central portion that represents the greater part of the cranial aspect of the transverse septum; this becomes the *central tendon* of the diaphragm; (2) dorsal, paired pleuroperitoneal membranes whose anterior margins become continuous with the posterodorsal edges of the central tendon; (3) a dorsal, unpaired portion from the dorsal esophageal mesentery which constitutes the medial part of the diaphragm; (4) circumferential portions derived from the lateral body wall which are added to the periphery of the pleuroperitoneal membranes as the lungs expand.

The muscular portion of the diaphragm is largely derived from the early migration (shortly after the early limb bud stage) of *myoblasts* or primitive muscle cells into the transverse septum and the pleuroperitoneal membranes. Presumably, the muscle cells originate from the hypaxial portions of the third, fourth, and fifth cervical myotomes since the motor and in part the sensory (*phrenic nerve*) innervations of the diaphragm are from the third, fourth, and fifth cervical nerves. There is also evidence that some muscle fibers may originate from mesenchyme cells in the transverse septum itself.

During the descent of the heart into the thoracic region and with the rapid enlargement of the lungs, the diaphragm undergoes an extensive movement in the caudal direction. This is clearly indicated by positional changes in the cervical nerves that pass to the muscular tissue of this partition. For example, the diaphragm lies opposite the third, fourth, and fifth cervical myotomes at approximately three weeks of development. By eight weeks, the dorsal parts of the diaphragm have moved far caudally, giving this partition a strong dome-shaped contour. The diaphragm eventually lies at the level of the lower thoracic or upper lumbar segments of the body.

THE PERITONEAL CAVITY

The peritoneal cavity is formed from that part of the intraembryonic coelom lying caudal to the transverse septum. Initially, the gut tube with its suspending mesentery separates the intraembryonic coelom into right and left halves (Fig. 17–7). With rupture of the ventral part of the mesentery, there results a large embryonic peritoneal cavity that extends from the thoracic to the pelvic region of the embryo.

THE MESENTERIES

During the transverse folding process that separates the embryo from the extraembryonic membranes (Fig. 17–7 A), the sheet of embryonic endoderm becomes rolled and fashioned into the gut tube (Fig. 17–7 B). Concurrently the splanchnic mesoderm from either side swings toward the midline and wraps around the endodermal tube to give rise to a double-layered partition known as the *primitive mesentery* (Fig. 17–7 C). Extending from the roof of the intraembryonic coelom to the midventral body wall, the primitive mesentery is interrupted by the early, straight gut tube to form upper (*dorsal mesentery*) and lower (*ventral mesentery*) components (Fig. 17–7 C). The dorsal mesentery tends to persist, but the ventral mesentery, as mentioned above, is quite temporary, and its degeneration leads to the confluence of the right and left coelomic cavities below the gut.

The double-layered dorsal mesentery will differentiate into a variety of structures. It will form connective tissue and a covering epithelium (*mesothelium*) that lines the peritoneal cavity. Where the mesentery continues around the endodermal tube of the gut, it will differentiate as the *serosa*. It will also contribute to the connective tissue, vascular tissue and smooth muscle tissue of the gut wall.

Derivatives of the Dorsal Mesentery

The gut tube is initially suspended throughout most of its length by a definitive dorsal mesentery. The mesentery extends in the mid-

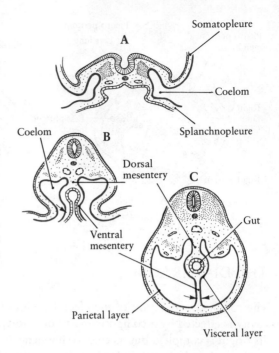

17–7 Schematic drawings to illustrate successive stages in the formation of the primitive mesentery in human embryos. The arrows indicate sites at which somatic and visceral layers of mesoderm join together. A, 2 mm; B, 4 mm; C, 8 mm.

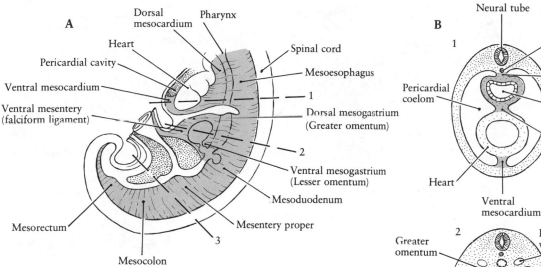

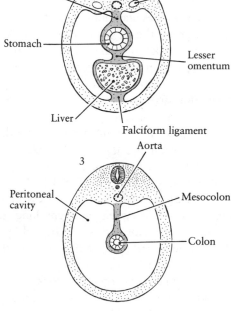

plane from the roof of the peritoneal cavity to the gastrointestinal tract and serves as a supporting vehicle for blood vessels and nerves passing to and from the gut. Commonly, distinctive names are given to the dorsal mesentery that support the different regions of the gut. Thus, there is the *dorsal mesogastrium* or *greater omentum* of the stomach, the *mesoduodenum* of the duodenum, the *dorsal mesentery proper* of jejunum and ileum, the *mesocolon,* and the *mesorectum.* The early relationships of some of these mesenteries are shown at several levels of the human embryo in Figure 17–8 A,B.

The pharynx and the upper portion of the esophagus lack a dorsal mesentery since the intraembryonic coelom does not normally extend this far cranially. The remainder of most of the esophagus, however, is supported by a thick, dorsal mesentery known as the *mesoesophagus* (Figs. 16–7; 17–6 B; 17–8 A). It will contribute to a thick, specialized medial septum in the adult termed the *mediastinum.* The mediastinum supports the early primary lung bud rudiments and the esophagus in its transit through the pleural cavities. Near its junction with the stomach, the mesoesophagus thins out into a typical mesentery.

The primitive, simple relationships of the dorsal mesentery behind the esophagus are quickly complicated as the gut undergoes growth, elongation, and folding to produce its adult configuration. Part of the dorsal mesentery becomes greatly exaggerated; other portions of the dorsal mesentery disappear or secondarily fuse with each other. Modification of the dorsal mesentery of the stomach in particular establishes new relationships for the spleen, the pancreas, and the duodenum.

17–8 A, left-side view to show the primitive mesenteries in the human embryo; B, relationships of the early human mesenteries as seen in cross section at levels 1 through 3 as indicated in A.

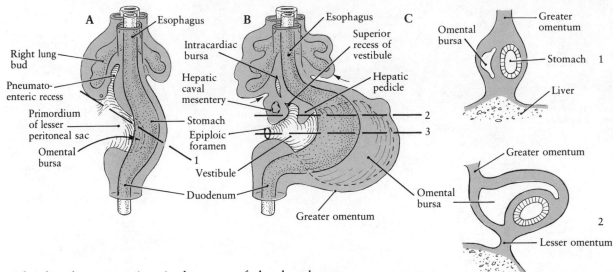

The dorsal mesogastrium is that part of the dorsal mesentery which suspends the stomach (Figs. 17–8 A,B; 17–12). Beginning at about four weeks of human development, a sacculation appears in the mesogastrium known as the *omental bursa* (Fig. 17–9 A). Although the formation of the bursa sac is often described as being an invagination dependent upon the rotation of the stomach, it more likely forms as the result of the coalescence of separate clefts that initially appear in the right surface of the dorsal mesogastrium (Fig. 17–9 C). Gradually, the saccular recess deepens toward the left behind the stomach, bringing about a shift in the attachment of the dorsal mesogastrium (Fig. 17–9 C). The finger-shaped projection termed the *pneumoenteric recess* is continuous with the bursa and extends craniad between the right lung and the esophagus (Fig. 17–9 A). Its anterior end is interrupted by the growing diaphragm to form a blind sac that often persists in the adult as the *infracardiac bursa* (Fig. 17–9 B).

As the stomach undergoes its clockwise rotation to bring the cardiac end of this organ to the left and the pyloric end to the right (Figs. 17–10; 17–11 A–C), the bursa expands transversely and comes to lie dorsal to the stomach and to the right of the esophagus (Fig. 17–9 C). Accompanying these axial changes in the orientation of the stomach is a marked extension of the dorsal mesogastrium to a point well beyond the greater curvature of the stomach (Fig. 17–11 A–E). Indeed, the dorsal mesogastrium appears as an apron-like, double-folded mesentery, the *greater omentum,* which sprawls over the small intestine. It is clearly distinguishable from the *lesser omentum,* which is the ventral mesentery passing between stomach and liver (Figs. 17–9 C; 17–10).

17–9   Development of the omental bursa in human embryos at four (A) and six (B) weeks, ventral views. C, transverse views at levels indicated in A and B. The large arrows indicate approximate level of transverse septum.

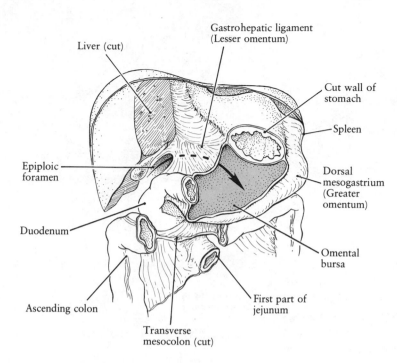

Liver (cut)

Gastrohepatic ligament
(Lesser omentum)

Cut wall of
stomach

Spleen

Epiploic
foramen

Dorsal
mesogastrium
(Greater
omentum)

Duodenum

Omental
bursa

Ascending colon

First part of
jejunum

Transverse
mesocolon (cut)

17–10 Model showing the relationships of the omental bursa to the peritoneal cavity and the surrounding viscera. (From L. Arey, 1974. Developmental Anatomy. W. B. Saunders Company, Philadelphia.)

The entire portion of the peritoneal cavity that becomes captured above the stomach and delineated above by the folded dorsal mesogastrium and below by the lesser omentum is called the *lesser peritoneal space* or *sac* (Fig. 17–9 A,B). Its organization can be dissected as follows. The omental bursa is that part of the lesser peritoneal space entirely bounded by the greater omentum of the stomach (Fig. 17–9 C). It opens into the *vestibule,* a chamber outlined below by the lesser omentum and above by the peritoneal wall and liplike fold of the dorsal mesentery (*caval mesentery*). The vestibule in turn communicates with the general peritoneal cavity by a slitlike aperture termed the *epiploic foramen* or the *foramen of Winslow* (Figs. 17–9 C; 17–10).

The caudal extension of the omental bursa establishes secondary attachments and greatly influences the growth and position of such structures as the spleen, pancreas, and duodenum. As the bursa expands caudally beyond the greater curvature of the stomach, it meets, adheres to, and fuses with the suspending dorsal mesentery of the transverse colon (Fig. 17–11 D). A double mesenterial sheet, the *gastrocolonic ligament,* thus joins together the stomach and the colon (Fig. 17–13). Beyond the colonic attachment, the walls of the bursa collapse and unite so that its cavity is obliterated (Fig. 17–13).

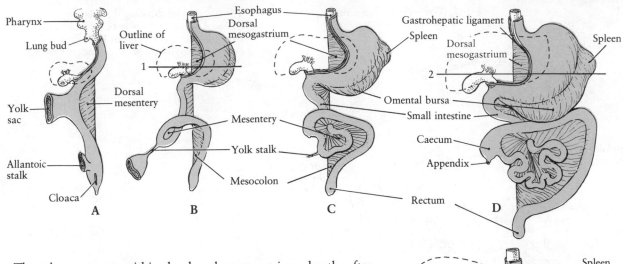

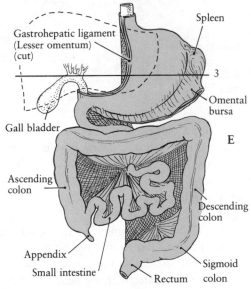

17–11 A series of schematic drawings in frontal view showing the major developmental changes in the position of the enteric tract and its associated mesenteries. The cross-hatched areas in E indicate the part of the dorsal mesentery of the duodenum and segments of the large intestine which become fused to the dorsal body wall. The heavy lines marked 1, 2, and 3 represent the locations of transverse sections shown in Figure 17–12. (From Human Embryology by B. M. Patten. Copyright © 1968 by McGraw-Hill, Inc. Used with permission of McGraw-Hill Book Company.)

The spleen appears within the dorsal mesogastrium shortly after the initial phases of the axial rotation of the stomach (Fig. 17–12 B). As the spleen enlarges and bulges from the left face of the dorsal mesogastrium, it reaches the dorsolateral wall and is pressed against it. That portion of the greater omentum between the stomach and the spleen is the *gastrosplenic ligament* (Fig. 17–12 C).

As pointed out in the chapter on the gastrointestinal tract, the pancreas initially begins to form between the two layers of the dorsal mesentery suspending the duodenum. Rather quickly the proliferating pancreatic tissue pushes into the greater omentum. As in the case of the spleen, the pancreas is carried dorsad against the body wall where the greater omentum contacts and fuses with the parietal peritoneum (Figs. 17–12 C; 17–13). Gradually, the fusion between the dorsal mesentery and the body wall becomes more extensive, leaving the pancreas tightly adherent to the dorsal body wall. The original right face of the dorsal mesogastrium now covers the surface of the pancreas.

Similar to the rest of the enteric tract, the duodenum initially has its own dorsal mesentery or *mesoduodenum*. Rotation of the stomach brings the duodenum closer to the dorsal body wall with consequent shortening of the mesoduodenum. By approximately the third month of human development, the duodenum comes to lie against the body wall and its own mesentery is completely resorbed (Fig. 17–13). In this new fixed, retroperitoneal position, most of the duodenum is situated between the transverse mesocolon and the more dorsal part of the mesogastrium (Fig. 17–11 E). These mesenteries, especially the mesocolon, secondarily form the peritoneal covering for the duodenum.

The dorsal mesentery of the remainder of the intestine is greatly affected by the rapid growth of this part of the enteric tract and its

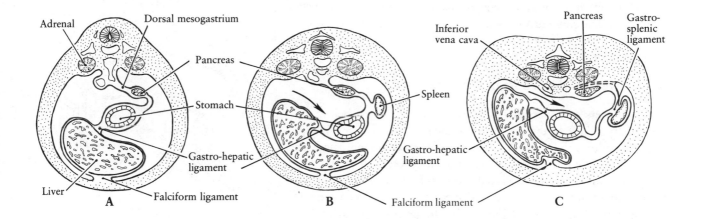

Adrenal — Dorsal mesogastrium

Pancreas

Stomach

Gastro-hepatic
ligament

Liver

Falciform ligament

A

Spleen

Gastro-hepatic
ligament

Falciform ligament

B

Inferior
vena cava — Pancreas — Gastrosplenic
ligament

C

herniation into the umbilical cord. The result is the production of
an elongate, rather fan-shaped appearing mesentery. In contrast to
the fixed position of the duodenum, the jejunum and the ileum portions of the small intestine remain freely movable within the peritoneal cavity and are supported by the folded *mesentery proper*.

Much of the embryonic suspending mesentery of the large intestine is lost as portions of this part of the gut become fixed to the
body wall. The free and obliterated portions of this mesentery are
illustrated in Figure 17–11 E. For example, the *ascending* and *descending mesocolons* become pressed against the dorsal body wall,
shorten, and progressively fuse with the adjacent peritoneum. Consequently, the ascending and descending segments of the colon are
fixed in this position. The *transverse mesocolon* remains largely

17–12 Transverse sections through the region
of the stomach to show the changes in the relationships between the mesenteries. Note the
changes in the position of the pancreas. The
arrows in B and C indicate position of the epiploic foramen. (From Human Embryology by B.
M. Patten. Copyright © 1968 by McGraw-Hill,
Inc. Used with permission of McGraw-Hill Book
Company.)

17–13 Schematic longitudinal sections of the
body to show the secondary associations of the
omental bursa in human embryos.

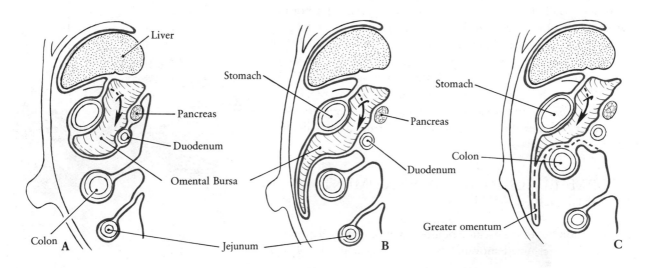

Liver

Pancreas

Duodenum

Omental Bursa

Colon **A**

Jejunum

Stomach

Pancreas

Duodenum

B

Stomach

Colon

Duodenum

Greater omentum

C

free, although it secondarily covers the duodenum as previously mentioned. The *sigmoid mesocolon* remains free, but the mesorectum disappears as the rectum becomes fixed against the body wall at the level of the sacrum.

Derivatives of the Ventral Mesentery

The two layers of the splanchnic mesoderm which meet below the gut and contribute to the formation of the primitive mesentery (Fig. 17–7) constitute the *ventral mesentery*. For most of the length of the intraembryonic coelom, the ventral mesentery is quite temporary and soon becomes obliterated (Fig. 17–8 B). At the level of the pleural cavity, this leaves the dorsal mesentery to enclose each enlarging lung as the *visceral pleura*. In the pericardial cavity, the splanchnic mesoderm beneath the foregut folds around the tubular heart and as such forms a specialized region of the ventral mesentery (Fig. 17–8). The portion of the ventral mesentery between the heart and the foregut constitutes the *dorsal mesocardium* (Fig. 17–8). It soon disappears leaving the heart without any permanent supporting mesentery. The portion of the ventral mesentery between the heart and the floor of the pericardial cavity is the *ventral mesocardium* (Fig. 17–8). This mesentery is also transitory.

The ventral mesentery persists in the vicinity of the stomach, upper duodenum, and liver and contributes to several special mesenterial supports called *ligaments*. A permanent ventral mesentery in this general region of the gut appears to arise secondarily as the result of the growth of the liver bud into the mesoderm of the transverse septum. As the stomach and liver draw away caudally, the splanchnic mesoderm is drawn into a definitive ventral mesentery that is continuous from the lesser curvature of the stomach to the ventral body wall. It can be divided into three parts: (1) a portion between the diaphragm and the liver (*coronary ligament*) and a portion between the ventral body wall and the liver (*falciform ligament*) (Figs. 17–8; 17–14); (2) a portion extending from the stomach and duodenum to the liver (lesser omentum) (Figs. 17–9; 17–10; 17–14); this in turn can be regionalized into a cranial *gastrohepatic ligament* and a caudal *hepatoduodenal ligament;* (3) a portion that becomes the enveloping capsule of the liver (Glisson's capsule).

ABNORMALITIES IN THE DEVELOPMENT OF COELOMIC CAVITIES

The formation of the musculotendinous diaphragm is dependent upon rigidly determined movements of the pleuropericardial and

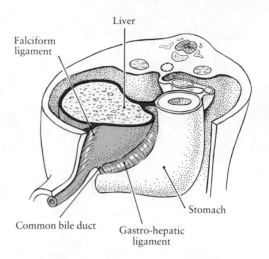

17–14 A drawing to show several derivatives of the ventral mesentery in the vicinity of the liver and the stomach in a 17 mm human embryo. A portion of the liver has been removed. (From W. Hamilton and H. Mossman, 1972. Human Embryology. Macmillan Press, London.)

17–15 Photograph of a transverse section through the thoracic region of a newborn infant to show a large left lateral posterolateral defect in the muscular diaphragm. (From K. L. Moore, 1977. The Developing Human: Clinically Oriented Embryology, 2nd ed. Courtesy of W. B. Saunders Company, Philadelphia.)

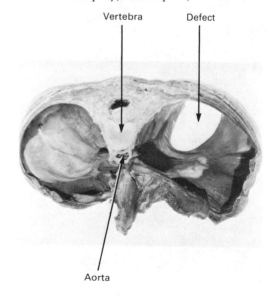

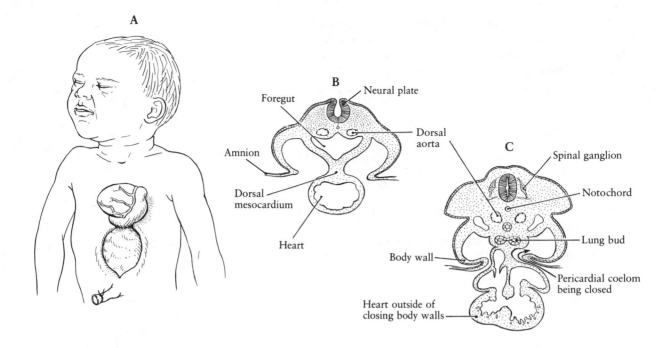

pleuroperitoneal membranes between six and seven weeks of development in the human embryo. *Diaphragmatic hernias* occur in approximately 0.08 percent of births and are abnormalities of the diaphragm resulting from defective formation, movement and/or fusion of the pleuroperitoneal membranes.

Posterolateral defect of the diaphragm, which occurs about once in 2200 births, appears as a large opening (the so-called foramen of Bochdalek) in the diaphragm because of a failure in closure of the pleuroperitoneal opening (Fig. 17–15). The defect appears to be more prevalent on the left side of the diaphragm than on the right side. The abdominal viscera, such as spleen, stomach, and small intestine, tend to herniate into the pleural cavity and thereby interfere with the normal function of both lungs and heart. If the herniation takes place before complete growth of the lung, the lung is often hypoplastic or greatly reduced in size. Although mortality is high in infants if diaphragmatic abnormalities are left untreated, surgical procedures are available which can be employed to restore normal relationships between the body cavities.

Defects in the separation of the pericardial cavity from the pleural cavities by the pleuropericardial membranes are less common than diphragmatic hernias. Failure to close the pleuropericardial opening, if present, is usually on the left side. Occasionally, the left atrium may herniate into the left pleural cavity upon atrial systole.

A rare but severe abnormality that usually results in postnatal death is *ectopia cordis* (Fig. 17–16). The heart lies outside of the body, a condition presumably arising because of faulty separation between extraembryonic and intraembryonic regions in the cardiac area as the ventral body walls of the embryo are closing (Fig. 17–16).

REFERENCES

Corliss, C. E. 1976. Patten's Human Embryology. Elements of Clinical Development, pp. 307–324. New York: McGraw-Hill.

Moore, K. L. 1977. The Developing Human, pp. 145–155. Philadelphia: W. B. Saunders.

Wells, L. J. 1954. Development of the human diaphragm and pleural sacs. Carnegie Contrib. Embryol. 35:107–143.

18

The Cardiovascular System

One of the first organ systems to become functional in the embryo is the cardiovascular system. This is not surprising when one bears in mind that the embryo cannot grow beyond a volume of a few cubic millimeters using processes of simple diffusion to meet critical metabolic requirements. When an embryo has reached a certain small size, therefore, an elaborate system of vascular channels is fashioned to provide for the nutritional, respiratory, and excretory needs of developing tissues and cells. As in the adult, the main blood vessels in the embryo tend to be associated with centers of intense metabolic activity such as the yolk and placenta. The circulating blood carries nutrients and oxygen from organs of absorption to sites of growing and differentiating cells. In turn, waste materials are picked up and transported to organs facilitating elimination or storage. By necessity, the topographical arrangement of blood vessels in the embryo (particularly the amniote embryo) is quite different from that of the adult because centers of metabolic activity shift during the development of the organism.

The embryo then is faced with a difficult task in the design of its cardiovascular system. It must not only construct a vascular system associated with the functional metabolic centers of the embryo, but it must also provide an arrangement of vessels which anticipates a shift in the sites where these metabolic activities are to be carried out in the posthatch or postnatal organism. In the case of the mammalian embryo, the activities of the placenta are at birth passed on to the digestive tract, lungs, and kidneys. Although accessory fetal organs such as the yolk sac and placenta are temporary, they possess an enormous circulating blood supply. Indeed, in order for the embryo proper to circulate blood to the extensive extraembryonic circulation, its heart and blood vessels must be many times larger, relative to body size, than the adult heart and vessels to adult body size. Greater absolute increase in fetal growth reduces this discrepancy after about the fifth month of gestation in the human embryo.

For purposes of convenience, the cardiovascular system can be divided into three major components: (1) the blood vascular system, including heart, arteries, and veins; (2) the hemopoietic or blood-forming organs; and (3) the lymphatic system. We will consider each of these, but place most of our emphasis on the blood

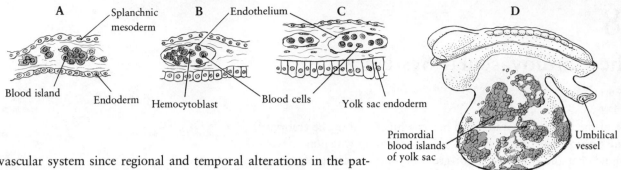

A Splanchnic mesoderm   B Endothelium   C   D

Blood island   Endoderm   Hemocytoblast   Blood cells   Yolk sac endoderm

Primordial blood islands of yolk sac   Umbilical vessel

vascular system since regional and temporal alterations in the pattern of developing blood vessels are more dramatic and interesting.

ANGIOGENESIS AND HEMOPOIESIS

Blood cells and blood vessels are specializations of mesenchyme. This important embryonic tissue fashions the epithelial lining, the collagenous and elastic tissues, and the smooth muscle that participate in the construction of arteries and veins.

The earliest formative vascular tissue to appear in the mammalian embryo is termed *angioblast* (or *hemangioblast*); the process of primitive blood vessel development is called *angiogenesis* (*hemangiogenesis*). The tissue is in the form of solid masses of cells located in the splanchnic mesoderm of the yolk sac (Fig. 18–1). These clusters of cells, or *blood islands,* hollow out (Fig. 18–1 A–C). In this process, the more peripheral cells of the blood island become organized as a flattened, vascular *endothelium.* The central cells remain as *primitive blood cells* that float in *primitive blood plasma* produced by cells of the blood island. Because these mesenchyme cells can differentiate into either primitive blood cells or vascular endothelium, they have been termed angioblasts or hemangioblasts. By growth and union of these hollowed-out cords of cells, the originally solid, isolated clusters of hemangioblastic tissue are converted into plexuses of blood vessels. These are present on the yolk sac, the body stalk, and the chorion of human embryos as early as the head process stage. Once the system of closed vessels is established, new extraembryonic vessels arise as outgrowths from preexisting vessels.

The first vessels within the embryo proper are detected during the period of early somite formation. These develop from islands of hemangioblastic tissue localized in the mesenchyme of the early organ primordia and form by the same processes as previously described for extraembryonic blood vessels. It was initially thought that the source of intraembryonic vessels was angioblastic tissue spreading from the yolk sac into the embryo. Experimental evidence

18–1   The development of primitive blood vessels and blood cells from yolk sac blood islands. A, aggregation of cells to form blood islands in human embryo in the fourth week; B, beginning of the differentiation of the endothelium and the primitive blood cells; C, a more advanced condition showing organized endothelium and primitive blood cells suspended in plasma; D, the Corner 10-somite embryo showing blood islands on the yolk sac.

now tends to support the concept that the intraembryonic endothelium differentiates in situ from intraembryonic mesenchyme. Only secondarily does the network of intraembryonic vessels join with that over the yolk sac. Once a primitive, closed system of embryonic vessels is established, new blood vessels arise primarily by sprouting from preexisting vessels.

Hemopoiesis or *hematopoiesis* is a term referring to the development of various blood cell types. In species that have been studied to date, including frog tadpole, chick, mouse, and man, blood cells form by the differentiation of mesenchyme tissue at different locations (particularly for red blood cells) in the embryo. In the frog embryo, for example, red blood cells develop and mature in the kidney and the liver. Following metamorphosis of the tadpole, the spleen becomes the center of red blood cell maturation. The sequence and time of appearance of hemopoietic centers in the human are: yolk sac (week 4); body mesenchyme and blood vessels (week 5); liver (week 6); spleen, thymus, and lymph glands (weeks 8 to 16); and bone marrow (week 16). At any of these sites, the mesenchymal cells round up, lose their typical mesenchymal intercellular junctional complexes, proliferate, and become free basophilic progenitors of the various blood cell types.

There is now an extensive body of literature that tends to support the concept that a single stem cell (the *hemocytoblast*) has the capacity to differentiate into erythropoietic (red blood cells), granulopoietic (granular white blood cells), and megakaryocytic (nongranular white blood cells) cells. Although the precise morphological identity of this stem cell has yet to be fully ascertained, it is thought to be large and lymphocytelike, possessing a granular, basophilic cytoplasm, and very mobile. How these pleuripotent stem cells are able to differentiate into specific hematopoetic cell lines, such as red or white blood cells, is a major unresolved question. It is suspected that somehow the stem cells selectively acquire a responsiveness to only those regulatory mechanisms that characterize and control the differentiated cell line.

The study of erythroid cell differentiation in the fetus has contributed substantially to our current understanding of the basic processes and regulatory mechanisms that prevail during normal and abnormal cell differentiation. There are several unique features of *erythropoiesis* that make it a suitable system for studies in cell differentiation. First, relatively large numbers of cells can be obtained from accessible sites in the embryo, cultured in vitro, and subjected to experimental manipulation. Second, hemoglobin, comprising about 90 percent of the protein synthesized in the red blood cell, is a biochemically and genetically well-characterized protein; it is a useful marker in examining the relationships between morphologi-

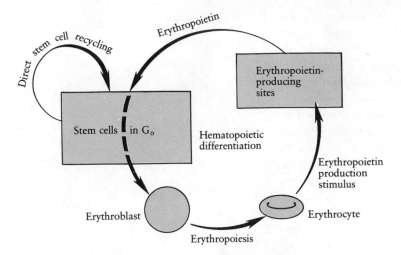

Stem cells in G_o

Direct stem cell recycling

Erythropoietin

Erythropoietin-producing sites

Hematopoietic differentiation

Erythropoietin production stimulus

Erythroblast

Erythrocyte

Erythropoiesis

18–2   A diagrammatic representation of a model showing the relationship between erythropoetin and red blood cell formation. (After J. Okunewick, 1970. Cell Differentiation, ed. by Ole A. Scheide and Jean De Vellis. (© 1970 by Litton Educational Publishing, Inc. Reprinted by permission of Van Nostrand Reinhold Company.)

cal and biochemical changes during erythroid cell differentiation. Third, erythroid cell production is stimulated by a hormone (*erythropoietin*) throughout postpartum life and possibly during embryogenesis as well.

The number of red blood cells produced from a precursor cell population and the amount of hemoglobin synthesized are regulated by the titer or level of circulating erythropoietin. In the adult, presumably in response to low tissue levels of oxygenation, the kidney either elaborates and releases erythropoietin itself or a renal activator of a plasma (liver) erythropoietin precursor. Several models have been proposed to show how erythropoietin stimulates red blood cell formation. One of these models is shown in Figure 18–2. It recognizes that there are two major compartments in the red blood cell system: the *stem cell compartment* and the circulating *erythrocyte cell compartment*. In the former compartment, erythropoietin acts to trigger sensitized, nondividing hemocytoblasts to proceed to differentiate into erythroid cells. Sudden removal of a segment of the stem cell population stimulates other stem cells to proliferate in order to replace those removed. Erythropoietin production is controlled by the number of cells in the circulating compartment and the amount of oxygen that they transport. The circulating erythrocyte compartment contains cells with a finite lifespan (110 to 120 days) and incapable of division.

The fetal mouse has been particularly useful in the examination of where and how red blood cells differentiate. The first population of red blood cells appears on the yolk sac during the seventh day of gestation. These are termed *erythroblasts* and enter the circulation several days later. Here the erythroblasts proliferate and undergo maturation until by the fifteenth day they can be considered mature, nucleated erythrocytes. The circulating lifespan of these early or

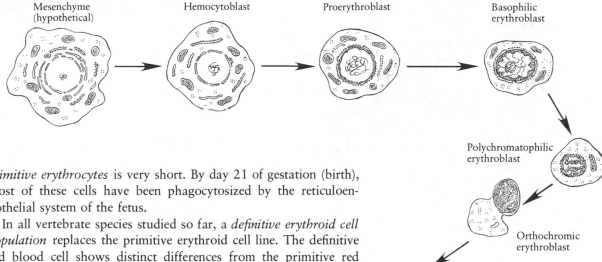

Mesenchyme (hypothetical)　　Hemocytoblast　　Proerythroblast　　Basophilic erythroblast

Polychromatophilic erythroblast

Orthochromic erythroblast

Reticulocyte

primitive erythrocytes is very short. By day 21 of gestation (birth), most of these cells have been phagocytosized by the reticuloendothelial system of the fetus.

In all vertebrate species studied so far, a *definitive erythroid cell population* replaces the primitive erythroid cell line. The definitive red blood cell shows distinct differences from the primitive red blood cell in details of its morphology and in the type of hemoglobin synthesized. Also, and in contrast to the primitive cell population, the definitive cell population is self-renewing.

The fetal liver is the first major site for the production of the definitive red blood cell type. The beginning of the differentiation of the definitive erythroid cell, characterized by a sequence of morphological cell transformations (Fig. 18–3), is detected in the mouse on day 10 of gestation. By about day 11, cells termed *proerythroblasts* are found between the cords of liver cells. These lack hemoglobin, but their nuclei show intense synthesis of rRNA. The accumulation of RNA in the cytoplasm is responsible for the basophilia of the stage of differentiation known as the *basophilic erythroblast.* Although it is difficult to detect hemoglobin cytochemically at this stage, it is suspected that the synthesis of this protein is initiated in this cell type. Hemoglobin is detectable by staining in the *polychromatophilic erythroblast.* Polychromatophilic cells are nucleated, show marked reduction in the rate of RNA synthesis, and intense accumulation of hemoglobin. In the *orthochromic erythroblast,* the nucleus becomes pynocytic and eventually is eliminated from the cell with a small amount of cytoplasm. The cell now enters the circulation on day 12 as an *anucleated reticulocyte.* Anucleated reticulocytes continue to make hemoglobin for a day or so. When hemoglobin synthesis is terminated, the cell becomes a mature erythrocyte.

The 13-day mouse liver, which contains the complete morphological series of red blood cell types, has been used by many investigators to determine the cellular and molecular basis for hemoglobin formation. The addition of erythropoietin to the fetal liver in vitro results in an acceleration of DNA synthesis within 20 minutes,

18–3 A suggested scheme for the differentiation of erythropoietic cells in the embryonic liver and in all adult erythropoietic tissues of a mammal. (After R. Rifkind, 1974. Concepts of Development. J. Lash and J. Whittaker, eds. Sinauer Associates, Sunderland, Mass.)

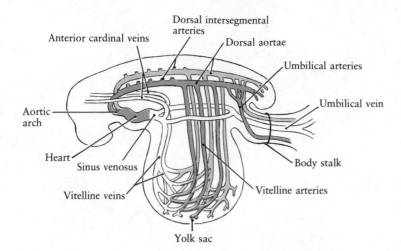

Anterior cardinal veins

Dorsal intersegmental arteries

Dorsal aortae

Umbilical arteries

Aortic arch

Umbilical vein

Heart

Sinus venosus

Body stalk

Vitelline veins

Vitelline arteries

Yolk sac

and of RNA and hemoglobin synthesis within approximately two hours. Hemoglobin synthesis and the increased DNA production are both inhibited by actinomycin D and puromycin. This suggests that, under hormonal stimulation, there is an initial, early transcription that results in the production of a protein. This protein is necessary for DNA replication. Following DNA replication, there is a second, later phase of transcription that produces the mRNA required for hemoglobin synthesis.

THE PRIMITIVE VASCULAR SYSTEM

Diffuse, capillary plexuses always precede the formation of arteries and veins in any given region of the embryo. Arteries and veins gradually become differentiated through the enlargement of individual capillaries and the fusion and confluence of adjacent ones. Capillaries from which the flow of blood is diverted during this process undergo regression and atrophy. Presumably, genetic background and local hemodynamic influences, such as the direction and velocity of the blood, control not only the selection of those channels that are to enlarge, but also the structural characteristics of their walls (i.e., whether they are to be arteries or veins).

The primitive vascular system in all vertebrate embryos consists of simple, paired, symmetrically arranged endothelial tubes. Initially, arteries and veins cannot be structurally distinguished; however, they are named in terms of their fate and relationship to the heart. Human embryos of about 12 somites clearly show the initial arrangement of definitive blood vessels (Fig. 18–4). Directly beneath the notochord are the paired *dorsal aortae*. These are con-

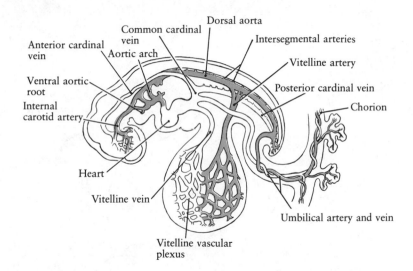

Anterior cardinal vein

Common cardinal vein

Aortic arch

Dorsal aorta

Intersegmental arteries

Vitelline artery

Ventral aortic root

Internal carotid artery

Posterior cardinal vein

Chorion

Heart

Vitelline vein

Umbilical artery and vein

Vitelline vascular plexus

18–5 A drawing to show the arrangement of the heart and blood vessels at the end of the first month in the human embryo. Left-side view.

tinued around the tip of the pharynx as the first pair of *aortic arches* where they then join the anterior end of the heart. Paired, dorsal *intersegmental arteries* spring from the dorsal aortae and pass between successive pairs of somites. Vessels passing to and from the yolk sac (*vitelline arteries* and *veins*) and placenta (*unbilical* or *allantoic arteries* and *veins*) are established and circulate blood extraembryonically shortly after the onset of contractions of the heart (about 26 days). A pair of *anterior cardinal veins* returns blood from the capillary plexuses of the head end of the embryo to the heart.

At slightly later stages of development (Fig. 18–5), additional aortic arches are sequentially added, the dorsal aortae fuse into a single, median vessel as far forward as the pharynx, and the posterior end of the embryo is drained by a pair of *posterior cardinal veins*. Each posterior cardinal vein joins with an anterior cardinal vein to form a short common vessel, the *common cardinal vein* (*duct of Cuvier*), which empties into the heart.

The arrangement of blood vessels described above undergoes substantial alteration during the course of development. Blood vessels fuse, hypertrophy, regress, or atrophy with shifts in patterns of blood flow and internal changes in the organization of the heart. For purposes of convenience, we will describe under separate subheadings the changes in the heart, arteries, and veins that result in the adult arrangement of the cardiovascular system. The student should keep in mind, however, that alterations in the organization of the heart and in the patterns of arteries and veins occur simultaneously and are interdependent.

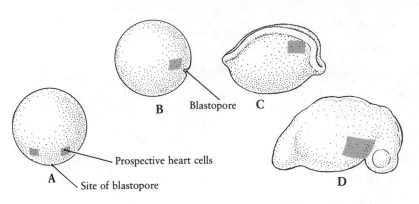

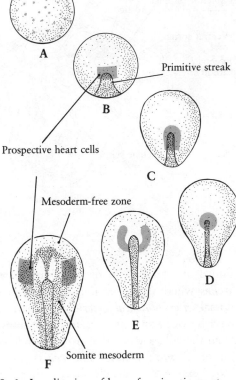

THE HEART

Localization and Induction of Heart-Forming Tissue

The primitive heart in most vertebrates is tubular and arises as the result of the fusion of a pair of cardiac primordia. This is particularly evident in forms such as the bony fishes, reptiles, and birds where the developing embryo is flattened and pressed against the yolk. Long before the heart is recognizable as a tubular structure, cells with heart-forming capacity can be localized using techniques of vital staining, extirpation, and transplantation.

The approximate locations of heart-forming mesodermal cells in the urodele at successive stages of development are shown in Figure 18–6. At the onset of gastrulation, the areas of presumptive heart tissue are located on either side of the dorsal lip of the blastopore (Figure 18–6 A,B). After passing through the dorsolateral lips of the blastopore, each cardiac area is located in the edge of the mesodermal mantle, rather high on the flank of the embryo adjacent to the presumptive hindbrain of the neural plate (Fig. 18–6 C). If one of these cardiac regions is dissected out at the tail bud stage (Fig. 18–6 D) and cultured in the proper medium, it will differentiate into an S-shaped, pulsating heart tube.

The position and extent of the presumptive cardiac regions at various stages in the chick embryo have been rather precisely mapped out by explanting fragments of the blastoderm to the chorioallantoic membrane of eight-to-nine-day host embryos (Fig. 18–7). Explants with heart tissue will differentiate into cellular vesicles of contractile activity. Hence, the capacity of these tissue fragments to self-differentiate into cardiac tissue has been a useful tool in constructing a fate map for the heart. At about the time that the primitive streak forms, the presumptive cardiac tissue is located in the mesoderm just lateral to the tip of the streak (Fig. 18–7 B,C). By

18–6 Localization of heart-forming tissue at various stages in a urodele embryo. A, gastrula, dorsal view; B, gastrula, left lateral view; C, neurula, left lateral view; D, tail bud, right lateral view. (After W. Copenhaver, 1955. Analyses of Development. B. Willier, P. Weiss, and V. Hamburger, eds. W. B. Saunders Company, Philadelphia.)

18–7 Localization of heart-forming tissues at progressively later stages in the chick embryo.

the definitive to late primitive streak stage, the cardiac regions are paired and appear anterolaterally to Hensen's node (Fig. 18–7 E,F).

There is some evidence that the heart-forming regions are determined in their cardiogenic potency by interactions with neighboring tissues, particularly the endoderm. Precardiac mesoderm appears to require the presence of endoderm for successful cardiac muscle differentiation. In the amphibian, for example, the presumptive heart mesoderm is in contact with the foregut endoderm during its movement after migration through the blastopore. Balinsky and others have shown that the extirpation of the entire endoderm from embryos at the neurula stage results in the complete absence of the heart. Also, fragments of presumptive cardiac mesoderm from salamander embryos at gastrula or early neurula stages typically produce well-formed hearts in culture only if explanted with endoderm. Jacobson and Duncan (1968) have shown that a particular fraction of endoderm, prepared by passing homogenized endoderm through a Sephadex column, can partially substitute for intact endoderm in culture. Hence, the formation of heart tissue would appear to be dependent upon inductive influences emanating from the endoderm.

The importance of the endoderm in the determination of heart-forming tissue is less clear in higher vertebrates. Studies by Waddington and his colleagues are inconclusive. Cultured chick embryos, following removal of the entire area pellucida endoderm (hypoblast) at the definitive primitive streak stage, generally showed an absence of well-formed hearts. However, one case was reported in which the embryo displayed an organized heart in the absence of endoderm. DeHaan removed the endoderm overlying the presumptive cardiac region from only one side of the primitive streak stage chick embryo. No heart appeared on the operated side of the embryo. When he cultured the fragments removed from the operated side of the embryo, approximately 70 percent of these developed masses of beating heart tissue. This demonstrated that extirpation techniques may remove not only the endoderm but also the mesoderm that contains presumptive heart tissue as well. The absence of heart tissue in Waddington's studies is probably related to the fact that the presumptive heart-forming tissue had been removed with the presumed inducer. Le Douarin and his collaborators have demonstrated that the avian precardiac mesoderm can differentiate in vitro to some extent in the absence of endoderm, but the development of mature cardiac cells was clearly retarded in the absence of this germ layer. Generally, it appears that the differentiating mesoderm will develop into a tubular organ only if endoderm is present in the culture. Manasek (1976) proposes that the normal morphogenesis of the heart can only take place if there is normal cytodifferentiation and maturation of cardiac tissue. He suggests that the basal lamina of the endoderm, perhaps through the synthesis of small molecules such as collagen or glycoproteins, mediates the interaction between the precardiac mesoderm and the endoderm.

Formation of the Primitive Tubular Heart

The heart can be viewed as a highly specialized blood vessel with very thick muscular walls. The heart follows a generally similar pattern of early embryonic development in most vertebrates. The formation of this organ in the amphibian embryo is rather simple and perhaps should be considered before that of other vertebartes (Fig. 18–8). Recall that by the end of neurulation the lateral plate mesoderm, lying on either side of the tubular gut, is split into parietal and visceral layers. At the end of neurulation, the free, ventromedial edges of the mesodermal mantle swing toward the midline and become noticeably thickened in the heart-forming regions (Fig. 18–8 A,B). Cells proliferate from the heart-forming regions, migrate beneath the gut, and become organized as a longitudinal, vascular strand of tissue. A lumen develops within the vascular strand, thus converting a solid cord of cells into an endothelial-lined tube (Fig. 18–8 C). The endothelial lining of the future heart cavity constitutes the rudiment of the *endocardium.*

As the endocardial tube is being formed, the edges of the lateral plate mesoderm continue to push toward the midline. Subsequently, the visceral layers of mesoderm from either side meet below and above the endocardial tube to form suspending partitions, the *ventral* and *dorsal mesocardia* (Fig. 18–8 C-E). The visceral mesoderm enveloping the endocardial tube will thicken and form the *epimyocardium* layer (Fig. 18–8 D,E). The epimyocardial rudiment will later differentiate into the cardiac muscle tissue and covering layer of the heart. The coelomic cavities on either side of the tubular heart will expand. With the disappearance of the ventral mesocardium, they join together as the *pericardial cavity* (Fig. 18–8 D,E).

The early stages in the development of the heart in bony fishes, reptiles, and birds are considerably more complicated owing to the fact that the postgastrulative embryo, organized as flat plates of cells, rests upon a large yolk mass. Consequently, the unpaired heart arises gradually as the two widely separated, lateral cardiac primordia swing toward the ventral midline with the lateral plate mesoderm and fuse below the foregut.

The heart begins to form in the chick embryo shortly after the head process stage (Fig. 18–9 A). At this time the heart-forming regions are indicated as thickenings in the splanchnic mesoderm on either side of the anterior intestinal portal (Fig. 18–9 E). Cells de-

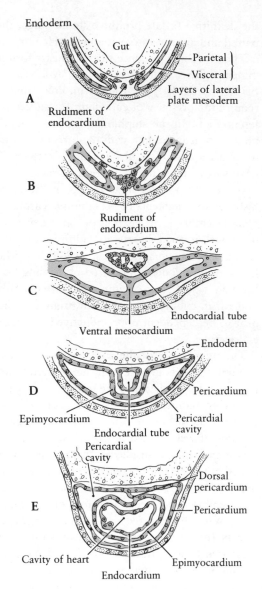

18–8 Formation of the primitive tubular heart in amphibians as seen in a series of transverse sections.

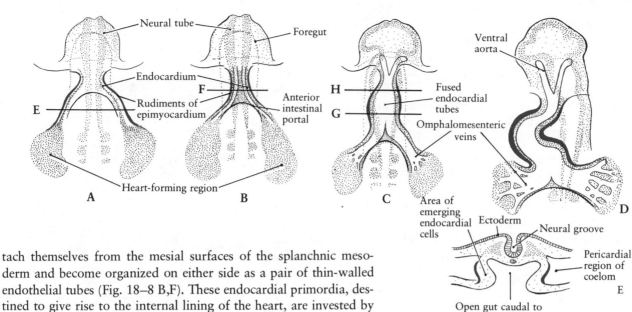

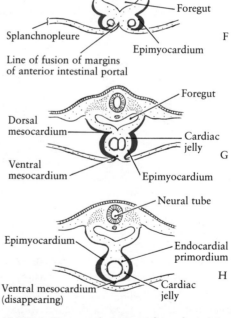

tach themselves from the mesial surfaces of the splanchnic mesoderm and become organized on either side as a pair of thin-walled
endothelial tubes (Fig. 18–8 B,F). These endocardial primordia, destined to give rise to the internal lining of the heart, are invested by
the thickened, intact splanchnic mesoderm or epimyocardial primordia (Fig. 18–9 E,F). As the body folds undercut the embryo and
separate it from the yolk, the ventral wall of the gut and the ventral
body wall of the embryo are completed. In this process, the endocardial tubes from the right and left sides are brought together
and fuse in the midline below the gut (Fig. 18–9 C,D,F,G). Simultaneously, the epimyocardial rudiments close around the endocardial
vessels, meeting initially below and then above them (Fig.
18–9 G). The double-layer of splanchnic mesoderm meeting above
the endocardial tubes constitutes the *dorsal mesocardium* and that
below the endocardial tubes the *ventral mesocardium*. The ventral
mesocardium is very transitory and disappears shortly after it forms
(Fig. 18–9 H), leaving the primitive tubular heart suspended in an
unpaired pericardial cavity by the dorsal mesocardium.

In the human embryo, the primordium for both the heart and the
pericardial cavity initially lies as a crescentic-shaped zone of mesoderm cephalic to the embryonic disc (Fig. 18–10). It is visible as
early as the primitive streak stage (15 days). At a slightly later stage
(17–18 days), the thickened mesoderm becomes split into parietal
and splanchnic layers through the appearance and coalescence of
many vesicular spaces, a process leading to the formation of the
pericardial cavity (Fig. 18–11 A,B). A U-shaped *cardiogenic plate* or
heart primordium now lies below the pericardial cavity (Fig. 18–11
B).

As the head of the embryo pushes rapidly forward, the limbs of
the cardiogenic plate are swept back on either side of the body following the curve of the foregut. Hence, the heart primordium is

18–9   A–D, ventral views to show the origin
and fusion of the paired cardiac primordia in the
chick embryo; E–H, transverse sections through
the heart region at locations indicated in A–C
above. (A–D, after R. DeHaan, 1965. Organogenesis. R. H. DeHaan and H. Ursprung, eds.
Holt, Rinehart and Winston, New York.)

reversed end-for-end with respect to its original orientation and thus comes to lie above the pericardial cavity (Fig. 18–11 C,D).

The earliest signs of heart formation are indicated by the appearance of clusters of cells that aggregate, on either side of the open gut, as a pair of elongated strands (cardiogenic cords) between the endoderm and the splanchnic mesoderm of the cardiogenic plate (Fig. 18–12 A). Each vascular cord then quickly becomes canalized or hollowed out to produce a thin-walled endocardial tube (Fig. 18–11 D; 18–12 B). As in the chick embryo, the splanchnic mesoderm on either side thickens as the epimyocardial rudiment where it lies adjacent to the endocardial tube (Fig. 18–12 B).

While these changes occur in the splanchnic mesoderm, the folding off of the embryonic body progresses concurrently with closure of the floor of the foregut. The paired endocardial tubes are brought closer together as the process of embryonic separation from extraembryonic tissues reaches the level of the heart (Fig. 18–13 A). The two tubes then fuse to form a single, endocardial tube lying in the midline (Fig. 18–12 C,D; 18–13 B,C). It is enveloped by a single, troughlike fold formed by the right and left epimyocardial rudiments (Fig. 18–12 D). The apposed layers of the splanchnic mesoderm meet above the endocardial tube as the dorsal mesentery of the heart or dorsal mesocardium (Fig. 18–12 D). No comparable structure is produced below the heart so that the originally paired right and left coelomic cavities become immediately confluent to form the definitive, unpaired pericardial cavity. A distinct extracellular space, filled with a loose, gelatinous reticulum or *cardiac jelly,* separates the endocardium and the epimyocardium of the primitive tubular heart (Fig. 18–12 C). The cardiac jelly is a gel with high viscosity and contains the glycosaminoglycans, hyaluronate and chondroitin sulfate. Most of these macromolecules of the cardiac jelly are synthesized by the developing epimyocardium. The production of these extracellular substances decreases as the heart matures. Fucose-containing glycoproteins also appear to be normal structural components of this extracellular matrix. These are probably synthesized by the endoderm and may represent the endoderm requirement for cardiac differentiation. Continued retreat of the anterior intestinal portal joins the paired cardiac primordia to the portion of the heart already formed. Fusion continues until the entire heart is a single organ.

Even before the paired cardiac halves have started to merge in the midline, each endocardial tube, partially invested by its epimyocardial mantle, shows a sequence of dilations which foreshadow the future chambers of the tubular heart (Fig. 18–14). Named in the order in which they transport blood through the heart, the primary divisions of the early embryonic heart are: *sinus venosus, atrium,*

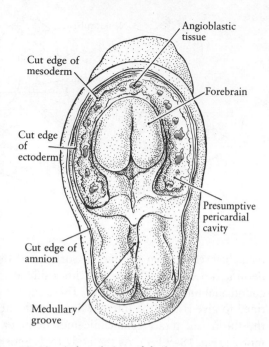

18–10   A dorsal view of the late presomite human embryo to show angioblastic tissue in the splanchnic mesoderm. The ectoderm and somatopleure have been removed. (From C. Davis, 1927. Carnegie Contributions to Embryology 19, 245.)

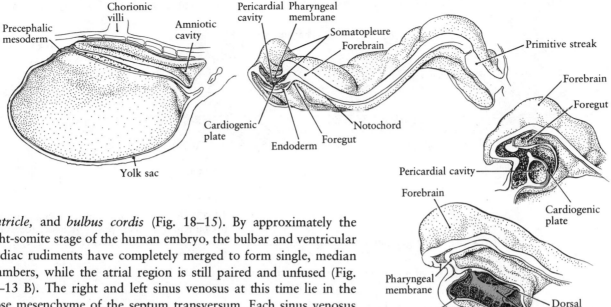

Labels for top figures:
Chorionic villi
Precephalic mesoderm
Amniotic cavity
Pericardial cavity
Pharyngeal membrane
Somatopleure
Forebrain
Primitive streak
Cardiogenic plate
Endoderm
Foregut
Notochord
Yolk sac
Forebrain
Foregut
Pericardial cavity
Cardiogenic plate
Forebrain
Pharyngeal membrane
Dorsal mesocardium
Endocardium
Epimyocardium
Pericardial cavity

ventricle, and *bulbus cordis* (Fig. 18–15). By approximately the eight-somite stage of the human embryo, the bulbar and ventricular cardiac rudiments have completely merged to form single, median chambers, while the atrial region is still paired and unfused (Fig. 18–13 B). The right and left sinus venosus at this time lie in the loose mesenchyme of the septum transversum. Each sinus venosus serves as the center of confluence for the cardinal, umbilical, and vitelline veins. Cephalically, the bulbus cordis continues into a short *truncus arteriosus* (Fig. 18–15). The truncus arteriosus is formed by the fusion of paired endothelial tubes that are fashioned from two strands of mesenchyme anterior to the level of the heart. Within the next several days, the paired atria and sinus venosuses will merge to

18–11 A series of drawings to show the early transformation of the cardiogenic plate in the human embryo. (From C. Davis, 1927. Carnegie Contributions to Embryology 19, 245.)

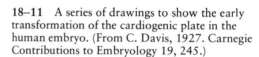

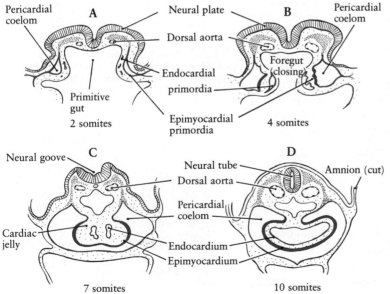

A — 2 somites
Pericardial coelom
Neural plate
Dorsal aorta
Endocardial primordia
Primitive gut
Epimyocardial primordia

B — 4 somites
Pericardial coelom
Foregut (closing)

C — 7 somites
Neural goove
Cardiac jelly

D — 10 somites
Neural tube
Dorsal aorta
Pericardial coelom
Amnion (cut)
Endocardium
Epimyocardium

18–12 Four stages in the fusion of the paired cardiac primordia of the human heart as seen in transverse section. (From Human Embryology by B. M. Patten. Copyright © 1968 by McGraw-Hill, Inc. Used with permission of McGraw-Hill Book Company.)

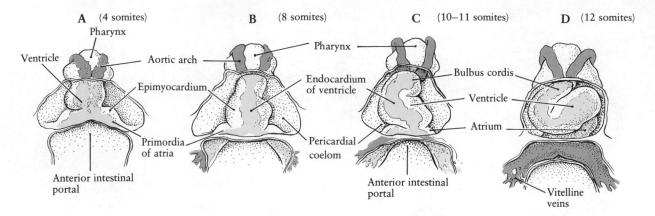

A (4 somites)
Pharynx
Ventricle
Aortic arch
Epimyocardium
Primordia of atria
Anterior intestinal portal

B (8 somites)
Pharynx
Endocardium of ventricle
Pericardial coelom

C (10–11 somites)
Bulbus cordis
Ventricle
Atrium
Anterior intestinal portal

D (12 somites)
Vitelline veins

complete formation of the primitive tubular heart (Figs. 18–13 D; 18–17 A,B; 18–18 A,B).

In short, the early tubular heart of all vertebrates consists of four chambers in sequence, each of which is composed of two layers (endocardium and epimyocardium) separated by cardiac jelly. Stellate-shaped cells subsequently appear in the cardiac jelly. These cells originate from the endocardium, proliferate in the extracellular matrix, and give rise to thickened pads of mesenchymatous tissue in the atrioventricular canal (*dorsal* and *ventral endocardial cushions*) and along the walls of the bulbus cordis (*bulbar ridges*) (Fig. 18–15). These ridges of endocardial connective tissue are the earliest signs of the future septa of the heart.

The convergence of the two lateral cardiac primordia in the ventral midline to produce a single, heart tube is a complex event. It appears to involve a series of different, but simultaneously occurring and coordinated morphogenetic cell movements. DeHaan and his colleagues have analyzed some of these movements in chick embryos using several techniques, including that of time-lapse cinematography. The movements that result in the union of the paired cardiac regions include: (1) folding movements of the endoderm to form the crescentic-shaped pouch of the anterior intestinal portal; (2) rapid, anteromesial migration of special clusters of cells (*precardiac clusters*) within the cardiac regions; and (3) ventral emigration movements of cells that lose their association with the splanchnic mesoderm to form the hemangioblast or presumptive endocardial layer.

The movements of the endoderm are of great importance in heart tube formation. Because of its cohesive properties, the endoderm adheres tightly to the overlying cardiac primordia. As the endoderm moves medially and obliquely backwards to complete the roof and

18–13 A–D, four stages in the formation of the human heart as exposed by dissection. Ventral views. (From C. Davis, 1927. Carnegie Contributions to Embryology 19, 245.)

18–14 The paired cardiac tubes showing regionalization into chambers in the six-somite human embryo. Ventral view. (From C. Davis, 1927. Carnegie Contributions to Embryology 19, 245.)

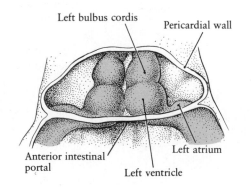

Left bulbus cordis
Pericardial wall
Anterior intestinal portal
Left ventricle
Left atrium

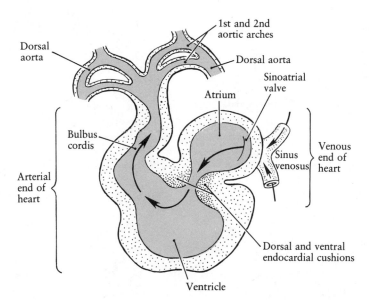

Dorsal
aorta

1st and 2nd
aortic arches

Dorsal aorta

Sinoatrial
valve

Atrium

Bulbus
cordis

Sinus
venosus

Venous
end of
heart

Arterial
end of
heart

Dorsal and ventral
endocardial cushions

Ventricle

18–15   A diagrammatic, sagittal section through the human heart (12-somite stage) showing the beginning of the formation of the bulbar ridges and endocardial cushions. Arrows indicate the direction of blood flow through the heart.

floor of the gut, the heart-forming regions are dragged passively toward the midline.

The heart-forming areas of the chick embryo are initially rather broad and diffuse, consisting of small clusters of tightly packed cells within an intact mesodermal epithelium. Both electron and light microscope observations show that the translocation of the cells of the cardiac epithelium is collective; that it, the mesodermal epithelium moves as a sheet. The cells of the cardiac epithelium will give rise to the cardiac muscle. By analyzing tracings of photographs made from time-lapse films, DeHaan has shown that the precardiac cell clusters actively migrate toward the anterior intestinal portal during heart tube formation and give rise to the endocardial cells (Fig. 18–16). Initially, the clusters exhibit random movements with no apparent relation to their "goal" of the anterior intestinal portal (Fig. 18–16 A,B). At a later stage, however, when the anterior ends of the cardiac regions begin to move forward and mesiad, the clusters become arranged in a stable configuration (Fig. 18–16 C). Subsequently, each cluster migrates anteromesially and joins the forming heart in the order of its position along the anteroposterior axis (Fig. 18–16 D,E). The sudden change in the migratory behavior of the precardiac clusters from random to oriented movements is probably related to influences emanating from the underlying endoderm. DeHaan has noted that the early embryonic endoderm consists of flattened, squamous cells organized as an epithelium. Shortly thereafter, a band of lunate, columnar-shaped cells differen-

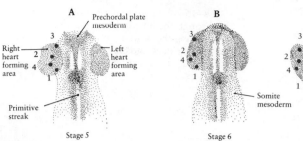
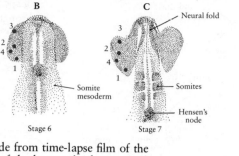
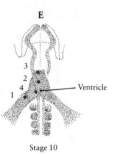

18-16 A–E, tracings of photographs made from time-lapse film of the chick embryo to show that the formation of the heart tube from paired heart-forming areas is accompanied by directed movements of clusters of precardiac cells. The precardiac cell clusters are numbered 1–4 and will give rise to the endocardium (After R. DeHaan, 1965. Organogenesis. R. H. DeHaan and H. Ursprung, eds. Holt, Rinehart and Winston, New York); F, micrograph of a section through the precardiac or heart-forming region at the time that the heart tube begins to form in the chick embryo. Arrows point to boundary between endoderm (EN) and heart-forming mesoderm. EC, presumptive epimyocardial cell. (From F. Manasek, 1976. The Cell Surface in Animal Embryology and Development. G. Poste and G. Nicolson, eds. North Holland Publishing Co., New York.)

tiates in the endoderm, running in a crescentic-shaped arc, directly beneath the cardiac regions. It is presumed that the precardiac clusters use the endoderm as a substratum and are oriented by the altered cell shape in this layer. Since glycoproteins are synthesized by the endoderm and accumulate in the basal lamina during the period of precardiac cell translocation, it is conceivable that these macromolecules provide directional cues to the precardiac cell clusters.

The Establishment of External Form for the Heart

The endocardial tube and its epimyocardial mantle are suspended from the roof of the pericardial cavity by the dorsal mesocardium (Fig. 18–12). By the 16-somite stage (day 24), this curtain of tissue has disappeared leaving most of the heart free and movable within the pericardial cavity. The arterial (cranial) and venous (caudal) ends of the heart tube remain fixed in place by the aortic arches and the major veins in the septum transversum, respectively. This arrangement allows the originally straight heart tube to change shape and position as it grows into an adult organ.

A primary factor changing the configuration of the primitive heart is its own rapid elongation within the pericardial cavity. Consequently, the heart is forced into a complex pattern of bends which enhances the regionalization of the cardiac chambers. The details involved in the formation of the cardiac loop are illustrated in Figure 18–17 and Figure 18–18. Note that it is primarily the midpor-

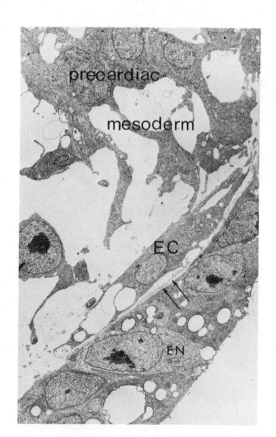

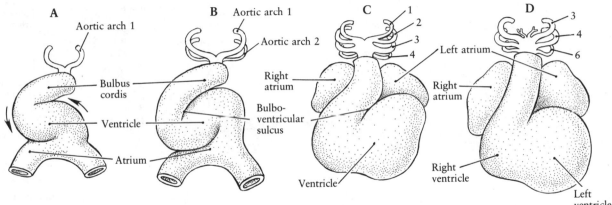

tion of the cardiac tube that undergoes extensive alteration in position.

Initially, the cardiac tube increases in length so much faster than the pericardial cavity that it is thrown into a U-shaped bend (*bulboventricular loop*) to the right (Figs. 18–17 A; 18–18 A). Later, the heart appears as a compound S-shaped loop that nearly fills the pericardial cavity (Fig. 18–13 D; 18–17 B). As the heart tube bends, the bulboventricular portion moves ventrad and caudad so that the ventricle, formerly situated cephalic to the common atrium, is brought to its characteristic adult position posterior to the atrium (Fig. 18–17 C,D). Because the common atrium is bounded below by the bulbus cordis and above by the sinus venosus, it enlarges primarily in the lateral and ventrolateral directions. The result is a pair of sacculations which foreshadows the future, definitive right and left atria. The undilated narrowed portion of the cardiac tube between the atrium and the ventricle is the *common atrioventricular canal* (Fig. 18–19 A). The sinus venosus remains anchored to the transverse septum during cardiac loop formation. It is a thin-walled chamber into which empty the major systemic, vitelline, and umbilical veins (Fig. 18–18 B,C). The sinus quickly becomes differentiated into three regions as its right side, owing to important shifts in the pattern of blood flow returning from the liver, undergoes enlargement (Fig. 18–18 C,D). These are the *right* and *left horns* of the *sinus venosus* and a narrow intervening *transverse portion* of the *sinus venosus*. The opening of the sinus venosus into the atrium by way of the *sinoatrial orifice* is concentrated on the right side of the common atrium (Fig. 18–19 A).

Continued growth of the cardiac tube stimulates several additional alterations in its external form. The proximal part of the bulbus cordis is absorbed into the right side of the common primitive ventricle. Presumably, this is related to a lag in the development

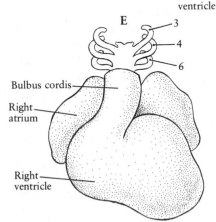

18–17 Ventral views of reconstructions of the hearts of young human embryos during successive stages in cardiac loop formation. (From T. Kramer, 1942. Am. J. Anat. 71, 343.)

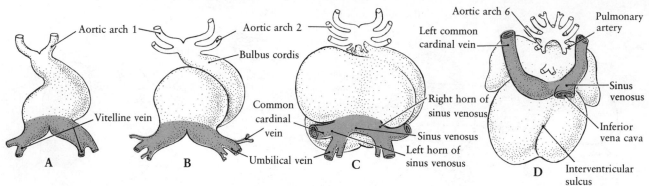

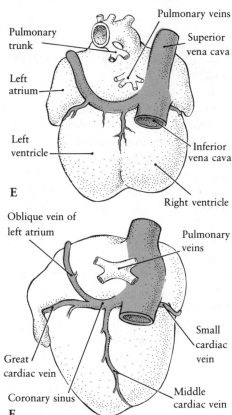

of the wall of the bulboventricular loop marked by the bulboventricular sulcus (Fig. 18–17 C,D). At about the same time the ventral surface of the ventricle shows a distinct, median longitudinal groove or *interventricular sulcus* (Figs. 18–17 C,D; 18–19 A). The sulcus marks the position of an internal, muscular partition beginning to divide the common ventricle into two chambers.

The S-shaped cardiac loop brings about an arrangement of chambers that is observed during cardiogenesis in most vertebrate embryos. In adult cartilaginous and bony fishes, the heart retains this configuration and functions as a single, tubular organ pumping venous blood to the gills for oxygenation. Substitution of lungs for internal gills in air-breathing vertebrates is associated with major internal alterations in heart structure and in the organization of the aortic arch arteries. The introduction of paired lungs into the vertebrate plan of organization requires the heart to act as a double pump, pumping one bloodstream (pulmonary) from the right side of the heart to the lungs and another bloodstream (systemic) from the left side of the heart to the general body circulation by way of the aorta. Conversion of the S-shaped, tubular heart into an elaborately valved, four-chambered, partitioned organ, which effects a complete separation of pulmonary and systemic bloodstreams, is achieved only in birds, mammals, and crocodiles. The amphibians and reptiles have advanced beyond the fishes in the sense that there is some internal subdivision of the atrium and ventricle.

The partitioning of the cardiac tube is certainly one of the most important and dramatic changes observed in the developing heart. Cardiac septa initially appear in the venous end of the heart and subsequently in the arterial end of the heart. They migrate toward the base of the ventricle where their fusion assures proper internal division into right and left functional compartments. One must remember that the heart continues its work of pumping blood despite major reorganization in its internal structure.

Little is known about the mechanisms underlying cardiac looping

18–18 A–F, dorsal views of successive stages in the development of the human heart, showing particularly the changing relations of the sinus venosus. (From Foundations of Embryology by B. Patten and B. Carlson. Copyright © 1974 by McGraw-Hill, Inc. Used with permission of the McGraw-Hill Book Company.)

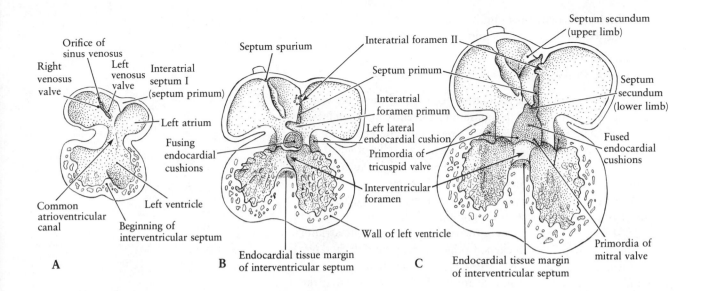

A

B

C

Orifice of sinus venosus

Right venosus valve

Left venosus valve

Interatrial septum I (septum primum)

Left atrium

Fusing endocardial cushions

Common atrioventricular canal

Left ventricle

Beginning of interventricular septum

Septum spurium

Interatrial foramen II

Septum primum

Interatrial foramen primum

Left lateral endocardial cushion

Primordia of tricuspid valve

Interventricular foramen

Wall of left ventricle

Endocardial tissue margin of interventricular septum

Septum secundum (upper limb)

Septum secundum (lower limb)

Fused endocardial cushions

Primordia of mitral valve

Endocardial tissue margin of interventricular septum

18–19 Semischematic drawings of the interior of the heart to show initial steps in partitioning. A, cardiac septa as they appear in human embryo at five weeks; B, cardiac septa as they appear at six weeks. Note that the interatrial foramen primum is nearly closed and the interatrial foramen secundum is beginning to appear; C, the interior of the heart at a stage when the foramen primum is closed and the septum secundum is established. (From B. Patten, 1960. Am. J. Anat. 107, 271.)

and the growth, position, and migration of the cardiac septa. For a number of years, it was assumed that the velocity and pressure of blood flowing through the cardiac tube were responsible for changes in external shape and the determination of where cardiac septa were located. Unfortunately, the design and execution of meaningful experiments on embryos to test the importance of this hypothesis have proved difficult. Early studies by Bacon using the frog showed that the embryonic heart tube when isolated in vitro was capable of curvature despite the absence of circulating blood. Llorca and Gill (1967) claim that in the chick curvature of the isolated heart can only take place in a coelomic cavity and even then its morphogenesis is always imperfect when compared with normal embryos. More recently, Manasek and his colleagues (1972) have concluded that formation of the early cardiac loop (i.e., formation of bulboventricular loop) is due to differences in the shapes of myocardial cells on two sides of the presumptive ventricle. Myocardial cells on the presumptive right or convex side of the heart change from cuboidal to a more flattened, squamous shape. This transformation in cell shape is accompanied by a substantial increase in apical surface area. Since the myocardial cells do not apparently change positions relative to one another, the sudden increase in surface area is accommodated by a change in the shape of the organ. The heart bends to the right. Hence, regional differences in myocardial cell shape and alignment appear to mediate cardiac looping. Factors regulating the rotation of the heart tube and consequently the direction of the looping are still poorly understood. Other studies, particularly by Rychter, have demonstrated that alteration in the bloodstreams passing into the venous end of the heart lead to a variety of disturbances, including septal defects.

Partitioning of the Venous End of the Heart

The venous end of the embryonic heart consists of the sinus venosus, the common atrium, and the common atrioventricular canal (Fig. 18–15). Initially, the sinus venosus opens into the center of the primitive atrium and the right and left horns are about of equal size (Fig. 18–18 C). Progressive enlargement of the right horn results from two left-to-right shunts of blood, which appear during the fourth week of development in human embryos. As this occurs, the sinoatrial opening moves to the right side of the common atrium (Figs. 18–18 D; 18–19 A). Where the orifice opens into the atrium, it is bounded by a pair of thickened ridges termed the *right* and *left venosus valves* (Fig. 18–19 A). These ridges typically merge on the cephalodorsal wall of the atrium to form a projection known as the *septum spurium* (Fig. 18–19 B). As its name implies, the septum spurium plays no direct role in septation of the heart.

At approximately the five-millimeter stage (32 days), a sickle-shaped, sagittal, muscular fold appears in the cranial wall of the atrium (Fig. 18–19 A). This *primary interatrial septum* (*septum primum; interatrial septum I*) grows downward toward the common atrioventricular canal, thereby separating the common atrium into *right* and *left atria* (*auricles*). The space between the free edge of the septum primum and the common atriventricular canal constitutes the *interatrial foramen primum* or *primary interatrial foramen* (Figs. 18–19 B; 18–26 A). It is normally obliterated as the septum primum reaches the dorsal and ventral endocardial cushions (Fig. 18–26 B).

By the time of the appearance of the primary interatrial septum, the dorsal and ventral endocardial cushions have noticeably thickened (Fig. 18–20 A). These fuse together in human embryos of about 38 days to form a sagittal partition known as the *septum intermedium* (Figs. 18–19 B,C; 18–20 B,C; 18–26 B). As a consequence, the common atrioventricular canal is split into the narrow *right* and *left atrioventricular canals* (Figs. 18–19 C; 18–20 C,D).

A very critical event occurs in the development of the human heart just prior to the fusion of the primary interatrial septum with the septum intermedium (Fig. 18–19 C). If the primary interatrial septum were to remain intact after fusion with the cushion complex, the right half of the venous end of the heart would be the only one to receive a substantial return of blood. The left half of the venous end of the heart would receive little because return from the lungs is scanty. To assure that the left atrium, and, indeed, the fu-

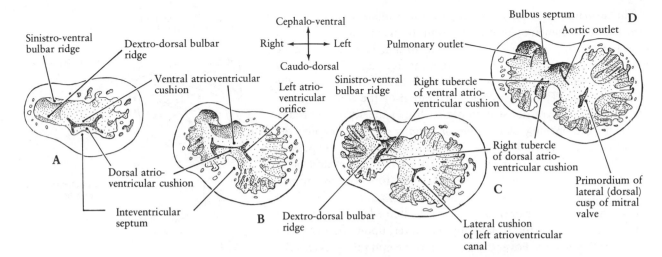

Cephalo-ventral

Right ← → Left

Caudo-dorsal

A — Sinistro-ventral bulbar ridge; Dextro-dorsal bulbar ridge; Ventral atrioventricular cushion; Dorsal atrioventricular cushion; Inteventricular septum

B — Left atrioventricular orifice; Sinistro-ventral bulbar ridge; Dextro-dorsal bulbar ridge

C — Right tubercle of ventral atrioventricular cushion; Right tubercle of dorsal atrioventricular cushion; Lateral cushion of left atrioventricular canal

D — Bulbus septum; Aortic outlet; Pulmonary outlet; Primordium of lateral (dorsal) cusp of mitral valve

ture systemic portion of the heart, receives adequate bloodflow during fetal life, a complicated valvular mechanism develops in the atrial compartment. A number of small perforations appear in the cranial portion of the primary interatrial septum (Fig. 18–19 B). These coalesce and a secondary communication, the *foramen secundum* or *secondary interatrial foramen,* is thus established between the right and left atria (Figs. 18–19 C; 18–26 B). The timing of the formation of the foramen secundum and the fusion of the primary interatrial septum with the dorsal and ventral endocardial cushions is critical. The acceleration of septa fusion or retardation in the formation of the secondary interatrial opening could severely distrub the distribution of blood within the cardiac tube and the eventual division of the common ventricle.

Closure of the primary interatrial foramen is followed by the formation of the second interatrial septum (*secondary interatrial septum* or *septum secundum*) along the right atrial wall between the attachments of the left venosus valve and the primary interatrial septum (Fig. 18–19 C). This fold from the ventrocranial wall is also crescentic-shaped, but its free edge tends to be directed toward the base of the sinoatrial orifice. The difference in the direction of growth of the septum secundum is compared with the septum primum in Figure 18–21. As the septum secundum migrates toward the septum intermedium, its free edge extends beyond the foramen secundum of the primary interatrial septum. A permanent opening, termed the *foramen ovale,* remains in the secondary interatrial septum (Fig. 18–28). Although the foramen ovale becomes smaller during the course of development, it will remain open until after birth (Fig. 18–22).

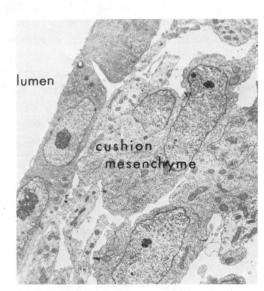

18–20   A–D, formation of the endocardial cushions and their fusion to form the septum intermedium in human embryos. Transverse views posterior to the atrioventricular canal. A, 8.8 mm; B, 11 mm; C, 13 mm; D, 14.5 mm. (From T. Kramer, 1942. Am. J. Anat. 71, 343); E, micrograph of forming endocardial cushion (mesenchyme) in the atrioventricular canal of the chick embryo. (From F. Manasek, 1976. The Cell Surface in Animal Embryogenesis and Development. G. Poste and G. Nicolson, eds. North Holland Publishing Co., New York.)

The structural relationships between the primary interatrial septum and the foramen ovale are important to the one-way passage of blood from the right atrium to the left atrium. Carefully examine Figures 18–22 and 18–28 and note that the free edge of the primary interatrial septum is situated opposite to the gap formed by the foramen ovale. The growth and orientation of the free margin of the secondary interatrial septum are such that the septum partially overrides the opening of the *inferior vena cava*. Functionally, the blood from this vessel becomes split into two streams, one passing directly through the foramen ovale into the left atrium and other into the right atrial chamber. Because of this function, the margin of the septum secundum is often called the *crista dividens*. As blood moves through the foramen ovale, the free, thin edge of the primary interatrial septum is forced laterally. However, upon atrial contraction, this flap is forced over the foramen ovale and thus prevents the regurgitation of blood back into the right atrium. The lower part of the primary interatrial septum is often referred to as the *valve of the foramen ovale*. After birth the cranial edge of the valve of the foramen ovale is pressed against the secondary interatrial septum owing in great measure to the progressive increase in the return of blood from the paired lungs. It fuses with the cephalic portion of the secondary interatrial septum to form the definitive interatrial septum. The foramen ovale is thereby obliterated.

During the partitioning of the common atrium and the common

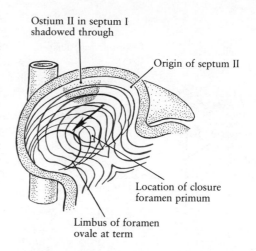

18–21 Schematic drawing showing by a series of contour lines the growth of the septum secundum. The direction of growth of the septum primum is indicated by curved solid black lines. (From B. Patten, 1960. Am. J. Anat. 107, 271.)

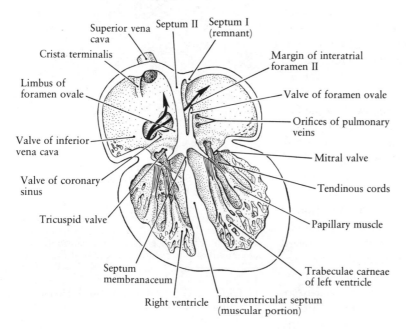

18–22 Semischematic drawing to show the relationships between the two interatrial septa during the latter part of fetal life. Note particularly the arrangement of the lower part of the septum primum. (From Foundations of Embryology by B. Patten and B. Carlson. Copyright © 1974 by McGraw-Hill, Inc. Used with permission of the McGraw-Hill Book Company.)

atrioventricular canal, much of the right horn of the sinus venosus is absorbed into the wall of the right atrium because it fails to keep pace with the rapid growth of the rest of the cardiac tube (Fig. 18–23 A,B). The smooth part of the right atrium or *sinus venarum* is derived from this part of the sinus venosus and is the site into which the major systemic veins empty (Fig. 18–23 B). The left horn dwindles and generally persists only as the stem of the *oblique vein* of the left atrium (Fig. 18–23 B). The transverse portion of the sinus remains as the *coronary sinus,* receiving the oblique vein and other cardiac veins. The loss of the functional importance of the sinus venosus causes the major systemic veins, the *superior vena cava* and the *inferior vena cava,* to open independently into the right atrium.

Important changes also occur in the right and left venosus valves guarding the sinoatrial orifice. The left valve gradually approaches and fuses with the cephalic extremity of the secondary interatrial septum. After becoming a prominent ridge in the right atrium, the right venosus valve becomes reduced and divided into two major components: (1) a cranial part known as the *crista terminalis,* a vertical ridge that separates the sinus venarum from the primitive atrium (Fig. 18–22); and (2) a caudal part that is divided into the *valve of the inferior vena cava,* located to the right of the ostium of the inferior vena cava, and a smaller, *caudal valve of the coronary sinus* (Fig. 18–22).

Thus, the venous limb of the primitive cardiac tube is greatly modified to produce the right and left atria, chambers separated in the adult heart by a continuous muscular interatrial septum fashioned from the embryonic septum primum and septum secundum. The right atrium is formed from the right half of the common atrium, the right half of the right atrioventricular canal, and a portion of the sinus venosus. The left atrium is formed from the left half of the common atrium, the left half of the common atrioventricular canal, and portions of the stems of the pulmonary veins. Most of the inner surface of both atria has a rough, trabeculated appearance due to the presence of thin, muscular projections known as the *pectinate muscles.*

The Atrioventricular Valves

The openings of the right and left atria into their corresponding ventricles are guarded by the *atrioventricular valves* (*tricuspid valve* on the right and *mitral valve* on the left). The flaps comprising these valves arise from localized proliferations of endocardial tissue on the lateral walls of the atrioventricular canal (*lateral endocardial cushions*) and from the dorsal and ventral endocardial cushions

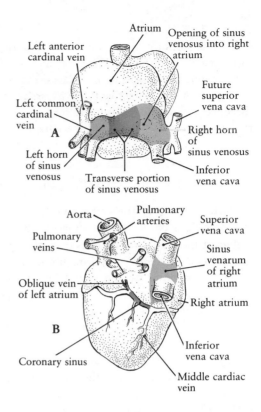

18–23 Diagrams illustrating the fate of the sinus venosus in the human embryo. A, dorsal view of the sinus venosus at about one month; B, dorsal view of the heart after transformation of the sinus venosus. The extraembryonic veins are not shown.

(Fig. 18–19 B,C). These soft cushions become hollowed out on their ventricular sides by the action of blood during ventricular contraction. Each flap differentiates as a mass of fibrous tissue and becomes connected to special muscles of the ventricle (*papillary muscles*) by cords of connective tissue (*chordae tendineae*) (Fig. 18–22). Three flaps or valvular cusps are formed around the right atrioventricular canal and two around the left.

Partitioning of the Arterial Limb of the Heart

The arterial limb of the embryonic heart consists of the ventricle and the bulbus cordis. Partitioning of this part of the heart, as well as that of the truncus arteriosus or *aortic sac* (see below), into pulmonary and systemic compartments occurs concurrently with the internal separation of the venous limb. Division of the arterial limb is very complex because of the rotation of the cardiac partition in the bulbus cordis.

As previously mentioned, the proximal portion of the bulbus cordis is incorporated into the wall of the right ventricle because of the laggard growth of this part of the heart. This part of the embryonic heart is represented in the adult organ by the *conus arteriosus* or *infundibulum* of the right ventricle.

The remainder of the bulbus cordis is divided into two channels, the *aorta* and the *pulmonary trunk,* by a spiral *aorticopulmonary* or *bulbar septum.* The rudiments of this septum are visible throughout the bulbus in human embryos of five millimeters in length. They appear as two prominent, opposed thickenings of subendocardial tissue termed the bulbar ridges (Figs. 18–24; 18–27 A). Similar ridges of tissue are found in the truncus arteriosus and are directly continuous with those of the bulbus cordis. Figure 18–24 B shows the spiral orientation of the bulbar ridges from the distal end to the proximal end of the bulbus cordis. The rotation of the ridges is presumably a reflection of the pattern of bloodstream flow through this part of the heart (Fig. 18–24 G). Proximally, the *right bulbar ridge* projects into the lumen of the ventricle just above the right atrioventricular canal. The *left bulbar ridge* lies opposite to the right one and adjacent to the forming septum of the ventricle (Figs. 18–26 A,B; 18–27 A).

The bulbar ridges by the eighth week have enlarged and fused distally to form the aorticopulmonary septum. It divides the lumen of the bulbus into a pulmonary trunk (dorsal) and a systemic trunk or aorta (ventral) (Figs. 18–24 D,F; 18–27 B,C). Partitioning of the bulbus continues a process initiated in the truncus arteriosus be-

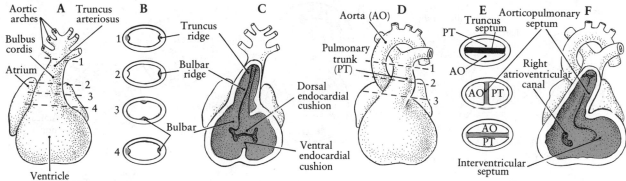

tween the ventral aortic roots of the fourth and sixth pairs of arches and involving the fusion of its own paired longitudinal ridges of tissue (Fig. 18–24 A–F). Fusion of the bulbar ridges along the free edge of the bulbar septum then continues toward the ventricle with the septum following the same spiral course as the rudiments from which it is formed. The result is that the aorta is continuous anteriorly with the third and fourth pair of aortic arches and the pulmonary trunk with the sixth pair of aortic arches (Fig. 18–24 H).

Following the internal, longitudinal subdivision of the bulbus, two furrows on the outer surface pinch in along the plane of the aorticopulmonary septum (Fig. 18–25 A,B). As the furrows deepen and eventually meet, the bulbus cordis disappears as such and is then represented by the pulmonary trunk and the ascending aorta (Fig. 18–25 C). Transverse sections through these vessels show that each is composed of three layers. The innermost layer is the *tunica intima* and differentiates from the embryonic endocardium. Both the middle (*tunica media*) and the outer (*tunica externa*) layers develop from the epimyocardial rudiment.

Division of the primitive ventricle into right and left chambers is first indicated by a ridge of loosely woven muscular fibers or *trabeculae carneae*. Gradually, these muscle fibers become consolidated into a crescentic-shaped muscular fold, the *interventricular septum*, which projects inward from the apex of the ventricle (Fig. 18–19 A,B). Most of the initial increase in length of the muscular interventricular septum results from the dilation of the ventricles on either side of it, a process that produces a furrow on the external surface known as the interventricular sulcus (Fig. 18–19 A,B). The dorsal limb of the interventricular septum extends toward the atrioventricular canal where it fuses with the *right tubercle* of the *dorsal endocardial cushion* (just to the left of the right atrioventricular canal) (Figs. 18–20 C,D; 18–26 A,B). The ventral limb of the parti-

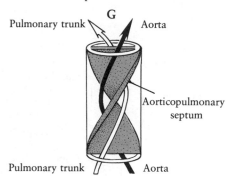

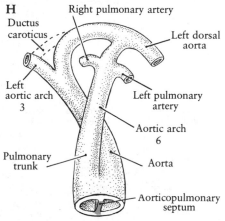

18–24 A series of diagrammatic drawings illustrating the division of the bulbus cordis and the truncus arteriosus. A, ventral view of the human heart at five weeks; B, transverse sections through the levels of the heart as indicated in A to show the truncal and bulbar ridges; C, ventral view of the heart to show the endocardial cushions; D, ventral view of the heart after the initiation of the division of the arterial limb; E, transverse sections through the bulbus (D) to show relationships between the aorticopulmonary septum, the aorta, and the pulmonary trunk; F, ventral view of the heart demonstrating the aorticopulmonary septum; G, diagram illustrating the spiral of the aorticopulmonary septum; H, diagram showing the two major arteries twisting around each other as they leave the heart.

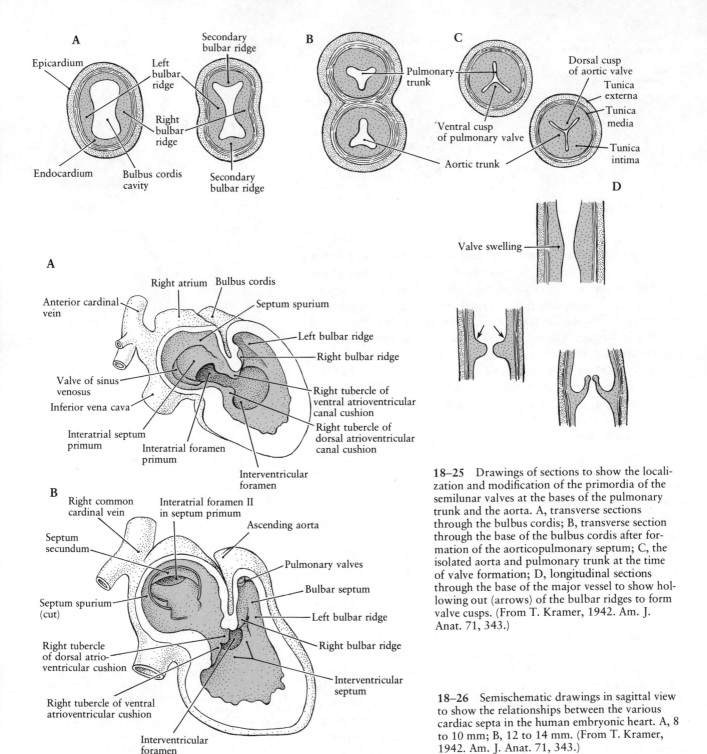

A

Epicardium
Left bulbar ridge
Right bulbar ridge
Endocardium
Bulbus cordis cavity
Secondary bulbar ridge
Secondary bulbar ridge

B

Pulmonary trunk
Aortic trunk

C

Dorsal cusp of aortic valve
Tunica externa
Tunica media
Tunica intima
Ventral cusp of pulmonary valve

D

Valve swelling

A

Anterior cardinal vein
Right atrium
Bulbus cordis
Septum spurium
Left bulbar ridge
Right bulbar ridge
Valve of sinus venosus
Inferior vena cava
Interatrial septum primum
Interatrial foramen primum
Right tubercle of ventral atrioventricular canal cushion
Right tubercle of dorsal atrioventricular canal cushion
Interventricular foramen

B

Right common cardinal vein
Interatrial foramen II in septum primum
Ascending aorta
Septum secundum
Pulmonary valves
Bulbar septum
Septum spurium (cut)
Left bulbar ridge
Right bulbar ridge
Right tubercle of dorsal atrioventricular cushion
Right tubercle of ventral atrioventricular cushion
Interventricular septum
Interventricular foramen

18–25 Drawings of sections to show the localization and modification of the primordia of the semilunar valves at the bases of the pulmonary trunk and the aorta. A, transverse sections through the bulbus cordis; B, transverse section through the base of the bulbus cordis after formation of the aorticopulmonary septum; C, the isolated aorta and pulmonary trunk at the time of valve formation; D, longitudinal sections through the base of the major vessel to show hollowing out (arrows) of the bulbar ridges to form valve cusps. (From T. Kramer, 1942. Am. J. Anat. 71, 343.)

18–26 Semischematic drawings in sagittal view to show the relationships between the various cardiac septa in the human embryonic heart. A, 8 to 10 mm; B, 12 to 14 mm. (From T. Kramer, 1942. Am. J. Anat. 71, 343.)

tion merges with the *right tubercle* of the *ventral endocardial cushion* (just to the right of the left atrioventricular canal) (Figs. 18–20 C,D; 18–26 A,B). The space bounded by the free edge of the interventricular septum and the fused endocardial cushions of the atrioventricular canal is the *interventricular foramen* (Fig. 18–26 A,B).

In contrast to the atrium, where closure between the right and left sides is delayed until birth, the interventricular foramen is rapidly obliterated so that by eight weeks there is little evidence of communication between the right and left ventricles. Closure of the space along the anterior margin of the interventricular septum is a complex process. It apparently results from the rapid growth of the ventricular cavities and the proliferation and active migration of pliable endocardial tissues from several sources, including the margin of the interventricular septum itself.

The details of the final steps in the partitioning of the ventricle are illustrated in Figure 18–27. Cells proliferated from the right side of the fused dorsal and ventral endocardial cushions move ventrally and caudally along the free margin of the interventricular septum, thus reducing the craniocaudal extent of the interventricular foramen. Simultaneously, the right bulbar ridge enlarges, fuses with the right tubercle of the ventral endocardial cushion, and then migrates ventrocaudally and to the left.

This effectively occludes the communication between the right atrium and the common ventricle through the ventral part of the atrioventricular canal. Similarly, the left bulbar ridge enlarges, fuses with the right tubercle of the dorsal cushion, and then migrates dorsocaudally and to the right. This effectively occludes the communication between the left atrium and the common ventricle through the dorsal part of the atrioventricular canal. The two bulbar ridges then fuse with each other and with the endocardial tissue along the margin of the interventricular septum to close the interventricular foramen. These activities join the right atrioventricular canal with the right ventricle and the pulmonary trunk, and the left atrioventricular canal with the left ventricle and the ascending aorta.

The definitive interventricular septum is thus composed of two sections. The muscular part originates from the coalescence of numerous muscular trabeculae. The base of the interventricular partition is initially formed by the soft endocardial tissue of the bulbar ridges and the endocardial cushions. This endocardial tissue gradually becomes converted into fibrous connective tissue to form the membranous part of the interventricular septum (the *pars membranacea septi*).

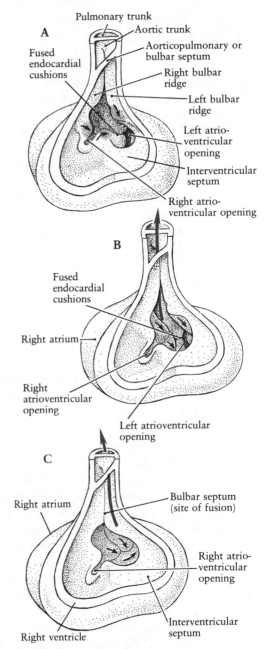

18–27   A series of drawings illustrating closure of the interventricular foramen and formation of the membranous part of the interventricular septum. A, division of the bulbus cordis and fusion of the atrioventricular cushions; B, reduction in the size of the interventricular foramen by the proliferation of endocardial tissues; C, completion of the bulbar and interventricular septa and closure of the interventricular foramen. (After W. Hamilton and H. Mossman, 1972. Human Embryology. Macmillan Press, London.)

Semilunar Valves of the Aorta
and Pulmonary Trunk

Valves develop in the arterial limb of the heart between the ventricles and the bases of their associated arterial vessels. These arise as specializations of bulbar endocardial tissue. In addition to the main bulbar ridges, two smaller asscessory ridges appear beneath the endocardium to extend throughout most of the bulbus (Fig. 18–25 A). After the physical separation of the bulbus along the aorticopulmonary septum, the base of each vessel contains one of the accessory ridges and half of each of the larger ridges (Fig. 18–25 B,C). Thus, three endocardial swellings guard the orifice of both the aorta and pulmonary artery. They soon become hollowed out on their distal sides to form the three cusps of the *semilunar valves* (Fig. 18–25 D).

The Cardiac Wall and the
Conducting System

The primitive cardiac tube is initially composed of two layers, an inner endocardium and an outer epimyocardium. These layers are separated by the relative large extracellular ground substance which is rich in glycosaminoglycans. As the heart becomes more convoluted, the cardiac jelly becomes thinner and thereby permits a closer approximation between the endocardium and the epimyocardium. Indeed, the endocardium even appears to penetrate the innermost layer of the developing epimyocardium.

Rather early in embryonic life, the epimyocardium differentiates and its cells are initially all functional cardiac myocytes. In most vertebrates, cardiac function begins shortly after the primitive streak stage. It is clearly associated with the acquisition of organized myofibrils by the cardiac muscle cells. Hence, the biochemical and morphological changes that lead to a functionally active heart must take place with great rapidity. Manasek (1976) states that all other noncardiac muscle cell types, such as those contributing to the connective tissue framework of the cardiac skeleton (fibroblasts), the epithelial and connective tissues of the epicardium, and the vascular smooth muscle tissue, are added during the course of heart development after the cytodifferentiation of cardiac muscle. Cell heterogeneity, therefore, in the outer embryonic heart layer increases during ontogeny as nonmuscle cell types assist in the architectural design of the heart. The cardiac muscle is initially a single, continuous layer throughout the heart tube. Gradually, however, it differentiates into a thin, superficial layer of dense muscle and a thick, spongy layer of loosely arranged muscular trabeculae. Spaces be-

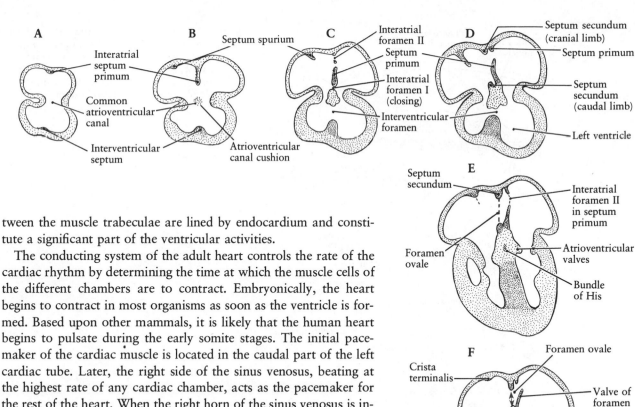

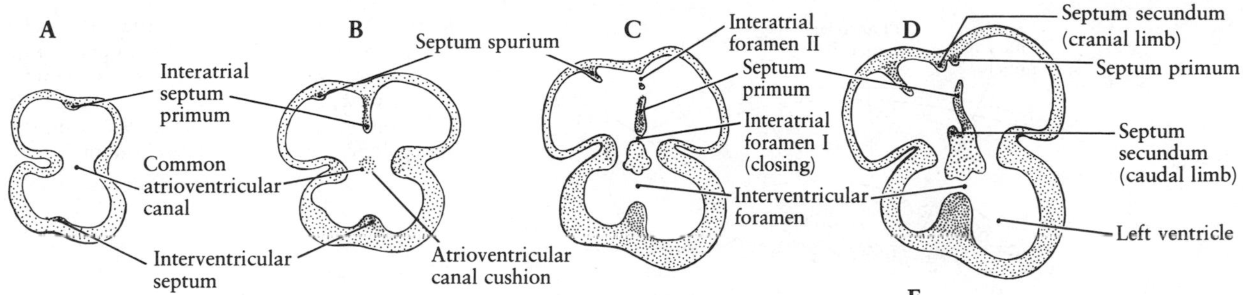
A
B
C
D
Septum spurium
Interatrial
septum
primum
Common
atrioventricular
canal
Interventricular
septum
Atrioventricular
canal cushion
Interatrial
foramen II
Septum
primum
Interatrial
foramen I
(closing)
Interventricular
foramen
Septum secundum
(cranial limb)
Septum primum
Septum
secundum
(caudal limb)
Left ventricle

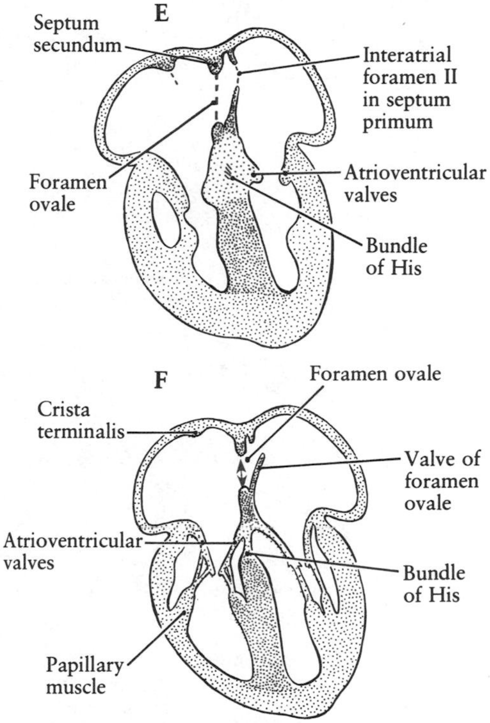
E
Septum
secundum
Interatrial
foramen II
in septum
primum
Foramen
ovale
Atrioventricular
valves
Bundle
of His
F
Foramen ovale
Crista
terminalis
Valve of
foramen
ovale
Atrioventricular
valves
Bundle
of His
Papillary
muscle

18–28 A–F, a series of drawings of human hearts to show the rate of progress of the cardiac septa. Frontal views. (From Foundations of Embryology by B. Patten and B. Carlson. Copyright © 1974 by McGraw-Hill, Inc. Used with permission of McGraw-Hill Book Company.)

tween the muscle trabeculae are lined by endocardium and constitute a significant part of the ventricular activities.

The conducting system of the adult heart controls the rate of the cardiac rhythm by determining the time at which the muscle cells of the different chambers are to contract. Embryonically, the heart begins to contract in most organisms as soon as the ventricle is formed. Based upon other mammals, it is likely that the human heart begins to pulsate during the early somite stages. The initial pacemaker of the cardiac muscle is located in the caudal part of the left cardiac tube. Later, the right side of the sinus venosus, beating at the highest rate of any cardiac chamber, acts as the pacemaker for the rest of the heart. When the right horn of the sinus venosus is incorporated into the right atrium, the pacemaker function is also transferred to this part of the heart in the form of the *sinoatrial node*. Some cells from the left wall of the sinus venosus become located in the base of the interatrial septum just anterior to the opening of the coronary sinus. These cells, together with special cells of the atrioventricular canal, make up the *atrioventricular node* and the *bundle of His* (Fig. 18–28 E,F). This specialized tissue is normally the only conducting pathway from the atria to the ventricles. A band of connective tissue grows in from the epicardium and subsequently interrupts muscle layer continuity between atria and ventricles.

Nerve fibers from both vagus nerves and sympathetic chains subsequently innervate the sinoatrial node, the atrioventricular node, and the bundle of His. Generally, the histological features of these various components of the conducting system cannot be delineated until birth.

THE ARTERIES

The primary arteries of the early vertebrate embryo are the *right* and the *left primitive aortae*. Each of these vessels can be readily

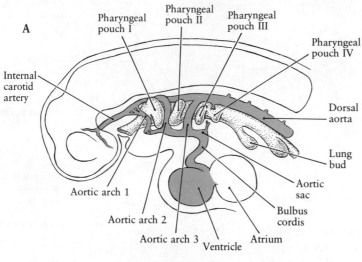

A

Pharyngeal pouch I
Pharyngeal pouch II
Pharyngeal pouch III
Pharyngeal pouch IV
Internal carotid artery
Dorsal aorta
Lung bud
Aortic sac
Aortic arch 1
Aortic arch 2
Aortic arch 3
Ventricle
Atrium
Bulbus cordis

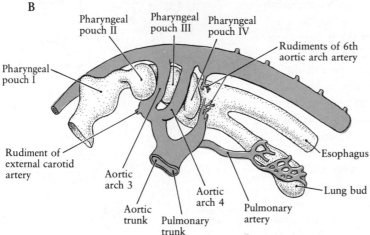

B

Pharyngeal pouch II
Pharyngeal pouch III
Pharyngeal pouch IV
Rudiments of 6th aortic arch artery
Pharyngeal pouch I
Rudiment of external carotid artery
Aortic arch 3
Aortic trunk
Pulmonary trunk
Aortic arch 4
Pulmonary artery
Esophagus
Lung bud

18–29   Drawings from reconstructed models of human embryos to show the development and transformation of the aortic arches. A, 4 mm, left-side view; B, 5–11 mm, left-side view. (After W. Hamilton and H. Mossman, 1972. Human Embryology. Macmillan Press, London.)

divided into three regions in early somite embryos (Fig. 18–4): (1) a short ventral segment continuous caudally with the endocardial tube of the heart; (2) a primitive branchial or aortic arch artery; and (3) a long dorsal segment (*dorsal aortae*), which distributes blood from the heart to various organs chiefly by way of the inter-segmental arteries, the vitelline arteries, and the umbilical arteries.

Following the formation of the primitive tubular heart, the short ventral sections of the primitive aortae fuse to form the midventral *truncus arteriosus* (Fig. 18–29). The truncus at its cranial end later becomes substantially dilated into the *aortic sac* (Fig. 18–29 A). From the cephalic portion of the aortic sac, the first pair of aortic arches bends around the rostral part of the pharynx to join the paired dorsal aortae. Successive pairs of aortic arches will differentiate in the mesenchyme of the visceral arches as the embryo continues to develop (Fig. 18–29 A–B).

The complicated adult plan of arteries is derived from this arrangement of truncus arteriosus, paired aortic arches, and paired dorsal aortae. Vertebrates such as teleost and elasmobranch fishes, in which respiration is at the level of the pharynx (i.e., gills), retain this simple arrangement of blood vessels. Each aortic arch artery, interrupted by the capillary network of the gill, becomes divided into *afferent* and *efferent branchial arteries*. Behind the pharynx, the dorsal aortae fuse into a single, median vessel, the *dorsal aorta*. The introduction of pulmonary respiration and the consequent partitioning of the heart results in major changes in the symmetrical pattern of embryonic arteries, particularly in higher vertebrates.

The Pharyngeal (Aortic) Arch Arteries

Six pairs of aortic arches, connecting the truncus arteriosus (or *ventral aorta*) with the dorsal aortae, develop in most vertebrate embryos. However, the entire set of aortic arch arteries are not all present at the same time. Generally, the first two pairs of arches involute and disappear rather quickly.

In human embryos, the primitive aortic arch pattern is laid down within the first four weeks of development. It is transformed into the basic adult arrangement of arteries during the period between six to eight weeks. The first and second pairs of aortic arches appear between the third and fourth weeks, but subsequently undergo regression and involution. Their atrophy is probably associated with the relative caudal migration of the heart and the aortic sac, making them less directly accessible to blood flow than the third and fourth pairs of aortic arches immediately behind them (Fig. 18–29 B). There is some evidence that parts of the first pair of arteries contribute to the *maxillary arteries* and the second pair to the *stapedial arteries*. The ventral portions of the first two aortic arches may also contribute to the *external carotid arteries* (Fig. 18–29 B).

The early degeneration of the first two pairs of aortic arches, as well as that of the fifth pair of arches (these appear in about 50 percent of embryos), leaves only the third, fourth, and sixth pairs along with their dorsal and ventral roots to play important roles in the construction of adult vessels (Figs. 18–29 B; 18–30). On either side, the portion of the dorsal aorta between the third and fourth arches (called the *ductus caroticus*) eventually disappears (Fig. 18–29 B). The third pair of aortic arches with contributions from the short cephalic extensions of the dorsal aortae form the primitive *internal carotid arteries* (Fig. 18–30 A,B). The *external carotid arteries* originate as vascular sprouts from the bases of the third arches. Con-

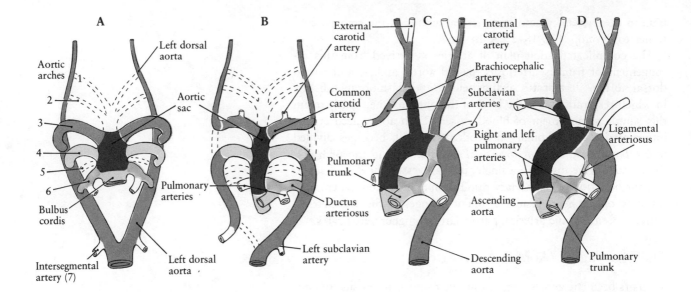

A

Aortic arches 1
2
3
4
5
6
Bulbus cordis
Intersegmental artery (7)
Left dorsal aorta
Aortic sac
Pulmonary arteries
Left dorsal aorta

B

External carotid artery
Common carotid artery
Pulmonary trunk
Ductus arteriosus
Left subclavian artery

C

Internal carotid artery
Brachiocephalic artery
Subclavian arteries
Right and left pulmonary arteries
Ascending aorta
Descending aorta

D

Ligamental arteriosus
Pulmonary trunk

tributions to these arteries are probably made by the vascular channels produced by the degeneration of the first two pairs of arches. The common stem of each third aortic arch, caudal to the origin of the external carotid artery, remains as the *common carotid artery* (Fig. 18–30 B).

Both of the fourth pairs of aortic arches persist, but their contribution to the adult organization of arteries is quite different. On the right, a ventral portion of the aortic sac elongates into the *brachiocephalic* or *innominate artery;* the latter serves as a common trunk for the right common carotid and right subclavian vessels (Fig. 18–30 C). The right subclavian artery is formed chiefly from the right fourth aortic arch and a short segment of the dorsal aorta (Fig. 18–30 B,C). Therefore, much of the right dorsal aorta, from its point of junction with the left dorsal aorta to the subclavian artery, undergoes regression and disappears. Concurrently, the portion of the right sixth aortic arch beyond the origin of the right pulmonary artery drops out. On the left side, the fourth aortic arch is retained as a major component of the systemic channel leading from the heart to the dorsal aorta. With contributions from the ascending aorta (i.e., divided truncus and bulbus) and the left dorsal aorta, it persists as the *arch of the aorta*. It is interesting to note that the right half of the fourth arch is retained in the bird as the main route to the dorsal aorta. As discussed later in this chapter, the *left subclavian artery* originates as an enlargement of a segmental branch of the left dorsal aorta near its union with the left fourth aortic arch. It is equivalent to only the distalmost part of the right subclavian artery.

18–30 Diagram summarizing the transformation of the aortic sac, bulbus cordis, aortic arches, and dorsal aortae into the adult arterial pattern. A, aortic arches at six weeks; B, seven weeks; C, eight weeks; D, the arterial vessels of a six-month-old infant. Broken lines indicate vessels that normally disappear.

The pulmonary or sixth arches begin as vascular sprouts from the dorsal aorta and the aortic sac (Fig. 18–29 B). The dorsal rudiment taps the extension from the aortic sac in such a way that a distal segment of the latter remains as the *pulmonary artery*. The right sixth arch loses its connection with the dorsal aorta, leaving its proximal part as the stem of the right pulmonary artery. The distal part of the left sixth arch persists as a shunt (the *ductus arteriosus* or *duct of Botallo*) until its atrophy at birth (Fig. 18–30 C,D). The remainder of the arch then constitutes the stem of the left pulmonary artery (Fig. 18–30 D).

The transformation of the aortic arches occurs simultaneously with the internal subdivision of the truncus arteriosus and bulbus cordis. The result is that the aorta opens into the third and fourth aortic arches (or its derivatives) while the pulmonary trunk is continuous with the left sixth aortic arch.

Branches of the Dorsal Aorta

Even before the dorsal aorta becomes a single, median vessel behind the pharynx, each of the endothelial tubes that contribute to its formation gives rise to several major sets of tributaries. A schematic arrangement of these vessels through the trunk of the embryo is shown in Figure 18–31. The most conspicuous of these vessels are the *dorsal, somatic intersegmental arteries*. These pass between adjacent or successive somites to become continuous with vascular plexuses developing in the somites, the lateral body wall, and the neural tube. *Lateral arteries* arise from the sides of the descending aorta and supply structures associated with the intermediate mesoderm. *Ventral, splanchnic arteries* are distributed to the gut and its accessory organs such as the yolk sac and allantois.

The dorsal intersegmental arteries initially arise as a series of dorsolateral, symmetrically arranged vessels extending from the level of the occipital somites to the somites of the sacral region. Although each artery is primitively associated with the neural tube, it gradually sends secondary branches out as adjacent structures grow and are added. For convenience, two tributaries of the original artery can be identified (Fig. 18–31). A dorsal tributary (or *dorsal ramus*) passes caudally between successive ribs and transverse processes supplying vessels to the spinal cord, the dorsal musculature, and the skin. A ventrolateral tributary (the *ventral ramus*) curves around the body wall, courses along the primary branches of the spinal nerves, and termintes ventrally in an anastomosis with the same vessel of the opposite side. The ventral branches of the intersegmental arteries persist in the thoracic and lumbar regions of the

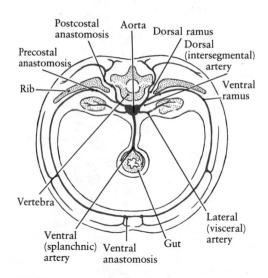

18–31 A schematic drawing in transverse view to illustrate the arrangement of the branches of the dorsal aorta. Longitudinal anastomoses are indicated as beadlike enlargements.

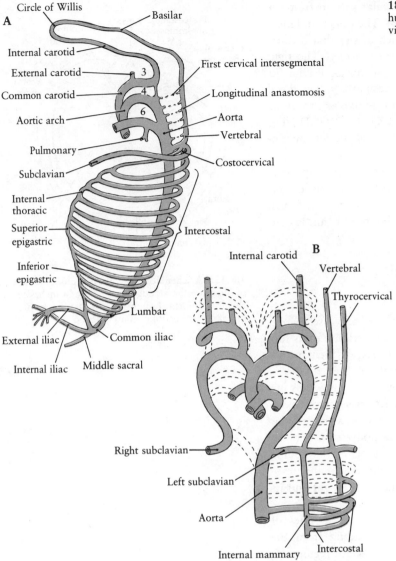

A

Circle of Willis

Basilar

Internal carotid

First cervical intersegmental

External carotid

3

Common carotid

4

Longitudinal anastomosis

6

Aorta

Aortic arch

Vertebral

Pulmonary

Costocervical

Subclavian

Internal thoracic

Superior epigastric

Intercostal

Inferior epigastric

Lumbar

External iliac

Common iliac

Internal iliac

Middle sacral

B

Internal carotid

Vertebral

Thyrocervical

Right subclavian

Left subclavian

Aorta

Internal mammary

Intercostal

18–32 Derivatives of the branches of the human dorsal aorta. A, left-side view; B, ventral view showing origin of several cranial arteries.

embryo as the serially arranged *intercostal* and *lumbar arteries* (Fig. 18–32).

At the occipital, cervical, and sacral regions of the embryo, there is an extensive reorganization of the intersegmental arteries. With definition of the neck and the forelimbs and with the loss of the ductus caroticus, longitudinal vascular connections appear just dorsal to the ribs (*postcostal anastomoses*) to join together the intersegmental arteries of the cervical region (Fig. 18–32). The roots of the first six cervical arteries then degenerate, leaving the dorsal branch of the seventh intersegmental artery and its longitudinal anastomosis on either side as the *vertebral artery* (Fig. 18–32 B).

The vertebral arteries then extend cranially and bend mesially just beneath the metencephalon. Here the vertebrals fuse to form the single, *basilar artery* (Figs. 18–32 A; 18–33). At approximately the level of the diencephalon, branches of the basilar artery unite with the internal carotid arteries to form the *circular arteriosus of Willis.* Hence, the carotid and the vertebral-basilar circulations are two separate routes of blood supply to the brain.

With the caudal descent of the heart and the elongation of the neck, the seventh intersegmental artery comes to lie opposite the dorsal end of the fourth pair of aortic arches (Fig. 18–30 B). Conveniently, this is the level at which the anterior limb bud begins to take shape during the fifth week of human development. It is not surprising, therefore, to find that the seventh intersegmental artery on either side enlarges to become the subclavian artery. Beyond the vertebral artery, the subclavian continues into the forelimb as the *axillary artery.*

The striking dissimilarity in the origin of the right and left subclavian arteries has been referred to under the aortic arches. It is directly related to the fate of the fourth pair of aortic arches. Since the left fourth arch is retained, the left subclavian artery is formed solely from the seventh' intersegmental artery. On the right, the aorta drops out behind the seventh intersegmental artery, leaving the right subclavian artery to be fashioned from the latter plus the portion annexed from the right fourth aortic arch.

Several additional branches from the subclavian arteries provide insight into the construction of other arteries. Longitudinal anastomoses between the tips of the ventral branches of intersegmental arteries in the thoracic and lumbar regions bring about the formation of the *internal thoracic (internal mammary), superior epigastric,* and *inferior epigastric arteries* (Fig. 18–32 A). The *thyrocervical arteries* develop on either side from longitudinal anastomoses below the ribs (*precostal anastomoses*) and between ventral rami of intersegmental arteries anterior to the subclavian arteries. The *costocervical arteries* develop in similar fashion but from the three ventral rami immediately caudal to the subclavian arteries.

The lateral branches of the dorsal aorta supply the organ derivatives of the intermediate mesoderm. Initially, these blood vessels develop in relationship to the paired mesonephric kidneys and are quite numerous (Fig. 18–34 A). Regression of the mesonephroi reduces the number of lateral arteries. They are represented in the adult by the *inferior phrenic, suprarenal, renal,* and *internal spermatic* or *internal ovarian arteries* (Fig. 18–34 B).

Of the three major types of branches of the dorsal aorta, the ven-

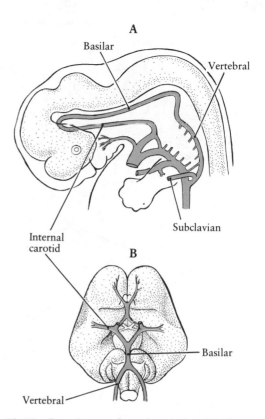

18–33 Drawings to show the relationships between the internal carotid and vertebral arteries. A, 6 weeks, left-side view; B, 14 weeks, ventral view of brain. (After L. Arey, 1974. Developmental Anatomy. W. B. Saunders Company, Philadelphia.)

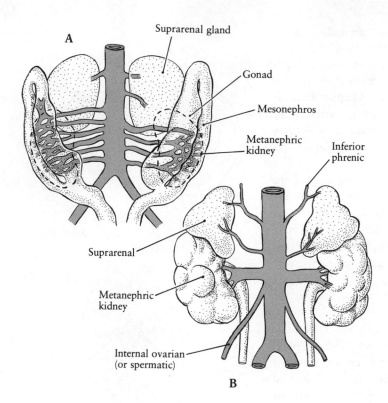

A

Suprarenal gland

Gonad

Mesonephros

Metanephric kidney

Inferior phrenic

Suprarenal

Metanephric kidney

Internal ovarian (or spermatic)

B

18–34 Ventral views of the lateral branches of the human aorta at seven weeks (A) and birth (B).

tral ones are the least segmental in nature. They are primitively represented by the paired *vitelline (omphalomesenteric) arteries* to the yolk sac and the paired *umbilical (allantoic) arteries* to the allantois (Fig. 18–35 A). Fusion of the dorsal aortae into a single vessel stimulates the consolidation of vitelline vessels into single, ventral blood vessels. Subsequently, three major arterial trunks, which pass by way of the dorsal mesentery to the gut, are visible. These are the *coeliac artery* (to stomach, duodenum, liver, pancreas, and spleen), the *superior mesenteric artery* (to small intestine and part of large intestine), and the *inferior mesenteric artery* (to the descending colon, sigmoid colon, and rectum) (Fig. 18–35 C). It has been suggested that these three arteries probably represent the original splanchnic vessels of the seventh cervical, third thoracic, and fifth thoracic segments, respectively.

The umbilical arteries are established very early in development and accompany the outgrowth of the allantois. As the embryo increases in length, these blood vessels, passing through the umbilical cord to the placenta, migrate caudally to the lower lumbar region. Here, on either side, an anastomosis forms between the umbilical artery and the fifth lumbar intersegmental artery.

The root of each umbilical artery then regresses, leaving the lumbar intersegmental artery to form the stem of the definitive umbilical artery. When at birth the placental circulation ceases, the umbilical arteries beyond the embryo proper begin to atrophy. Within the embryo, the stem of each umbilical artery is retained as the *common iliac artery* (Fig. 18–35 B). Beyond the origin of the *external iliac artery,* which is a new vessel supplying the hindlimb bud, the umbilical artery persists as the *internal iliac artery* (Fig. 18–35 B).

Caudal to the level of the umbilical arteries, the dorsal aorta becomes diminished in size. It continues toward the tail as the slender *caudal artery* or *middle sacral artery.*

Both the anterior and posterior limb buds are well established in human embryos of three days. Each limb bud is a simple swelling of ectoderm which encloses closely packed cells originating from the adjacent mesoderm. As each appendage bud enlarges, it acquires a vascular plexus supplied by several intersegmental branches of the dorsal aorta. In the case of the forelimb, the lateral branch of the seventh cervical intersegmental artery forms the *axillary artery.* The axillary artery is initially continued into the upper arm as the *brachial artery* and into the forearm as the *interosseous artery* (Fig. 18–36 A). The most prominent vessels of the forearm, the *radial* and *ulnar arteries,* arise as branches of the brachial artery.

The main artery of the early hindlimb is the *sciatic artery* (Fig. 18–36 B). It accompanies the sciatic nerve of the lower extremity and originates as a branch from the future internal iliac artery. Subsequently, this vessel is largely replaced by the *femoral artery,* which springs from the external iliac artery. The sciatic artery is reduced to the *inferior gluteal artery* (proximally) and the *popliteal* and *peroneal arteries* (distally). The major vessels of the foot, the *anterior* and *posterior tibial arteries,* are specializations of the sciatic and femoral arteries, respectively.

THE VEINS

The veins of the early amniote embryo can easily be grouped into three systems (Fig. 18–5): (1) the vitelline system consisting of the right and left *vitelline veins (omphalomesenteric veins),* which arise in the splanchnic mesoderm of the yolk sac; (2) the umbilical system consisting of the right and left *umbilical veins (allantoic veins),* which drain the capillaries of the chorionic villi or allantois; and (3) the cardinal system, which initially consists of the *anterior* and *posterior cardinal* veins. Subsequently, paired *subcardinal* and *supracardinal veins* appear to supplement and gradually replace the postcardinal veins by participating in the formation of the inferior vena cava.

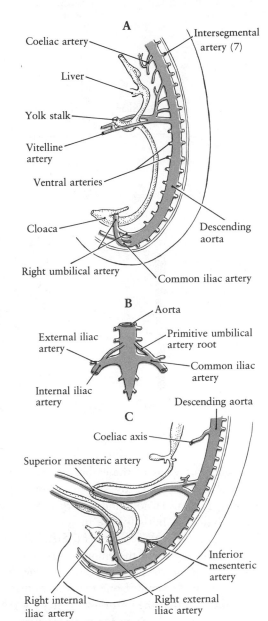

18–35 Derivatives of the ventral branches of the human aorta. A, 5 mm, right-side view; B, 5 mm, ventral view of the terminal end of the aorta; C, 9 mm, right-side view.

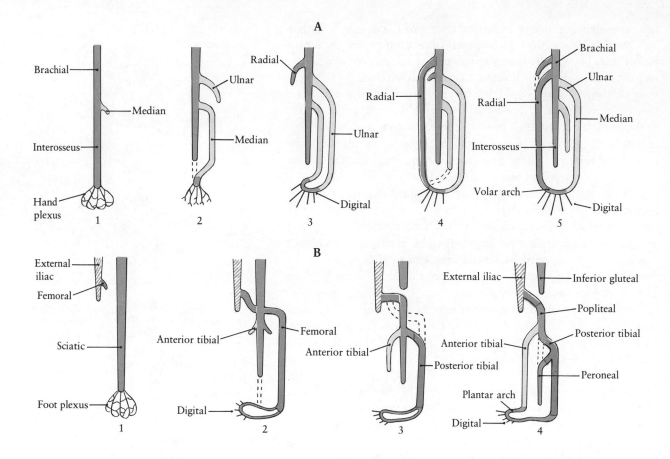

A

1 Brachial / Median / Interosseus / Hand plexus

2 Radial / Ulnar / Median

3 Radial / Ulnar / Digital

4 Radial

5 Brachial / Ulnar / Radial / Interosseus / Median / Volar arch / Digital

B

1 External iliac / Femoral / Sciatic / Foot plexus

2 Anterior tibial / Femoral / Digital

3 Anterior tibial / Posterior tibial

4 External iliac / Inferior gluteal / Popliteal / Anterior tibial / Posterior tibial / Peroneal / Plantar arch / Digital

18–36 Stages in the development of the arteries of the human arm (A) and leg (B). (From L. Arey, 1974. Developmental Anatomy. W. B. Saunders Company, Philadelphia.)

Most of the veins of the embryo arise as capillary plexuses that increase in complexity by sprouting and anastomosing with adjacent plexuses. Fusion and enlargement give rise to fewer but larger channels. Initially, the major vessels of the venous system show a symmetrical arrangement. Striking alterations, particularly in the trunk region of the embryo, substantially modify this primitive organization of the veins. Such changes in the vascular pattern are easy to understand if one remembers that the young vessels are plexiform and that the natural tendency for the blood is to seek the most direct route back to the heart. Central to giving shape to the final, asymmetrical venous pattern in mammalian embryos are two dramatic shifts in the position and direction of blood flow. The first is a left-to-right shunt of blood that results from the transformation of the vitelline and umbilical veins within the liver. The second is a left-to-right shunt of blood brought about by an oblique cross-connection between the left and right anterior cardinal veins. With the right half of the atrium designed to receive blood of the systemic

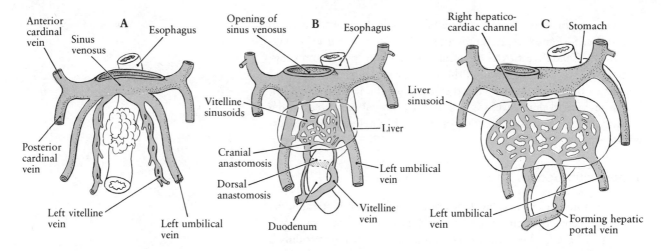

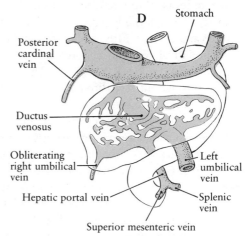

18–37 A series of schematic drawings (A–D) to show the transformation of the vitelline and umbilical veins within the developing liver.

circulation, there is a distinct tendency to emphasize those venous channels on the right side of the embryo.

Transformation of the Vitelline Veins

The fate of the vitelline veins, as with the umbilical veins, is intimately tied to the growth and differentiation of the liver. The paired vitelline veins initially pass on either side of the anterior intestinal portal and course through the septum transversum to empty into the sinus venosus (Fig. 18–37 A). The continuity is interrupted by the growth ventrally of the liver primordium. The endothelium of the two vessels breaks up into the primitive *hepatic sinusoids* of the liver (Fig. 18–37 B). The stems of the vitelline vessels between the liver and the sinus venosus are then retained as the *right* and *left hepatic veins (hepaticocardiac channels)* (Fig. 18–37 B,C). The right hepatic vein will eventually enlarge and contribute to the proximal end of the inferior vena cava.

The distal segments of the paired vitelline veins become joined together by three cross anastomoses (cranial, middle, caudal) with the middle connection lying dorsal to the duodenum (Fig. 18–37 B). When the stomach and duodenum elongate and rotate from their original midsagittal position, the most direct route to the liver for the venous blood is not by way of the original right and left vitelline veins, but rather from one vessel to the other via the interconnecting anastomoses (Fig. 18–37 C). The blood from the right vitelline vein tends to flow across the caudal (ventral) anastomosis to the left vitelline vein, and then across the middle interconnecting plexus to the hepatic end of the persistent part of the right vitelline vein. The intervening portions of the two vitelline vessels drop out, leaving a composite, S-shaped vessel known as the *hepatic portal vein* (Fig. 18–37 D). Caudally, it extends to the union of the splenic and superior mesenteric veins. Although the *superior mesenteric vein* would appear to be represented by the distal part of the left vitelline vein, it is a new vessel that develops in situ in the dorsal mesentery of the intestinal loop. The distalmost segments of the vitelline veins regress with decline of the yolk sac.

Transformation of the Umbilical Veins

As the primitive right and left lobes of the liver expand laterally, the umbilical veins become enmeshed and broken up into sinusoids (Fig. 18–37 B,C). The stems of the umbilical veins persist for only a short time as blood returning from the placenta is progressively diverted through the hepatic sinusoids in its return to the heart. By approximately the fifth week of human development, the entire right umbilical vein and the proximal stem of the left umbilical vein have dropped out (Fig. 18–37 D). The left umbilical vein then continues throughout fetal life as the major blood vessel carrying oxygenated blood from the placenta toward the heart.

Initially, the blood from the left umbilical vein crosses the liver into the sinusoids formed by the right proximal vitelline vein. This route becomes very circuitous as the right lobe of the liver continues to enlarge. Gradually, therefore, the hepatic sinusoids between the point of entry of the left vitelline vein into the liver and the right hepatic vein enlarge and merge to form a large intrahepatic channel known as the *ductus venosus* (Fig. 18–37 D). The ductus venosus passes into the enlarging right horn of the sinus venosus by way of the right hepatic vein. A sphincter mechanism in the ductus venosus regulates the flow of umbilical blood into the liver.

Formation of the Superior Vena Cava

The right and left anterior cardinal veins are the main venous drainage channels from the cranial and neck regions of the early embryo (Fig. 18–5). Each runs caudally to join the corresponding posterior cardinal vein at the level of the common cardinal vein. Frequently, the cephalic portion of the anterior cardinal vein is termed the *primary head vein* because it eventually receives smaller vessels from the deeper (*cerebral veins*) and more superficial (*dural sinuses*) parts of the brain.

With definition of the neck region and descent of the heart, the anterior cardinal veins become elongated. At approximately eight

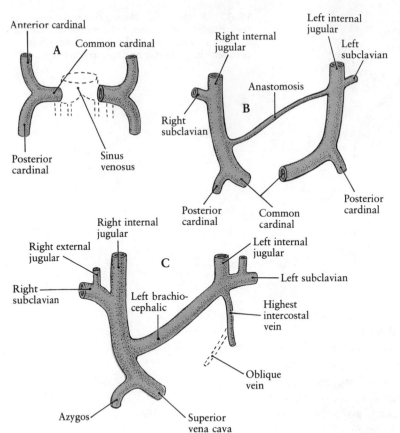

Anterior cardinal

A

Common cardinal

Posterior cardinal

Sinus venosus

Left internal jugular

Right internal jugular

Left subclavian

Anastomosis

B

Right subclavian

Posterior cardinal

Common cardinal

Posterior cardinal

Right internal jugular

Right external jugular

C

Right subclavian

Left brachio-cephalic

Left internal jugular

Left subclavian

Highest intercostal vein

Oblique vein

Azygos

Superior vena cava

18–38   Transformation of the anterior and posterior cardinal veins in the human embryo. A, six weeks; B, eight weeks; C, adult.

weeks of development, an oblique, transverse anastomosis joins the left anterior cardinal to the base of the right anterior cardinal vein (Fig. 18–38 A,B). The proximal part of the left anterior cardinal then regresses to persist as part of the *highest intercostal vein* (Fig. 18–38 C). The left common cardinal vein, no longer an important vessel in the return of blood, contributes to the formation of the *oblique vein* of the left atrium. The intercardinal anastomosis itself forms the *left brachiocephalic vein* (Fig. 18–38 C).

The right common cardinal vein and the base of the right anterior cardinal vein (to the union with the left brachiocephalic vein) constitute the *superior vena cava,* a vessel destined to serve as the major channel draining the head, neck, and anterior appendages (Fig. 18–38 C). Each anterior cardinal vein beyond the level of the external jugular and subclavian veins becomes the *internal jugular vein.* The *external jugular vein* on either rise originates as a secondary channel from a capillary plexus in the facial region.

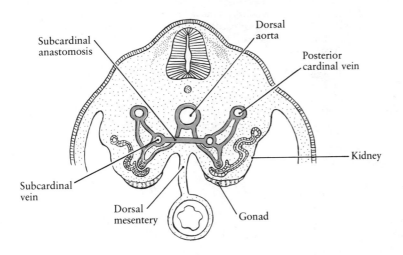

Subcardinal anastomosis

Dorsal aorta

Posterior cardinal vein

Subcardinal vein

Kidney

Dorsal mesentery

Gonad

18–39 A schematic drawing of a transverse section through the posterior abdominal wall of the early human embryo to show the relationships between the posterior and subcardinal veins.

Formation of the Inferior Vena Cava

The formation of the inferior vena cava or *postcaval vein* is very complex. It involves major alterations in the three pairs of cardinal veins that appear in succession to drain the body wall, the viscera, and the lower limbs. The posterior cardinal veins appear slightly later than the anterior cardinals and arise as two longitudnal vessels dorsolateral to the urogenital fold (Fig. 18–39). They are concerned primarily with the drainage of the lateral body wall, the meso-nephric kidneys, and the hindlimb buds. Subsequently, the paired *subcardinal veins* differentiate on the ventromedial surfaces of the mesonephroi (Fig. 18–39). They terminate cranially in the posterior cardinal veins. Numerous transverse anastomoses through the vascular sinus of the kidneys also join the posterior and subcardinal vessels. Finally, a third set of longitudnal veins, the *supracardinal veins,* develops dorsomedial to the posterior cardinal complex. On either side, each supracardinal is continuous anteriorly and posteriorly with the posterior cardinal vein (Fig. 18–40).

Between the sixth and eighth weeks of development, enlargement, atrophy, and fusion between these cardinal vessels lead to the emergence of a single, unpaired vessel or inferior vena cava. The origin of this vessel requires additional description (Fig. 18–40). Initially the systemic circulation on either side of the embryo is drained toward the common cardinal veins by both the posterior and subcardinal vessels (Fig. 18–40 A). Shortly, thereafter, the right subcardinal vein becomes connected to the right hepatic vein (or proximal right vitelline vein) by a vascular plexus that develops in the *caval mesentery*. The caval mesentery is a thickening of the dorsal body wall just to the right of the dorsal mesentery; it effectively

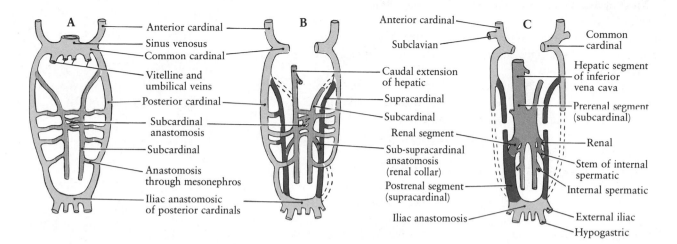

A — Anterior cardinal — B — Anterior cardinal — C — Common cardinal
Sinus venosus
Common cardinal
Subclavian
Vitelline and umbilical veins
Caudal extension of hepatic — Hepatic segment of inferior vena cava
Posterior cardinal
Supracardinal — Prerenal segment (subcardinal)
Subcardinal anastomosis
Subcardinal
Renal segment — Renal
Subcardinal
Sub-supracardinal ansatomosis (renal collar) — Stem of internal spermatic
Anastomosis through mesonephros
Postrenal segment (supracardinal) — Internal spermatic
Iliac anastomosic of posterior cardinals
Iliac anastomosis — External iliac
Hypogastric

acts as a bridge between the right lobe of the liver and the right mesonephros. Since this is a very direct route to the heart, enlargement of this new channel proceeds rapidly. The right proximal vitelline vein forms the *hepatic segment* of the inferior vena cava. The cephalic end of the right subcardinal vein becomes the *prerenal* or *mesenteric segment* of the inferior vena cava (Fig. 18–40 B,C).

The consolidation and enlargement of the hepatic and prerenal portions of the inferior vena cava indirectly hastens the degeneration of the posterior cardinal veins. On the right, a portion of the right posterior cardinal vein persists to contribute to the *azygous vein* (Fig. 18–38 C).

As more blood from the caudal part of the body is collected and passed through the mesonephroi, an extensive *subcardinal anastomosis* develops between the kidneys (Fig. 18–40 B). Gradually, a single, main channel emerges within this anastomosis of irregular venous spaces. Since this channel comes to lie between the metanephric kidneys, it contributes to the *interrenal segment* or *renal segment* of the inferior vena cava (Fig. 18–40 C,D).

Elimination of the need for passing blood through the kidney on its return to the heart is effected by a special connection (known as the *renal collar* or *renal anastomosis*) between the right supracardinal vein and the interrenal segment of the inferior vena cava (Fig. 18–40 B). Behind this connection, the right supracardinal vein forms the *postrenal segment* of the inferior vena cava. The chief vessels opening into this part of the inferior vena cava are the *common, external,* and *internal iliac veins.* All of these vessels are fashioned from an early *iliac anastomosis* between the right and left posterior cardinal veins at the level of the hindlimbs (Fig. 18–40 B–D).

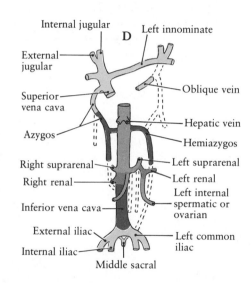

Internal jugular — D — Left innominate
External jugular
Oblique vein
Superior vena cava
Hepatic vein
Azygos
Hemiazygos
Right suprarenal — Left suprarenal
Right renal — Left renal
Left internal spermatic or ovarian
Inferior vena cava
External iliac — Left common iliac
Internal iliac
Middle sacral

18–40 Transformation of the primitive veins of the trunk of the human embryo to show formation of the inferior vena cava. Ventral views. A, six weeks; B, seven weeks; C, eight weeks; D, adult. (From L. Arey, 1974. Developmental Anatomy. W. B. Saunders Company, Philadelphia.)

Most of the left supracardinal vein drops out, although a prerenal portion may persist as the *hemiazygous vein* (Fig. 18–40 D). A short cross-connection unites it with the azygous vein. A short anterior portion of the right supracardinal vein contributes to the formation of the azygous vein.

Several additional tributaries of the inferior vena cava should be mentioned because they reflect the differences that take place in vascular reorganization on the right and left sides of the embryo. The metanephric kidneys are drained by the *renal veins*. The origin of the right renal vein is simple; it represents a consolidation of vascular channels which joins directly the renal anastomosis (Fig. 18–40 C,D). The left renal vein is more complicated because the renal anastomosis on the left is not incorporated into the inferior vena cava. Hence, it is a consolidation of a primitive renal vein, the left renal anastomosis, and a fused portion of the subcardinal anastomosis (Fig. 18–40 C,D). The *right* and *left suprarenal veins* are also not homologous vessels as Figure 18–40 illustrates. The *spermatic* and *ovarian veins* represent portions of the subcardinal veins that persist caudal to the kidneys.

The Pulmonary Veins

From the left atrium, the primitive pulmonary vein arises as a sprout of endothelium, which joins the pulmonary capillary plexus on the endodermal primordia of the lungs. As the sinus venous is being absorbed into the right atrium, the stem of this single pulmonary vein, as well as the bases of the right and left pulmonary veins, are absorbed into the wall of the left atrium. Four separate pulmonary venous orifices come to open into the dorsal wall of the left atrium (Figs. 18–22; 18–41).

The Veins of the Limbs

From the capillary plexus that develops in the mesoderm of the limb buds, there emerges a *border vein* that acts as the early drainage channel of blood brought in by the axillary artery. In the forelimb, the border vein initially opens into the posterior cardinal vein. Secondarily, however, it is transferred to the anterior cardinal vein as a result of the caudal descent of the heart. The *subclavian veins,* the *axillary veins,* and the *basilar veins* develop from the embryonic border vein. In the hindlimb, the major vein (*femoral vein*) develops as a vessel from the posterior cardinal vein. Within the hindlimb proper, the border vein differentiates into the *anterior tibial, small saphenous,* and *inferior gluteal veins.*

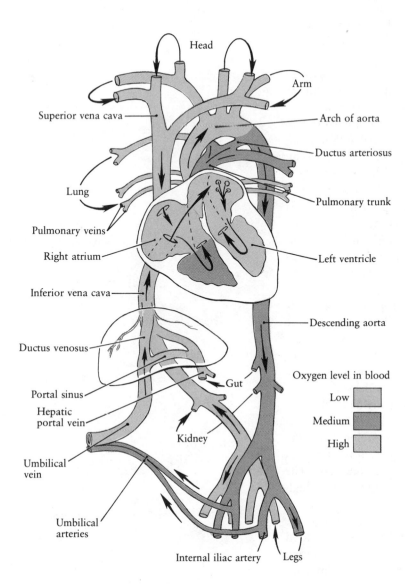

Head

Arm

Superior vena cava

Arch of aorta

Ductus arteriosus

Lung

Pulmonary trunk

Pulmonary veins

Right atrium

Left ventricle

Inferior vena cava

Descending aorta

Ductus venosus

Gut

Oxygen level in blood

Portal sinus

Low

Hepatic
portal vein

Medium

Kidney

High

Umbilical
vein

Umbilical
arteries

Internal iliac artery   Legs

18–41   The pattern of circulation in the human fetus. Arrows indicate the direction of blood flow and colors the approximate levels of oxygen saturation.

THE FETAL AND NEONATAL CIRCULATIONS

The fetal cardiovascular system is designed primarily to serve prenatal requirements and to permit those modifications at birth which quickly establish the postnatal circulatory pattern. Although birth requires immediate changes in the flow of blood, the particular arrangement of the fetal blood vessels allows the neonate to accomplish this transition with relative ease.

As pointed out previously, the placenta acts as an organ of

transfer of oxygen and nutritive material from the maternal bloodstream to the fetal circulation, and of carbon dioxide and nitrogenous wastes of metabolism from the fetal to the maternal circulation. Some knowledge of the fetal circulation is necessary in order to appreciate the abrupt changes that occur with the shift at birth in the sites where these various activities are carried out.

A simplified scheme of the fetal circulation is diagrammed in Figure 18–41. Blood, approximately 80 percent saturated with oxygen, returns from the placenta to the liver by way of the umbilical vein. Using special techniques (*angiocardiography*) which permit analysis of the distribution patterns and oxygenation of the fetal blood, it has been demonstrated that about half of the placental return is diverted through the hepatic sinusoids, whereas the other half bypasses the liver and courses through the ductus venosus into the inferior vena cava. A muscular sphincter at the junction of the ductus venosus and the umbilical vein regulates the flow into each of these vascular pathways.

Blood from both the ductus venosus and the hepatic portal circulation is collected by the inferior vena cava and emptied into the right atrium. Since the inferior vena cava already contains deoxygenated blood from the caudal regions of the fetus, its level of oxygenation is not so high as that in the umbilical vein. Most of the blood flow from the inferior vena cava is diverted by the lower margin of the septum secundum (i.e., the crista dividens) through the foramen ovale into the left atrium (Fig. 18–22). Here there is some mixture with the deoxygenated blood returning from the lungs. In this way, most of the blood returning from the placenta bypasses the lungs and is shunted to the left side of the heart. The vessels of the heart, head, and neck thus receive blood with a high level of oxygen tension.

A small stream from the inferior vena cava passes through the right atrium and mixes with a large volume of deoxygenated blood from the superior vena cava and the coronary sinus. After entering the right ventricle, this blood courses by way of the pulmonary trunk through the ductus arteriosus and into the descending aorta. Initially, probably less than 10 percent of the right ventricular blood flow goes to the lungs. Flow to the lungs does appear to steadily increase in later stages of fetal life. A large portion of the mixed blood in the dorsal aorta passes out into the umbilical arteries for reoxygenation in the capillaries of the chorionic villi.

Major adjustments occur in the pattern of circulation within minutes of the transfer of respiration function from the placenta to the lungs (Fig. 18–42). An immediate response to the first breath of the neonate is a contraction of the two umbilical arteries to prevent further blood from circulating to the placenta. This is followed by con-

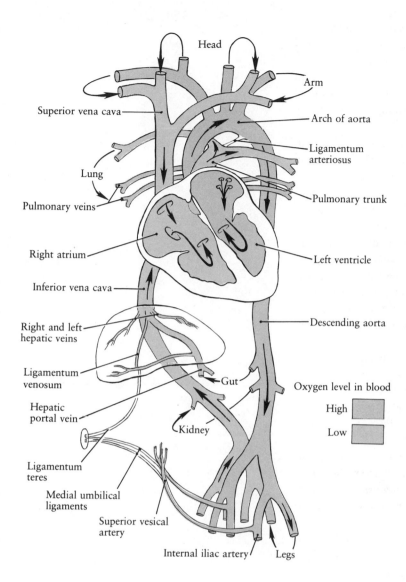

18–42 The pattern of circulation in the human neonate. Arrows indicate the direction of blood flow. The derivatives of fetal vessels are also shown.

striction of the umbilical vein and the ductus venosus. If the umbilical cord is not tied for several minutes, there is some transfer of blood from the placenta to the neonate.

Alterations in the umbilical arteries, the umbilical vein, and the ductus venosus occur simultaneously with a narrowing of the ductus arteriosus. Closure of the ductus arteriosus is an essential step in the shift from the fetal to the neonatal pattern of circulation. In contrast to earlier views, it is now agreed that complete closure of this shunt takes place over a period of several months. Initially, however, there is a *functional closure* of the ductus arteriosus within the first several minutes of birth. This involves the contraction of the muscular tissue in the wall of the ductus, a process presumably mediated under the influence of a substance (*bradykinin*) released by the lungs upon their initial inflation. A consequence of this reduction of the ductus arteriosus is marked increase in blood flow to the lungs. *Anatomical closure* of the ductus is achieved by the proliferation of the tunica intima.

The sudden increase in the volume of the lungs is associated with a sharp reduction in pulmonary vascular resistance. The increase in pulmonary blood flow leads to a sharp rise in the pressure of the left atrium. Since the pressure in the right atrium is decreased with the sudden occlusion of the placental circulation, there is a cessation of blood flow through the foramen ovale (*transatrial flow*) as the valve of the foramen is forced against the septum secundum. Hence, the foramen ovale may be regarded as functionally closed. Anatomical closure of the foramen ovale is effected through the proliferation and hypertrophy of endothelial and connective tissues around the opening, a process that also requires several months for completion. As long as pulmonary blood flow is normal and the pressure in the left atrium is at least equal to that in the right atrium, the fact that there is a structural opening between the two chambers for some time is of little importance.

Vessels no longer required in the postnatal pattern of circulation eventually become obliterated (i.e., their lumens disappear due to hypertrophy of the tunica intima). However, the fibrous connective tissue of the walls of these vessels commonly persists as *ligaments* in the adult (Fig. 18–42). The intra-abdominal portion of the umbilical vein forms the *ligamentum teres,* which extends from the umbilicus to the hepatic portal vein. The *ligamentum venosum,* a remant of the ductus venosus, passes through the liver and joins the inferior vena cava and the hepatic portal vein. The ductus arteriosus becomes the *ligamentum arteriosum,* which passes from the left pulmonary artery to the arch of the aorta. Much of the intra-abdominal portion of the umbilical arteries remains as the *medial umbilical ligaments.*

THE LYMPHATIC SYSTEM

The lymphatic system is a network of terminally closed vessels that return tissue fluids to the venous system. It begins to develop in the human embryo shortly after the appearance of the primitive cardiovascular system.

There are differences of opinion on the precise method of origin of the lymph vessels. The older view is that the lymph channels

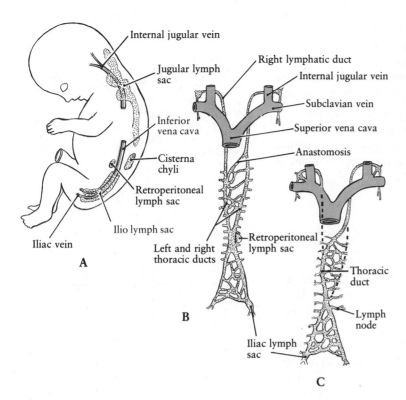

18–43 Diagrams showing the development of the human lymphatic system. A, lymphatic system at seven weeks, left lateral view; B, ventral view of the lymphatic system at nine weeks showing the paired thoracic ducts; C, formation of the adult thoracic and right lymphatic ducts. (After K. L. Moore, 1977. The Developing Human: Clinically Oriented Embryology, 2nd ed. Courtesy of W. B. Saunders Company, Philadelphia.)

arise in a manner similar to that previously described for blood vessels (i.e., progressive coalescence of mesenchymal-lined spaces). A current view is that the earliest lymph vessels originate as capillary sprouts from the endothelium of embryonic veins.

The early lymph channels tend to be distributed along the main venous trunks. Dilations of these vessels give rise to six lymph sacs (Fig. 18–43 A): (1) two *jugular lymph sacs* near the union of the subclavian and anterior cardinal veins; (2) two *iliac lymph sacs* near the union of iliac and posterior cardinal veins; (3) an unpaired *retroperitoneal sac* in the base of the dorsal mesentery near the suprarenal glands; and (4) the *cisterna chyli* dorsal to the retroperitoneal sac. By continuous elongation, centrifugal growth, and branching, lymph vessels extend out from these lymph sacs to most of the tissues of the body.

At a slightly later stage in development, two large lymph channels (the *right* and *left thoracic ducts*) join the cephalic jugular sacs with the caudal cisterna chyli (Fig. 18–43 B). The adult *thoracic duct* originates from the cranial end of the left lymph duct, the interconnecting anastomosis between the two lymph ducts, and the caudal part of the right lymph duct (Fig. 18–43 C). It opens into the venous system by way of the left jugular sac at the junction of the internal jugular and subclavian veins. The *right lymphatic duct* is derived from the cranial part of the right thoracic duct (Fig. 18–43 C).

Most of the lymph sacs become transformed into lymph nodes during the early fetal period. Mesenchyme cells invade the sac and subdivide its cavity into a network of *lymph sinuses.* Proliferation and differentiation of the mesenchymal tissue lead to the formation of clusters of lymphoid masses. Lymph nodules and germinal centers of lymphocyte production do not appear in these lymphoid masses until just before or shortly after birth.

ANOMALIES OF THE CARDIOVASCULAR SYSTEM

Disturbances in the development of the heart and in the usual arrangement of the blood vessels are among the commonest of developmental anomalies. The overall incidence of congenital malformations of the heart and of its associated major vessels is about 0.7 percent of live births in humans. In view of the complexity of the events leading to the formation of the four-chambered heart and the striking rearrangements in the vascular pathways that occur with the definition of the final vascular pattern of vessels, it is indeed surprising that malformations of the cardiovascular system are not more common.

Congenital defects, particularly those of the heart, are interesting embryologically. Clinically, these disturbances run the gamut from variations in vascular routes that are functionally insignificant to abnormalities that are serious and life threatening. The gravity of defects is generally determined by the extent to which they interfere with the pulmonary circulation, particularly with respect to the efficiency of the oxygenation of the blood and the sufficiency of the blood being returned from the lungs for delivery into the systemic circulation from the left ventricle. A few of the more common disturbances in the cardiovascular system are described below.

Heterotaxis (Reverse Rotation) and Displacement of the Heart

Normally, the cardiac tube is thrown into a loop to the right (Fig. 18–44 A). If the tube bends to the left, there is a transposition in which the heart and its two major vessels are reversed left-to-right (Fig. 18–44 B). This so-called left looping results in a positional abnormality of the heart known as *dextrocardia.* Interestingly, if dex-

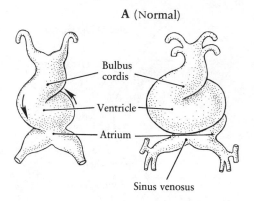

A (Normal)

Bulbus cordis

Ventricle

Atrium

Sinus venosus

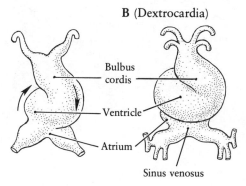

B (Dextrocardia)

Bulbus cordis

Ventricle

Atrium

Sinus venosus

18–44 Sketches of the cardiac tube to show right looping (A) and left looping resulting in dextrocardia (B).

trocardia is accompanied by transposition of the viscera (*situs inversus*), there are few associated cardiac defects and the heart can function in a normal way.

In *ectopia cordis,* the heart lies outside of the pericardial cavity owing to defective developments of the mediastinum and the pericardium. *Extrathoracic ectopia cordis* is an extreme condition in which the heart protrudes through the chest wall because of a failure of the lateral body folds to meet and fuse properly.

Failure of the aorticopulmonary septum to pursue its normal spiral course can result in complete transposition of the major vessels (Fig. 18–45). In typical cases, the aorta lies anterior to the pulmonary trunk and springs from the right ventricle; the pulmonary trunk originates from the left ventricle. For survival, there must be associated defects in the cardiac septa and persistence of the ductus arteriosus so that some exchange between the pulmonary and systemic circuits can take place.

Malformations Due to Arrest of Development

A number of cardiac defects can be traced to failures in processes relating to the growth, migration, and/or degeneration of septa or their primordia. This is well illustrated with examples of the defective closure of fetal openings in the heart.

Atrial septal and ventricular septal defects are among the most common congenital heart anomalies. The most frequent type of atrial septal defects is *persistent* or *patent foramen ovale* (Fig. 18–46). Patent foramen ovale usually arises from an abnormal resorption of the septum primum (valve of the foramen ovale) during the formation of the foramen secundum. For example, if the septum primum is excessively resorbed, the future valve of the foramen ovale is too short to blanket the foramen ovale (Fig. 18–46 B). Also, if the septum secundum is too short, resulting in an abnormally large foramen ovale, the septum primum is unable to close at birth (Fig. 18–46 C). A large percentage (25%) of persons have a condition known as *probe patent foramen ovale.* The presence of this functional opening in the interatrial septum can be demonstrated by passing a probe obliquely from one atrium to the other atrium. Unless the patent foramen ovale is forced open because of other defects in the heart, this condition is not considered to be pathological.

Other clinically significant atrial septal defects include *patent foramen primum, persistent atrioventricular canal* (owing to failure of the fusion of the dorsal and ventral endocardial cushions), and *common atrium* (owing to failure of the septum primum and septum secundum to develop). Generally, interatrial septal defects at

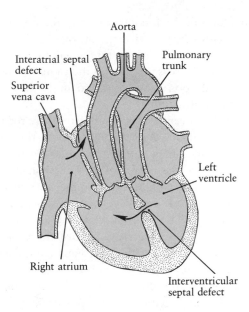

18–45   A sketch showing complete transposition of the aorta and pulmonary trunk.

the level of the foramen ovale or the foramen primum are compatible with life, provided the atrioventricular canal is normally partitioned and guarded by functional valves. Commonly, these hearts show an increase in size on the right side because of the extra load imposed upon it by blood moving from the left to right with each atrial contraction.

Isolated ventricular septal defects are the most frequent of all cardiac anomalies. As one might expect, these defects typically involve the formation of the membranous portion of the interventricular septum and the closure of the interventricular foramen. Endocardial tissues of the bulbar ridges, the cushions of the atrioventricular canal, and the free edge of the muscular interventricular septum must meet at the right time and in the right place to complete division of the ventricle. Failure to accomplish this task is commonly associated with disturbances in the partitioning of the bulbus cordis. Complete absence of the interventricular septum is very rare and results in a three-chambered heart (*cor triloculare biatriatum*).

The bulbus cordis is the site of several anomalous conditions, most of which can be traced to disturbances in its partitioning by the aorticopulmonary septum. *Persistent bulbus cordis* results from the failure of the aorticopulmonary septum to develop and divide the bulbus into pulmonary trunk and the aorta. Both ventricles then pump blood into a common outlet with free mingling of the blood from the two sides of the heart. The inefficiency of this pattern of circulation is obvious and must be corrected if there is to be postnatal survival.

Typically, the bulbus cordis is equally subdivided into an aorta and pulmonary trunk. Occasionally, this part of the arterial outlet is partitioned unequally, presumably owing to disturbances in the position of the bulbar ridges that fuse to form the aorticopulmonary septum. According to the direction of the malplacement, what results is either a large pulmonary trunk and a small aorta or a small pulmonary trunk and a large aorta (Fig. 18–47 A). If the aorta is narrowed, the condition is *aortic stenosis;* if the pulmonary trunk is constricted, it is *pulmonary stenosis*. In either case, the aorticopulmonary septum cannot properly fuse with the interventricular septum and a ventricular septal defect results. Commonly, the larger of the two vessels will override the septal defect in the ventricle (Fig. 18–47 B). The complete absence of a lumen in the aorta or pulmonary trunk leads to a condition known as *atresia*.

Several of the above examples indicate that disturbances in the development of one part of the heart are invariably accompanied by the formation of defects in another part of the heart. A classic example of this is the *tetralogy of Fallot*. Four defects constitute this condition (Fig. 18–47 B): (1) pulmonary stenosis; (2) ventricular

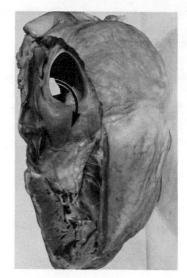

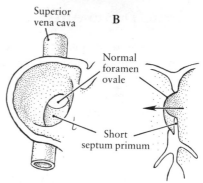

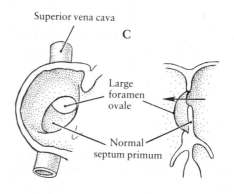

18–46   Patent foramen ovale. A, photograph of an adult heart as seen from the right side; B, a sketch from the right aspect of the interatrial septum showing defect due to excessive resorption of the septum primum; C, a sketch from the right aspect of the interatrial septum showing defect due to a short septum secundum. (From K. L. Moore, 1977. The Developing Human: Clinically Oriented Embryology, 2nd ed. Courtesy of W. B. Saunders Company, Philadelphia.)

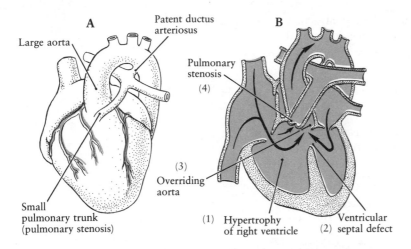

A

Large aorta

Patent ductus arteriosus

B

Pulmonary stenosis (4)

(3) Overriding aorta

Small pulmonary trunk (pulmonary stenosis)

(1) Hypertrophy of right ventricle

(2) Ventricular septal defect

18–47   A, a sketch of an infant's heart to show a narrowed pulmonary trunk (pulmonary stenosis) and a large aorta resulting from unequal partitioning of the bulbus cordis; B, a frontal section through a heart to show the tetralogy of Fallot.

18–48   Coarctation of the aorta below the ductus arteriosus (A) and the common routes of collateral circulation that develop in association with the defect (B).

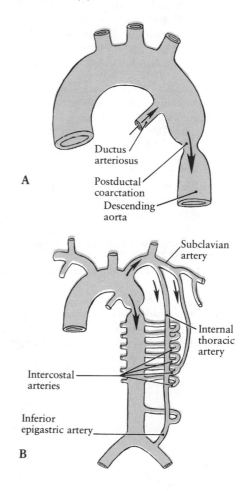

A

Ductus arteriosus

Postductal coarctation

Descending aorta

Subclavian artery

Internal thoracic artery

Intercostal arteries

Inferior epigastric artery

B

septal defect; (3) aorta overriding the septal defect; and (4) hypertrophy of the right ventricle. These conditions result in little blood reaching the lungs for aeration. The lack of oxygen in the peripheral circulation gives a bluish tinge (cyanosis) to the skin and the lips. If the ductus arteriosus remains open, blood flow from the aorta to the pulmonary artery can supply sufficient blood to the lungs to support life. Several surgical methods are available to correct deficiencies in the pulmonary circulation if the ductus arteriosus closes. The Blalock and Taussig technique involves anastomosing the brachiocephalic artery to the right pulmonary artery or the left subclavian artery to the left pulmonary artery. Another technique involves the coupling of the end of the right pulmonary artery to the side of the superior vena cava. These vascular connections are designed as shunts to increase pulmonary flow.

Aortic Arch Anomalies

The transformation of the embryonic arrangement of the aortic arches can be accompanied by several types of variations. Disturbances include the persistence of vessels that normally disappear (i.e., right aortic arch) or the disappearance of a vessel that is normally retained (i.e., left aortic arch). A common malformation is *coarctation of the aorta* in which there is stenosis of the aorta just above or below the ductus arteriosus (Fig. 18–48 A). When the aorta is constricted below the ductus, an extensive collateral circulation often develops to assist with the movement of blood to the peripheral parts of the body (Fig. 18–48 B).

Failure of the distal portion of the sixth aortic arch to involute at birth to form the ligamentum arteriosum leads to *patent ductus ar-*

teriosus. The primary cause of patency is failure of the contraction of the musculature surrounding the ductus. It is a defect associated with maternal rubella infection during early pregnancy.

REFERENCES

Davis, C. L. 1927. Development of the human heart from its first appearance to the stage found in embryos of twenty paired somites. Carnegie Contrib. Embryol. 19:245–284.

DeHaan, R. L. 1963. Organization of the cardiogenic plate in the early chick embryo. Acta Embryol. Morphol. Exp. 6:26–38.

DeHaan, R. L. 1963. Regional organization of prepacemaker cells in the cardiac primordia of the early chick embryo. J. Embryol. Exp. Morphol. 11:65–76.

DeHaan, R. L. 1965. Morphogenesis of the vertebrate heart. Organogenesis. Eds., R. L. DeHaan and H. Ursprung. New York: Holt, Rinehart, and Winston.

DeVries, P. A. and J. B. de C. M. Saunders. 1962. Development of the ventricle and spiral outflow tract in the human heart. A contribution to the development of the human heart from age group IX to age group XV. Carnegie Contrib. Embryol. 37:87–114.

Jacobson, A. G. and J. T. Duncan. 1968. Heart induction in salamanders. J. Exp. Zool. 167:79–103.

Kramer, T. C. 1942. The partitioning of the truncus and conus and the formation of the membranous portion of the interventricular septum in the human heart. Am. J. Anat. 71:343–370.

Llorca, F. and D. Gill. 1967. A causal analysis of the heart curvature in the chick embryo. Wilhelm Roux Arch. Entwicklungsmech. Org. 158:52–63.

Manasek, F. 1976. Heart development: Interactions involved in cardiac morphogenesis. In: The Cell Surface in Animal Embryogenesis and Development, pp. 545–598. Eds., G. Poste and G. L. Nicolson. New York: Elsevier/North-Holland Biomedical Press.

Manasek, F. J., M. Burnside, and R. Waterman. 1972. Myocardial cell shape change as a mechanism of embryonic heart looping. Dev. Biol. 29:349–371.

Patten, B. 1960. Persistent interatrial foramen primum. Am. J. Anat. 107:271–280.

Rawles, M. E. 1943. The heart-forming areas of the early chick blastoderm. Physiol. Zool. 16:22–43.

Rychter, Z. 1962. Experimental morphology of the aortic arches and the heart loop in chick embryos. Adv. Morphog. 2:333–371.

Waddington, C. H. 1932. Experiments on the development of chick and duck embryos cultivated *in vitro.* Trans. Philos. Roy. Soc. Lond. Ser. B. 221:179–230.

19

The Urogenital System

The excretory and the reproductive systems are closely associated anatomically, developmentally, and functionally—a fact implied by the use of the term urogenital system. Both systems develop from a common mesodermal ridge that runs longitudinally along the posterior abdominal wall, lateral to the dorsal mesentery of the gut. The ducts of both systems open into the same cavity, the cloaca. In addition, in the male, parts of the functional excretory system of the embryo, when they lose their excretory responsibilities, do not degenerate but are converted into parts of the functional reproductive system of the adult. Both systems in the adult male share a common excretory pathway, the urethra.

However, although they develop in close association with each other, for descriptive purposes we will consider the two systems separately.

THE EXCRETORY SYSTEM

The Intermediate Mesoderm

When the embryonic mesoderm first appears, it is concentrated around the notochordal process where it it is known as the paraxial mesoderm. From here it spreads out laterally between the ectoderm and the endoderm as the lateral plate mesoderm (Fig. 19–1 A). Shortly after its appearance, the paraxial mesoderm begins to form segmentally arranged somites proceeding in a craniocaudal direction. The lateral mesoderm splits into two layers to surround the coelom: somatic mesoderm associated with the ectoderm—together termed the somatopleure—and splanchnic mesoderm associated with the endoderm—together termed the splanchnopleure. The region of the lateral mesoderm between the somite and the coelom is the intermediate mesoderm (Fig. 19–1 B). The intermediate mesoderm will give rise to the excretory system.

During the development of the mammalian excretory system, three different types of kidneys appear. These are the *pronephros*, the *mesonephros*, and the *metanephros*. They develop in a temporal sequence as well as in a spatial craniocaudal sequence (Fig. 19–2). Since all three types develop from the same longitudinal ridge of

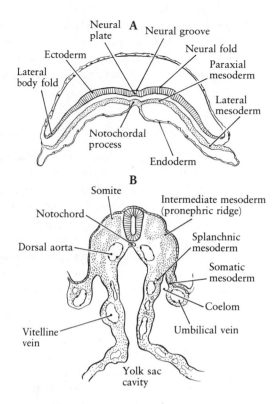

19–1 A, section through the neural plate of an 18-day-old presomite human embryo. Mesoderm lateral to the notochord subdivided into paraxial and lateral portions; B, section through the somite region of a 22-day-old 10-somite human embryo. The intermediate mesoderm, here differentiating into pronephros and called the pronephric ridge, is located between the somite mesoderm and the coelom.

451

nephrogenic tissue—often with no definite boundaries between them—there is some justification for considering all three as parts of a single unit which develop in different regions and at different times, as a progressive differentiation along a continuum.

The Pronephros

The pronephros or head kidney, never functional in man, is the functional kidney of some lower vertebrates. A functional pronephros (Fig. 19–3) consists of paired pronephric tubules developed from the nephrogenous tissue. One end of each tubule opens into the coelom, the other into a longitudinally running duct, the pronephric duct, uniting the lateral ends of successive pronephric tubules. A branch of the dorsal aorta indents either the pronephric tubule or the coelom close to the point where the pronephric tubule opens into it. The former is termed an *internal glomerulus,* the latter an *external glomerulus.* The glomerulus is covered by a thin layer of epithelium through which wastes are filtered either into the tubule or into the coelom. Wastes in the coelom move into the tubule through the *peritoneal funnel.* Wastes that are filtered through the internal glomerulus enter an expanded portion of the pronephric tubule, the *nephrocoele,* from which they pass into a more lateral portion of the tubule through the *nephrostome.* The tubules drain into the pronephric duct, the excretory duct opening into the cloaca.

In the human embryo, the pronephros is made up of 7 to 10 pairs of solid "tubules" that develop from the nephrogenic cord in the cervical region during week three. The exact caudal limit of the pronephros is not well defined since it overlaps the territory of the mesonephros. Pronephric tubules are present for only a short period of time, the more anterior degenerating while the more posterior are still developing. By the five-millimeter stage, all of the tubules have degenerated. As a part of the pronephros, a pronephric duct is formed by the joining of segmental delaminations from the nephrogenic ridge. Below the region of the pronephros, the blind end of the pronephric duct grows caudally as a solid rod of cells which subsequently hollows out. It opens into the cloaca. The rudimentary pronephric tubules do not establish any connection with the pronephric duct. Although the tubules quickly degenerate, the pronephric duct persists and becomes the functional excretory duct of the mesonephros when this structure develops. In the male, it eventually forms a part of the reproductive tract when the mesonephros degenerates.

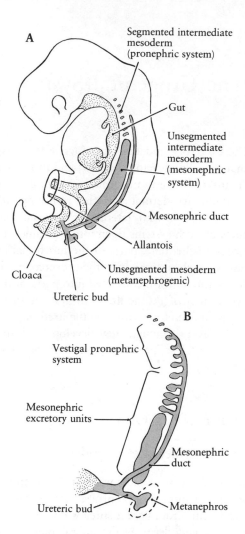

19–2 Diagram showing the development of the proneophros, the mesonephros, and the metanephros from the intermediate mesoderm (nephrogenic ridge) in a craniocaudal sequence.

The Mesonephros

The mesonephros in the human embryo extends from about the 10th to the 26th somite (fourth lumbar). The mesonephric tubules arise from the nephrogenic cord in a caudally running progression. Mesonephric tubules are not segmentally arranged, and as many as three to four per segment may be present. When this organ reaches its maximum development during month two, approximately 35 to 49 tubules are present. Each tubule connects laterally to what was originally the pronephric duct but which is now termed the meso-nephric or *Wolffian duct* (Fig. 19–4 A). The medial end of each tubule becomes invaginated by a glomerulus around which forms a thin-walled double epithelial membrane, *Bowman's capsule*. The capsule and the glomerulus together make up the mesonephric or *renal corpuscle* (Fig. 19–4 B). The tubule becomes S-shaped and a

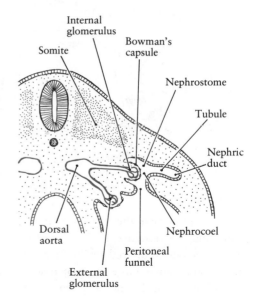

19–3   Schematic drawing of a functional pro-nephros showing the relationship of the two types of glomeruli to the coelom.

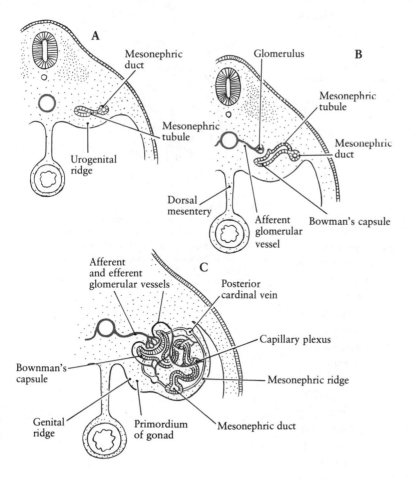

19–4   Successive stages in the development of the human mesonephros during the fifth and sixth weeks. A, connection of a mesonephric tubule to the mesonephric duct; B, medial end of a mesonephric tubule being invaginated by a glomerulus to form a renal corpuscle; C, renal corpuscle, mesonephric tubule and mesonephric duct differentiated. Genital ridge forming medial to the mesonephric tissue.

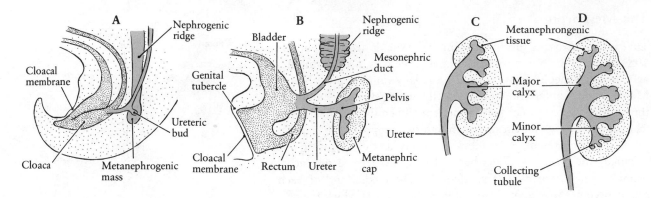

secretory region near the capsule and an excretory region toward the duct may be recognized. The size of the human mesonephros is somewhat small compared to the large organ developed in the pig or the rabbit, but is large in comparison to that of the rat or the mouse. The size of the mesonephros appears to bear some relation to the permeability of the placenta.

As the mesonephric tubules increase in size, the mesonephros cannot be accommodated in the body wall, and it bulges into the coelom as a longitudinal ridge lateral to the dorsal mesentery. Since the gonad also develops from this tissue, it is called the *urogenital ridge*. It is suspended from the dorsal body wall by the *urogenital mesentery*. The urogenital ridge soon divides into a medial *genital ridge* and a lateral *mesonephric ridge* (Fig. 19–4 C).

The Metanephros

The metanephros is the last of the three types of excretory organs to appear, and it will develop into the functional kidney of the adult. It has a dual origin: (1) the collecting system develops from an outgrowth of the mesonephric duct; (2) the excretory system develops from the nephrogenic ridge caudal to the mesonephros.

The *metanephric diverticulum (ureteric bud)* appears as an outgrowth from the dorsomesial wall of the mesonephric duct just before it enters the cloaca (Fig. 19–5 A). The diverticulum grows first dorsally and then cranially, forming an elongated duct, the *ureter*. The distal blind end of this duct expands to form the *renal pelvis*. It pushes into the caudal end of the nephrogenic ridge, which then becomes molded about it as the *metanephric cap* (Fig. 19–5 B). The renal pelvis divides to form two or three primary tubules that are the future *major calyces* (Fig. 19–5 C). Each primary tubule further subdivides and forms secondary tubules that represent the future *minor calyces* (Fig. 19–5 D). Two to four open into each major calyx. The secondary tubules continue to subdivide until approxi-

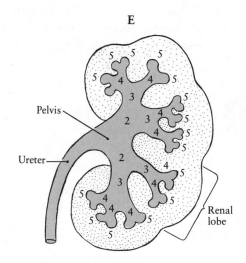

19–5 Origin of the human metanephric duct (ureteric bud) from the mesonephric duct and its combination with the nephrogenic ridge tissue (metanephrogenic mass) to form the kidney. A, 5 mm; B, 11 mm; C, D, development of the distal end of the ureteric bud into the renal pelvis, calyces, and the duct system of the kidney—C, 15 mm; D, 20 mm.

mately 13 to 14 generations of tubules are formed. As each tubule divides, the metanephric cap is also subdivided so that the end of each tubule always retains an individual covering of me-tanephrogenic tissue. As the secondary tubules enlarge and develop into the minor calyces, they absorb the third and fourth generation tubules so that the tubules of the fifth order, some 10 to 25 in number, open into each minor calyx. These are the *papillary ducts* of the adult kidney. Tubules of higher orders form the collecting tubules that converge on the papillary ducts forming the renal pyramids (Fig. 19–5 D).

The metanephric cap moves laterally and forms clusters of tissue on each side of the collecting tubule. These metanephric vesicles appear first in the 18 to 20 millimeter embryo during month two (Fig. 19–6 A,B). The vesicle enlarges and becomes S-shaped. The limb of the S away from the collecting tubule is invaginated by a tuft of capillaries, the glomerulus, to form the renal corpuscle (Fig. 19–6 C). Both ends of the S-shaped vesicle remain relatively fixed in position and secondary curvatures and histological modification of the tissue between these points produce the complicated twisting nephric tubule. Convolutions near the glomerulus and near the collecting tubule form the *proximal* and *distal convoluted tubules,* respectively (Fig. 19–6 D,E). Between these two regions, the remaining portion of the nephron develops into the thin-walled *loop of Henle* (Fig. 19–6 D,E). The glomerulus and the convoluted tubules become part of the *cortex* of the kidney and the collecting tubules draining into the minor calyces form a part of the *medulla.* The loops of Henle dip down into the medulla (Fig. 19–7).

The kidney is unusual in that it undergoes a cranial migration, from its original pelvic location to a position opposite the first lumbar vertebra. This positional change, which brings the cranial pole of the kidney into contact with the caudally migrating suprarenal gland, is due in part to an active migration and in part to the straightening of the lumbar curvature.

Dependent Differentiation

Neither the mesonephric nor the metanephric tubules are self-differentiating, the former needing the presence of the mesonephric (pronephric) duct, the latter needing the presence of the ureteric bud. If the pronephric duct is transected at any level, its further caudal extension is effectively blocked (Fig. 19–8 A). If the caudal extension of the pronephric duct is prevented from reaching the mesonephric level of the nephrogenic cord, mesonephric tubules do not differentiate (Fig. 19–8 B). In addition, if the ureteric bud is prevented from reaching the metanephrogenic region of the

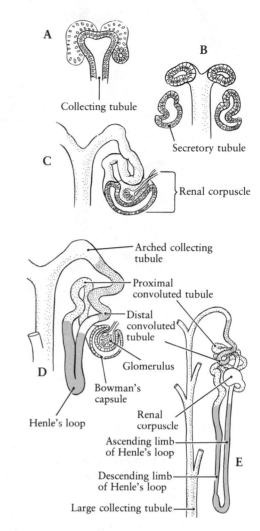

19–6 Differentiation of the uriniferous tubule (nephron) from the metanephrogenic tissue.

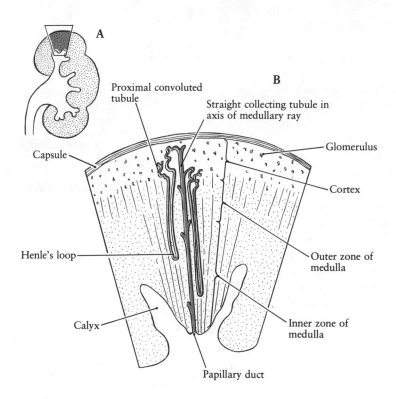

B

Proximal convoluted
tubule

Straight collecting tubule in
axis of medullary ray

Glomerulus

Capsule

Cortex

Henle's loop

Outer zone of
medulla

Calyx

Inner zone of
medulla

Papillary duct

19–7 Drawing of a lobe of the kidney of a six-month-old embryo showing the relationship of the uriniferous tubules and glomeruli to the medulla and cortex. Inset, relationship of lobule drawn to the entire kidney.

nephrogenic cord, a metanephrogenic blastema may form, but tubules will not differentiate. However, in both the chick and the mammal, central nervous system tissue will promote tubule formation in mesonephrogenic and metanephrogenic mesenchyme; the action is thus more comparable to evocation and is not the result of a specific induction. However, an entirely normal mesonephros is never formed in the presence of nervous tissue only, and thus some of the determination of the structure must be attributed to the influence of the pronephric duct beyond its action as an evocator. In the light of the interrelationship of the kidney and the mesonephric duct, it is not surprising that, in the human male, kidney agenesis on one side is accompanied by the absence of the vas deferens on the same side, since the vas deferens develops from the mesonephric duct.

The Bladder and the Urethra

The caudal portion of the hindgut to which the allantois is connected and into which the pronephric duct originally opens is the *cloaca* (Fig. 19–9). A cloacal membrane separates the cloaca from the proctodeum. At about the five-millimeter stage, near the end of

19–8 A, absence of the nephric duct on the right side of a chick embryo following transection of the duct at a more cranial level; B, failure of the mesonephric tubules to form on the right side of a chick embryo in the absence of the left nephric duct. Only a formless blastema is present. (After C. H. Waddington, 1938.)

Nephric
duct

A

B

Blastema

Tubule

Nephric
duct

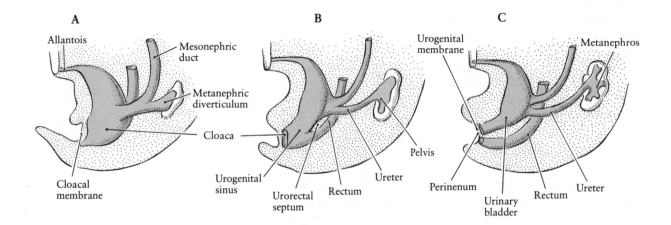

A
Allantois
Mesonephric duct
Metanephric diverticulum
Cloaca
Cloacal membrane

B
Urogenital sinus
Urorectal septum
Rectum
Ureter
Pelvis

C
Urogenital membrane
Metanephros
Perinenum
Urinary bladder
Rectum
Ureter

the first month, a mesodermal partition, the *urorectal septum,* begins to form at the cranial angle between the allantois and the hindgut (Fig. 19–9 A). During the second month, the urorectal septum grows toward and fuses with the cloacal membrane, partitioning the cloaca into an anterior *urogenital sinus* and *bladder* and a posterior *rectum* (Fig. 19–9 B,C). At the point of fusion of the urorectal septum and the cloacal membrane, the *perineal body* is formed; the cloacal membrane is now divided into a urogenital membrane and an anal membrane, indicating the separate openings to the outside of the urogenital and the gastrointestinal systems. Between them is the *perineum.*

As the urorectal septum develops, the mesonephric ducts, from which the ureteric buds are developing, now open into the urogenital sinus (Fig. 19–9 B). Growth of the region of the urogenital sinus, into which the mesonephric ducts open, imposes marked changes on the relationship of the mesonephric and metanephric ducts (Fig. 19–10). The caudal ends of the mesonephric ducts are gradually absorbed by the expanding urogenital sinus and the mesonephric and metanephric ducts each now obtain their own individual openings into the urogenital sinus (Fig. 19–10 B). A cranial movement of the metanephric duct openings and a movement of the openings of the mesonephric ducts medially toward each other results in the definitive configuration of a triangle, the base of which is craniad and is represented by the openings of the metanephric ducts while the apex is caudal and represented by the openings of the mesonephric ducts (Fig. 19–10 C,D). This is the *trigone* of the adult. The mesonephric ducts open on an elevation on the posterior wall of the urogenital sinus, which is called *Müller's tubercle.*

The bladder develops from the anterior part of the former cloaca, craniad of the openings of the mesonephric ducts. It is thus mainly

19–9 Diagrams of the formation of the urorectal septum and the separation of the coaca into the urogenital sinus and the rectum. A, four weeks; B, five weeks, C, six weeks.

formed by the expansion of the proximal part of the allantois, although the urogenital sinus makes some contribution. The allantois distal to the part that forms the bladder becomes reduced in size and its lumen is occluded. It remains as a cord connecting the cranial end of the bladder to the umbilicus. In the fetus it is called the *urachus*. In the adult it is the *middle umbilical ligament*. Uncommonly the distal portion of the allantois, between the bladder and the umbilicus, remains patent establishing a *urachal fistula* through which urine may escape.

The urogenital sinus may be separated into a cranial (pelvic) portion nearest to the bladder, receiving the openings of the mesonephric ducts, and a more caudal (phallic) portion. Depending upon the sex of the individual, the fates of these two parts of the urogenital sinus differ as will be described more completely in the section on the reproductive system. In brief, in the male, the urogenital sinus forms a long *urethra* whose channel is extended to an opening at the tip of the penis (Fig. 19–11 A). In the female, a short urethra forms corresponding only to the extent of the male urethra from the base of the bladder to Müller's tubercle. The remainder of the pelvic (plus all of the phallic) portions unite to form a shallow *vestibule* into which both the urinary and the genital ducts open (Fig. 19–11 B).

THE GENITAL SYSTEM

As mentioned in the previous section, the gonads develop in close association with the mesonephros as a part of a longitudinally running thickened ridge, the urogenital ridge, developed from the intermediate mesoderm and located on the dorsal body wall lateral to the dorsal mesentery. During the fifth week, the common ridge begins to separate into two and a ventromedial thickening, the genital ridge, represents the portion of the structure which will develop into the gonad (Fig. 19–4).

The Primordial Germ Cells

Chapter 2 introduced the concept of the germ plasm, the material that is usually relegated to a few cells in the early embryo, which are then known as the primordial germ cells and represent the stem cells of the germ line. That a specialized cytoplasmic substance could direct the differentiation of cells into the germ line was first discovered in studies on insects. At about the middle of the 19th century, it was known that the cells which occupy the posterior pole of the insect egg are those destined to become the germ cells.

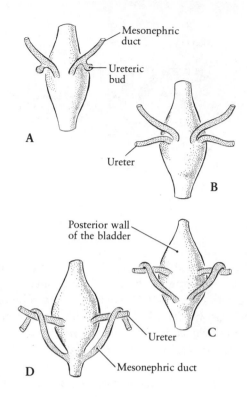

19–10 Dorsal view of the bladder showing the relationship of the mesonephric ducts and the ureter. The two systems attain separate openings and the ureters move craniad and the mesonephric ducts caudad.

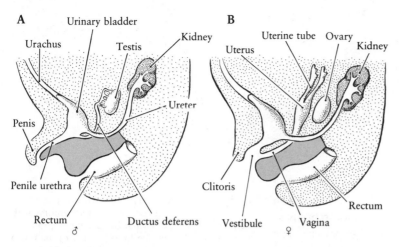

A
Urinary bladder
Urachus   Testis   Kidney
Penis   Ureter
Penile urethra
Rectum   Ductus deferens
♂

B
Uterine tube   Ovary
Uterus   Kidney
Clitoris
Rectum
Vestibule   Vagina
♀

19–11 Diagrams of 12-week-old male and female urogenital systems. In the male, the urethra is long and extends to the tip of the penis. The short female urethra opens into the vestibule.

Shortly after the turn of the century, Hegnar proposed that the granules observed in the pole plasm are, in fact, the germinal determinants. Since that time, numerous experiments have shown that the cytoplasm of the posterior pole of the dipterans and the coleopterans possesses some factor which determines that the nuclei which colonize it will differentiate into germ cells while those which do not will become somatic cells. A brief discussion of some of the experimental analyses of the role of the pole plasm has been presented in Chapter 11.

The Germ Plasm in Anurans
Studies on the germ plasm and the germ cells of the anurans have yielded strikingly similar results to those on the insects. In *Xenopus* the primordial germ cells may be distinguished on the basis of microscopically recognizable cytoplasmic inclusions, the germ plasm. The germ plasm is found at the vegetal pole of the egg and in the two-cell stage it is aggregated in small patches extending several millimeters away from the pole (Fig. 19–12 A). As the two-cell stage divides, the aggregates move toward the cleavage furrow, coalescing as they do so (Fig. 19–12 B), and in the majority of the eggs each of the four cells of the four-cell stage has a single aggregate located close to the cleavage furrow (Fig. 19–12 C). The average number of cells containing germ plasm granules in all embryos studied increased only slightly to about five in the blastula stage. This is not due to the fact that cells containing germ plasm do not divide. They do, as can be seen by the progressive decrease in size of the cells that are found to have germ plasm granules. However, the germ plasm is located at the polar region of each cell in which it appears and, therefore, in the process of normal cleavage it

19–12 Diagrams of the location and state of aggregation of the germ plasm granules during the first two cleavages in *Xenopus*. A, two-celled stage showing individual aggregates in the vegetal pole region; B, beginning of the second cleavage. Aggregates moving toward the cleavage furrow and coalescing; C, section of a four-celled embryo. Granules in a single aggregate along the cleavage furrow. (After P. McD. Whitington and R. E. Dixon, 1975. J. Embryol. Exp. Morphol. 33, 57.)

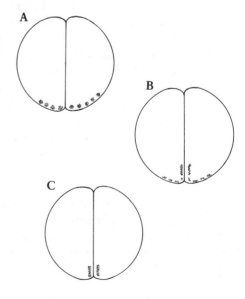

A
B
C

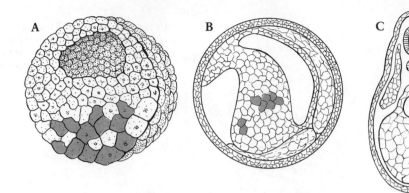

is passed on to only one of the two daughter cells. An increase in the number of cells containing pole plasm in some embryos is merely due to the inherent variability of the cleavage pattern. The number of germ plasm containing cells in the early gastrula depends solely on the relative positions of the cleavage planes and the germ plasm. During gastrulation the germ plasm migrates from the polar region of the cell to a position capping or ringing the nucleus. From this time on until the early tadpole stage, when the primordial germ cells begin their migration out of the endoderm, each goes through two to three divisions. These, as are all other successive divisions, are now cloning, and each of the daughter cells receives some germ plasm, although not in the exact same amount.

Because of the original position of the germ plasm, the primordial germ cells are located above and around the vegetal pole through the blastula stage (Fig. 19–13 A). During gastrulation they participate in the same morphogenetic movements as the surrounding endoderm cells as a part of the invaginating endoderm. At the end of gastrulation and during the tail bud stages, they are located in the deep floor of the archenteron near the blastopore (Fig. 19–13 B,C). In the early tadpole stage they undergo a dramatic change in position and are now found in the most dorsal region of the endoderm of the gut (Fig. 19–14 A). When the two sheets of lateral mesoderm which are moving dorsally to surround the gut meet, the primordial germ cells leave the endoderm and lie below this sheet of mesoderm (Fig. 19–14 B). When this mesoderm then forms the dorsal mesentery, the primordial germ cells become embedded in it (Fig. 19–14 C), and from here they migrate dorsally through the dorsal mesoderm and then laterally into the genital ridges. The movement of the primordial germ cells from the deep endoderm to the superficial dorsal endoderm, to the dorsal mesentery, and to the genital ridges is through the active ameboid movement of the cells themselves. During this rather extensive migration the cells do not divide. However, once established in the developing gonad, they begin to divide again.

19–13 Diagrams to represent the position of the primordial germ cells in *Xenopus* embryos of different ages. A, blastula; B, gastrula; C, tail bud. Germ cells may be found at any of the positions marked by the asterisks. (After P. McD. Whitington and R. E. Dixon, 1974. J. Embryol. Exp. Morphol. 33, 57.)

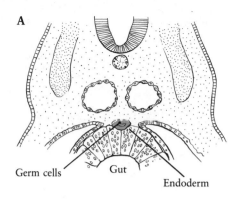

A

Germ cells · Gut · Endoderm

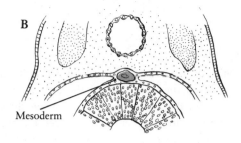

B

Mesoderm

Primordial Germ Cells in the Urodeles

That the primordial germ cells represent the progenitors of the entire germ line has been proven in a number of different experiments. The belly endoderm of one species of *Xenopus* in which the nuclei contain two nucleoli may be replaced by that of another strain in which the nuclei have only a single nucleolus. Following this, the germ cells of the host will then all contain only one nucleolus, and this characteristic of the graft will also be found in all of the host's offspring. Thus, the primordial germ cells grafted into the host in the belly endoderm are the sole basis for the establishment of the germ line.

A similar type of experiment has been performed in the urodele amphibians. In this class of amphibians germ plasm cannot be seen at the ventral pole of the cleaving egg, and primordial germ cells are not delineated until the gastrula stage, when they may be distinguished among the cells of the lateral mesoderm. Neither removal of cytoplasm at the vegetal pole of the undivided egg nor removal or transplantation of blastomeres at the vegetal pole of the blastula has any effect on the number of germ cells in the larva. Nor does removal in the gastrula stage of the presumptive endoderm that will form the caudal part of the gut have any effect on the germ cells. The transplantation of belly endoderm between two species of urodeles whose germ cells are distinguishable on the basis of pigment granule content has the opposite result from the experiment just described using *Xenopus*. The germ cells are always characteristic of the host. These experiments all demonstrate that neither the germ plasm nor the primordial germ cells are associated with the endoderm in these species. However, if the lateral mesoderm is removed, almost all of the larvae develop gonads lacking germ cells. Grafts of lateral and ventral lip mesoderm (which will form the lateral mesoderm) between *Triturus cristatus* and *Amblystoma mexicanum,* where differences in pigment granules distinguish the cells

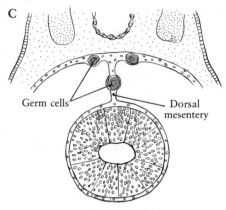

C

Germ cells · Dorsal mesentery

19–14 Migration of the primordial germ cells from the endoderm into the dorsal mesentery. A, germ cells at the most dorsal part of the endoderm of the gut before the two migrating mesodermal sheets meet in the dorsal midline; B, germ cells have left the endoderm and lie beneath the sheet of mesoderm; C, as the dorsal mesentery forms, the germ cells migrate into it and then toward the genital ridges. (After P. McD. Whitington and R. E. Dixon, 1975. J. Embryol. Exp. Morphol. 33, 57.)

of the two species, result in the formation of graft-type germ cells. Again, the primordial germ cells, although they appear later and in a different germ layer, are shown to be the forerunners of the entire germ line.

Primordial Germ Cells in the Chick

In the chick embryo, about 20 primordial germ cells may be distinguished uniformly distributed in the blastodisc of the unincubated egg, presumably separated from the somatic cells during the cleavage stages. These cells increase in number and in later blastula stages become localized along the anterior and lateral borders of the blastodisc. In the primitive streak stage, they form a crescentic-shaped group of cells anterior to the primitive streak in the extraembryonic area at the juncture of the area opaca and the area pellucida, forming what is known as the *germinal crescent* (Fig. 19–15). Depriving the embryo of any interaction with this germinal crescent, either by destroying it by cauterization or radiation or by explanting the embryo and not the germinal crescent, results in the formation of sterile gonads. Here again we have clear proof of the origin of all of the germ cells from a group of primordial germ cells segregated from the somatic cells early in development.

Interestingly, in the chick the primordial germ cells move to the developing gonads by the way of the vitelline circulation, which they enter by active migration between the endoderm cells at approximately 33 to 38 hours of incubation. Two embryos may be explanted side by side, one of which has been "sterilized" by the removal of the germinal crescent. Unless circulatory connection is established between the explants, the operated embryo will remain sterile. But if a connection does develop, primordial germ cells pass from the normal to the operated embryo and colonize its gonads and produce germ cells. The unoperated embryo, of course, always develops a normal complement of germ cells since its own primordial germ cells pass to the gonads in the embryo's own circulatory system.

Relation of the Germ Plasm to the Primordial Germ Cells

From the above experiments we may conclude that there is clear evidence that cells with specific distinguishing characteristics are set aside early in the development of many species, cells that will later migrate into and populate the genital ridges. Experimental analysis by destruction and transplantation supplements the descriptive work on their migration and establishes the fact that these cells represent the stem cells of the entire germ line. But what is the relation of the germ plasm to the primordial germ cells?

In the anurans, where the germ plasm is situated at a specific

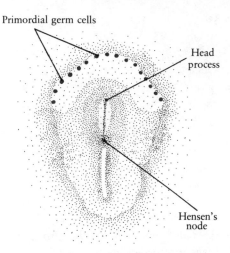

19–15 Position of the primordial germ cells in the chick embryo between the area opaca and area pellucida forming the germinal crescent craniad of the head process.

location in the cleaving egg, we have the opportunity to perform the same kinds of experiments that we have described in the insects. Irradiation of the vegetal hemisphere of the frog egg (*Rana pipiens*) at the beginning of the first cleavage with a UV dose of 8000 ergs per mm² results in the development of larvae lacking germ cells completely. Lower doses have less of an effect but even a dose as low as 2600 ergs per mm² results in an easily observable reduction in the number of germ cells. Irradiation of the animal hemisphere has no effect on germ cell production. UV irradiation of *Xenopus* eggs at the beginning of the first cleavage has the same effect. With a UV dose rate of 150 ergs per mm², as the time of irradiation increases the number of germ cells decrease and no primordial germ cells develop when the total dose is 4500 ergs per mm² or higher (Fig. 19–16).

Microsurgical operations, where a portion of the cytoplasm at the vegetal pole of the embryo is removed, also often result in a total or partial absence of germ cells. Although such experiments obviously indicate the importance of the germ plasm, it is hard to define either qualitatively or quantitatively exactly what was removed.

If we sterilize a frog embryo by irradiating it at the beginning of the first cleavage, what will happen if we inject cytoplasm from the vegetal pole of an unirradiated egg into the irradiated egg? In one such experiment, when vegetal cytoplasm from an unirradiated fertilized egg was injected into four-cell embryos that had been irradiated at the beginning of the first cleavage, about 50 percent of the eggs developed into larvae with germ cells, although in smaller numbers than normal. Transfer of animal pole cytoplasm into irradiated eggs had no effect on germ cell development and all of the irradiated eggs developed into larvae without germ cells.

There seems to be little doubt then that the substance at the vegetal pole which can be histologically identified in the cleaving anuran egg and traced into cells that will develop into primordial germ cells is, in fact, responsible for inducing these cells to differentiate into germ line stem cells. Can we define the nature of this material? Unfortunately, as is the case in another important factor in the development of the amphibian, the organizer, we cannot do so precisely. There are, however, a number of indications that it may be a nucleic acid. There is good correspondence between the UV absorption spectrum for nucleic acids and the relative efficiency of UV irradiation of different wavelengths in germ cell reduction. Since DNA and RNA absorption spectra are the same, this correlation does not distinguish between them. However, the cluster of dense granules found in the vegetal cytoplasm and considered to be a part of the germ plasm stain positively for RNA. In addition, these gran-

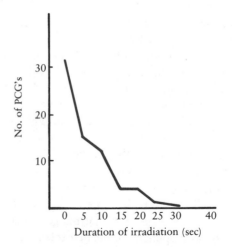

19–16 Average number of primordial germ cells (PGCs) per tadpole following UV irradiation of the *Xenopus* egg at the time of the first cleavage with 150 egs/mm²/sec for increasing lengths of time. (From K. Tanabe and M. Kotani, 1974. J. Embryol. Exp. Morphol. 31, 89.)

ules resemble those found in the pole plasm of the insects that also stain positively for RNA.

Despite all of the evidence relating the germ plasm to the primordial germ cells, the exact role of the germ plasm in controlling germ cell differentiation is poorly defined. In the anurans the few cells that contain the germ plasm behave exactly as do the other endodermal cells up to gastrulation. They divide and undergo the same morphogenetic movements. The first indication of any difference is seen when they begin to show an active migration from the deep endoderm to the roof of the gut. Interestingly, this migration coincides with the movement of the germ plasm from the pole of the cell to the region of the nucleus. This intracellular shifting has led to the suggestion that the germ plasm may well be inactive in early development and its first role in germ cell formation may be to direct the migration of the primordial germ cells from the deep endoderm into the genital ridges. It may also play a role in the initiation of mitotic division of the germ cells after they populate the gonads and the initiation of meiotic divisions of the gonial cells.

Primordial Germ Cells in the Mammal

In mammals, including man, cells that segregate early in development and later migrate into the genital ridges have also been described and identified as primordial germ cells. They show various distinguishing features depending upon the staining techniques employed. When stained with hematoxylin and eosin, they have a clear cytoplasm, but when stained by the azur A method for nucleic acids, the cytoplasm is strongly basophilic. In the mouse, they have also been shown to have at the EM level of observation a number of features which distinguish them from other cells. These include many ribosomes and polysomes, dense granulofibrillar bodies, and annulate cisternae. Also, their nuclei contain compact masses of granules and fibrils, evidence that nuclear metabolic activity is high, perhaps related to the large numbers of ribosomes and polysomes in the cytoplasm. The cells are also distinguished by the small amount of endoplasmic reticulum and Golgi complex that they contain.

In the eight-to-nine-day mouse embryo, the primordial germ cells may be found distributed among the endoderm cells of the allantoic diverticulum, the yolk sac, and the hind gut and midgut. In man, large primordial germ cells with round nuclei, large nucleoli, and clear cytoplasm are seen in the endoderm of the yolk sac of the 13-somite embryo. From here they migrate into the endoderm of the hindgut (Fig. 19–17) and at the 25-somite stage start to leave the hindgut to move to the genital ridges by way of the dorsal mesentery (Fig. 19–18 A,B). They form lobate and filiform pseudopodia

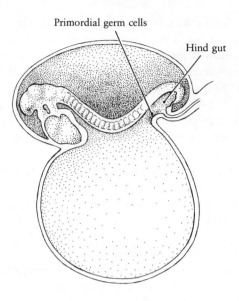

Primordial germ cells

Hind gut

19–17 Diagram of a 16-somite human embryo showing the location of the primordial germ cells in the endoderm of the yolk sac and hindgut. (After E. Witschi, 1948. Carnegie Contributions to Embryology 32, 67.)

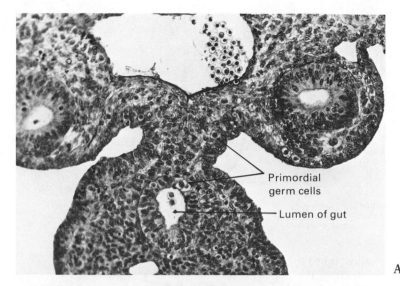

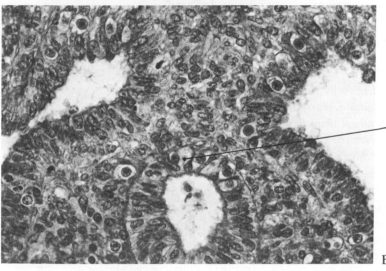

Primordial
germ cells

Lumen of gut

A

19–18   A, cross section through the lower part of the gut of a 32-somite human embryo with primordial germ cells in the dorsal endodermal epithelium, the gut mesenchyme, and the coelomic angles; B, higher power view of two primordial germ cells in the gut epithelium. The cell on the right has broken down the basement membrane and is migrating into the mesenchyme. (From E. Witschi, 1948. Courtesy of the Carnegie Institution of Washington, Davis Division.)

Primordial
germ cell
migrating from
gut endoderm
into the
mesenchyme

B

and the migration is thus due to the active movements of the individual cells.

The Indifferent Gonad

Although the sex of the individual is determined genetically at the time of fertilization, it is not possible to determine the sex of the embryo morphologically until after the age of six weeks. Up until this time, differentiation of the genital ridge is exactly the same in the male and female, and the potential testis and ovary are indistin-

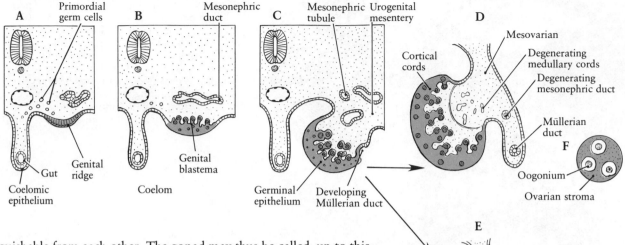

During the fifth week, the thickening *germinal epithelium* proliferates cells into the underlying mesenchyme. The first cells to be
proliferated occupy the deepest position—next to the mesonephros—and form the *rete blastema*. Further proliferation of the
germinal epithelium forms irregular cords of cells, the *primary sex
cords*. They surround the migrating primordial germ cells and constitute the *genital blastema* (Fig. 19–19 B). The indifferent gonad
may be divided into a *primary cortex,* the germinal epithelium, and
a *primary medulla,* the *genital blastema* (primary sex cords) and the
rete blastema. However, there is no actual separation between any
of these parts of the gonad.

The indifferent gonad bulges into the coelom, as the medial part
of the urogenital ridge, connected to the dorsal body wall by a
mesentery that it shares in common with the mesonephros, the
urogenital mesentery (Fig. 19–19 C). As the gonad increases in size,
it separates from the mesonephros and acquires its own separate
mesentery—the *mesorchium* in the male, and *mesovarium* in the
female (Fig. 19–19 D,E).

19–19 Early differentiation of the ovary and
the testis. A, B, primordial germ cells migrating
from the dorsal mesentery into the germinal blastema; C, the indifferent gonad at the age of six
weeks; D, differentiation of the ovary by the proliferation of the secondary sex cords (cortical
cords); E, differentiation of the testis by the proliferation of the primary sex cords (medullary
cords); F, G, diagrams of sections through the
gonads.

Development of the Testis

During the seventh week, two events occur to distinguish a testis
from an ovary. Both of these events occur in the indifferent gonad
destined to become a testis. Their failure to occur at this time
thereby distinguishes an ovary. The changes that take place in the
prospective testis are: first, a continuing proliferation of the primary
sex cords; and second, the formation of a connective tissue layer,
the *tunica albuginea,* between the cortex and the medulla (Fig.
19–19 E).

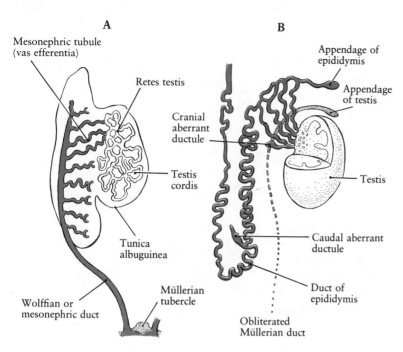

A   B

Mesonephric tubule
(vas efferentia)

Retes testis

Cranial
aberrant
ductule

Testis
cordis

Tunica
albuginea

Wolffian or
mesonephric duct

Müllerian
tubercle

Appendage of
epididymis

Appendage
of testis

Testis

Caudal aberrant
ductule

Duct of
epididymis

Obliterated
Müllerian duct

19–20 A, diagram of the male genital ducts in the fourth month of development. The Müllerian system has regressed;, B, diagram of the male genital ducts showing the vestigial remnants of the Wolffian and Müllerian systems. (After L. B. Arey, 1974. Developmental Anatomy. W. B. Saunders Company, Philadelphia.)

The primary sex cords of the genital blastema continue to proliferate and form branched strands of cells, the *medullary sex cords*. These will form the *seminiferous tubules* of the testis. The seminiferous tubules are lined with an epithelium consisting of two types of cells: primordial germ cells that will differentiate into spermatogonia; cells derived from the germinal epithelium that will form the sustentacular or *Sertoli cells*. The early sex cords are composed primarily of Sertoli cells.

The rete blastema differentiates into a network of channels, the *rete testis*, which establishes connection with the seminiferous tubules through the straight tubules, *tubuli recti*. The general topography of the testis is well marked by the middle of pregnancy and the duct system is well organized (Fig. 19–20). However, the duct system is not completely canalized, and the sperm are not differentiated until puberty.

The mesenchymal portion of the medulla forms the connective tissue components. Between the seminiferous tubules, it forms septa that partition the testis into over 200 lobules. The septa converge toward the mesorchium to form the *mediastinum* where the rete testis is located. Peripherally, the septa extend to the tunica albuginea, which by about 10 weeks completely envelopes the testis. The tunica albuginea separates the cortex from the medulla and effectively prevents any further participation of the original germinal epithelium in the differentiation of the testis. The germinal epithelium flattens out to form the mesothelium and the tunica albuginea forms the underlying capsule.

In addition to connective tissue, the mesenchymal cells of the medulla also differentiate into interstitial or *Leydig cells.* Leydig cells reach a maximum number in the fetus at about the end of the fifth month; after this period they decline. As they fall off in numbers, the rate of the differentiation of the seminiferous tubules increases. However, a causal relationship between these two events has not been established.

Development of the Ovary

In the indifferent gonad destined to become an ovary, the primary sex cords do not continue to proliferate after the sixth week, nor does a tunica albuginea develop at this time, Rather, the primary sex cords remain indistinct and are intermingled with connective tissue that does not form septa. Their fate is to form a rudimentary *rete ovarii* (homologous to the rete testis) and the medullary tissue of the ovary.

The development of the cortical portion of the gonad distinguishes the ovary from the testis. At about 10 weeks the coelomic germinal epithelium undergoes a secondary proliferation (Fig. 19–19 D). This proliferation forms cortical sex cords or *secondary sex cords,* a process that has no counterpart in the male. These cords penetrate the underlying mesenchyme but remain close to the surface. During the fourth month, isolated masses of the cortical sex cords surround individual primordial germ cells forming primordial follicles. A primordial (primary) follicle consists of a single layer of flattened cells, follicular cells, derived from the secondary sex cords, surrounding an oogonium, which is the derivative of a primordial germ cell (Fig. 19–19 G). Ovarian follicle cells and testicular Sertoli cells are homologous to each other. The mitotic activity of the primordial germ cells continues throughout most of fetal life, and the proliferation of the germinal epithelium also continues until a thin tunica albuginea is formed during the eighth month. The primary (medullary) sex cords and the primordial germ cells associated with them in the indifferent gonad do not contribute to the formation of ovarian follicles. They degenerate and are replaced by a vascular, fibrous connective tissue stroma that forms the definitive medulla of the ovary.

Proliferative activity in the ovary ceases before birth and the formation of new or additional germ cells does not ever take place again. Thus, the human female at birth contains in her ovaries all of the germ cells that she will ever produce. Contrast this to the male where the major function of the postpuberal testis is the continual production of many millions of new spermatogonia.

Although some of the primary follicles in the fetal ovary may respond to increased estrogen secretion in late fetal life by forming antra, these follicles do not mature but become atretic. Most of the primary follicles remain in their undifferentiated stage until, at puberty, they respond to hormonal stimulation by developing into mature follicles.

The Reproductive Duct System

The sex ducts and the sex accessory glands develop from discrete primordia in each sex. However, in all embryos, no matter what the sex, there is a time when the primordia of the duct systems of both sexes are present. The male appropriates as its major sex duct the mesonephric (Wolffian) ducts. The major portion of the female duct system develops from the *paramesonephric (Müllerian)* ducts, which first appear as infoldings of the coelomic epithelium of the urogenital ridge lateral to the mesonephric ducts.

The development of the duct system of both sexes is complicated by the fact that in each sex remnants of the system of the opposite sex persist and form nonfunctional vestigial structures.

The Male
The germinal epithelium of the seminiferous tubules is the site of sperm production and from this location, the sperm must find their way to the outside. The development of the passageways for the first stage in this journey, from the seminiferous tubules to tubuli recti to rete testis—all derivatives of the primary sex cords—has already been described.

It has been noted that the male appropriates the mesonephric duct to form the vas deferens. A connection between the vas deferens and the rete testis must then be established. This connection is made through the mesonephric tubules at the level of the developing testis. As the mesonephros degenerates, the tubules in the region of the testis become shortened and somewhat disorganized, and the glomeruli become fibrous and are extruded from the glomerular capsule. The rete testis is in close contact with the blind ends of these tubules. The rete testis establishes connections with them, and they become canalized and form the *vas efferentia,* the passage from the testis to the mesonephric duct (Fig. 19–20 A). The region of the mesonephric duct just below the point where the vas efferentia open becomes elongated and highly convoluted and forms the *epididymis.* The remainder of the Wolffian duct caudad of the epididymis acquires a thick coat of smooth muscle and develops into the vas deferens. The vas deferens opens into the urogenital sinus at a point marked by Müller's tubercle as has been previously described. Just before the point where the vas deferens opens into the urogenital sinus a sacculation appears at about three months, representing the beginning of the development of the *seminal vesicles.* The short portion of the vas deferens between the point of origin of the seminal vesicles and its entrance into the urogenital sinus (urethra) is known as the *ejaculatory duct.*

Some parts of the mesonephros not forming functional sections of the male duct system fail to degenerate completely and persist as vestigial structures (Fig. 19–20 B). The blind cranial end of the mesonephric duct forms the *appendix epididymis.* Some of the cranial group of mesonephric tubules, which form the vas efferens, end blindly and become the *cranial aberrant ductules.* A caudal group of tubules, which never form any functional component of the system, also persist as the *paradidymis* and the *caudal aberrant ductule.*

The Female

The paramesonephric (Müllerian) ducts form the *uterine tubes* (oviducts, Fallopian tubes), the *uterus,* and part of the *vagina.* These ducts first appear during the fifth week as bilateral thickenings of the coelomic epithelium on the anterolateral surface of the urogenital ridge near its cranial pole (Fig. 19–21 A).

Each thickening sinks in to form a groove (Fig. 19–21 B) whose lips then close over to form a duct, which, however, remains open at its cranial end. The Müllerian ducts grow caudally in close relationship with the mesonephric ducts. As they approach the cloaca, they move medially, anterior to the mesonephric ducts, and fuse into a common *uterovaginal canal* (Fig. 19–22). Fusion of the two Müllerian ducts also brings together the two folds of peritoneum in

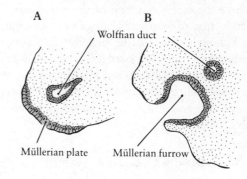

19–21 A, early development of the Müllerian duct as a thickening of the coelomic epithelium lateral to the Wolffian duct; B, the plate invaginates to form a groove.

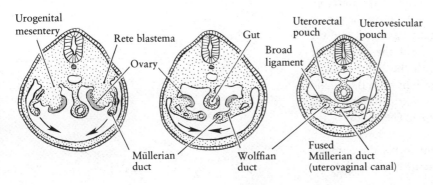

19–22 Anteromedial movement and fusion of the Müllerian ducts represented by diagrams drawn of successively more caudal levels. Ovary becomes positioned on the posterior aspect of the two folds of mesentery (future broad ligaments) in which the Müllerian ducts lie.

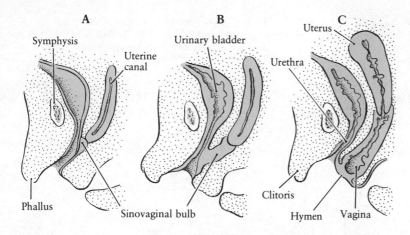

A — Symphysis, Uterine canal, Phallus, Sinovaginal bulb

B — Urinary bladder

C — Uterus, Urethra, Clitoris, Hymen, Vagina

19–23 Diagram of the development of the uterus and the vagina. A, nine weeks; B, end of the third month. Sinovaginal bulbs between the urogenital sinus and the uterus. Solid at first (upper cross section), they begin to hollow out (lower cross section); C, at birth. The vagina is separated from the vestibule by an incomplete hymen.

which they lie. The fused uterovaginal canal is thus connected on either side by a broad sheet of tissue to the posterior body wall. This sheet is the *broad ligament*. The uterovaginal canal and the broad ligament divide the peritoneal cavity in this region into an anterior *vesicouterine pouch* and a posterior *rectouterine pouch* (of Douglas) Figs. 19–22 C; 19–23). The uterovaginal canal ends blindly in contact with the urogenital sinus (Figs. 19–23; 19–24), and at this site is formed the elevation on the posterior inner wall of the sinus known as *Müller's tubercle* (Fig. 19–24).

The unfused cranial portions of the Müllerian ducts form the paired uterine tubes. The funnel-shaped opening at the cranial end of the tube becomes the abdominal ostium and develops fringes or fimbriae surrounding the opening into the uterine tube.

The fused portion of the ducts forms the *corpus* and the *cervix* of the uterus. The juncture between the two Müllerian ducts is at first Y-shaped and the uterus is thus bicornuate up until the third month (Fig. 19–24 A). Thereafter, a secondary cranial extension of this area occurs so that the original angular junction of the Müllerian tubes now becomes dome-shaped, forming the *fundus* (Fig. 19–24 B,C). The mesenchyme surrounding the uterus becomes greatly thickened to form the uterine myometrium, the muscular wall of the uterus.

At the point where the blind end of the uterovaginal canal approaches the urogenital sinus, a pair of solid masses of tissue grows out of the urogenital sinus into the caudal end of the uteroveginal canal. These are the *sinovaginal bulbs* (Fig. 19–24). They form a solid plate of cells, the vaginal plate, which proliferates rapidly and increases the distance between the urogenital sinus and the primordium of the uterus. Later, the central core of this plate breaks down and forms the vaginal lumen. By the fifth month, the vagina is en-

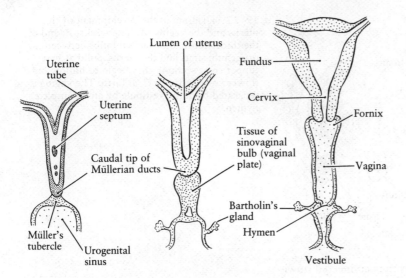

Uterine tube

Uterine septum

Caudal tip of Müllerian ducts

Müller's tubercle

Urogenital sinus

Lumen of uterus

Fundus

Cervix

Tissue of sinovaginal bulb (vaginal plate)

Bartholin's gland

Hymen

Fornix

Vagina

Vestibule

19–24 Diagrams of frontal sections of the stages shown in Figure 19–17. Bartholin's glands develop as outgrowths of the urogenital sinus. They open into the vestibule.

tirely canalized and winglike extensions surround the uterine cervix forming the vaginal *fornices.* Although the uterovaginal bulbs form the vaginal epithelium, the fibromuscular coat of the organ develops from the uterovaginal primordium. The vagina is separated from the urogenital sinus by a fold of tissue, the *hymen,* which persists to varying degrees postnatally as an incomplete partition over the entrance to the vagina.

Heterosexual Remnants of the Duct System

The Male
The Müllerian system in the male atrophies during the third month of development with the exception of cranial and caudal remnants. The cranial remnant becomes the *appendix testis.* The caudal remnant persists as a small pouch on the dorsal wall of the urethra, the *prostatic utricle* or *vagina masculina* (Fig. 19–20 B).

The Female
Portions of both the cranial and the caudal groups of mesonephric tubules persist as vestigal structures in the female (Fig. 19–25 B). The cranial tubules form a number of tiny canals attached to a short remnant of the mesonephric duct, which in the male forms the epididymis. Collectively, these tubules, located within the broad ligament, form the *epoöphoron.* A few of the cranial tubules become the cystic *aberrant tubules.* Remnants of the caudal group of tubules form the *paroöphoron.* Isolated remnants of the mesonephric duct, corresponding to regions that form the vas deferens in the

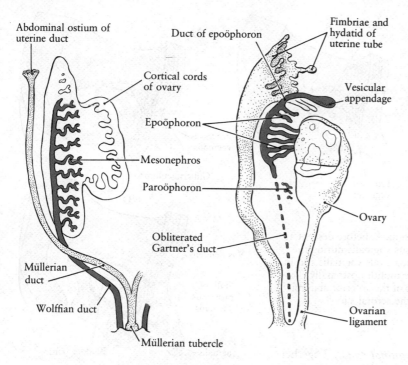

Abdominal ostium of
uterine duct

Duct of epoöphoron

Fimbriae and
hydatid of
uterine tube

Cortical cords
of ovary

Vesicular
appendage

Epoöphoron

Mesonephros

Paroöphoron

Ovary

Obliterated
Gartner's duct

Müllerian
duct

Wolffian duct

Ovarian
ligament

Müllerian tubercle

19–25 A, diagram of the duct system of the female in the second month of development. Fused
Müllerian ducts meet the urogenital sinus at a
point marked by Müller's tubercle. B, Vestigial
remnants of the mesonephric tubules and mesonephros in the female. (After L. B. Arey, 1974.
Developmental Anatomy. W. B. Saunders Company, Philadelphia.)

male, may persist in the broad ligament lateral to the uterus or in
the walls of the vagina as the *duct of Gartner*.

Genital Ligaments and the Descent of the Gonads

The Male

The developing gonad and the mesonephros are attached to the
posterior body wall by the urogenital mesentery (Fig. 19–19 C). As
the mesonephros degenerates, this broad connection narrows and
becomes the mesentery of the gonad, which in the case of the testis
is called the *mesorchium* (Fig. 19–19 E). The cranial pole of the
testis is continuous with the mesonephros and the urogenital mesentery that extends up to the diaphragm. Both of these structures
degenerate completely, after which the cranial pole of the testis does
not have any ligamentous attachment. However, the peritoneal fold
attached to the caudal pole of the testis persists and, reinforced by
mesoderm and parts of the degenerating mesonephros, becomes the
caudal genital ligament (Fig. 19–26 A). The caudal genital ligament
extends from the caudal pole of the testis to the region where the
urogenital ridge bends toward the midline. From this bend, a new
ligament makes connection with the adjacent body wall and is, in
turn, continuous with a mesenchymal condensation extending
through the abdominal wall into the genital (scrotal) swellings. The

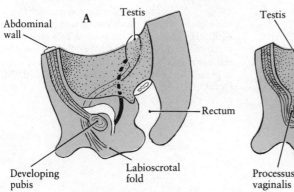
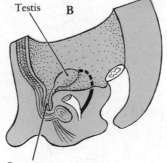
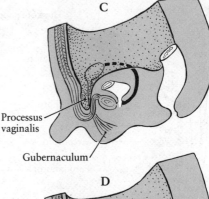

A — Abdominal wall, Testis, Developing pubis, Labioscrotal fold, Rectum

B — Testis, Processus vaginalis

C — Processus vaginalis, Gubernaculum

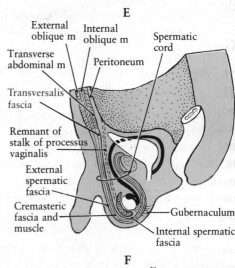

D — Vas deferens, Stalk of processus vaginalis, Processus vaginalis, Bladder (cut)

E — External oblique m, Internal oblique m, Spermatic cord, Transverse abdominal m, Peritoneum, Transversalis fascia, Remnant of stalk of processus vaginalis, External spermatic fascia, Cremasteric fascia and muscle, Gubernaculum, Internal spermatic fascia

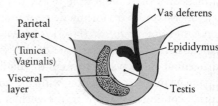

F — Parietal layer (Tunica Vaginalis), Visceral layer, Vas deferens, Epididymus, Testis

19–26 Descent of the testis shown in sagittal section. A, before descent at about seven weeks; B, C, passage into the processus vaginalis during the seventh month; D, fully descended but with the processus vaginalis still in communication with the abdominal cavity; E, one month postnatally. Processus vaginalis closed off. All of the muscle layers of the anterior abdominal wall are represented by muscle and fascia of the scrotal sac.

passage through the abdominal wall is the *inguinal canal*. Together these three tissue cords connecting the caudal pole of the testis to the scrotum constitute the *gubernaculum testis*. As the abdominal cavity increases in cross-sectional and longitudinal directions, the testis remains attached to the scrotum by the gubernaculum. The gubernaculum does not keep pace with the growth of the abdominal region and thus the testes undergoes an apparent caudal migration so that by the end of the third month they no longer are found in the abdominal cavity but are in the pelvic cavity close to the area of the inguinal canals.

At the beginning of the third month, a bilateral evagination of the coelom forms just anterior to each gubernaculum. Each peritoneally lined extension of the coelom is known as a *processus vaginalis*. Each sac evaginates into the anterior abdominal wall and follows the course of the gubernaculum through the inguinal canal into the scrotal swelling (Fig. 19–26). The herniation of the vaginal process is covered by the muscular and connective tissue components found in this region of the anterior abdominal wall. They will form coverings of the testis, each of which can be related to its corresponding layer in the abdominal wall.

The testes remain in the pelvic cavity in close proximity to the processus vaginalis until the eleventh month. At this time, the testes descend through the inguinal canal into the scrotum (Fig. 19–26 D). The testes and the gubernaculum always lie beneath the peritoneal lining of the processus vaginalis. The epididymis, vas deferens, and the blood vessels and nerves supplying the testes are carried into the vaginal process with the testes. These ducts, vessels, and nerves passing back into the peritoneal cavity through the inguinal canal collectively constitute the *spermatic cord*. The original broad opening between the vaginal process and the peritoneal cavity becomes narrower and is obliterated before birth. Within the scrotum, a remnant of the vaginal process persists. The lining of this cavity is the parietal layer of the *tunica vaginalis* that becomes, where it covers the testis, the visceral layer of the tunica vaginalis (Fig. 19–26 E).

The final descent of the testes from the peritoneal cavity into the scrotal sacs is accompanied by a marked shortening of the gubernaculum. However, whether or not this is responsible for the descent of the testes is not known. There is good evidence that androgens and gonadotrophins play a role in the descent of the testis, and this is supported by clinical applications.

The Female

In the female, both the cranial and the caudal poles of the ovary are connected to ligamentous remnants of the urogenital region, forming the *suspensory ligament* of the ovary and *ovarian (proper) ligaments,* respectively. The ovarian ligament attaches the ovary to the broad ligament. A caudal extension connects the broad ligament and the uterus to the labia majora. This is the *round ligament*. Thus, the ovarian ligament and the round ligament together are homologous to the gubernaculum of the male. The male has no homologue of the suspensory ligament. The ovary undergoes a descent but does not normally pass through the inguinal canal into the genital swellings although a small processus vaginalis is formed. It is usually obliterated but may persist as a small diverticulum of the peritoneum, the *canal of Nuck*.

The ovary is connected to the posterior wall of the broad ligament by the *mesovarium,* a persistent part of the original urogenital ligament. The uterine tubes are connected to the broad ligament by the mesosalpinx, connective tissue remnants of the mesonephros.

External Genitalia

The primorida of the external genitalia represent, as do those of the gonads, a true case of ambisexuality in which there is present at an early stage a set of structures that have the potentiality of differentiating in either a male or a female direction.

During the third week of development, a pair of elevated folds of mesoderm develop on either side of the cloacal membrane. These are the *cloacal folds*. During the fourth week, these folds meet an-

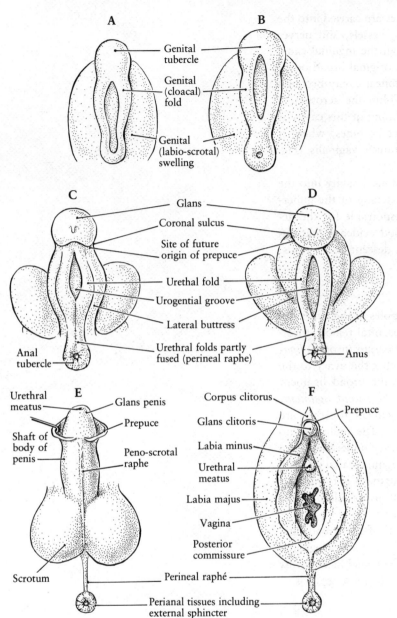

A

Genital tubercle

Genital (cloacal) fold

Genital (labio-scrotal) swelling

B

C

Glans

Coronal sulcus

Site of future origin of prepuce

Urethal fold

Urogential groove

Lateral buttress

Anal tubercle

Urethral folds partly fused (perineal raphe)

D

Anus

E

Urethral meatus

Glans penis

Prepuce

Shaft of body of penis

Peno-scrotal raphe

Scrotum

F

Corpus clitorus

Prepuce

Glans clitoris

Labia minus

Urethral meatus

Labia majus

Vagina

Posterior commissure

Perineal raphé

Perianal tissues including external sphincter

19–27 Development of the male and female genitalia from a perineal view. A, B, indifferent stages at 4 and 7 weeks; C, E, male at about 9 and 12 weeks; D, F, female at about 9 and 12 weeks.

teriorly at the site of a median elevation, the *genital tubercle* (Fig. 19–27 A, B). At the same time, a second pair of rather indistinct elevations, the *genital (labioscrotal) swellings* appear (Fig. 19–27 A, B). They surround both the genital tubercle and the cloacal folds. When the urorectal septum fuses with the cloacal membrane, it divides it into an anterior urogenital membrane and a posterior anal membrane surrounded by the urogenital folds and the anal folds, respectively. Up to this time, six weeks, the appearance of the external genitalia in the male and the female is identical.

The Male

During the third month, a male is characterized by a marked enlargement and elongation of the genital tubercle (phallus) as it begins to develop into the *penis* (Fig. 19–27 C). As the phallus elongates, it pulls the urogenital folds anteriorly, and they form an elongated pair of folds stretching along the underside of the developing penis. The urogenital sinus has now broken through and appears as a deep groove, the *urogenital (urethral) groove* between the urogenital folds but not reaching all the way to the tip of the penis (Fig. 19–27 C). The urethral groove is lined by the endoderm of the phallic portion of the urogenital sinus.

The urethral folds grow toward each other and at the end of the third month they fuse along the midventral axis of the penis. The urethral groove is thus converted into a canal, the *penile urethra*. The most distal part of the definitive penile urethra, however, is not a derivative of the urogenital groove, but is formed by canalization of a cord of ectodermal cells, which grows inward from the tip of the glans to meet the portion of the urethra formed from the urethral groove (Fig. 19–28). The *external urethral meatus* and the *navicular fossa* (glandular part of the urethra) are derivatives of the ectodermal cord. The skin at the distal margin of the penis grows forward over the *glans penis* to form the *prepuce*. Initially the prepuce fuses with the glans but separates from it during infancy.

The genital swellings become the *scrotal swellings* and grow toward and fuse with each other to form the scrotum. The line of fusion is marked by the *scrotal raphe* (Fig. 19–27 E).

The *corpus cavernosum urethrae* (*corpus spongiosum*) surrounding the penile urethra and the paired *corpora cavernosa penis* develop from the mesenchymal tissue of the shaft of the penis.

The Female

The changes that occur in the female are not so profound as those in the male. The phallus enlarges only slightly and bends caudally to form the *clitoris*. It has a *glans clitoris* and a *prepuce*. The urethral folds do not fuse and form the *labia minora*. They flank a shallow cavity, the *vestibule*, which represents the urethral portion of the urogenital sinus (Fig. 19–27 D). Nor do the genital swellings fuse, except posteriorly where they form the posterior commisure. They enlarge to become the horseshoe-shaped *labia majora* (Fig. 19–27 F).

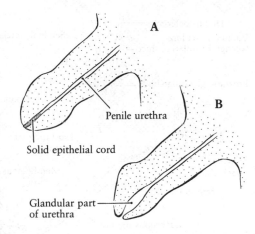

19–28   Development of the penile urethra.

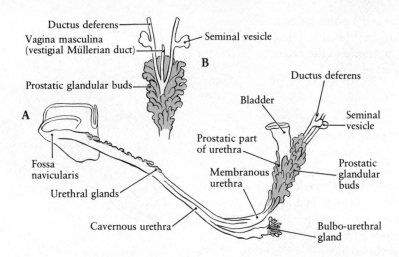

Ductus deferens

Vagina masculina
(vestigial Müllerian duct)

Seminal vesicle

B

Prostatic glandular buds

A

Ductus deferens

Bladder

Seminal
vesicle

Prostatic part
of urethra

Fossa
navicularis

Prostatic
glandular
buds

Urethral glands

Membranous
urethra

Cavernous urethra

Bulbo-urethral
gland

19–29 Vas deferens, urethra, and related structures at about midterm. A, lateral view; B, posterior view.

The Accessory Sex Glands

The Male

Accessory sex glands are more highly developed in the male. The origin of the seminal vesicles from the lower ends of the mesonephric ducts has been described. The mesoderm into which they grow forms the muscle of their walls.

Three other glands, all derivatives of the urethral epithelium, also develop, the *prostate,* the *bulbourethral* (Cowper's) glands and the *urethral glands* (of Littré). The large prostate develops as a multiple outgrowth of the urethra above and below the openings of the mesonephric ducts (Fig. 19–29). These differentiate into the glandular epithelium of the organ while the surrounding mesoderm forms their muscle and connective tissue components. The bulbourethral glands arise as a pair of solid outgrowths at the beginning of the penile urethra, from the portion that will form the membranous urethra. They extend a short distance posteriorly paralleling the urethra and pick up their muscle and connective tissue coats from the surrounding mesoderm. The numerous small glands of Littré develop as buds from the cavernous urethra.

The Female

Since the seminal vesicles are outgrowths of the mesonephric ducts it is understandable that the female, in which these ducts degenerate, forms no homologue of these glands. However, homologues of the three derivatives of the urethral epithelium do develop. In the female, the sex accessory glands are all considerably smaller than the male homologues. The *urethral* and *paraurethral glands* (of Skene) correspond to the prostate. Outgrowths of the urogenital sinus form the *major vestibular glands* (of Bartholin) and the *minor vestibular glands* both opening into the vestibule. They are the homologues of the bulbourethral glands and the urethral glands of Littré, respectively.

HORMONAL CONTROL OF THE DIFFERENTIATION OF THE REPRODUCTIVE SYSTEM

As described in the previous sections, parts of both the male and the female reproductive systems differentiate from embryonic structures that at one stage in development are common to both sexes (ambisexuality—gonad, external genitalia). On the other hand, other parts develop from discrete primordia (bisexuality—duct system). In addition, the reproductive system in the adult is an important part of the endocrine system, synthesizing in both sexes potent hormones that are responsible for the maintenance and function of the reproductive organs. Since the adult system is so markedly influenced by the sex hormones, it is not surprising that there has been considerable investigation of the role of sex hormones in the development of the system. This is particularly interesting in respect to the genetic control of sex and the presence of ambisexual and bisexual primordia.

The genetic sex of an individual is determined at the time of fertilization. In man, the male is the heterogametic sex with 22 pairs of autosomes and a pair of unmatched sex chromosomes (XY). The female has the same number of autosomes but a matched pair of sex chromosomes (XX). Normally, the genetic sex expresses itself in the development of either a typical male or a typical female.

Genetic control of the development of the reproductive system, however, is not absolute. In fact, it can be reversed. Generally, the lower one goes on the evolutionary scale, the more easily can sexual development be modified. In fact, so labile is genetic sex determination in the platyfish (a favorite viviparous fish of aquarium fanciers) that about 1 percent of these fish normally develop into functional adults of a sex opposite to their genotype. Experimental sex reversal, using sex hormones, can easily be accomplished in many teleosts. In the amphibians, while there are differences between species, sex reversal following experimental exposure of the embryos to steroid hormones of the opposite sex has been reported often. In *Rana* and *Hyla*, the female is homogametic and may be completely masculinized by androgen treatment. In *Xenopus*, lifelong sex reversal of the male toad may be induced by adding estrogens for only three days to the aquarium water containing the larvae. In *Xenopus*, the male is the homogametic sex (ZZ). Mating these sex-reversed ZZ females to normal males should, and does, result in entirely male offspring.

Birds and toads present somewhat of a special situation in which genetic sex may be reversed surgically owing to the presence in the adult of gonadal remnants of the opposite sex which are stimulated to differentiate when the normal gonads are removed. Bidder's organ in the male toad is a cortical remnant, a rudimentary ovary, located at the cranial pole of each testis. Following removal of the testes, Bidder's organ enlarges and develops into a functional ovary. In the female chicken, the right gonad remains rudimentary. It consists mainly of medullary tissue and, if the functional left ovary is removed, the right rudimentary gonad will develop into a testis in which spermatogenesis proceeds normally. However, since in the female the Wolffian duct system has regressed, there is no way for the sperm to reach the outside.

Development of the Gonad

One method of studying the effect of hormones on the development of the gonad is through parabiosis. Parabiotic union of salamander larvae before the sex of the larvae can be determined will result in about 50 percent of the unions being between individuals of the opposite sex. In such heterosexual pairs, the testes develop normally but the ovaries are inhibited. The parabiosed females are sterile and may later develop testicular nodules in the sterile gonad which show spermatogenesis and produce mature sperm. From the results of such parabiosis experiments, it has been concluded that the testes differentiate earlier than the ovaries and secrete male hormones that pass across to the female larva and inhibit the development of its gonad. Although union of larvae of the opposite sex of the same age results in male dominance, the opposite effect—the female inhibiting male differentiation—may result from the union of older or more rapidly developing females with younger or more slowly developing males.

Other experiments in fish, amphibians, and birds could be cited, including hormone administration and gonad transplantation, which demonstrate control of the differentiation of the gonad by the sex hormones in these phyla.

With few exceptions, the situation in the mammal is not the same and the gonad not only develops according to the genetic sex without any stimulation from the sex hormones but also is generally refractory to hormonal influence whether it occurs naturally or by experimental design. One exception is the freemartin, a masculinized heifer that develops as a twin of a normal male. During development, the fetal membranes of the twins are united in such a manner that they provide cross circulation between the male and the female fetuses. In the freemartin, the ovary is inhibited to a greater or lesser degree, the most masculinizing effect being the development of sterile seminiferous tubules.

Numerous attempts have been made to duplicate nature's freemartin "experiment" and to demonstrate an inhibitory effect of sex hormones on the differentiation of the gonads in mammals. The results have almost always been negative. Injection of the mother or the fetus with steroid hormones does not result in any effect on the developing gonad, although, as will be discussed in the next section, effects on the duct system and external genitalia do occur. One exception is the opossum. The opossum is born at an early stage of development when the reproductive system is still undifferentiated and spends the last part of what should be its intrauterine life attached to a nipple in its mother's pouch. Injection of estradiol into newborn male opossums stimulates the development of the cortical region of the testis, forming an ovatestis in which oocytes may differentiate.

Although steroid hormone injections usually do not modify gonad differentiation, if fetal gonads of the opposite sex are placed in close proximity to each other, the influence is much greater. Transplants of heterosexual rat gonads where the ovary is taken from a fetus older (16 days) than that which provides the testis transplant (13 days) have shown that the older fetal ovary can suppress, but not reverse, the differentiation of the younger testis. However, in heterosexual transplants of gonads from embryos of the same age, the testis appears to exert a greater influence than the ovary. When ovaries and testes from mouse embryos of the same age are transplanted together below the kidney capsule, the ovaries develop into ovatestes. In this situation, potential female germ cells form spermatogonia.

It has been suggested that the fetal testis secretes a hormone different from that of the adult testis, one that can inhibit the differentiation of the cortical tissue of the developing gonad. However, such a hormone has never been identified nor synthesized, and the concept remains controversial. Despite the small number of cases in which it has been shown that sex hormones may influence the differentiation of the gonad, the conclusion is generally reached that under normal conditions the gonad in mammals differentiates according to its genetic constitution and is not influenced by hormonal factors.

Development of the Duct System and the External Genitalia

The development of the duct system and the external genitalia presents a different story; here it has been shown that the secretions of the developing gonads—in particular the testes—control the direction of differentiation. One method of determining the effect of the gonad is to remove it. In the castrated male fetus, the Wolffian duct system either does not differentiate or regresses, the Müllerian system persists, and the external genitalia remain undifferentiated and femalelike. In the castrated female fetus, the Müllerian system and the external genitalia develop normally, and the Wolffian system does not differentiate or regresses. These effects indicate that the male reproductive tract requires the stimulation of hormones from the developing testes while the Müllerian derivatives can develop normally without any hormonal influence. This conclusion is supported by tissue culture experiments. The Wolffian duct will develop and differentiate in tissue culture only if testicular material is present. Contrary to this, the Müllerian ducts develop whether ovarian tissue is present or not.

If the male system differentiates only in the presence of testicular hormones and the female system needs no hormonal stimulation, this readily explains why, in the female fetus, the Wolffian system regresses and the Müllerian system differentiates. But why, in the male fetus, does the Müllerian system regress? It would be logical to expect that substances from the fetal testes, in addition to stimulating the male system might also inhibit the female. In the normal male fetus and in the castrated male fetus into which a fetal testis has been transplanted, the Wolffian system differentiates and the Müllerian system regresses. However, in the castrated male fetus injected with androgens, although the Wolffian system persists, so does the Müllerian. It would appear that the testicular substance responsible for the regression of the Müllerian system is not an androgen. This is further supported by the fact that if an antiandrogen is given to a normal male fetus, the Wolffian ducts will regress but so will the Müllerian.

The general conclusion, then, is that in the male two different substances secreted by the developing testes are needed for the differentiation of the male reproductive tract and the regression of the female tract, respectively. The first is an androgen. The second has not been identified—except that it is not an adrogen. In the female, in the absence of any stimulating androgenic effect, the Wolffian system regresses and in the absence of an inhibitory signal from testicular tissue, the Müllerian system differentiates.

The period of time during which a testis can exert its influence is limited to that period during which the reproductive structures are differentiating. There is then what may be called a "critical period," and only during this time can testicular hormones be effective. Once any part of the Wolffian system has developed, it escapes from the influence of the male hormone and will not regress if the androgenic influence is withdrawn. The same holds true for the Müllerian system. Once it has differentiated, it will not regress. Equally important, once either system has regressed, it can no longer be called back into existence and is lost forever. It follows that, if the Wolffian system is stimulated by the male hormone during only part of the critical period and then the stimulus is removed, its differentiation will be incomplete, stopping at the time the male hormone is withdrawn but not regressing to a more undifferentiated level.

GENETIC DETERMINATION OF GONADAL DIFFERENTIATION

In mammals, the XX/XY scheme of sex determination exists with the male being the heterogametic sex. Since the disparity between the number of X chromosomes between the male and the female is eliminated by an X-inactivation mechanism (which will be further described in the following section), the only significant genetic difference between the sexes is due to the Y chromosome, which is male specific. In the fetus that carries an XY set of sex chromosomes, the gonads will differentiate into testes that then synthesize and secrete the hormones controlling the differentiation of a male reproductive tract and accessory sex glands and external genitalia.

It is the Y chromosome that is responsible for the organization of a testis, and this function is considered to be due to the production of a Y-linked histocompatibility antigen (H-Y), a plasma membrane protein. Investigation of the H-Y antigen began in 1955 when it was discovered that female mice unexpectedly rejected skin grafts from male mice of the same inbred strain. Humoral antibody against the H-Y antigen can be produced in female mice sensitized with male skin grafts. This antibody is cytotoxic for mouse sperm and dissociated male epithelial cells. These effects provide the opportunity to test for the presence of H-Y antigen in other species by absorbing the antibody with cells of the other species and then testing for residual cytotoxic activity. It has been demonstrated that male cells of all mammalian species tested, including man, specifically absorbed the H-Y antigen while female cells did not. The occurrence of this antigen in all male species and its absence in all female species tested suggested that it might, in fact, be the testis-organizing plasma membrane protein by which the Y chromosome exerted its effect on gonadal differentiation.

The experimental evidence supports this proposal. If a suspension of cells from a mouse testis is allowed to reaggregate in culture, the cells will form numerous short, seminiferous tubulelike structures. However, if these same cells, before they are allowed to reaggregate, are first subjected to an excess of H-Y antibody—which effectively strips them of the H-Y antigen—they now form folliclelike structures in which a single male primordial germ cell is surrounded by what appear to be follicular cells. Thus, tubular organization is the function of the H-Y antigen, and in its absence testis cells that presumably would have become Sertoli cells now form follicle cells.

The differentiation of the indifferent gonad into a testis thus depends upon the expression of H-Y antigen, which is usually dependent upon the presence of a Y chromosome. However, in certain cases, maleness may be expressed in the absence of a Y chromosome. XX males occur in a frequency of about one to several thousand and have been shown to express H-Y antigen. In fact, in the mole-vole, *Eliobus lutescens,* the Y chromosome has been permanently eliminated, and the sex chromosome constitution is XO in both sexes. The males, however, all express the H-Y antigen and the females do not. In this species then the H-Y gene is probably linked to the X chromosome. The direction of the differentiation of the fetal gonad then should be considered to depend solely on the presence or absence of the expression of the H-Y antigen.

Conversely, some individuals with a Y chromosome may show a female phenotype. In one instance, this has been found to be due to a mutation of the X-linked gene, which specifies the production of the androgen-receptor protein. In the absence of a receptor protein, the tissues fail to respond to any androgen present. This illustrates that the sole function of the H-Y antigen in determining maleness is to organize testicular material. In this mutant the antigen fulfills its testis-determining role, but other factors intervene to prevent the action of the male hormone. A different situation occurs in the wood lemming (*Mypopus schistocolor*). In this species, some females produce all female progeny when mated to normal XY males. This has been determined to be due to a mutation on the X chromosome of the female. In the presence of this mutation XY lemmings develop into completely normal females that, in turn, never produce anything but female progeny. Here, the H-Y antigen is itself repressed and never gets the opportunity to exercise its function.

The H-Y antigen has also been shown to be present in species other than mammals and evidence for the presence of an antigen identical or showing cross-reaction with mouse H-Y has been presented both in species in which the male is the heterogametic species (the frog, *Rana pipiens*) and in which the female is the heterogametic sex (the white leghorn chicken, *Gallus domesticus* and the South African clawed frog, *Xenopus laevis*). When the female is heterogametic, the H-Y (H-W) antigen is found in the female. Thus, the mouse H-Y antigen is a cell surface component, which over an evolutionary span of several hundred millions of years, has functioned to direct the indifferent fetal gonad to differentiate in the direction typified by the heterogametic sex of the particular species in question (testes in XY males and ovaries in ZW females).

Intersexuality

On the basis of the above description of the control of the differentiation of the reproductive system, it is apparent that serious abnormalities of this system result either from the failure of the male gonad to exert its normal influence on the male fetus or from the influence of androgens on the female fetus during the development of its reproductive system. Timing is critical: when a stimulus is applied or is lacking is of utmost importance. The strength of the stimulus is also a factor. In man, a large number of reproductive system abnormalities presents evidence of the variety of effects that may result when the normal hormonal levels are not maintained.

In studying abnormalities of the reproductive system it is often difficult to determine the actual (genetic) sex of the individual by a physical examination, so complex are the abnormalities that present themselves. Of considerable value in this respect was the discovery of the sexual dimorphism of the interphasic nuclei of somatic cells; the female has been shown to have and the male to lack a special chromocenter, the *sex chromatin* or *Barr body*. The Barr body is the condensed chromatin of one inactivated X chromosome. The specific genetic sex may be determined by the examination of leucocytes obtained from blood smears.

Genital abnormalities that result in intersexual individuals present a bewildering variety of differences that are often difficult to classify. Indeed, new classifications are introduced frequently. These are important for clinical purposes, but we will not attempt to present any system of classification; instead, we will examine only a few of the types of known intersexual variations.

Hermaphrodism

A *true hermaphrodite* possesses both testicular and ovarian tissues. This is a rare condition in humans and, since the time of the first description of a true hermaphrodite in the medical literature in 1899

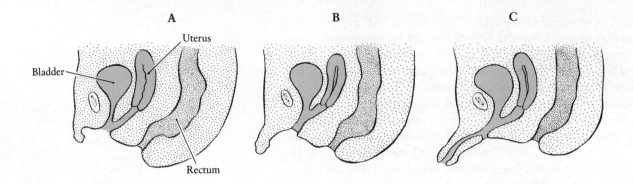

A   B   C

Bladder

Uterus

Rectum

until 1974, only 302 cases have been reported. The gonadal tissue may appear as a separate testis and ovary or as a combined ovatestis. Sterility is the rule and only in rare cases is germ cell maturation completed. An ovatestis is the combination most characteristic. Approximately one third of the cases show a testis on one side and an ovary on the other. The latter condition is usually accompanied by the presence of sex ducts that are different on each side, conforming to the type of gonad found there. The external genitalia range from malelike to femalelike (Fig. 19–30). A common condition is *hypospadia* where, owing to hypoplasia of the inferior portion of the phallus, the urethra does not extend to the tip of the penis but opens somewhere along the inferior aspect (Fig. 19–30 C).

Although externally apparent malformations may be noted from the time of birth, hermaphrodites are generally raised as being members of one particular sex—that which most closely fits the appearance of the genitalia. The failure to undergo the normal morphological changes that occur at the time of puberty then results in a medical examination and a determination of the true status of the individual.

Pseudohermaphrodism

Male and *female pseudohermaphrodism* are conditions much more common than true hermaphrodism. A male pseudohermaphrodite is an individual whose gonad is a testis but whose sex ducts, genitalia, and secondary sexual characteristics resemble more closely those of the female sex. In agreement with the presence of only testicular tissue, these individuals have no Barr bodies and an XY chromosome configuration. Although many male pseudohermaphrodites may have malelike genitalia, hypospadia is common. In addition, the sex ducts show a much greater development of the Müllerian derivatives, usually with a well-developed uterus and uterine tubes, with

19–30 Some types of urogenital structures developed in hermaphrodites ranging from A, external genitalia that are femalelike with a common external opening for the urethra and the vagina, to B, an opening into a urogenital sinus, and C, development of a penis with hypospadia.

the testes often occupying the position where the ovaries would be expected (Fig. 19–31).

Female pseudohermaphrodism is a much rarer condition in which the individual is genetically female, is chromatin positive, and has ovarian tissue although she shows modifications of the urogenital system in a male direction. Not to be confused with this condition are others, including the *adrenogenital syndrome,* where genetic females develop malelike structures whose cause is extragonadal. Most commonly, female pseudohermaphrodites have an enlarged phallus resembling a penis which, however, is hypospadic. Otherwise, the external genitalia are femalelike. In many cases, the vagina is short and narrow and opens into a urogenital sinus as does the urethra. The uterus and the uterine tubes are more or less normal.

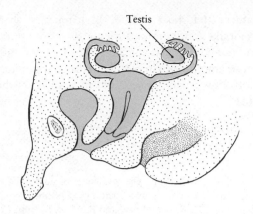

19–31 Urogenital system in a male pseudohermaphrodite.

Gonadal Dysgenesis
As the name implies, this is a condition in which the gonad fails to develop. As would then be expected, since the genital system develops without any influence from the gonad, the sex ducts and genitalia are normally and completely female, although immature. The genetic sex may be XX, XY, or XO. Their stature is generally small and a webbed neck is typical. Gonadal remnants are present and distinguish this condition from true agonadism, a very rare occurrence in which the gonad never develops at all.

Klinefelter's Syndrome
True Klinefelter's syndrome is applied to chromatin positive but phenotypic males, with an XXY chromosomal configuration. They resemble normal males with hypogonadism, are often mentally retarded, and show enlarged breasts (gynecomastia). It is estimated that the incidence of this condition is one in every thousand males.

The Adrenogenital Syndrome
This syndrome is characterized by a masculinization of the genitalia and the physique owing to an oversecretion of androgens from the adrenal glands. A variety of conditions are seen in this syndrome, depending upon the genetic sex of the individual and the time when the increased secretion of androgens occurs. If the individual is male and the condition is congenital, the reproductive system develops normally although the penis may be slightly enlarged. On the other hand, congenital occurrence in a female results in masculinization of the genital organs. The external genitalia show a wide variety of conditions depending upon the amount of androgen secreted by the adrenal glands. Postnatal development in males with the syndrome is characterized by precocious puberty, strong muscu-

lature, and short stature. In females, virilization of the external genitalia continues and they also show precocious development of pubic and axillary hair and are short and muscular. Owing to the large amount of circulating androgen, pituitary secretions of gonadotropins is suppressed, and in both sexes the gonads do not mature.

REFERENCES

Boczkowski, K. 1968. The syndrome of pure gonadal dysgenesis. In: Medical Gynaecology and Sociology. Oxford: Pergamon Press.

Brunet, J., R. R. Mowbray, and P. M. F. Bishop. 1968. Management of the undescended testis. Br. Med. J. 1:1367–1372.

Bulmar, G. 1957. The development of the human vagina. J. Anat. 91: 490–502.

Gillman, J. 1948. The development of the gonads in man, with a consideration of the role of the fetal endocrines and histogenesis of ovarian tumors. Carnegie Contrib. Embryol. 32:81–131.

Glenister, T. W. A. 1954. The origin of the urethral plate in man. J. Anat. 88:413–425.

Gruenwald, P. 1952. Development of the excretory system. Ann. N.Y. Acad. Sci. 55:142–146.

O'Connor, R. J. 1939. Experiments on the development of the amphibian metanephros. J. Anat. 74:34–44.

Ohno, S. 1978. The role of H-Y antigen in primary sex determination. J. Am. Med. Assoc. 239:217–220.

Tanabe, K. and M. Kotani. 1974. Relationship between the amount of the "germinal plasm" and the number of primordial germ cells in Xenopus laevis. J. Embryol. Exp. Morphol. 31:89–98.

Torrey, T. W. 1954. The early development of the human nephros. Carnegie Contrib. Embryol. 35:175–197.

Torrey, W. 1965. Morphogenesis of the vertebrate kidney. In: Organogenesis. Eds., R. L. DeHaan and H. Ursprung. New York: Holt, Rinehart and Winston.

Waddington, C. H. 1938. The morphogenic function of a vestigial organ in the chick. J. Exp. Zool. 15:371–377.

Whitington, P. McD and K. E. Dixon. 1975. Quantitative studies of germ plasm and germ cells during early embryogenesis of Xenopus laevis. J. Embryol. Exp. Morphol. 33:57–74.

Witschi, E. 1948. Migrations of germ cells of human embryos from the yolk sac to the primitive folds. Carnegie Contrib. Embryol. 32:67–80.

20

The Nervous System

The nervous system may be divided into the *central nervous system*—the brain and its caudal continuation, the spinal cord—and the *peripheral nervous system* made up of millions of nerve fibers that connect the central nervous system to all parts of the body. The part of the nervous system that innervates visceral structures—smooth muscle and glands of the viscera and the integument—is called the *autonomic nervous system*. The autonomic nervous system is not a separate system but merely that part of the nervous system which functions in the involuntary control of visceral organs. The autonomic nervous system is, in turn, subdivided into *sympathetic* and *parasympathetic* divisions. The sympathetic division has the cell bodies of its motor fibers located in the thoracic and upper lumbar regions of the spinal cord. The parasympathetic division has nerve fibers that are associated with cranial nerves III, VII, IX, X, and XI and with cell bodies in the sacral region of the spinal cord. Because of the distinct anatomical locations of these divisions, they are also termed the *thoracicolumbar* and the *craniosacral* divisions.

The basic unit of the nervous system is the nerve cell or *neuron*. Each neuron consists of a cell body containing the nucleus and a number of processes that transmit the nerve impulse. *Dendrites* transmit impulses toward the cell body, and *axons* transmit impulses away from the cell body. Each neuron has a single axon but may have a number of dendrites.

The early development of the nervous system, which involves the formation of the neural tube, has been described previously. Further development consists of considerable modification of this originally more or less straight tubular structure, the most marked changes and the greatest growth taking place at the cranial (rostral) end, resulting in the formation of the brain. Caudad of the brain, the neural tube retains a fairly uniform diameter and since the developmental changes that occur here are much less complicated than those that occur in the brain, the histogenesis and morphogenesis of the nervous system will first be examined in the spinal cord.

THE SPINAL CORD

Histogenesis of the Spinal Cord—*Neurogenesis*

Neurogenesis involves three processes—proliferation, migration, and maturation. When the neural plate first forms, it consists of a single layer of columnar cells. These cells proliferate so rapidly that by the time the neural tube is formed, it consists of many more cells, which appear to be arranged in a number of layers (Fig. 20–1). A basement membrane, the *external limiting membrane,* covers the surface of the neural tube and the lumen of the tube, the central canal, is lined by a thin *internal limiting membrane*. At this stage of development, the cells of the tube are not actually arranged in layers but are pseudostratified. The nuclei appear to be located at essentially two different levels. One level consists of oval nuclei below the external limiting membrane contained in wedge-shaped cells with slender cytoplasmic processes extending to the internal limiting membrane, where they are interconnected by terminal bars (Fig. 20–1). This is the layer that is usually termed the mantle layer, but recently the name *intermediate layer* has been suggested for it. The second layer consists of round cells in various stages of mitosis with broad contact with the internal limiting membrane. Since mitotic figures are seen only in this region close to the lumen of the tube, it has been termed the germinal layer on the assumption that this layer of proliferating cells functions to supply cells to the outer layers. However, more accurate studies of histological preparations, reported in the midthirties and confirmed experimentally in the fifties and sixties by colchicine treatment, by tritiated thymidine uptake, and by electron microscope studies, have presented a different interpretation. What appear to be two layers of different kinds of cells actually represent different stages in the cell cycle of the same type of cell, the *neuroepithelial cell* (Fig. 20–2 A). During the synthetic phase of the cell cycle, the nuclei are found in the wedge-shaped cells at different levels below the external limiting membrane. The nuclei, as they enter the mitotic stage of the cell cycle, now move toward the lumen to take up a position in what is now termed the *ventricular layer*. The broad dividing cells squeeze the cytoplasmic processes of the wedge-shaped cells into slender strips. In the early stages of neurogenesis, the mitotic spindles are arranged parallel to the internal limiting membrane. Division completed, the daughter nuclei move away from the lumen to occupy their positions in the intermediate layer. They repeat the migration when they divide again.

Sometime after the closure of the neural tube, there appear close to the external limiting membrane cells that are histologically dif-

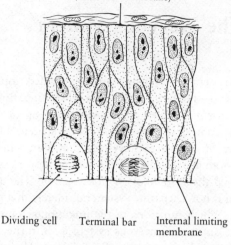

External limiting membrane (Basement membrane)

Dividing cell   Terminal bar   Internal limiting membrane

20–1 Drawing of a cross section of the neural tube of an early chick embryo. Although the position of the nuclei presents a layered appearance, the neural tube at this stage is a pseudostratified columnar epithelium. (After J. Langman, R. L. Guerrant and B. G. Freeman, 1966. J. Comp. Neurol. 127, 399.)

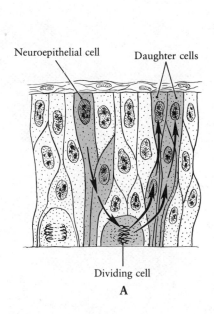

Neuroepithelial cell   Daughter cells

Dividing cell

A

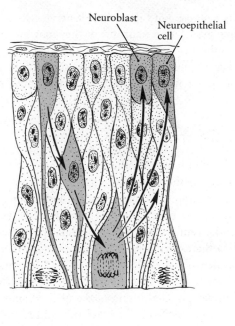

Neuroblast   Neuroepithelial cell

B

ferent from the neuroepithelial cells and that, in addition, do not synthesize DNA. These cells are *neuroblasts* and represent the first stage in the differentiation of the neuron. At the time the first neuroblasts appear, it has been observed that some of the dividing neuroepithelial cells have their spindles oriented perpendicular to the internal limiting membrane. It has been proposed that this would represent a possible mechanism for the release of one of the daughter cells, the one away from the lumen would be freed from its terminal bar connections and thus able to migrate to the outermost level of the neural tube (Fig. 20–2 B).

During its further differentiation, the neuroblast passes successively through apolar, bipolar, and unipolar to multipolar stages (Fig. 20–3). The persisting process of the unipolar stage grows out of the intermediate layer to become a part of the *marginal* layer below the external limiting membrane. This process becomes the axon of the nerve cell. On the side of the cell opposite the axon, the appearance of a number of small, branched processes marks the beginning of dendrite formation. Further differentiation involves the appearance of fine neurofibrils in the cytoplasm of the cell and its processes and, considerably later, the appearance of RNA-rich Nissl bodies in the cell. The dendrites make synaptic connections with the axons of adjacent neurons. The axons running in the

20–2   A, schematic drawing of the wall of the chick neural fold. The nuclei of the cells synthesizing DNA are located in a region at a distance from the internal limiting membrane but move toward it when they start to divide. Following division, the daughter nuclei again move away from the lumen; B, schematic drawing of the chick neural tube. The tube has increased in thickness over A. Some mitotic figures in the ventricular zone are now oriented parallel to the lumen. One daughter cell from such a dividing neuroepithelial cell loses its terminal bar connections and migrates into the outer portion of the intermediate zone as a primitive neuroblast. (After J. Langman, R. L. Guerrant and B. G. Freeman, 1966. J. Comp. Neurol. 127, 399.)

marginal zone may synapse with dendrites of nerve cells within the spinal cord, forming association neurons; or they may pierce the external limiting membrane and leave the central nervous system, many axons at each segmental level forming the *motor (anterior, ventral) root* of a spinal nerve that becomes associated with the myotome at that level.

Histogenesis in the Spinal Cord: Gliogenesis

The next cells to differentiate from the neuroepithelial cells are the *glioblasts,* forerunners of the *neuroglia,* the supportive cells of the nervous system. Some supportive elements can be recognized early in the development of the neural tube. These are *ependymal* cells whose nuclei lie in the ventricular layer and whose processes extend from the internal to the external limiting membrane. After the disappearance of the neuroepithelial cells—as they differentiate into the forerunners of the neurons and the neuroglia—ependymal cells persist as the definitive epithelial lining of the neural canal.

The glioblasts are the precursors of *astrocytes* and *oligodendroglia* cells (Fig. 20–3). Astrocytes may be either *fibrous* or *protoplasmic,* the former most prevalent in the white matter, the latter in the grey. The ends of the processes of the astrocytes often develop expansions that become closely associated with nervous system membranes and blood vessels. In addition to their supportive function, astrocytes are also concerned with the supply of nutrients to the nervous elements. The oligodengroglia develop fewer and less delicate processes than the astrocytes. They are found in both the white and grey matter of the nervous system but are more common in the white, where they function in the formation of myelin sheathes around the axons of the nerve cells. Delicate extensions of these cells are seen closely related to the myelin sheath.

Another type of glial cell, *microglia,* appears late in development; its origin and identification are controversial. Since it appears at the time that the blood vessels are invading the nervous tissue, it is often suggested that the mesodermal connective tissue of the walls of the blood vessels may be the precursors of the microglia. A different interpretation has been offered. It recognizes a small glioblast, a derivative of the neuroepithelial cells, which may differentiate directly into a microglial cell or, by growth, become a precursor of the larger glial cells, the astrocytes and oligodendroglia. Microglia cells generally appear inactive, but following injury to nervous tissue, they proliferate rapidly and become phagocytic.

Neuroglia cells differ from the connective tissue cells of mesodermal origin in two respects. They are not stained by the usual connective tissue staining methods but do show up clearly following

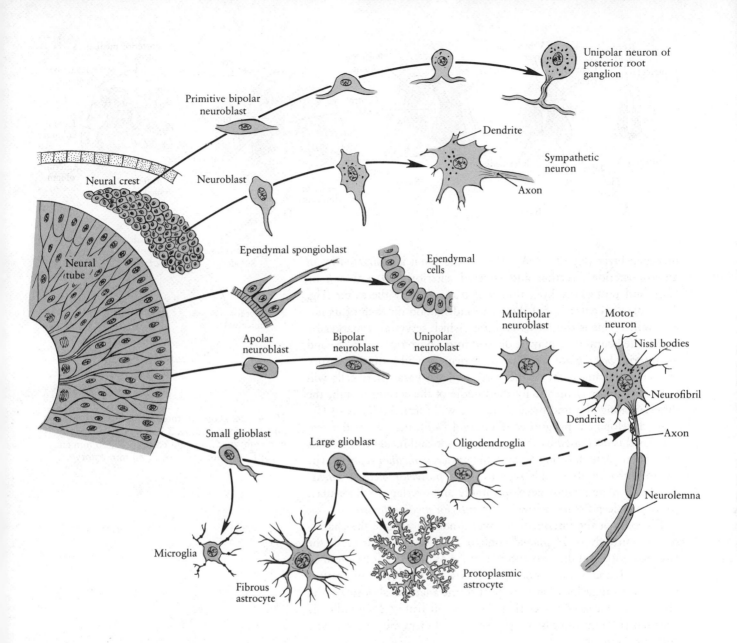

Unipolar neuron of posterior root ganglion

Primitive bipolar neuroblast

Neural crest

Neuroblast

Dendrite

Sympathetic neuron

Axon

Neural tube

Ependymal spongioblast

Ependymal cells

Multipolar neuroblast

Motor neuron

Apolar neuroblast

Bipolar neuroblast

Unipolar neuroblast

Nissl bodies

Neurofibril

Dendrite

Axon

Small glioblast

Large glioblast

Oligodendroglia

Neurolemna

Microglia

Fibrous astrocyte

Protoplasmic astrocyte

silver impregnation, as is characteristic of all nerve cells and their processes. In addition, they do not form intercellular fibrous elements.

Further Development of the Spinal Cord

In man, by the end of the first month of development, the spinal cord shows a thick intermediate zone outside of which is seen a thin

20–3   Diagram showing the types of neurons and neuroglia developed from the neuroepithelial cells of the neural tube and from the neural crest.

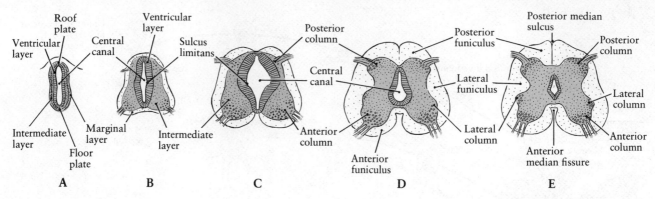

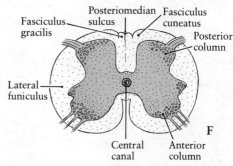

20-4 Six stages in the development of the human spinal cord. A, 3.7 mm embryo; B, 10 mm embryo; C, 11 mm embryo; D, 30 mm embryo; E, 45 mm embryo; F, 80 mm embryo.

marginal layer (Fig. 20–4 A). The central canal is elongated in an anteroposterior direction and covered anteriorly by a thin *floor plate* and posteriorly by a thin *roof plate*. Shortly thereafter (Fig. 20–4 B), the central canal shows an indentation on each of its lateral walls. This is the *sulcus limitans,* which serves as a marker by which the neural tube may be divided into a posterior *alar plate* and an anterior *basal plate.* The alar plate neurons will form the sensory and coordinating parts of the cord, and the basal plate cells will form the motor elements. By the middle of the second month, the differentiating alar and basal plates are well formed (Fig. 20–4 C).

As development progresses (Fig. 20–4 D–F), the size of the central canal is decreased by the approximation and fusion of the walls of the alar plate, forming a seam, the *posterior median septum.* The shallow groove above this septum is the *posterior median sulcus.* The basal plate regions develop rapidly and overlap the floor plate to form a deep fissure below it, the *anterior median fissure.*

The cells of the intermediate layer gradually assume the characteristic butterfly or H-shaped configuration of the adult cord; the two posterior and the two anterior limbs of the H are often termed the dorsal and ventral horns, respectively. However, in conformance with their location in respect to the anatomical position and also to emphasize the fact that they are, in reality, longitudinally oriented columns of cells, we prefer to label them the *posterior* and *anterior columns.*

The neurons of the posterior column are associated with sensory (afferent) impulses. Fibers from the sensory receptors (exteroceptors in the integument, proprioceptors in muscles and tendons, and interoceptors in the visceral organs) return to the spinal cord where they make synaptic connections with the dendrites of the neurons in the posterior column.

The neurons of the anterior column are associated with motor

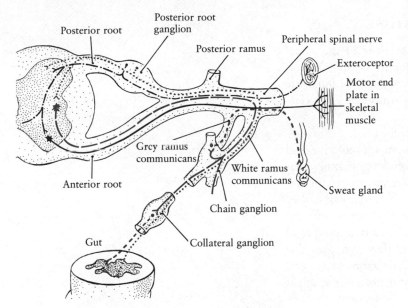

20–5   Diagram of a spinal nerve and its anterior (motor) and posterior (sensory) roots. The chain ganglia of the sympathetic division of the autonomic nervous system are connected to the spinal cord by the grey ramus communicans and the white ramus communicans. The functional types of fibers, their location, and their central and peripheral connections are shown. Somatic efferent —, visceral efferent preganglionic ———, visceral efferent postganglionic ------, somatic afferent — · — · —, visceral afferent · · · · · ·.

(efferent) impulses. Their axons grow out of the spinal cord to make peripheral connections with effectors that are both somatic (skeletal muscle) and visceral in nature.

The marginal region of the cord consists mainly of longitudinally running fiber tracts carrying sensory impulses upward from the spinal cord to the brain and motor impulses downward from the brain to the cord. On the basis of their location, three regions of the marginal zone are designated as the *posterior, lateral,* and *anterior funiculi* (Fig. 20–4 D,E).

20–6   The effect of somite excision and somite transplantation on the development of the spinal ganglia and nerve roots. A, incomplete segmentation of ganglia on the right side after excision of somites 2, 3, 4, and 5; B, three somites (3, 4, and 5) on the right side were excised and replaced with four somites. Note the presence of a supernumerary ganglion and nerve (3A) associated with the additional somite. (After P. Weiss, 1955. Analysis of Development, eds. B. J. Willier, P. Weiss and V. Hamburger. W. B. Saunders Company, Philadelphia.)

THE SPINAL NERVES

Thirty-one pairs of segmentally arranged spinal nerves develop. Each consists of an *anterior* (motor) *root* and a *posterior* (sensory) *root* whose junction forms the spinal nerve (Fig. 20–5). The segmental arrangement of the spinal nerves and their ganglia is not intrinsic to the nervous system but dependent upon the segmental arrangement of the somites. If the somites on one side of a salamander embryo are removed, the spinal nerves and ganglia on that side will show an incomplete haphazard segmentation (Fig. 20–6 A). If additional somites are transplanted to an area, supernumerary nerves and ganglia will develop (Fig. 20–6 B).

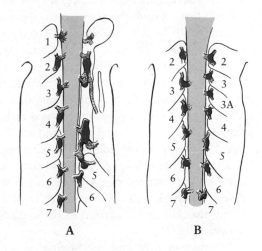

A   B

The Anterior Roots of the Spinal Nerves

Most of the fibers that make up the anterior roots of the spinal nerves are the axons of neurons, which develop in the anterior column of the spinal cord. These are motor fibers that will innervate the large skeletal muscle masses, and for this reason they are classified functionally as *somatic efferent fibers*.

In the thoracic and upper lumbar regions of the cord, a third column develops, a small *lateral column*, between the anterior and posterior columns. The neurons in this column develop axons that also leave the cord to make up a part of the anterior root of the spinal nerve, but soon after becoming a part of the spinal nerve, they leave it and grow toward one of a number of different efferent ganglia (accumulations of nerve cell bodies) located in a number of different positions in the trunk area. Here, they synapse. The neurons with which they synapse now send their axons to visceral effectors. This two-neuron chain, with the first neuron in the spinal cord and the second in a ganglion, represents the sympathetic division of the autonomic nervous system. Similarly, the neurons of the parasympathetic division of the autonomic nervous system, which are located in the brain stem and the sacral region of the spinal cord, develop preganglionic fibers that synapse in different ganglia. Postganglionic fibers from the neurons in these ganglia then send their axons to the appropriate visceral effectors. The motor ganglia in which all of the preganglionic fibers of the autonomic nervous system syanpse are derivatives of the neural crest.

The Neural Crest

The early development of the neural crest was described in Chapter 8. When first formed, the neural crest appears as two longitudinally running bands of cells on either side of the spinal cord, between it and the somites. The cells of the neural crest soon migrate away from their original locations and become widely distributed throughout the body, contributing to the formation of a number of different structures. In the head region, neural crest cells give rise to the skeleton of the face and the visceral arches; part of the sensory ganglion of the fifth cranial nerve and all of the sensory ganglia of cranial nerves VII, IX, and X; the parasympathetic ganglia in the head region; the Schwann cells; and the pigment cells. The spinal neural crest forms the posterior sensory root ganglia of the spinal nerves; the trunk and collateral ganglia of the autonomic nervous system; the cells of the adrenal medulla; the Schwann cells; and the pigment cells.

The physiological and morphological diversity of neural crest derivatives and their widespread distribution present many unanswered questions concerning the control of their morphogenesis and migration. At the time the cells migrate out of the neural crest, they are still undifferentiated and only go through their final stages of differentiation after they have reached their precise location in the developing embryo. There is no evidence that the cells, although undifferentiated during their migration, are actually already determined and move along selective pathways. Also, the evidence is against a spatiotemporal determination, since replacing neural crest of young chicks with transplants from old chicks results in the development of normal neural crest derivatives. What appears to be important is the interaction of the neural crest cells with the tissue environment in which they eventually become located. If the part of the neural crest in the chick embryo which normally supplies cells that form the enteric intestinal ganglia of the parasympathetic system is transplanted to a location from which its cells will migrate into the regions where sympathetic chain ganglia develop, it will differentiate completely functional sympathetic neurons. This developmental sequence involves a major physiological shift from a cholinergic to an adrenergic type of neurotransmission. There is no specific attraction of the end organ for any predetermined type of neural crest cell. The cells migrate along pathways according to the pattern and structure of the tissue in which they find themselves when they are released. Once they end up in some particular area, the tissue interactions in this area determine their final differentiation.

Cells migrate away from the neural crest in two streams. The first is dorsolateral into the superficial ectoderm dorsal to the neural tube and the somites. Most of these cells will form pigment cells. The second is ventral between the neural tube and the somites. These cells will form both the sensory ganglia of the posterior roots of the spinal nerves and the ganglia of the autonomic nervous system in the neck and trunk area.

The Autonomic Nervous System Ganglia

Generally, the first cells to leave the neural crest end up in locations the farthest away from their original position. The three groups of cells that migrate the greatest distances all become ganglia of the autonomic nervous system, whose axons (postganglionic) carry impulses to smooth muscles and glands of the viscera.

Those that migrate the farthest ventrally locate within the walls of the alimentary tract, and there they develop into the *enteric plexuses*. They form a part of the parasympathetic division of the autonomic nervous system, whose preganglionic supply is mainly through the tenth cranial nerve.

Other groups of neural crest cells use as pathways the branches of the dorsal aorta supplying visceral structures. They reach locations within the abdomen, and there they form a number of plexuses called *collateral ganglia* (Fig. 20–5). The postganglionic fibers that grow out of these plexuses are efferent fibers of the sympathetic division of the autonomic nervous system.

A third group does not migrate very far ventrally and forms a chain of ganglia along the dorsolateral length of the aorta. These *chain ganglia* (Fig. 20–5) are also a part of the sympathetic division.

Certain preganglionic fibers from the neurons in the lateral column grow out of the spinal cord into the anterior roots of the spinal nerves. They then leave the spinal nerves and grow into the chain ganglia where some of them synapse. The postganglionic fibers from the chain ganglia may grow back to the spinal nerve and pass with it to sympathetic effectors in the integument such as those found in piloerector muscle and sweat glands. Other fibers may pass through the chain ganglia without synapsing and grow into a collateral ganglion before they synapse. The postganglionic fibers from the collateral ganglia supply effectors in the viscera.

All these preganglionic and postganglionic fibers of both divisions of the autonomic nervous system are classified on a functional basis as *visceral efferent*—motor fibers innervating visceral structures.

Posterior Root Ganglia

The group of neural crest cells that remain closest to the spinal cord form the sensory *posterior root ganglia* (Fig. 20–5). The neural crest cells migrate more easily through than between the somites, which may be one reason why the segmental arrangement of the somites is reflected in the segmental arrangement of the posterior root ganglia. Each of the 31 pairs of spinal nerves develops a posterior root ganglion.

The axons and dendrites that grow out of the posterior root ganglia form the fibers making up the posterior roots of the spinal nerves. The neurons in the spinal ganglia at first show two processes leaving the cell. These later fuse to form a single process that branches at some distance from the cell body (Fig. 20–3). One branch of this process grows peripherally and becomes functionally linked with a sensory receptor. The other branch grows centrally into the spinal cord. The fibers that make connections with *exteroceptors* (touch, pain, temperature receptors) and *proprioceptors* (neuromuscular and neurotendonous receptors) are classified functionally as *somatic afferent*. Those that connect to *enteroceptors* in the visceral organs are classified as *visceral afferent*. Thus, the cells of the spinal ganglia develop the sensory or afferent components of

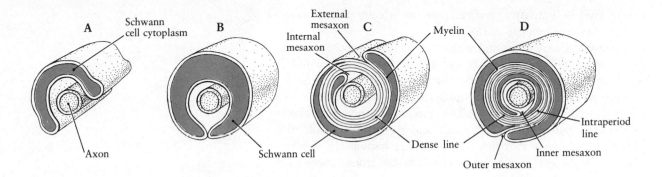

the spinal nerves carrying impulses from the numerous somatic and visceral sensory receptors into the central nervous system.

Schwann Cells

All peripheral nerves are surrounded by a delicate sheath or *neurolemma* made up of what are known as *Schwann cells*. These cells are neural crest derivatives. The Schwann cells migrate from the neural crest to the growing nerve fiber and then grow peripherally along with the fiber continuing to divide as they do so.

The one known function of the Schwann cells is the formation of the myelin sheath of some of the peripheral nerve fibers. During the process of myelinization, the naked nerve fiber settles into a groove in the surface of the Schwann cell and gradually the Schwann cell encircles it (Fig. 20–7 A,B). The point where the two folds of the Schwann cell meet is called the *mesaxon*. Envelopment continues and the Schwann cell forms scroll-like layers around the nerve fiber. At first these layers contain Schwann cell cytoplasm, but this then disappears and is found only at the innermost and outermost regions of the cell. The loss of the cytoplasm brings into contact the two inner layers of the Schwann cell membrane to form a dense line, the *major dense line* (Fig. 20–7 C). Contact of the outer surfaces of the Schwann cell membrane forms a thinner line, the *intraperiod line*. Thus, myelin is nothing more than the apposed membranes of the lamellae of the Schwann cell wrapped around the nerve fiber.

Whether or not a nerve fiber will be myelinated depends upon its size. In mammals, peripheral nerve fibers less than one micron in diameter are unmyelinated, although they still have a Schwann cell sheath. In myelinated fibers, the number of lamellae increases with the diameter of the fiber. Myelinization is not necessary for nerve impulse conduction—which occurs in the embryo before the forma-

20–7 Diagram showing the formation of the myelin sheath. A, axon being enveloped by a Schwann cell; B, axon completely enveloped. The mesaxon is the channel formed where the folds of a Schwann cell meet, opening to the extracellular space; C, lamellae of a Schwann cell wrapped around the axon forming the myelin. A dense line results from the loss of cytoplasm and the apposition of the inner surfaces of the lamellae and an intraperiod line results from the apposition of the outer surfaces.

tion of myelin—but, after myelinization, the velocity of the conduction of the nerve impulse increases.

Schwann cells are not found within the central nervous system although many fibers in the brain and spinal cord are myelinated. It was logical to propose that one of the glia cells was responsible for myelinization in the central nervous system, although exactly which one it was not known. Recently, EM studies have shown a continuity between the oligodendroglia cell and the myelin sheath thus proving conclusively that this cell is the one responsible. A single oligodendroglia cell may form myelin lamellae around more than one nerve fiber, but the process of myelinization and the end result is essentially the same as in the peripheral nerve fibers.

Adrenal Gland
Neural crest cells also form a part of the adrenal (suprarenal) gland. The adrenal glands of higher vertebrates are formed by two primordia of widely different origin, which combine secondarily into a single organ. The adrenal cortex is of mesodermal origin, and it encloses a medulla derived from ectodermal neural crest tissue. In some lower vertebrates the cortical and medullary parts of the gland normally remain as separate organs.

The adrenal cortex first appears as a group of cells in the angle of the posterior abdominal wall between the dorsal mesentery and the developing genital ridge at the level of the cranial end of the mesonephros (Fig. 20–8 A,B). The cells are derived from the coelomic mesoderm as are those of the gonad. The adrenal cortical cells separate from the mesothelium and proliferate to form, by the end of the second month, a cluster of large acidophilic cells enclosed in a connective tissue capsule. A second proliferation of cells from the coelomic mesothelium is added to the original mass at a later stage but the main portion of the adrenal cortex at birth is made up of the original group of cells, termed the fetal cortex.

During the second month of development, migrating neural crest cells reach the medial aspect of the adrenal anlagen by way of the sympathetic ganglia. These cells, which will form the medulla of the gland, form a mass on the medial aspect of the cortical cells (Fig. 20–8 C). They are gradually encapsulated by the cortex and give up their function as nerve cells and differentiate into endocrine elements. Owing to the presence of the hormones epinephrine and norepinephrine in these cells, they stain brown with chrome salts and are thus part of what is known as the chromaffin system, of which the adrenal medulla represents the major portion. Other chromaffin cells are found as clusters (paraganglia) associated with autonomic nervous system ganglia and also as clusters located along the course of the dorsal aorta.

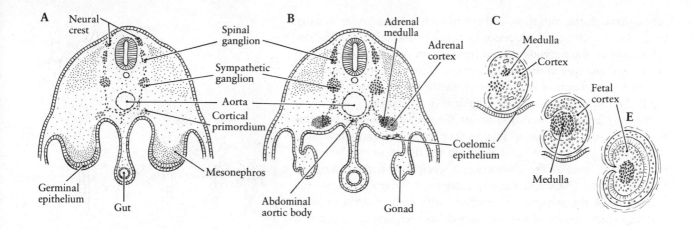

A — Neural crest / Spinal ganglion / Sympathetic ganglion / Aorta / Cortical primordium / Mesonephros / Germinal epithelium / Gut

B — Adrenal medulla / Adrenal cortex / Coelomic epithelium / Abdominal aortic body / Gonad

C — Medulla / Cortex / Fetal cortex / E / Medulla

20–8   Diagram showing the origin of the cortex and the medulla of the adrenal gland from the mesothelium and the neural crest, respectively.

At birth the adrenal gland is a comparatively large organ, almost one third the size of the kidney. However, a large part of the adrenal at this time consists of the primary or fetal cortex located between the definitive cortex and the medulla. Postnatally, the fetal cortex involutes and the gland decreases both actually and relatively in size. In the adult it is about 1/30th of the size of the kidney. The function of the fetal cortex is not known, although studies have shown that it is capable of secreting steroid hormones. The possible role of the adrenal in parturition has been discussed in Chapter 5.

The double origin of the cortex and the medulla is reflected in differences in function of these two parts of the gland in the adult. The cells of the medulla elaborate epinephrine or norephinephrine and function in relation to the sympathetic nervous system, being primarily concerned with emotional adjustments. The adrenal cortex secretes steroid hormones that function in carbohydrate and protein metabolism and the control of water and electrolyte balance. In addition, both androgens and estrogens are synthesized by the adrenal cortex.

ESTABLISHMENT OF PATTERN IN THE NERVOUS SYSTEM

In no other system in the animal are the cell patterns as complicated and the interconnections between cells as important as in the nervous system. The adult nervous system presents an amazingly complex network of billions of cells whose synaptic interconnections must be so patterned that they can function in the control of activities, which range from the seemingly uncomplicated spinal reflex through the initiation and coordination of muscular activity to the little understood processes of thought and learning. The development of the nervous system involves an orderly succession of events and changes in the multiplication, differentiation, migration, and interconnection of its cellular elements whose proper functioning is the result of a strict topographical organization.

We may ask many question about the neural ontogeny but, unfortunately, our experiments give us very few specific answers. How do nerve fibers grow? What determines the direction in which they grow? What controls the connection of peripheral nerve endings to specific muscle fibers and sensory receptors? What determines the formation of the synaptic connections within the central nervous system, which results in the correlation between sensory input and motor output?

Axon Growth

The mechanism of axon growth was still in dispute at the end of the 19th century. A number of possibilities had been suggested. The noted cell biologist, Schwann, proposed that a chain of individual cells, the Schwann cells, which form the axon sheath, also fused together to form the nerve fiber. This theory was readily disproved when it was shown that, following the removal of the neural crest, the axon developed normally in the complete absence of Schwann cells. In fact, as described previously, the axon develops before the Schwann cells reach it.

Another theory, based on faulty histology, stated that the early nervous system was a syncytium interconnected by filaments that later developed into the nerve fibers. More accurate histology prevailed against this proposal.

A third theory, that of the neuroanatomist Ramón y Cajal, proposed that the axon developed as an outgrowth of the cytoplasm of the young neuron. The actual outgrowth of nerve processes from the neuron was first described by Harrison in 1907 using the tissue culture technique he invented. Harrison pictured the outgrowth of nerve processes from neurons of the spinal cord of the frog as being ameboid in nature, the fibers putting out and retracting pseudopodia until one became dominant and then repeating the process (Fig. 20–9).

The axon grows out of the neuron in a consistent direction, that is, toward the periphery of the spinal cord. This orientation appears to be due to some innate polarization of the neuron rather than to any external influence exerted at the time of outgrowth. The polarization may be the result of its original attachment to the inner surface of the neural tube, and it can be recognized by a change in the

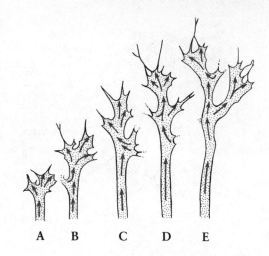

20–9 Diagram of five stages in the amoeboid-like growth of a nerve fiber. Dotted areas represent extensions that were put out and then withdrawn.

ultrastructure of the neuron before any outgrowth appears. Golgi bodies and rough endoplasmic reticulum, which are scanty in the young neuron, accumulate in increasing quantities in the region of the future outgrowth. This implies a timed gene activation switching on the synthetic activity necessary for the formation of the materials needed for axon growth followed by their differential distribution to the region of the cell where they will be utilized.

After the initial outgrowth, new materials for continued growth and maintenance are synthesized in the cell body and transported to the axon and are also synthesized in the axon itself. Although the cell body has large numbers of ribosomes, none are found in the axoplasm. The many mitochondria located in the axon, then, must be the site for RNA and protein synthesis in the nerve fiber itself.

Influence of Peripheral Structures on Neuroblast Proliferation and Fiber Outgrowth

Numerous experiments involving removal, addition, and transplantation of organs have shown that the size of the peripheral area to be innervated has a direct effect on the number of neurons in the areas supplying these structures. If the size of the peripheral field is reduced or increased, the number of neurons whose fibers supply the field is reduced or increased. This applies to motor neurons located in the anterior column of the spinal cord and to sensory neurons located in the posterior root ganglia.

Motor Neurons and Peripheral Organs

If a forelimb bud is removed early in development, a hypoplasia of the spinal cord motor column and the posterior root ganglia at the level of the spinal cord normally supplying the forelimb results (Fig. 20–10 A,B). Conversely a limb bud transplanted to a location opposite a region of the spinal cord which does not normally supply nerves to a limb will cause a hyperplasia of this region of the cord (Fig. 20–10 C,D). Most of these types of experiments have been done on amphibians and chicks, but the few examples for mammals support the same conclusions. Hypoplasia of corresponding nerve centers has been reported in man in cases of abrachia and other congenital limb abnormalities.

The reduction in the number of neurons following limb bud removal is due not to a failure of the normal proliferation of neurons but to an abnormal amount of cell death following normal proliferation. Peripheral structures apparently have no effect on the proliferation and differentiation of neuroblasts nor on the initial outgrowth of their axons. However, the absence of the peripheral organs that the nerve fibers would normally supply results in a mas-

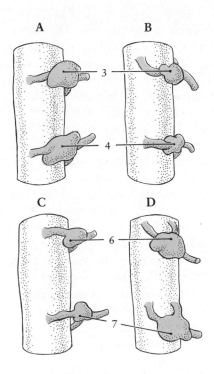

20–10 Hypoplasia and hyperplasia of spinal ganglia associated with limb excision and limb transplantation. A, left third and fourth spinal ganglia connected with a normal limb; B, hypoplasia of right third and fourth spinal ganglia following excision of the right forelimb primordium; C, normal sixth and seventh spinal ganglia, which have no connection with a limb; D, hyperplasia of right sixth and seventh spinal ganglia following connection with a transplanted limb bud. (From S. R. Detwiler, 1936. Neuroembryology. Hafner Publishing Company.)

sive death of the neurons. The motor column opposite the region where a limb bud has been removed shows only about 10 to 20 percent of the normal number of neurons.

The peak of cell death coincides with the time of establishment of neuromuscular connections and the onset of limb movement. This leads to the conclusion that the establishment of a connection to a muscle fiber and the formation of a motor endplate is essential for the continued growth and maintenance of the neuron. In fact, death of neurons in the anterior column is a part of normal development. This is due to the fact that there is always an overproduction of neurons that differentiate and send out axons toward the periphery. This is then followed by the death of those neurons whose axons fail to make connections with muscle fibers. In *Xenopus* it has been estimated that from three to eight neurons die for each one that survives. The number surviving, then, represents the number that are sufficient to "saturate" the periphery. The reason the periphery can be saturated is that each muscle fiber will accept only a single motor axon terminal in mammals and only a limited number in submammalian species. Only the uninnervated membrane of the muscle fiber is receptive to a nerve fiber. Once innervated, the muscle fiber membrane is no longer receptive. This phenomenon, which reminds one of the change in the egg membrane that prevents polyspermy, may be due to the release of acetylcholine by the motor endplate. If the muscle is poisoned with botulinus toxin—which prevents the release of acetylcholine—muscle fibers will now accept additional axon fiber connections.

Thus, autonomous proliferation, differentiation, and axon outgrowth are followed by the selective death of those neurons whose axons fail to establish functional connection with a muscle fiber. Theories about the mechanism causing the death of the neurons are speculative. It has been proposed that, once a functional connection has been made, this information is transferred from the muscle to the axon and then relayed back to the nerve cell body. The information could be in the form of some "material" that is necessary for the continued growth of the neuron.

Communication between the muscle fiber and its nerve supply is thought to have other consequences. If a limb muscle is transplanted near a normal limb in an amphibian tadpole and provided with motor innervation by diverting nerve fibers to the transplant from the nerve supply to the normal limb, the supernumerary muscle will contract simultaneously with the muscle of the same name in the normal limb. The same result applies for several supernumerary muscles or even for an entire limb, each transplanted muscle acting in concert with the corresponding muscle of the normal limb. Under the conditions of these experiments, the same nerve fibers do not always innervate the same supernumerary muscles, since the fibers are diverted to the transplant either as a matter of chance or at the choice of the experimentor. Thus, the conclusion may be reached that no matter what nerve fiber establishes connection with a muscle, that muscle in some way is able to convey its name to the fiber, imprinting it with the specific character (biochemical?) of the particular muscle. Once the axon is modulated by the specific character of its peripheral connection, this is conveyed to the nerve cell body, which then makes central connections in accordance with its acquired specificity. Thus, all nerve fibers reaching a biceps muscle—normal or transplanted—are stamped with the brand "biceps" and subsequently acquire the same central connections, which insure they will contract in synchrony.

The dendrites of motor column neurons also do not appear until after the axons of these cells have established their muscle connections. Thus, it seems that both dendrite outgrowth and the formation of the proper central synaptic connections are under the control of the peripheral connection.

Sperry has proposed a somewhat different concept but one that still entails a biochemical specificity between the muscle fiber, the axon, and the synaptic connection within the central nervous system. He suggests that matching specificities develop independently both in the muscle and the presynaptic central neuron. When the motor fiber makes its connection with the muscle fiber, the muscle's specificity is transferred to the axon and relayed back to the neuron. Following this, synapses can only be made between presynaptic and postsynaptic fibers with matching affinities. Although both proposals assume that the specificity of central connections is based upon biochemical affinity, there may certainly be other as yet undetermined factors involved.

Guidance of Axon Growth

In the adult, the path of a motor fiber from its central origin to its peripheral connection may be long and tortuous, leading to the consideration that indeed some extremely potent force must have been at work to guide the fiber along the proper path. However, we must consider that axon outgrowth takes place in the early embryo where distances are shorter and paths more direct. The first fibers that grow into the limb bud pass over these relatively short straight paths to connect to developing muscle. These "pioneering" fibers may now be passively towed along as the muscle with which they connect differentiates, grows, and migrates. In addition, the pioneering fibers now provide a pathway that fibers developing later may follow.

Nevertheless, some sort of directional guidance is probably exerted by the developing peripheral organs, and that it does occur is nicely illustrated from the results of transplantation experiments. If a barrier such as a small sliver of mica is placed between the spinal cord and the developing limb bud of a salamander, the brachial nerve fibers from segments three, four, and five, which normally supply the limb, will grow up to the barrier and then deviate from their course and grow around the barrier to reach the limb bud. If a frog limb bud is removed and transplanted a short distance caudal from its normal site, the brachial nerve fibers from segments three, four, and five will deviate from their usual routes and grow toward the transplant. However, if the limb bud is transplanted too far away from its normal site, it can no longer attract motor fibers from the normal spinal level of supply. Instead, fibers from the cord at the level of the transplant now grow toward the limb. Although the limb may be innervated by some fibers from levels other than its normal source of supply, it will not now show coordinated movements.

The attraction of peripheral organs for motor nerve fibers has been shown to be nonspecific. A transplanted optic cup or nasal placode will exert the same effect. Thus, nerve fibers are attracted or guided toward rapidly growing structures in a nonspecific manner. What is the nature of this attractive force? It has been proposed that the attraction may be either chemical (a chemotropism) or electrical (a galvanotropism) in nature. Theories of chemotropism and galvanotropism, however, are generally based on a priori reasoning and lack any substantive evidence in their support.

Another possible mechanism was suggested on the basis of observations of nerve fiber growth in vitro. We have already described it as ameboid in nature, the nerve fiber extending and retracting pseudopodiallike processes as it progresses. However, the analogy of nerve fiber growth to ameboid movement may give the erroneous impression that nerve fibers can move freely through tissue spaces and fluids. They cannot. Fiber growth can proceed only along interfaces such as solid–liquid, liquid–gas, or two immiscible liquids. The major interfaces available to the growing nerve fiber in the embryo are apparently those formed by the numerous fibrous units that make up a large part of the amorphous ground substance of tissues. It seems probable that the directional growth of the nerve fiber may well depend on the fact that these tissue units are not arranged haphazardly but have a definite orientation. Weiss (1934) was able to obtain directional nerve fiber growth in tissue culture by stretching the blood clot substratum. The previous random growth of the fibers now became oriented in the direction of the stretching of the fibrous units of the substratum. Nerve fibers growing in vitro on a mica coverslip scored with a pattern of scratches followed these pathways exclusively. Weiss termed this type of behavior *contact guidance*. To what extent this theory can explain the growth of the nerve fiber in the embryo is problematical. In what way could an oriented ground substance develop in the embryo in such a pattern that the nerve fibers could use it as a pathway? The fibrous units in the embryo might be oriented through stretching as the result of differential growth. It is possible that dehydration around rapidly growing organs could stretch the ground substance fibers in their direction and provide a guidance system directing the nerve fibers toward the proliferating structure. Over the years the contact guidance system has neither been proved nor disproved but still remains at the present as a plausible explanation.

Sensory Nerves and Sensory Receptors

During development, the sensory fibers growing out of sensory ganglia always grow into the sensory field before the development of any sensory receptors, suggesting that the differentiation of the receptors may depend upon some stimulus brought in by the sensory fibers. There are many different types of receptors responding to different kinds of chemical, thermal, and mechanical stimuli. Each receptor can respond only to a single kind of stimulus, and the question then arises whether, in addition to inducing the development of the receptor, the nerve fiber also controls its specificity. Most of the experiments on this subject have been done on postembryonic stages, but the results have obvious implications for the role of the sensory nerve fiber in the differentiation of its receptor.

All types of receptors degenerate when they are denervated and regenerate after their nerve supply is restored. A classic example of this trophic effect is seen in the dependence of taste buds on their sensory innervation. In the rat and the rabbit, a reduction in the size of the taste buds is seen eight hours after denervation, and they completely disappear in five to seven days. The taste buds on the posterior part of the tongue are supplied by cranial nerve IX and degenerate when this nerve is cut. They will regenerate if supplied by fibers from cranial nerve IX, but will also regenerate if supplied by fibers from cranial nerves VII or X. These are the three cranial nerves that normally supply sensory fibers to taste buds: VII to those on the anterior region of the tongue, IX to those on the posterior region, and X to buds in the larynx and pharynx. The taste buds will not regenerate if they are supplied by cranial nerve XII, which is a purely motor nerve to the skeletal muscle of the tongue, thus establishing a specificity at least between sensory fibers and sensory receptors. However, the specificity goes even further than this. Denervated taste buds will not regenerate if supplied by sensory fibers from branches of cranial nerve V. Thus, the trophic stimulus for the maintenance of taste buds is supplied only by sensory nerves, but only by sensory nerves that contain gustatory fibers.

A further aspect of this relationship is seen in the results from another experiment. The taste buds on the anterior and posterior regions of the tongue, which we have seen are supplied by cranial nerves VII and IX, respectively differ in their responses to different chemicals, and these differences can be detected on the basis of electrical response measured in the nerves that supply these regions. If cranial nerves VII and IX are switched so that VII supplies the posterior and IX the anterior region of the tongue, the electrical responses in the switched nerves are reversed and correspond to the region of the tongue the nerves supply. Thus, the precise functional specificity of the taste receptors is an inherent property of the epithelium in which they develop and the nerves exert a nonspecific morphogenetic action that calls for the maintenance of gustatory receptors in general, but does not determine their exact specificity.

Another example of epithelial control over the specificity of the receptor is seen when the skin of the beak and tongue of the duck, which contains certain specific types of mechanoreceptors, is grafted to the foot. These receptors, which are normally supplied by a branch of the Vth cranial nerve, degenerate when grafted but regenerate when sensory nerve fibers of the foot innervate the graft. Here, the sensory nerve fibers from the spinal cord are capable of stimulating the development of head sensory receptors normally supplied by cranial nerve fibers, but the specific nature of the receptors is inherent in the head epithelium.

Central Connections of Sensory Nerves

How are the central connections of sensory fibers determined? Are they specified by the function and location of the receptor or does the sensory fiber receive its specificity from the center and then make the appropriate peripheral connections? The evidence seems to be in favor of the first supposition.

If a hindlimb bud is grafted into the back region of a frog tadpole, it will develop, and the adult frog now carries an extra hindlimb in this abnormal position. Under the conditions of this experiment, motor nerves do not innervate the graft, which does serve, however, as a sensory field for sensory nerves growing out of the adjacent spinal ganglia. If the limb is stimulated, it does not move; instead, the corresponding normal hindlimb responds to the stimulus, as if it had been stimulated itself. The explanation is that the trunk sensory nerves supplying the grafted limb have received the imprint of the hindlimb sensory field and have thus made the appropriate central connections for sensory fibers from hindlimb receptors.

Another experiment that illustrates the same principle involves removing a strip of skin from the belly and the back of a frog tadpole and transplanting it with its dorsoventral axes reversed. Belly skin is now found on the back and back skin on the belly. After metamorphosis, when the grafted area now on the back is stimulated, the frog responds by wiping at the belly area with its limb and, when the grafted belly skin is stimulated, the frog scratches its back. After being transplanted in a new position, the sensory receptors of the skin still signal their old position to the central nervous system. Some quality in the skin determines the pattern of the reflexes set up in the central nervous system. Once determined, this pattern is permanent.

A final example of the specificity of peripheral to central connections involves experiments done mainly on frogs and fish on the growth of the optic tract nerve fibers centrally from the retina to their connections with the tectum of the midbrain—the visual center in these forms. Electrophysiological experiments in which the regional electrical activity of the tectum is recorded following stimulation of the retina with a spot of light show that there is a specific point-to-point projection of the retina back to the optic tectum. If the optic tract is cut, it will regenerate and, when it does, normal visuomotor coordination is restored and the pattern of the point-to-point electrophysiological mapping is the same as it was before the tract was severed. The regenerating optic fibers thus made their connections with the original positions in the tectum.

The specificity of these connections is nicely illustrated by the introduction of a number of surgical rearrangements of the eye after the optic tract has been cut. If the eye is rotated 180°, the optic tract fibers will still regenerate and vision will be restored. However, the visuomotor reflexes are now reversed and objects in the nasal field of vision are now seen as being in the temporal field of vision, since they are now seen by the part of the retina that, before rotation, saw the temporal field of vision, which now still projects back to its original temporal field of the tectum. The frog strikes at a fly as if it is in the direction just opposite to the one it actually is. This defect is permanent and no amount of experience ever corrects it. The optic fibers grow back to their original specific points of connection in the tectum, no matter what the orientation of the eye from which they originate.

It is not known why the fibers grow back to their original positions during regeneration nor, in fact, how the retinotectal connections form in the embryo in the first place. Some kind of guidance must be necessary for the fibers as they leave the retina: first, to get into the correct position in the optic tract which will take them to the proper tectum; second, to get into the proper branch that will end up in the correct general region of the tectum; and, third, to make the correct connections with the tectal cells.

Although the mechanism for the guidance of the fibers back to the tectum is not known, there is some indication that the final connections are specified by the retinal cells. Rotation of the optic cup in the adult, which produces a reversal of the visuomotor reflexes, results in perfectly normal vision if the operation is performed in *Amblystoma* any time before embryonic stage 34 (a time when the forelimb bud is just forming) in the tadpole. If the eye is reversed in stages 34 to 36, the operation results in greater and greater mixups of the visuomotor reflexes and, if performed after stage 36, complete reversal results. Thus, there is a time in development when the retinal cells change from an unspecified to a permanently specified condition. This specificity occurs in *Amblystoma* just before the tectal connections are made (stage 38). In *Xenopus,* specification occurs earlier, some 20 hours before the outgrowth of axons from the retinal cells. In both species, specification does not take place throughout the entire retina at the same time but, as in the limb, the anteroposterior axis is determined before the dorsoventral axis. Specification of the retinal cells is not accompanied by any as yet recognizable morphological or ultrastructural changes in the cells. However, DNA synthesis stops just before specificity appears.

Experiments in which the optic cups from two different *Xenopus* embryos were cut in half and then re-fused so that the resulting eyes consisted of two nsasal or two temporal halves have added more information to the problem of retinotectal connections. Following such an operation, electrophysiological mapping shows that the corresponding halves of double nasal or double temporal eyes both project back to the same tectal positions—as one might expect. However, unexpectedly, each nasal half or temporal half projected not to half of the tectum, as it normally would, but its fibers spread out over the entire tectum (Fig. 20–11). In addition, when the optic chiasma was uncrossed in these operated animals so that the optic fibers from a double eye were directed to a tectum previously connected to a normal eye and vice versa, the projection from each half of the double eye still spread out to occupy all of the previously normal tectum, and the fibers from the normal eye took up their normal projections to the tectum previously connected with the double eye. Thus, parts of the tectum that had previously been connected to the temporal half of the normal eye were still capable of forming connections to double nasal eyes having no temporal fibers

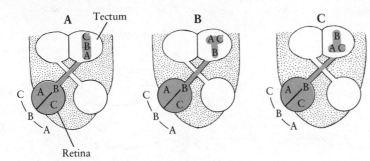

20–11 The relationship between the visual field, the retina, and the projection of the retina to the tectum in *Xenopus* in normal, double-nasal and double-temporal eyes. (From R. M. Gaze, 1963. J. Physiol. 165, 484.)

at all. Also, parts of the tectum previously connected to the nasal half of a double nasal eye were still capable of forming connections to the temporal part of a normal eye. Thus, the retinotectal connections do not direct that the tectum assume a permanent and fixed map of specifications. What is important is the topographical relation between the optic tract fibers as they project to the tectum. If it is the relative position of the optic tract fibers which is important, it is possible that the timing of the development of fibers from different parts of the retina could be translated into a corresponding orderly formation of tectal connections. If axonal outgrowth occurs in a spatiotemporal order, this would determine a spatiotemporal pattern of arrival of axons in the tectum and could be the mechanism determining the pattern of tectal connections. Development of a permanent specificity following these connections could result from the later formation of biochemical affinities between the connected cells.

As stated in the beginning of this section, much of the search for the reason for the establishment of the proper nervous system interconnections and the development of coordinated activity do not really give us many specific answers to the questions raised. In view of the tremendous complexity of this system, this lack of detailed knowledge is not surprising. Yet, we have been dealing with such relatively simple aspects as the connections between axons and muscle fibers, between sensory receptors and their nerve fibers, and as the establishment of simple central synapses. One cannot fail to appreciate how much more bewildering a problem is presented in an attempt to understand the connections and mechanisms controlling memory, learning, and thought processes.

THE BRAIN

From the beginning, the rostral part of the neural plate—the part that will form the brain—is the largest part of the developing central nervous system. Within the brain region itself, the further rostrally one goes, the more complicated the differentiation becomes

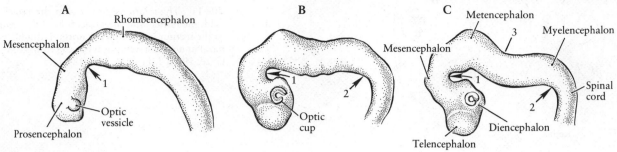

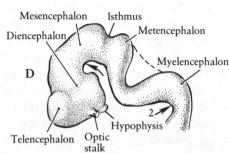

and the further the structures depart from the relatively simple organization of the spinal cord.

External Form

The cranial end of the neural tube at about day 25 shows three regional enlargements separated by two constrictions. These are the primary brain vesicles, the *prosencephalon* (forebrain), the *mesencephalon* (midbrain), and the *rhombencephalon* (hindbrain) (Fig. 20–12 A). At the time the three primary vesicles are formed, the originally straight neural tube, owing largely to the greater growth of the posterior portion of the mesencephalon, shows a bending or flexure in the middle of the brain. This is the *cephalic flexure* (Fig. 20–12 A). Shortly after the appearance of the cephalic flexure, a second bend develops approximately in the region of the juncture of the brain and the spinal cord. This is the *cervical flexure* (Fig. 20–13 B).

Two of the three primary brain vesicles, the prosencephalon and the rhombencephalon, subdivide so that the nine-millimeter embryo, early in the second month, shows five major brain regions (Fig. 20–12 C). These were named by His in 1893 the *telencephalon, diencephalon, mesencephalon, metencephalon,* and *myelencephalon* proceeding in a rostral to a caudal direction. Shortly after the five divisions are recognizable, a third flexure appears between the myelencephalon and the metencephalon. This is the *pontine flexure* (Fig. 20–12 C). The pontine flexure bends in a direction opposite to the first two flexures. In the 11-millimeter embryo (Fig. 20–12 D), the five brain divisions and the three flexures are easily recognized. A well-defined posterior constriction separates the telencephalon from the diencephalon. The developing optic cup and the hypophysis are two landmarks in the diencephalon. The cervical flexure marks the middle of the mesencephalon and a constriction, the *isthmus,* separates the mesencephalon and the metencephalon. The three flexures gradually become less pronounced and eventually the pontine and cervical flexures completely disappear. The cephalic

20–12 Four stages showing the external configuration of the brain during its early development. A, about 25 days showing the three primary divisions and the cephalic flexure (3.5 mm); B, about 30 days (5 mm); C, about 36 days (9 mm); D, about 39 days (11 mm). 1, cephalic flexure; 2, cervical flexure; 3, pontine flexure.

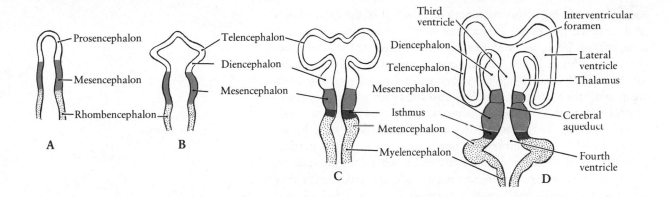

20–13   Expansion of the central canal in the region of the brain to form the ventricular system. (After E. L. House and B. Pansky, 1967. A Functional Approach to Neuroanatomy. Mc-Graw-Hill Book Company, New York.)

flexure, however, persists, and since this occurs in the region of the midbrain, the diencephalon and the telencephalon are permanently set at a slight angle to the rest of the brain.

The central canal of the spinal cord runs the length of the neural tube, and in that part of the tube that will form the brain, it undergoes modifications in accordance with the regional specializations of the brain to form a number of local enlargements known as *ventricles* (Fig. 20–13). The first and second ventricles lie within the telencephalon and become greatly enlarged as the cerebral hemispheres expand. The third lies within the diencephalon and is connected to the ventricles of the telencephalon by a narrow canal, the *foramen of Monro (interventricular foramen)*. The fourth ventricle develops in the rhombencephalon and later shows a wide lateral expansion. It is connected to the third by a narrow passage through the mesencephalon, the *aqueduct of Sylvius*.

Internal Configuration

In the brain, the characteristic H-shaped pattern formed by the cell bodies of the neurons in the spinal cord is found only in the most caudal region of the myelencephalon. Elsewhere, the histological appearance of the brain bears little resemblance to that of the spinal cord. This is the result of a number of factors: (1) the development of important fiber tracts which impinge on the cellular area that represents the intermediate area of the cord; (2) the migration of neurons from the intermediate layer into the outer marginal layer of the brain; and (3) the accumulation of groups of neurons in particular regions of the brain to form what are known as *cranial nuclei*.

The Functional Classification of Cranial Nerve Nuclei and Fibers
Many of the nuclei in the brain are associated with the cranial nerves. The neurons of cranial nerve nuclei form groups of cells,

each group serving a specific function. Thus, all of the motor fibers of the cranial nerves are axons from specific cranial nuclei sending their efferent impulses away from the brain stem. At the same time, the sensory fibers in the various cranial nerves, whose cell bodies are located in cranial nerve sensory ganglia outside of the brain stem, send their afferent impulses into the brain where they make central synapses with specific sensory nuclei. Very often a single cranial nucleus, be it motor or sensory in function, may be associated with fibers in more than one cranial nerve. This is particularly true for the sensory cranial nerve nuclei where, for instance, all of the visceral afferent fibers, no matter which cranial nerve they are found in, make their central synapses with the same nucleus. However, any single cranial nerve nucleus is always associated with only one functional type of nerve fiber.

We have seen that we can group the spinal nerve fibers into four classes or types on the basis of their function. These same four functional types are also found in the cranial nerves. However, the cranial nerves have three additional (special) types of fibers, and we are then concerned with seven different types of fibers in the cranial nerves. Any one cranial nerve may have one or more than one type of fiber associated with it. The efferent fibers are outgrowth of nuclei derived from the basal plate of different regions of the brain, and the sensory fibers make their central connections with nuclei, which are alar plate derivatives. The alar and the basal plates each give rise to three functional types of cranial nerve nuclei. Some of these nuclei are found at only one level of the brain while others may be present as long bands of cell bodies stretching through many levels. In the early embryo, these six types of nuclei show a regular arrangement (Fig. 20–14) but later migrations and disturbances from developing fiber tracts result in considerable rearrangement. The functional types of the cranial nerve nuclei are as follows:

1. *Somatic Efferent* (SE)—as in the spinal cord, motor neurons whose fibers supply skeletal muscle derived from somatic mesoderm.

2. *General Visceral Efferent* (GVE)—as in the spinal cord, motor nuclei whose fibers are preganglionic to structures of visceral origin such as the lungs, the heart, and the alimentary tract—a part of the parasympathetic division of the autonomic nervous system. In this division, the ganglia are located close to the structures they supply (even within the walls, as is the case with the enteric ganglia previously considered) and the postganglionic fibers are correspondingly short.

3. *Special Visceral Efferent* (SVE)—contrary to the implication

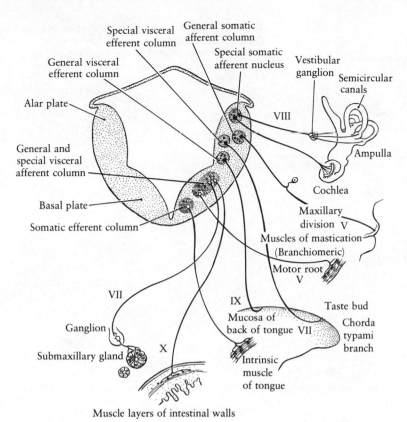

Special visceral
efferent column

General somatic
afferent column

General visceral
efferent column

Special somatic
afferent nucleus

Vestibular
ganglion

Semicircular
canals

Alar plate

VIII

General and
special visceral
afferent column

Ampulla

Cochlea

Basal plate

Maxillary
division V

Somatic efferent column

Muscles of mastication
(Branchiomeric)

Motor root
V

VII

IX

Taste bud

Mucosa of
back of tongue VII

Chorda
typami
branch

Ganglion

Submaxillary gland

X

Intrinsic
muscle
of tongue

Muscle layers of intestinal walls

of the name, the fibers of these nuclei are not a special part of the autonomic nervous system supplying visceral organs. Instead, they are efferent fibers to skeletal muscle. However, the muscles these fibers supply are derived from head or visceral arch mesoderm. The skeletal muscles formed from this type of mesoderm are histologically and functionally exactly the same as those formed from somatic mesoderm. They differ in only one thing—their embryonic origin. Because of this origin, their cranial nerve motor fibers are given this particular functional classification.

4. and 5. *General and Special Visceral Afferent (GVA, SVA)*—all of the visceral afferent fibers in the cranial nerves (with the exception of those in the olfactory nerve) make their central connections with the same cranial sensory nucleus. The general visceral fibers are connected peripherally to general visceral receptors. The special visceral fibers are connected to what are considered special visceral receptors—taste buds and olfactory receptors.

6. *General Somatic Afferent (GSA)*—nuclei receiving sensory input from peripheral somatic sensory receptors in the head region.

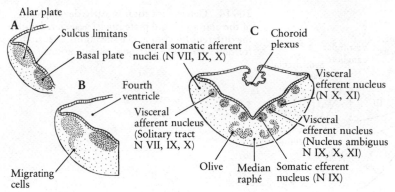

Alar plate

A

Sulcus limitans

Basal plate

B

Fourth ventricle

General somatic afferent nuclei (N VII, IX, X)

C Choroid plexus

Visceral efferent nucleus (N X, XI)

Visceral afferent nucleus (Solitary tract N VII, IX, X)

Visceral efferent nucleus (Nucleus ambiguus N IX, X, XI)

Olive Median raphé Somatic efferent nucleus (N IX)

Migrating cells

20–15 Three stages in the early development of the myelencephalon showing the lateral expansion of the fourth ventricle, the formation of the alar and basal plate nuclei and the development of the choroid plexus.

7. *Special Somatic Afferent* (SSA)—nuclei receiving sensory input from special sense organs of ectodermal origin—the eye and the ear.

Development of the Myelencephalon

The myelencephalon shows the least variation from the spinal cord. Early in development a change in the H-shaped pattern of the cord is seen. It is due primarily to two events (1) the expansion of the fourth ventricle and, as a consequence of this, the separation of the alar plates; and (2) the develpment of the brain nuclei.

The fourth ventricle is already a large cavity in the early embryo. When the pontine flexure develops, the fourth ventricle is expanded laterally. In this process the alar plates become separated and the roof plate stretches to form a thin ependymal layer roofing over the fourth ventricle and joining the right and left alar plates (Fig. 20–15). When the pia mater—the innermost meninx of the brain—develops, it forms a vascular plexus the *tela choroidea,* in a T-shaped pattern over the roof of the ventricle. This plexus of blood vessels, covered by the ependymal epithelium, then invaginates into the fourth ventricle forming the *choroid plexus* of that ventricle whose function is the secretion of cerebrospinal fluid into the ventricular system.

The lateral walls of the fourth ventricle show well-defined thick alar and basal plates marked off from each other by a distinct groove, the sulcus limitans (Fig. 20–15 A). The cell bodies of neurons serving a common function move to specific areas of the alar and basal plates where they accumulate as groups of cells collectively called a nucleus. The pattern made by these nuclei is characteristic of the region of the brain examined. Often the ultimate position of a nucleus may be the result of extensive migration of its individual neurons. One example of this is the migration of alar plate neurons of the myelencephalon into the basal plate to form the sensory way station, the *olivary nucleus* (Fig. 20–15).

As in the spinal cord, the neuroblasts derived from the basal plate send out fibers to form the efferent components of the cranial nerves, and those from the alar plate form the central nervous system connections (or way stations) for afferent impulses. Some derivatives of the basal plate of the myelencephalon are the *nucleus ambiguus,* which is the point of origin of of the special visceral efferent fibers running in cranial nerves IX, X, and XI, the *dorsal motor nucleus* of the Xth nerve (GVE), and the motor nucleus of the XIIth (hypoglossal) nerve (SE) (Fig. 20–15 C). From the alar plates are derived the *solitary nucleus,* which receives the visceral sensory fibers from cranial nerves VII, IX, and X; the *nucleus gracilis* and *nucleus cuneatus,* which are relay stations for proprioceptive impulses ascending from the spinal cord to the cerebellum and cerebrum.

The floor plate of the myelencephalon forms a nonnervous median raphe.

Development of the Metencephalon

The metencephalon consists of three parts: (1) a primary axial portion, the *tegmentum,* a continuation rostrally of the general structure of the myelencephalon; (2) a specialized expansion of the most posterior regions of the alar plates to form the *cerebellum;* and (3) a basal portion, the *pons,* containing a group of nuclei, the *pontine nuclei,* and the fibers connecting these nuclei to other parts of the central nervous system, particularly the cerebrum and the cerebellum. Regions two and three are both phylogenetically newer acquisitions and develop later than the tegmental region of the metencephalon.

The primary axial portion forms the floor of the metencephalic part of the fourth ventricle and shows the characteristic alar and basal plates separated by the sulcus limitans (Fig. 20–16 A). The lateral expansion of the middle of the fourth ventricle gives it a diamond-shaped appearance and the floor of the fourth ventricle, including the part formed by the myelencephalon, is known as the *rhomboid fossa.* The basal plates of the metencephalon form motor nuclei associated with cranial nerves V (SVE), VI (SE), and VII (GVE, SVE). Nuclei developing in the alar plates provide sensory connections for cranial nerves V (GSA), VII (GVA, SVA), and VII (SSA) (Fig. 20–16 C).

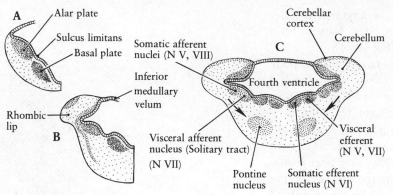

The Cerebellum

The most posterior parts of the alar plates rostral to the lateral recesses, which are separated from each other medially by the roof plate, become thickened to form the *rhombic lips* (Fig. 20–16 B). Progressing rostrally, the fourth vesicle narrows and the rhombic lips arroach and fuse with each other. Proliferation of the rhombic lips gives rise to the *cerebellar swellings* or *plates,* which are recognizable in the seven- to eight-millimeter embryo early in the second month (Fig. 20–17). During the second month each cerebellar plate thickens rapidly and forms a pair of bulges projecting into the fourth ventricle, which soon join medially to form a single dumb-bell-shaped cerebellum (Fig. 20–18).

During the third and fourth months, there is a rapid growth of the cerebellum and fissures appear on its surface which serve as landmarks to delineate its principal lobes. The first to appear is the *posterolateral fissure.* This sets off a region caudal to this fissure, the *flocculonodular* lobe. The part of the cerebellum rostral to the fissure is called the *corpus cerebelli* (Fig. 20–19 A). The median flocculus and the paired lateral nodular lobes are thus the most caudal part of the cerebellum, lying just cranial to the lateral recesses, and they are the first part of the cerebellum to differentiate. As is the general rule, the first part of a system to differentiate is the oldest part phylogenetically. Functionally, the flocculonodular lobe is concerned with the maintenance of equilibrium. The coordinating functions of the cerebellum, functions that are phylogentically more recently acquired, develop in the corpus cerebelli.

The *fissure prima* develops late in the fourth month, dividing the corpus cerebelli into anterior and posterior lobes (Fig. 20–19 B) and shortly thereafter a *fissure secunda* appears in the posterior lobe (Fig. 20–19 C). The part of the cerebellum just rostral to the fissure secunda, particularly its lateral aspects, is the last part to develop.

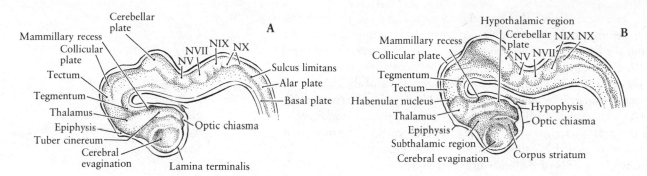

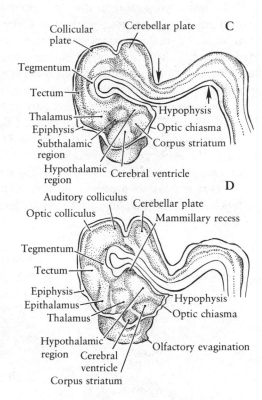

In man, this undergoes a marked expansion to form the lateral hemispheres. This newest part of the cerebellum receives the name *neocerebellum*. Functionally it is concerned with the integration of the muscular activity initiated by the phylogenetically newest part of the cerebrum, the neopallium. Both of these parts of the brain show their greatest development in the primates.

As development proceeds, many more subdivisions appear, and the adult cerebellum shows a complex pattern of fissures and lobules to which cumbersome and often fanciful names have been given. However, the fundamental divisions of embryological and functional significance are those outlined above. In their order of development, we may thus recognize three regions whose major functions differ—although there is certainly some overlap among them: (1) the flocculonodular lobe, termed the *archicerebellum,* which functions to maintain equilibrium; (2) the part of the body of the cerebellum anterior to the primary fissure, the anterior lobe, and the part of the body of the cerebellum between the posterolateral fissure and the fissure secunda. Collectively, these parts are termed the *paleocerebellum* and function to maintain muscle tone and posture. And (3) the region between the fissure prima and the fissure secunda, termed the *neocerebellum,* which functions to coordinate muscular activity. All three regions have essentially different connections to the medullary nuclei of the cerebellum and to other parts of the brain in accordance with the functions they serve.

Histogenesis of the cerebellum. The migration of the neuroepithelial cells and the neuroblasts of the cerebellum differs from that described for the spinal cord. The cerebellar plate at first shows the same characteristic three-layered (ventricular, intermediate, marginal) pattern as the spinal cord. However, as the cerebellar plate thickens, neuroepithelial cells move out of their position next to the lumen of the fourth ventricle and migrate to the periphery of the marginal zone to form what is termed the *external granular layer* (Fig. 20–20 A). Later, an *internal granular layer* develops in

20–17 Drawings of reconstructions of the brain of four human embryos early in the second month. A, about 31 days (7–8 mm); B, about 33 days (9–10 mm); C, about 35 days (12 mm); D, about 37 days (14.6 mm). (From G. L. Streeter, 1948. Carnegie Contributions to Embryology 32, 133.)

the marginal layer through the outward migration of other neuroepithelial derivatives and also by the inward migration of cells from the external granular layer (Fig. 20–20 B). Large, flask-shaped cells, *Purkinje cells,* mark the border between these two granular layers (Fig. 20–20 C). In later development, most of the cells of the outer granular layer migrate inward and end up in the inner granular layer, leaving a cell-poor layer, now called the *molecular layer,* as the most superficial part of the cerebellar cortex. The molecular layer is occupied by the dendrites of the Purkinje cells and the axons of the cells of the inner granular layer.

Other neuroepithelial derivatives remain in the deeper part of the cerebellum. They form four pairs of *medullary nuclei* and through their dendrites make synaptic connections with the axons of the Purkinje cells. The medullary nuclei relay impulses from the cerebellar cortex to other parts of the central nervous system. The first medullary nuclei to differentiate are the most medially located, and their connections are with the oldest part of the cortex, the flocculonodular lobe. The most lateral, which are the largest and the last to develop, are the *dentate nuclei* (Fig. 20–21), whose connections are with the Purkinje cells of the neocerebellum. Efferent impulses from the dentate nuclei are carried cranially into the mesencephalon by fibers that make up the major portions of the *superior cerebellar peduncles,* one of the three pathways to and from the cerebellar cortex.

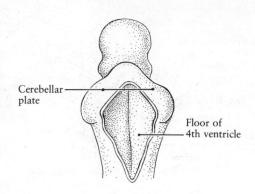

20–18 Fusion of the right and left cerebellar plates.

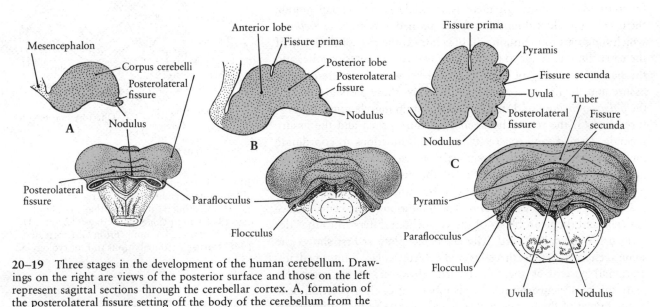

20–19 Three stages in the development of the human cerebellum. Drawings on the right are views of the posterior surface and those on the left represent sagittal sections through the cerebellar cortex. A, formation of the posterolateral fissure setting off the body of the cerebellum from the flocculonodular node; B, formation of the primary fissure in the body of the cerebellum; C, later development of the lobes of the cerebellum (about five months).

The roof plate in the region between the cerebellar plates is absorbed in the expansion of the cortex, but cranially and caudally it persists as the *superior* and *inferior medullary velum,* respectively (Fig. 20–21).

The Basilar Portion of the Pons

This portion of the metencephalon develops in connection with a group of nuclei, the pontine nuclei. Although these nuclei are located in the most anterior (basal) portion of the pons, they are derived from neuroblasts that have migrated to this position and are actually of alar plate origin (Fig. 20–16). The pontine nuclei are associated with the neocerebellum, to which they are connected by fibers that cross over in the most basilar region of the pons and ascend to the cerebellum by way of the *middle cerebellar penduncle* (*brachium pontis*). The pontine nuclei receive impulses from the cerebral cortex and thus form a link by way of which the newest part of the cerebellar cortex may interact with the newest part of the cerebral cortex in the coordination of muscular activity.

Development of the Mesencephalon

The mesencephalon does not show any striking modifications or expansions and is soon overshadowed by the cerbral cortex and the cerebellum. Three regions of the mesencephalon may be recognized: (1) the *tegmentum,* developed from the basal plates; (2) the *tectum,*

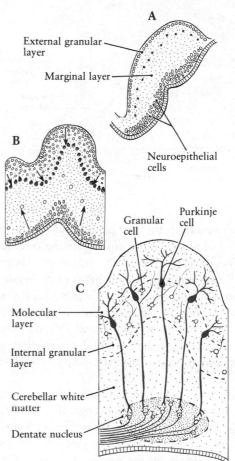

20–20 Histogenesis of the cerebellar cortex. Arrows indicate the direction of migration of the cells.

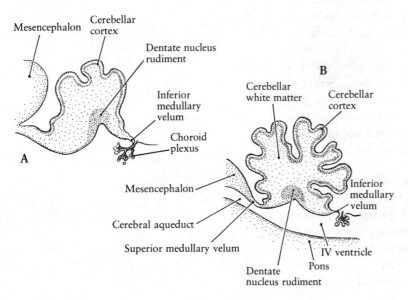

20–21 Sagittal sections of the developing human cerebellum. A, during the fourth month (100 mm); B, during the fifth month (150 mm). (After W. J. Hamilton and H. W. Mossman, 1972. Macmillan Press, London.)

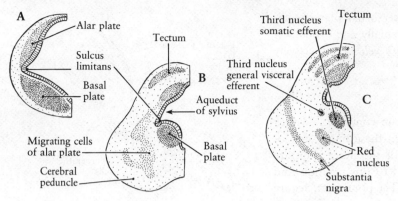

A

Alar plate

Sulcus
limitans

Basal
plate

Tectum

B

Migrating cells
of alar plate

Cerebral
peduncle

Aqueduct
of sylvius

Basal
plate

Third nucleus
somatic efferent

Tectum

Third nucleus
general visceral
efferent

C

Red
nucleus

Substantia
nigra

20–22 Three stages in the differentiation of the mesencephalon.

developed from the alar plates; and (3) the *cerebral peduncles* consisting of fiber tracts mainly from the cerebrum (Fig. 20–22).

The development of the tegmentum begins late in month one (3–5 mm embryo) as the basal plate begins to thicken. As is the general rule, the basal plate begins its differentiation before the alar plate. During the second month it gives rise to the somatic efferent nuclei of cranial nerves III and IV. Associated with the nucleus of the IIIrd nerve is a cranial component whose fibers are preganglionic fibers of the parasympathetic division of the autonomic nervous system (Fig. 20–22 C).

At the time the tegmentum is developing, the tectum is still undifferentiated. Not until the beginning of month three (24–27 mm embryos) does the alar plate region show any significant expansion. At this time the alar plates thicken and form two longitudinally running ridges on the posterior aspect of the mesencephalon, the *collicular plates* (Figs. 20–22; 20–17 C). Later, each ridge is divided transversely forming a rostral and a caudal pair of swellings, the *superior* and *inferior colliculi*, respectively (Fig. 20–23 B). Collectively, the colliculi are called the *corpora quadregemina*. As they increase in size, they obscure the roof plate. In the development of the tectum, neuroblasts migrate toward the surface, where they form peripheral tectal nuclei (Fig. 20–22 B,C); the colliculi thus resemble the cerebellar cortex in the reversal of white and grey matter. The superior colliculi are centers for visual reflexes; the interior colliculi are centers for auditory reflexes.

Two pairs of prominent nuclei develop in the tegmental area: the *red nucleus* and the *substantia nigra* (Fig. 20–22 C). Although their origin is not completely agreed upon, they are generally considered to be alar plate derivatives that migrate into the tegmental region.

The cerebral peduncles (*basic pedunculi*) make up the most anterior region of the mesencephalon. They consist of nerve fibers running longitudinally through the marginal layer of the tegmen-

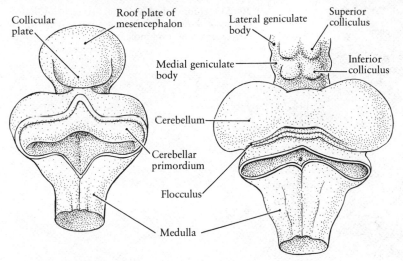

Collicular plate

Roof plate of mesencephalon

Lateral geniculate body

Superior colliculus

Medial geniculate body

Inferior colliculus

Cerebellum

Cerebellar primordium

Flocculus

Medulla

20–23 A, dorsal view of the hindbrain and the midbrain in a two-month-old human embryo; B, same view in a four-month-old embryo.

tum. They contain fibers from cerebral cortex nuclei passing to lower brain and spinal regions. *corticopontine, corticobulbar,* and *corticospinal* tracts.

As the basal and alar plates expand, they bulge into the ventricle of the mesencephalon and the mesocoele becomes progressively smaller ending up as a narrow channel, the *aqueduct of Sylvius,* connecting the fourth ventricle of the hindbrain to the third ventricle of the diencephalon. The floor plate is lacking. It is considered to terminate at the level of the rostral end of the metencephalon.

Development of the Diencephalon

Early in the development of the prosencephalon a lateral diverticulum appears on either side. These are the *optic vesicles* (Figs.20–12 A; 20–24) that will develop into the major portions of the eye. The optic vesicles are connected to the ventricle of the diencephalon by the hollow *optic stalk* (Fig. 20–24 B). They mark the rostral end of the diencephalon. The diencephalon is prominent during the middle of the second month, at which time the boundaries between it and the telencephalon are easily distinguished. Later it becomes overshadowed by the cerebral hemispheres, and the walls of the diencephalon and the telencephalon become closely connected.

Figure 20–25 shows the developing forebrain during the seventh week, at which time all of the primordia of the future diencephalic structures are recognizable. The diencephalon consists of three major subdivisions: the *epithalamus,* the *thalamus,* and the *hypothalamus.* The most anterior and the first to develop, the hypothala-

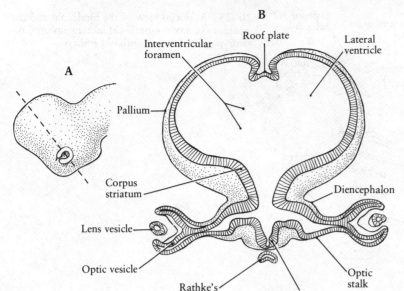

B

Interventricular foramen

Roof plate

Lateral ventricle

Pallium

Corpus striatum

Diencephalon

Lens vesicle

Optic vesicle

Rathke's pouch

Infundibulum

Optic stalk

A

20–24 Human diencephalon (10 mm). A, lateral view showing developing optic vesicle; B, cross section at level indicated in A.

mus, is marked off from the thalamus by the *hypothalamic sulcus*. The hypothalamic sulcus is not a continuation of the sulcus limitans, which stops in the mesencephalon, and thus does not divide the diencephalon into alar and basal plates. All of the forebrain, with the exception of roof plate derivatives, is formed from alar plate material. The *optic chiasma,* the *infundibulum,* and the *mammillary bodies* are hypothalamic derivatives (Fig. 20–17; 20–25). The optic chiasma represents the crossing over of parts of the optic tracts from one side to the other, the infundibulum will develop into the neural parts of the pituitary gland and the mammillary bodies will develop nuclei functioning as olfactory way stations. The neuroblasts of the intermediate layer of the hypothalamus will differentiate into a series of nuclei concerned with visceral functions, the brain center of the autonomic nervous system.

The epithalamus is the next area to differentiate. The cells of the intermediate layer in this region develop into the *habenular nuclei,* which are associated with olfactory impulses and lie adjacent to a dorsal evagination of the roof of the diencephalon, the *epiphysis* (Fig. 20–17 B; 20–25 B). The epiphysis will form the *pineal body.* Two commissures develop in the region, the *habenular commissure,* cranial to the epiphysis and the *posterior commissure,* caudal to the epiphysis.

The thalamus consists of an older portion, the *ventral thalamus (subthalamus),* which is an important transitional zone from the mesencephalon. A newer portion, the *dorsal thalamus,* which

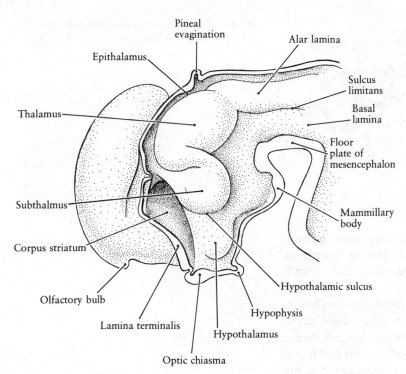

Pineal
evagination

Alar lamina

Epithalamus

Thalamus

Sulcus
limitans

Basal
lamina

Floor
plate of
mesencephalon

Subthalmus

Mammillary
body

Corpus striatum

Hypothalamic sulcus

Olfactory bulb

Hypophysis

Lamina terminalis

Hypothalamus

Optic chiasma

20–25 View of the medial surface of a reconstruction of the forebrain of a 19 mm human embryo.

reaches its highest development in man, differentiates important
nuclear masses that become association and relay centers for impulses to and from the cerebral cortex. The late-developing thalami
grow rapidly, bulge into the third ventricle, and join to form the *intermediate mass.*

The most posterior part of the thalamus differentiates the *lateral*
and *medial geniculate bodies,* the former associated with the superior and the latter with the inferior colliculi of the mesencephalon
(Fig. 20–23). This region of the thalamus is sometimes called the
metathalamus.

In addition to forming the epiphysis, the roof plate also forms the
thin ependymal tela choroidea, which becomes a part of the choroid
plexus of the third ventricle (Fig. 20–26 B).

Development of the Telencephalon

The differentiation of the telencephalon begins later than that of
other regions of the brain, but its rapid development, once started,
gives rise to a structure that far overshadows the rest of the brain.
This is accomplished by the tremendous expansion of the lateral
and posterior walls of the prosencephalic cavity. At first, the expanded lateral ventricles retain a wide connection with the cavity of

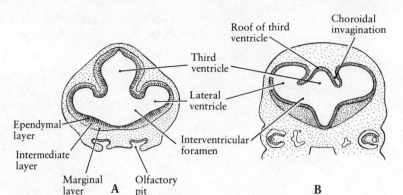

Roof of third
ventricle

Choroidal
invagination

Third
ventricle

Lateral
ventricle

Ependymal
layer

Intermediate
layer

Interventricular
foramen

Marginal
layer

Olfactory
pit

A

B

the third ventricle (Figs. 20–24; 20–26), but this cavity becomes progressively smaller as development proceeds. During its early expansion, the cerebrum extends laterally, posteriorly, and caudally but only slightly cranially.

During the second month, extension in a cranial direction begins; by the middle of that month, the *lamina terminalis*—which marks the most rostral end of the original brain stem and was still located at the most rostral position in the brain at the end of the first month (Figs. 20–27 A; 20–28 B)—is now found to be about in the middle of the expanding hemispheres (Figs. 20–27 B; 20–28 C). Caudally, the lamina terminalis is set off from the optic chiasma by the *optic recess,* which marks the boundary between the telencephalon and the diencephalon (Fig. 20–27 B). At this time, the optic chiasma is one of three important commissures found in this region of the brain. The other two are the *anterior commissure* and the *hippocampal commissure,* which are located in the lamina terminalis (Fig. 20–28). Since the lamina terminalis retains its original position while the cerebral hemispheres expand rostrally to it, these two commissures appear to be located in the middle of the cerebrum in later stages of development (Fig. 20–28). Posteriorly and caudally, the lamina terminalis connects to the roof of the diencephalon.

Further development during the second month consists of the continued expansion of the cerebral hemispheres, which will eventually extend far enough caudally to cover the lateral aspects of parts of the metencephalon, and of the beginning of the differentiation in its walls. The caudal expansion of the cerebral vesicles brings their medial walls into contact with the walls of the diencephalon with which they fuse. The early differentiation of the walls of the cerebral vesicles is seen in Figure 20–29 B. A marked thickening of the anterolateral wall differentiates first and represents the beginning of the formation of the *corpus striatum.* Next,

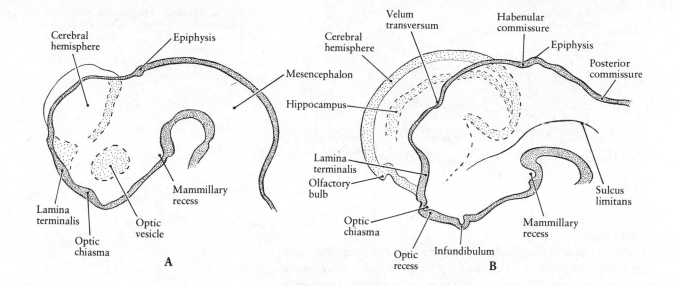

the medial wall differentiates to form the *hippocampus*. The medial wall posterior to the hippocampus, the posterior wall, and the suprastrial region of the wall (i.e., all of the wall of the cerebral vesicle between the hippocampus and the corpus striatum) is the primordium of the *neopallium,* the newest part of the cerebral cortex.

Medially, along its postcromcdial attachment to the diencephalon, the ependymal layer of the roof plate projects laterally into each ventricle to contribute to the formation of the choroid plexus of the first and second ventricles. It is convenient to consider the development of the three parts of the cerebrum—the corpus striatum, the hippocampus and the neopallium—separately.

20–27   Diagrams of midsagittal sections of the brains of human embryos during the fifth and sixth weeks of development. A, 7.5 mm; B, 19 mm. (After G. W. Bartelmez and A. S. Dekeban, 1962. Carnegie Contributions to Embryology 37, 13.)

20–28   Sagittal sections through the brain stem of three human embryos showing the development of the commissures. A, 9 mm; B, 25 mm; C, 65 mm. (After W. J. Hamilton and H. W. Mossman, 1972. Human Embryology. Macmillan Press, London.)

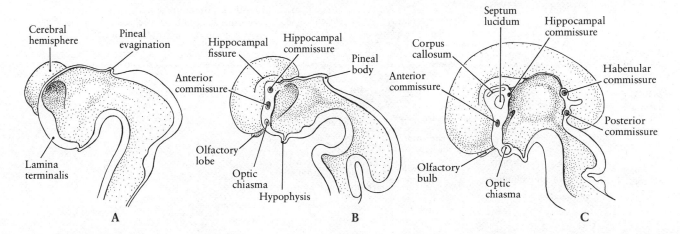

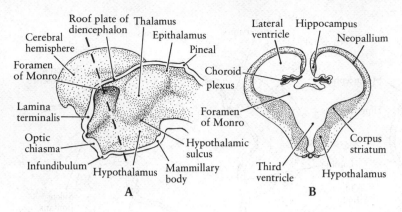

A

Cerebral hemisphere
Foramen of Monro
Roof plate of diencephalon
Thalamus
Epithalamus
Pineal
Choroid plexus
Lamina terminalis
Optic chiasma
Infundibulum
Hypothalamus
Mammillary body
Hypothalamic sulcus
Foramen of Monro

B

Lateral ventricle
Hippocampus
Neopallium
Choroid plexus
Corpus striatum
Third ventricle
Hypothalamus

20–29   A, drawing of the medial surface of a reconstruction of the forebrain of a seven-week-old human embryo; B, cross section through A at the level indicated. (From J. Langman 1963. Medical Embryology. Williams and Wilkins Company, Baltimore.)

Corpus Striatum

The corpus striatum can be separated into a medial accumulation of cells which retains its proximity to the ventricle and a more lateral region which gradually moves away from the ventricle. The former will develop into the *caudate nucleus;* the latter into the *lentiform nucleus* (Fig. 20–30).

As the cerebral cortex continues to expand caudally and then bends anteriorly, the corpus striatum is drawn out into a longitudinally running, comma-shaped ridge that is closely associated with the thalamus of the diencephalon (Fig. 20–31). The arched tail of the caudate nucleus ends in an accumulation of nerve cells termed the *amygdaloid nucleus.* Fiber tracts running in both directions between the developing neopallium and the thalamus appear on both sides of the lentiform nucleus. This thick bundle of fibers, in the form of a V that is open laterally, is called the *internal capsule.* The lentiform nucleus lies in the cavity of the V so that it is separated by the posterior limb of the internal capsule from the caudate

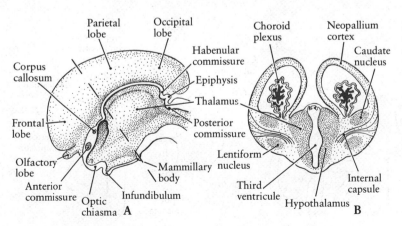

Parietal lobe
Occipital lobe
Corpus callosum
Habenular commissure
Epiphysis
Thalamus
Frontal lobe
Posterior commissure
Olfactory lobe
Anterior commissure
Optic chiasma
Infundibulum
Mammillary body
A

Choroid plexus
Neopallium cortex
Caudate nucleus
Lentiform nucleus
Third ventricle
Hypothalamus
Internal capsule
B

20–30   A, diagram of a sagittal section of the cerebrum at about 10 weeks; B, drawing of a cross section through A at the level indicated.

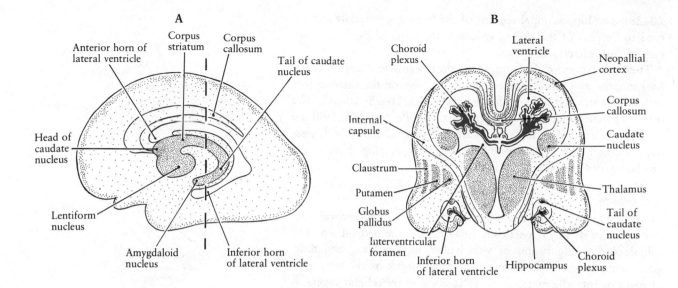

A

Anterior horn of lateral ventricle

Corpus striatum

Corpus callosum

Tail of caudate nucleus

Head of caudate nucleus

Lentiform nucleus

Amygdaloid nucleus

Inferior horn of lateral ventricle

B

Choroid plexus

Lateral ventricle

Neopallial cortex

Corpus callosum

Caudate nucleus

Internal capsule

Claustrum

Putamen

Globus pallidus

Interventricular foramen

Inferior horn of lateral ventricle

Hippocampus

Choroid plexus

Thalamus

Tail of caudate nucleus

20–31   A, diagram of a sagittal section through a human cerebrum of approximately 21 weeks; B, cross section through A at the level indicated. (From J. Langman, 1963. Medical Embryology. Williams and Wilkins Company, Baltimore.)

nucleus and by the anterior limb from the thalamus (Figs. 20–30; 20–31). The caudate nucleus and the thalamus thus come into direct contact. The lentiform nucleus divides into a lateral group of closely packed neurons, the *putamen,* and a medial protion, the *globus pallidus.* Another group of neurons develops lateral to the putamen to form the *claustrum,* the most superficial of the striatal nuclei (Fig. 20–31 B). The claustrum lies beneath an area of the cerebral cortex called the *insula,* a part of the cortex that develops more slowly than other regions and is overgrown by them so that it forms no part of the visible surface of the cortex but is hidden under the other lobes. Collectively, in the adult, the caudate nucleus, the lentiform nucleus, and the internal capsule are known as the *corpus striatum,* the highest center of the brain to develop in the lower vertebrates. Even in the birds, no substantial neopallium develops, and the corpus striatum is the center for correlation of sensory impulses and control of motor activity.

Hippocampal Cortex and Olfactory Complex

The hippocampal pallium is carried caudally and anterolaterally with the growth of the temporal lobes of the telencephalon. It appears on the medial wall of the cerebral vesicle as a curved area parallel to the choroidal fissure between it and the neopallium (Fig. 20–29 B). Much of the hippocampal structure undergoes retrogressive changes. The rostral parts of the hippocampal region are interconnected by a commisure, the *hippocampal commissure,* which develops in the posterior portion of the lamina terminalis (Fig.

20–28). The hippocampal regions of the brain are generally considered to be part of the *rhinencephalon*, the parts of the brain concerned with olfaction.

The major part of the rhinencephalon begins to form at about four months as a projection, the *olfactory lobe*, on the anterior rostral surface of each cerebral hemisphere (Figs. 20–28; 20–30). The olfactory lobe divides into a rostral part, the *olfactory bulb*, and the *olfactory stalk*. Fibers from the neurons in the olfactory bulb pass back through the olfactory stalk to centers developed from the caudal part of the olfactory lobe.

Neopallium

By far the most extensive changes in the walls of the cerebral vesicles occur in its phylogenetically newest part, the neopallium. The spinal cord configuration of ventricular, intermediate, and marginal layers is interrupted during the third month by the migration of neurons into the marginal layer to form outer cellular layers as in the cerebellum and the corpora quadrigemina. As the neopallial walls increase in thickness, these outer cellular layers also become much thicker, and its neurons become stratified. By the end of the seventh month, six layers of neurons make up the basic pattern of the neopallium. This pattern is modified in different regions of the cortex and about 100 different variations of the basic pattern have been described, each characteristic of a particular region.

The area of the cortex becomes greatly increased by the formation of numerous folds (*gyri*) and grooves (*sulci*) (Fig. 20–32). The gyri and sulci form a pattern on the surface of the cerebral hemispheres by means of which it may be divided into a number of different lobes. The *central sulcus* separates the *frontal* and *parietal* lobes. A *parietooccipital sulcus*, more prominent on the medial surface, and a line connecting it to the preoccipital notch defines the parietal and *occipital lobes*. The *lateral* (Sylvian) *fissure* separates the frontal and *temporal lobes*, and a line connecting the lateral fissue to the parietooccipital sulcus further defines the temporal lobe. The slower growing insula lies under the juncture of the temporal, parietal, and frontal lobes.

Commissures

The two sides of the cerebrum are interconnected by three commissures that develop in relation to the thickened area of the lamina terminalis known as the commissural plate (Figs. 20–28; 20–33). The first to develop is the anterior commissure followed shortly by the hippocampal commissure as has already been described. The anterior commissure contains fibers connecting olfactory bulb derivatives. The last commissure to develop, and the largest, is the *corpus*

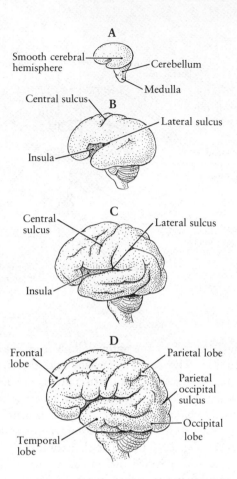

20–32 Diagram of successive stages in the development of the surface of the cerebrum. A, 13 weeks; B, 26 weeks; C, 35 weeks; D, newborn.

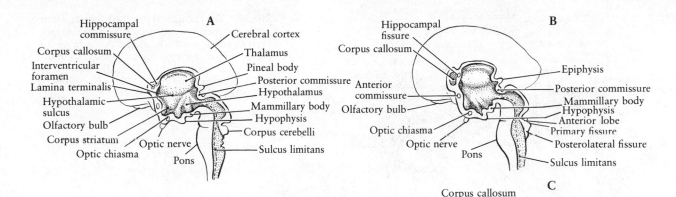

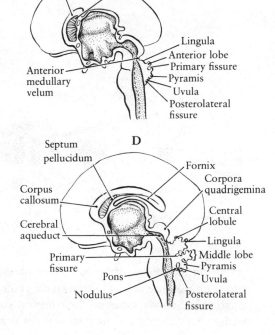

callosum (Fig. 20–28 C; 20–33). Its fibers are from the neopallium, crossing over just posterior to the hippocampal commissure. With the increase in the size of the neopallium and its continued expansion, the corpus callosum also increases rapidly in size and expands both cranially and caudally to form a large C-shaped structure in the center of the cerebrum (Fig. 20–33 C,D). The hippocampal commissure is carried caudally by the expanding corpus callosum and ends up in a position far caudad of that in which it originally appeared.

THE CRANIAL NERVES

As in the spinal cord, neurons in the rostral end of the nervous system establish peripheral connections through their fiber outgrowths. These peripheral extensions are the cranial nerves. Fundamentally, cranial nerves are similar to spinal nerves already discussed. Cranial motor fibers, which carry efferent impulses peripherally, are the axons of nerve cells in the brain stem. Cranial sensory fibers, which carry impulses centrally from sensory receptors, are the dendrites of nerve cells. The cell bodies of the afferent nerve fibers are not located within the brain stem but are found in cranial nerve ganglia just as the afferent fibers in the spinal nerve are parts of neurons located in the posterior root ganglia. Fibers growing centrally from the cranial nerve ganglia make connections with specific cranial nuclei within the central nervous system. The cranial nerves differ from the spinal nerves in that they are not segmentally arranged; nor do they have anterior and posterior roots.

There are 12 pairs of cranial nerves, any one of which may carry one or more kinds of nerve fibers with different functional classifications. It is appropriate to look at the large nerve trunks that constitute the cranial nerves as convenient pathways over which nerve fibers associated with the cranial nuclei arrive at their appro-

20–33 Diagrams of sagittal sections through the brains of human embryos during the third to the fifth months of development. A, 11 weeks; B, 4 months; C, 4½ months; D, 5 months. (After E. L. House and B. Pansky, 1967. A Functional Approach to Neuroanatomy. McGraw-Hill Book Company, New York.)

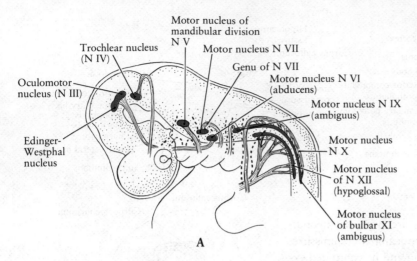

Motor nucleus of
mandibular division
N V

Trochlear nucleus
(N IV)

Motor nucleus N VII

Genu of N VII

Oculomotor
nucleus (N III)

Motor nucleus N VI
(abducens)

Motor nucleus N IX
(ambiguus)

Edinger-
Westphal
nucleus

Motor nucleus
N X

Motor nucleus
of N XII
(hypoglossal)

Motor nucleus
of bulbar XI
(ambiguus)

A

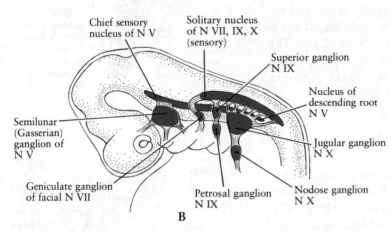

Chief sensory
nucleus of N V

Solitary nucleus
of N VII, IX, X
(sensory)

Superior ganglion
N IX

Nucleus of
descending root
N V

Semilunar
(Gasserian)
ganglion of
N V

Jugular ganglion
N X

Geniculate ganglion
of facial N VII

Petrosal ganglion
N IX

Nodose ganglion
N X

B

20–34 The cranial nerves, their central connections and their sensory ganglia in a human embryo of about six weeks of age. A, nuclei giving rise to motor fibers; B, nuclei with which sensory fibers make central connections. (After B. Patten, 1947. Human Embryology. McGraw-Hill Book Company, New York.)

priate terminations. Although fibers of different functional classification may use the same convenient route to their peripheral destination, when we examine their central connections we find that within the central nervous system there is a more strict separation into functional components and central nervous system nuclei or tracts are segregated to serve only one or at the most two functional classifications. By central connections for efferent fibers we mean the cranial nerve nuclei from which the efferent nerve fibers take origin. Central connections of afferent fibers are those nuclei to which sensory fibers return carrying impulses into the central nervous system from their peripheral receptors.

In the human embryo, the cranial nerves, their sensory ganglia, and their central connections are apparent early in the second month of development in the 10-millimeter embryo (Fig. 20–34). In discussing the cranial nerves, we will not take them up sequentially according to their number, but will consider them in relation to the functional classification of the fibers they carry. The peripheral pathways over which these fibers pass are of obvious importance and must be thoroughly learned in neuroanatomy. However, a study of the early development of the fibers and the establishment of their central and peripheral connections allows the embryologist to appreciate the functional aspect of the cranial nerves at a time when these connections are relatively unobscured.

The names and numbers of the cranial nerves and their sensory ganglia, when they are present, are listed below for reference:

Nerve Number	Name	Ganglion
I	Olfactory	
II	Optic	
III	Oculomotor	
IV	Trochlear	
V	Trigeminal	Semilunar (Gasserian)
VI	Abducens	
VII	Facial	
VIII	Acoustic	Acoustic and Vestibular
IX	Glossopharyngeal	Superior and Petrosal
X	Vagus	Jugular and Nodose
XI	Accessory	
XII	Hypoglossal	

Figure 20–34, to which continual reference should be made while studying the cranial nerves, is a diagrammatic representation of the cranial nerves in the 10-millimeter human embryo.

General Somatic Efferent

There are four cranial nerves that carry this type of fiber—III, IV, VI, and XII. The nuclei of origin of the somatic efferent fibers may be considered to represent a rostral extension of the anterior column of the spinal cord into the brain stem. This is particularly evident when considering the hypoglossal nerve whose rootlets can be seen emerging from the anterolateral sulcus in a position corresponding to the emergence of the anterior roots of the spinal nerves. The cranial nerve nuclei of the somatic efferent fibers, although they are considerably separated in their longitudinal aspect, are found to occupy similar positions in the brain stem close to the midline in the basal plate near the ventricular cavities.

Oculomotor Nerve (III)

The nucleus of origin of the third nerve is found in the basal plate of the mesencephalon at the level of the superior colliculus. Fibers emerge from the base of the mesencephalon in the region of the cephalic flexure and form a single trunk that passes to the developing muscle mass in the region of the orbit. As its name implies, the oculomotor nerve innervates the extrinsic eye muscles. Of the six eye muscles, it supplies the superior, inferior, and medial recti and the inferior oblique.

Trochlear Nerve (IV)
The nucleus of origin of the trochlear nerve also develops in the basal plate of the mesencephalon, but caudal to the motor nucleus of the third nerve—at the level of the inferior colliculus. The fibers from motor nucleus IV do not leave the brain stem directly but pass dorsally around the cerebral aqueduct, decussate in the dorsal part of the mesencephalon, and leave the midbrain in the region of the isthmus. The trochlear nerve is a slender nerve that innervates the superior oblique eye muscle.

Abducens Nerve (VI)
The abducens nucleus is the most caudal of those nuclei giving rise to fibers that pass to the extrinsic eye muscles. It lies in the floor of the fourth ventricle, and its fibers form a nerve that emerges just caudad of the pons and passes to the lateral rectus eye muscle. The name of the nerve indicates the action of this muscle.

Hypoglossal Nerve (XII)
The XIIth cranial nerve arises from a long slender nucleus located close to the midline stretching all through the myelencephalon. The rootlets of the hypoglossal nerve emerge all along the sides of the medulla to form the main trunk of the nerve, which supplies all of the intrinsic and most of the extrinsic muscles of the tongue.

Special Visceral Efferent

The cranial nerve nuclei, which in the embryo are just lateral to the somatic efferent nuclei, form a broken longitudinal column lying in the anterolateral region of the pons and the medulla. They are the nuclei of origin of the special visceral efferent fibers found in cranial nerves V, VII, IX, X and XI.

Trigeminal Nerve (V)
Cranial nerve V supplies motor fibers to the muscles derived from the first visceral arch. These muscles will develop into the muscles of mastication; in the adult, all of the masticator muscles are supplied by the Vth nerve. The special visceral efferent fibers of this

nerve arise in the motor nucleus of the trigeminal nerve developed in the reticular formation of the pons. They run in the mandibular division of the nerve.

Facial Nerve (VII)

Cranial nerve VII supplies motor fibers to muscles formed from the second visceral arch. Collectively, they form the muscles of facial expression. The motor nucleus of the VIIth cranial nerve is located in the caudal region of the pons. The nucleus of the facial nerve first develops caudad of the nucleus of the abducens nerve but then undergoes a change in position relative to the abducens nucleus, moving dorsally and cranially. As a result of this migration the motor fibers of the facial nerve pursue an arched course around the abducens nucleus, forming what is known as the *genu* of the facial nerve.

Glossopharyngeal, Vagus, and Spinal Accessory Nerves (IX, X, and XI)

The special visceral efferent fibers of these three nerves arise from a single nucleus, the nucleus ambiguus, extending throughout the length of the myelencephalon. Fibers running in the glossopharyngeal nerve supply muscles of the pharynx derived from the third visceral arch. Fibers of the vagus nerve supply muscles of the pharynx and larynx derived from the fourth and fifth arches, and the spinal accessory nerve supplies certain neck and shoulder muscles.

The vagus and spinal accessory nerves, considered separate nerves in the adult, form part of a single complex in the embryo. The accessory nerve has both a bulbar and a spinal portion. Fibers from the bulbar portion arise from the nucleus ambiguus and are distributed with the fibers of the vagus nerve to muscles derived from the caudal visceral arches. Fibers of the spinal portion of the nerve arise in the lateral part of the anterior grey column of the first five or six cervical segments of the spinal cord. The fibers from these segments emerge from the lateral surface of the cord, ascend alongside the cord through the foramen magnum and, joining the fibers of the bulbar division, emerge with them from the cranial cavity. However, they soon leave the common trunk as the external branch of the spinal accessory nerve and supply the sternocleidomastoid and trapezius muscles. These muscles are considered to be of branchiomeric origin and, therefore, the fibers in the accessory nerve supplying them are classified as special visceral efferent.

General Visceral Efferent

General visceral efferent fibers in the cranial nerves are a part of the parasympathetic division of the autonomic nervous system. As do the autonomic nervous system fibers of the spinal nerves, these fibers arising in the brain represent the first or preganglionic fibers of a two-neuron relay to the structure innervated. Preganglionic fibers of the parasympathetic nervous system are found in cranial nerves III, VII, IX, X, and XI.

Oculomotor Nerve (III)
The origin of the preganglionic fibers is in a special nucleus that lies in the rostral part of the motor nucleus of the oculomotor nerve in the basal plate of the mesencephalon. These fibers run in the IIIrd nerve to the *ciliary ganglion* from which postganglionic fibers supply the circular muscles of the iris and the ciliary muscle of the lens.

Facial Nerve (VII)
These fibers originate in the *superior salivatory nucleus* and supply the lacrimal gland and the submaxillary and sublingual salivary glands. The *sphenopalatine ganglion* contains the cell bodies of the postganglionic fibers to the lacrimal gland, and the *submaxillary ganglion* contains those whose fibers supply the salivary glands.

Glossopharyngeal Nerve (IX)
These fibers supply the parotid gland. Preganglionic fibers arising in the *inferior salivatory nucleus* in the basal plate of the myelencephalon pass to the *otic ganglion,* whose postganglionic fibers then run to the salivary gland.

Vagus and Spinal Accessory Nerves (X, XI)
The dorsal motor nucleus of the vagus nerve in the basal plate of the myelencephalon is the point of origin for the preganglionic fibers running in these nerves to be distributed to the thoracic and abdominal viscera.

General and Special Visceral Afferent

These are sensory fibers from visceral organs, and they run in cranial nerves I, VII, IX, and X. Visceral afferent fibers in nerves VII, IX, and X include: (1) fibers from the taste buds, mainly in VII and IX but a few in X, classified as special visceral afferent; and (2) fibers from the alimentary tract and other thoracic and abdominal viscera, classified as general visceral afferent. All of the visceral afferent fibers in these three nerves (VII, IX, and X) enter the solitary tract in the rhombencephalon and terminate in the nucleus of the solitary tract. The nucleus of the solitary tract starts in the myelencephalon and extends as far rostrad as the motor nucleus of the Vth nerve.

Facial Nerve (VII)

The sensory ganglion of the seventh nerve is the *geniculate* ganglion. Special visceral afferent fibers from it supply the taste buds on the anterior two thirds of the tongue. General visceral afferent fibers from the geniculate ganglion neurons supply the oral and pharyngeal mucosa.

Glossopharyngeal Nerve (IX)

Cranial nerve IX has two sensory ganglia. The one lying closer to the brain is the *superior* and the more distal one is the *petrosal.* The latter contains the cell bodies of origin of the special visceral afferent fibers to the taste buds on the posterior third of the tongue and the general visceral afferent fibers from visceral receptors in the pharyngeal mucosa. The central connections of the VIIth and IXth nerves are with the most rostral portions of the nucleus of the solitary tract.

Vagus Nerve (X)

The vagus nerve also has two ganglia along its trunk, a proximal *jugular* and a more distal *nodose,* of which the latter contains the cell bodies of origin of the visceral afferent fibers. A few fibers of the vagus nerve supply the taste buds of the pharyngeal mucosa and the epiglottis (special visceral afferent), but the vast majority of the vagus fibers convey general visceral afferent fibers from the alimentary tract and the thoracic and abdominal viscera. All central connections are to the solitary tract and its nucleus.

Olfactory Nerve (I)

Although the nasal placode from which the olfactory organ develops is of ectodermal origin, the Ist nerve is classified as special visceral afferent because of the general connection of the sense of smell with other mainly alimentary functions. However, the central terminations of the olfactory fibers are not with the nucleus of the solitary tract, but are in the olfactory bulb in the most rostral part of the telencephalon. Unlike other sensory nerves, the olfactory nerve does not have a ganglion. Its fibers develop from bipolar cells in the olfactory epithelium of the nose. The distal processes of these fibers protrude as bristles above the epithelial surface, and the proximal processes pass through the ethmoid bone to the olfactory bulb where they synapse with the dendrites of *mitral cells* (Fig. 20–35). Mitral cells are the second neurons in a chain conveying olfactory stimuli. Their axons pass through the olfactory tract to various terminations within the rhinencephalon.

General Somatic Afferent

General somatic afferent nerve fibers carry sensations from somatic receptors of the head region to their central connections within the brain stem. These fibers are found in cranial nerves V, IX, and X. The general somatic afferent fibers in all four of these cranial nerves terminate in the sensory nucleus of the Vth nerve.

Trigeminal

The trigeminal is the main general somatic sensory cranial nerve. It has a large ganglion, the *trigeminal,* distad of which the nerve splits into its three divisions, the *mandibular,* the *maxillary,* and the *ophthalmic.* Centrally, the nerve fibers from the trigeminal ganglion terminate either in the main sensory nucleus of the Vth nerve in the pons or, after descending in the spinal tract of the Vth nerve, in the nucleus of the spinal tract, which is continuous cranially with the main sensory nucleus in the brain. Caudally, the nucleus of the spinal tract is continuous with the part of the posterior column of the spinal cord, which receives somatic sensations from the neck and body regions.

Facial, Glossopharyngeal and Vagus Nerves (VII, IX, and X)

These three cranial nerves each carry a few general somatic afferent fibers from the region of the external auditory meatus and the ear. The ganglia in which their cell bodies are located are the geniculate, the superior, and the jugular, respectively.

Special Somatic Afferent

These fibers convey sensations from the organs of special sense of the head region, which are of ectodermal origin. Their fibers are found in cranial nerves II and VIII.

Optic Tract (II)

Since the sensory receptor of the eye, the retina, is actually an extension of the brain, the optic nerve is really a tract within the brain itself. Fibers in the optic tract are those from the third set of neurons in the visual chain and they carry visual impulses from the rods and cones to terminations mainly in the lateral geniculate body

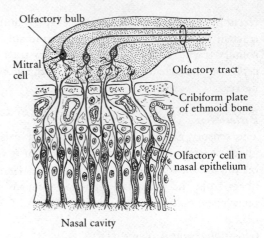

20–35 Diagram of the fibers from the olfactory epithelium passing through the cribiform plate of the ethmoid bone to synapse, in the olfactory bulb, with dendrites of the mitral cells. The axons of the mitral cells form the olfactory tract.

and the superior colliculi. The development of the eye and its visual receptors will be considered in the next chapter.

Acoustic Nerve (VIII)

The acoustic nerve carries fibers both from the organ of hearing, the *cochlea*, and the organ of equilibrium, the *semicircular canals*. Fibers from the cochlea have their cells located in the *spiral ganglion* closely associated with the cochlear duct and make central connections with the cochlear nucleus in the hindbrain. Those nerve fibers that carry impulses from the semicircular canals arise in the *vestibular ganglion* located in the internal auditory meatus and make central connections with a number of vestibular nuclei located in the myelencephalon and the metencephalon. Further consideration will be given to this nerve in the discussion of the development of the ear and the semicircular canals.

REFERENCES

Angevine, J. B., Jr., D. Bodian, A. J. Coulombre, M. V. Edds, Jr., V. Hamburger, M. Jacobson, K. M. Lyser, M. C. Prestige, R. L. Sidman, S. Varon, and P. A. Weiss. 1970 Embryonic vertebrate central nervous system: Revised terminology. Anat. Rec. 166:257–262.

Detwiler, S. R. 1936. Neuroembryology. New York: Macmillan.

Duncan, D. 1957. An electron microscope study of the embryonic neural tube and notochord. Texas Rep. Biol. Med. 15:367–377.

Harrison, R. G. 1907. Observations on the living developing nerve fiber. Anat. Rec. 1:116–118.

Hunt, R. K. and M. Jacobson. 1974. Neural specificity revisited. Curr. Topics Dev. Biol. 8:203–259.

Jacobson, M. and R. K. Hunt. 1973. The origin of nerve cell specificity. Sci. Am. 228:26–35.

Langman, J., R. L. Guerront, and B. G. Freeman. 1966. Behavior of neuropithelial cells during the closure of the neural tube. J. Comp. Neurol. 127:399–412.

Sauer, F. C. 1935. Mitosis in the neural tube. J. Comp. Neurol. 62:377–405.

Sperry, R. W. 1959. The growth of nerve circuits. Sci. Am. 201:68–75.

Vaughn, J. E. and A. Peters. 1971. The morphology and development of neuroglia cells. In: Cellular Aspects of Neural Growth and Differentiation, pp. 103–140. Ed., D. C. Pease. Los Angeles: University of California Press.

Watterson, R. L., P. Veneziano, and A. Barth. 1956. Absence of a true germinal zone in neural tube of young chick embryos as demonstrated by the colchicine technique. Anat. Rec. 124:379.

Weiss, P. 1934. In vitro experiments on the factors determining the course of the outgrowing nerve fiber. J. Exp. Zool. 68:393–448.

Weiss, P. 1936. Selectivity controlling the central-peripheral relations in the nervous system. Biol. Rev. 11:4949–531.

Weiss, P. 1955. Neurogenesis. In: Analysis of Development. Eds., B. H. Willier, P. Weiss, and V. Hamburger. Philadelphia: W. B. Saudners.

21

The Sense Organs

THE EYE

The development of the eye presents a fascinating but at the same time a complicated picture in that its component parts are of diverse origin. The optic cup and its sensory receptor area, the *retina,* are actually a part of the brain (an evagination of the forebrain), and as was mentioned in the discussion of the cranial nerves, the optic nerve then is really a tract within the brain. The *lens,* which focuses the light rays on the retina, is formed as an ingrowth from the ectoderm overlying the optic cup. Head mesoderm forms the tough fibrous coat, the *sclera* (which gives the eyeball its shape) and the vascular *choroid coat* as well as the transparent *cornea.* Mesoderm, which corresponds to head somite mesoderm of lower forms, develops the extrinsic eye muscles that attach to the sclera and move the eyeball. Finally, the eyelids are formed from folds of the skin after most of the other parts of the eye have been established. These heterogeneous components must be integrated into a definitive visual organ whose parts must match precisely. It is not surprising that during this process we will find some excellent samples of dependent differentiation, which we will discuss after we have described the morphogenesis of the eye.

Optic Vesicle and Early Optic Cup

The neural part of the eye first appears early in the third week as a pair of *optic grooves* on either side of the midline at the expanded cranial end of the still open neural folds (Fig. 21–1 A). As the neural folds close, the optic grooves deepen to form the *optic vesicles* as lateral evaginations of the brain wall, each with a cavity continuous with the central canal of the neural tube (Fig. 21–1 B).

During the fourth week, the optic vesicle closely approaches the surface ectoderm and its outer (distal) wall thickens and begins to invaginate, the first step in the conversion of the optic vesicle into the *optic cup* (Fig. 21–1 C). The distal portion of the optic vesicle as it invaginates then becomes the inner layer of the optic cup, the portion that will form the *retinal layer* of the eye. A constriction develops between the optic cup and the brain marking the beginning of the *optic stalk* (Fig. 21–1 C,D).

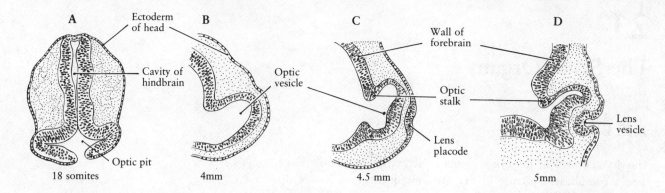

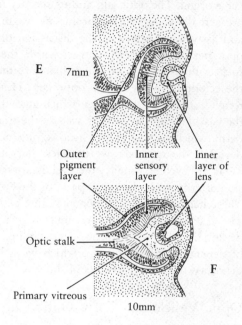

21–1 Early development of the lens and the optic cup. (From I. Mann, 1964. The Development of the Human Eye. British Medical Journal, London.)

When the optic vesicle approaches the surface, the ectoderm overlying it thickens to form the *lens placode*. This thickening occurs early in month two (4.5 mm), at which time the lens placode consists of a number of layers of cells (Fig. 21–1 C). When the optic cup forms, the lens placode invaginates into it to form the *lens vesicle* (Fig. 21–1 D). Shortly thereafter, the lens vesicle becomes closed (Fig. 21–1 E); by the sixth week it breaks away from the surface epithelium and appears as a rounded vesicle lying within the cavity of the optic cup. By the end of the sixth week, the cavity of the lens vesicle is excentrally placed owing to the beginning of the differentiation of the deeper (inner) region of the lens vesicle (Fig. 21–1 F).

The invagination that converts the optic vesicle into the optic cup does not occur in the exact center but is also extended to the midventral line. Because this invagination is excentric and because the distal ventral portion of the optic vesicle stops growing while the other margins continue to expand, the midventral wall of the optic cup shows a defect, the *optic (retinal) fissure* (Fig. 21–2). Blood vessels that develop in the nearby mesenchyme form the *hyaloid artery*, which enters the optic fissure to supply the inner surface of the optic cup and the lens. The hyaloid vein drains these areas. These vessels provide an intraocular vascular system for the developing eye (Fig. 21–3). However, this sytem atrophies completely at a later time and a new intraocular supply develops. In addition to allowing entrance to blood vessels, the optic fissure provides a short cut for the return of the axons of the retinal neurons to the diencephalon. Without benefit of this ventral defect, the nerves would have to reach the optic stalk by running out to the margin of the optic cup (Fig. 21–4). The optic fissure is not a permanent fixture but is obliterated during the second month of development by the overgrowth of its margins, first in the optic cup and later in the optic stalk.

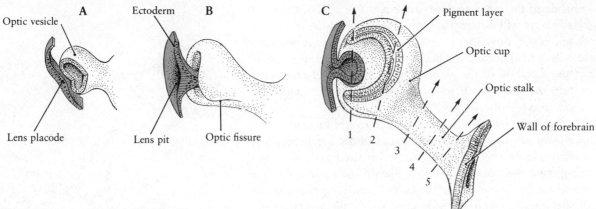

A — Optic vesicle — Ectoderm — B — C — Pigment layer — Optic cup — Optic stalk — Wall of forebrain — Lens placode — Lens pit — Optic fissure

Differentiation of the Optic Cup

At the end of the fifth week, the double-walled optic cup extends only a short distance past the equator of the lens (Fig. 21–2). The inner layer differentiates just like the wall of the neural tube—which, of course, it is. Owing to the invagination that has taken place, however, its layers are reversed: the ependymal layer being outermost and the mantle layer innermost. Further forward growth of the outer margin of the optic cup over the lens marks the beginning of the formation of a circumferential, marginal, nonnervous part of the cup that will overlay the outer region of the lens. This thinner nonnervous area is called the *pars caeca retinae* and it is separated from the nervous, light-sensitive region of the retina, the *pars optica retinae,* by a depression, the *ora serrata* (Fig. 21–5). The gap made by the outer circumference of the optic cup is the *pupil.*

The outer layer of the optic cup is always much thinner than the inner layer; early in its development it acquires granules and soon becomes densely pigmented. This pigmented layer extends all the way to the pupillary margin of the cup covering both the pars optica retinae and the pars caeca retinae (Fig. 21–5).

Histogenesis of the Pars Optica Retinae

The pars optica retinae is surrounded by a cavity that corresponds to the lumen of the neural tube; thus, its outer layer represents the ependymal and ventricular layers of the neural tube, and its inner layer corresponds to the marginal layer of the tube. Toward the end of month two (17 mm), cells from the outer layer start to migrate into the inner layer to form an *inner neuroblastic layer.* This migration begins first in the region of the posterior pole; the cells that remain in the outer layer form the *outer neuroblastic layer* (Fig. 21–6). A basement membrane (external limiting membrane) is

21–2 Models of the lens and the optic cup showing the formation of the optic fissure. The lens is shown as sectioned. In A and C part of the optic cup has been cut away. A, 4.5 mm; B, 5.5 mm; C, 7.5 mm. Arrows and number refer to Figure 21–3. From I. Mann, 1964. The Development of the Human Eye. British Medical Journal, London.)

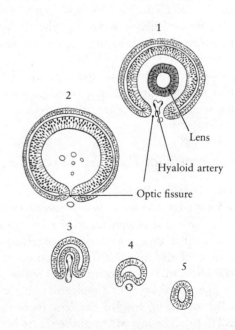

21–3 Cross sections of the optic cup and lens at the levels indicated by the arrows in Figure 21–2. (From I. Mann, 1964. The Development of the Human Eye. British Medical Journal, London.)

found outside of the inner neuroblastic layer. The cells of the outer neuroblastic layer will differentiate into cells whose outer ends form the *rods* and *cones,* the visual receptors. The protoplasmic processes of these cells extend beyond the limits of the external limiting membrane in the direction of the pigment layer. By the end of the seventh month, the shape of these processes serves to distinguish between the two types of cells (Fig. 21–7).

Some cells of the inner nuclear layer migrate still further inward to form a layer of ganglion cells. The axons of these ganglion cells form a fibrous layer over the inner surface of the retina, the fibers converging from their points of origin toward the optic stalk. The cells remaining in the inner nuclear layer become bipolar neurons that conduct impulses from the rods and cones to the ganglion cells. A schematic representation of this system is diagrammed in Figure 21–8. The region of the retina that lies in the direct visual axis is known as the *macula.* In the macula, only cones are present. The macula lies in the center of a shallow depression, the *fovea centralis.*

The cavity of the original optic vesicle, between the inner and outer layers, is gradually obliterated. These layers become closely associated with each other, with protoplasmic processes from the pigment layer interspersed about the processes of the rods and cones. The pigment granules migrate into and out of the processes of the pigment cells, to screen the photoreceptors from bright light in the former case and to allow maximum sensitivity in dim light in the latter. Despite this close association, the two layers do not fuse and a potential intraretinal space persists as a remnant of the ventricular system representing a potential plane of cleavage in which retinal separation can occur following injury to the eye.

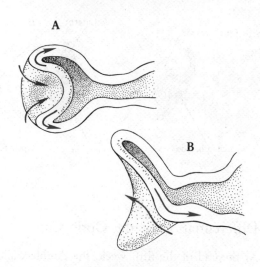

21–4 A, course the optic nerve fibers and blood vessels would have to take in the absence of an optic fissure. Both would have to run around the margin of the optic cup; B, when the optic fissure develops, the nerve fibers and the blood vessels can take the shortcut indicated by the arrows.

Development of the Pars Caeca Retinae

The Pars Ciliaris Retinae
The double-layered *pars ciliaris retinae* is the region of the pars caeca retinae just peripheral to the ora serrata. During the third month, as it is invaginated by the overlying mesoderm during the formation of the *ciliary body,* it becomes thrown into folds (Fig. 21–9). These folds, each consisting of an inner unpigmented and an outer pigmented layer of simple columnar cells, become arranged radially projecting toward the lens to form the *ciliary processes* (Fig. 21–10). The mesoderm of the ciliary body develops the ciliary muscle fibers. Contraction of the ciliary muscle acts to modify (thicken) the lens by relaxing the tension of the *suspensory liga-*

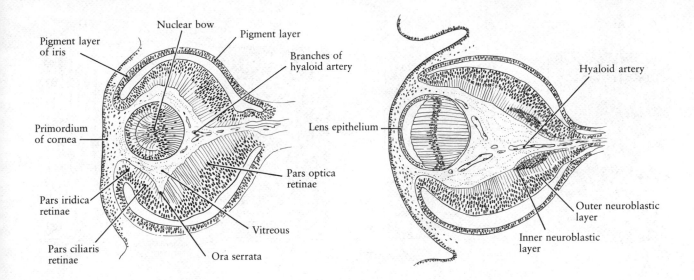

21–5 Section of the eye of a human embryo during the sixth week of development (11.5 mm). The ora serrata divides the nervous from the non-nervous region of the optic cup. (After A. Fischel, 1929.)

21–6 Section through the eye of a human embryo at seven weeks of development (17mm). The inner neuroblastic layer of the retina is beginning to form in the region of the optic stalk. (From I. Mann, 1964. The Development of the Human Eye. British Medical Journal, London.)

ment, which connects the tips of the ciliary processes to the capsule of the lens.

The Pars Iridica Retinae

Peripheral to the ciliary body is the *pars iridica retinae.* Both of its layers become pigmented, and the pars iridica retinae, plus the mesoderm associated with it, differentiates into the *iris.* A thin layer of mesoderm adherent to the outer layer of the pars iridica retinae extends beyond the inner margin of the iris over the surface of the lens forming the *pupillary membrane* (Fig. 21–9). This membrane is resorbed before birth. Smooth muscle fibers develop outside of the pars iridica retinae in the mesoderm covering it. Eventually, they differentiate into the dilator and constrictor muscles of the iris. They have long been considered to be formed from the outer layer of the pars iridica retinae rather than from the overlying mesoderm. In this case, this constitutes one of the few exceptions to the general condition that muscle tissue is of mesodermal origin. The sphincter muscles form a group close to the margin of the iris and the dilator muscles form a group of radially oriented muscles closer to the ciliary body (Fig. 21–10).

21–7 Section showing developing rods and cones at about seven months. (After I. Mann, 1969. The Development of the Human Eye. British Medical Journal, London.)

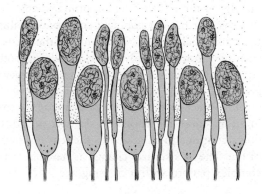

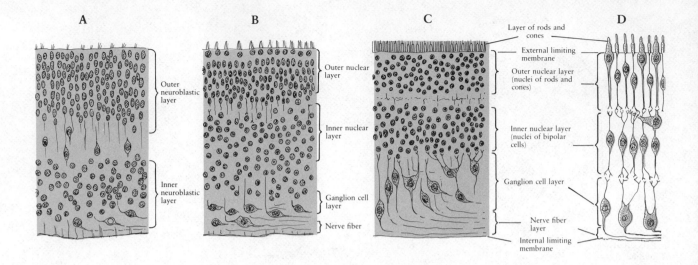

Outer
neuroblastic
layer

Inner
neuroblastic
layer

Outer nuclear
layer

Inner nuclear
layer

Ganglion cell
layer

Nerve fiber

Layer of rods and
cones

External limiting
membrane

Outer nuclear layer
(nuclei of rods and
cones)

Inner nuclear layer
(nuclei of bipolar
cells)

Ganglion cell layer

Nerve fiber
layer

Internal limiting
membrane

Development of the Lens

We have followed the development of the lens from the formation
of the lens placode up to the time when it forms a lens vesicle cut
off from its ectodermal origin, lying within the opening of the optic
cup. The beginning of the differentiation of the lens fibers was indicated as taking place during the sixth week when the cells of the
inner wall of the lens vesicle grow toward the outer wall, gradually
obliterating the cavity of the lens vesicle (Fig. 21–1 F). Only the
cells of the inner portion of the lens vesicle undergo this differentiation to form the *primary lens fibers*. The cells of the outer wall
remain as a simple cuboidal epithelium forming the *anterior lens
epithelium*. The nuclei of the primary lens fibers move to the equator of the lens and form a line that is convex outwardly, the *nuclear
bow* (Fig. 21–11). Each fiber is a single cell that stretches from the
inner to the outer pole of the lens, with its nucleus resting approximately on the equator. These primary lens fibers form the core of
the lens. Further development consists of multiplication of nuclei in
the equatorial region, which forms the *secondary lens fibers*. As
each fiber forms, it grows meridionally in both directions from its
equatorial nucleus toward either pole. However, new fibers fail to
grow the complete distance toward each pole, and, as a result, the
meeting place of the lens fibers is not at the two opposite poles but
in an irregular line known as the *lens suture* (Fig. 21–9). New lens
fibers continue to be added to the lens up until about the 20th year
of life. The lens sutures change as new fibers are added and show a
complex pattern with increasing age.

21–8 Stages in the histogenesis of the retina. A,
about 7 weeks (17 mm); B, about 11 weeks (65
mm); C, about 27 weeks (250 mm). (From
I. Mann, 1969. The Development of the Human
Eye. British Medical Journal, London.)

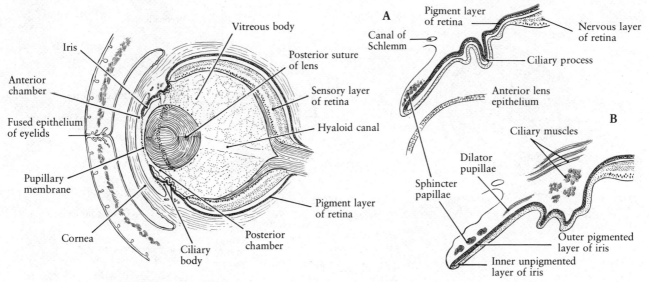

21–9 Cross section of an eye from a fetus of about 19 weeks (174 mm) showing fused eyelids and developing eyelashes.

21–10 Development of the pars caeca and the muscles of the iris and the ciliary body.

Accessory Structures

The Choroid and Sclera

When the optic vesicle first forms, the mesoderm surrounding it is loosely arranged as a network of mesenchymal cells showing no differentiation into cartilage, muscle, or connective tissue. The first sign of differentiation is the appearance of a vascular network formed as a continuation of the developing internal ophthalmic artery (a branch of the internal carotid). A part of the vascular bed develops into the hyaloid artery, already described as entering the optic fissure forming the intraocular vascular system. An extraocular system also develops and during the second month shows conspicuous blood vessels. This vascular layer, completely covering the optic cup, constitutes the *choroid coat* (Fig. 21–12).

Outside of the vascular choroid, the *sclera* develops as a fibrous connective tissue covering condensed from the surrounding mesenchyme. The sclera is continuous with the dura mater of the brain centrally over the optic tract. This tough connective tissue layer molds the eyeball and also provides attachment for the extrinsic eye muscles (Fig. 21–12).

The Vitreous Body

The area between the lens and the inner wall of the optic cup is occupied in the adult by a network of fibers whose interstitial spaces

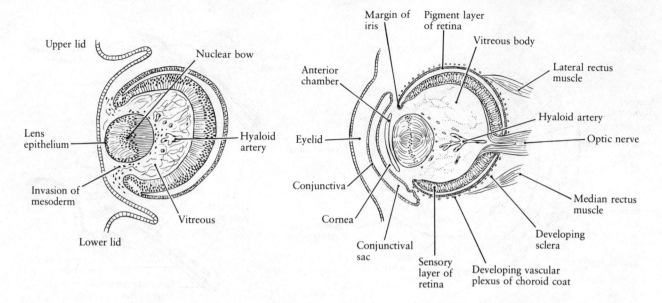

Upper lid

Nuclear bow

Lens
epithelium

Hyaloid
artery

Invasion of
mesoderm

Vitreous

Lower lid

Margin of
iris

Pigment layer
of retina

Vitreous body

Anterior
chamber

Lateral rectus
muscle

Hyaloid artery

Eyelid

Optic nerve

Conjunctiva

Median rectus
muscle

Cornea

Developing
sclera

Conjunctival
sac

Sensory
layer of
retina

Developing vascular
plexus of choroid coat

21–11 Eye of a human embryo of about seven
weeks (17 mm) at the time the eyelids are
beginning to develop. (After A. Fischel, 1929.)

21–12 Section of the eye of a human fetus at
about 11 weeks (48 mm).

are filled with a gelatinous material. This is the *vitreous body* (Fig.
21–12). Very early in the formation of the lens placode and the
optic cup, the space between them is occupied by a few mesodermal
cells (Fig. 21–1 D). As the lens vesicle and the optic cup develop
further, the space between them becomes larger and contains a few
mesodermal cells interspersed between fibrils connecting the lens
and the optic cup. Later, when blood vessels appear in this area, the
ectodermal lens fibrils and the mesodermal cells become associated
with the blood vessels to form the primary vitreous (Fig. 21–1 D,E).
It is not possible to distinguish whether the primary vitreous is of
ectodermal or mesodermal origin, or both. Later, when the space
between the lens and the optic cup enlarges further, the definitive
secondary vitreous forms. Again, it appears that it is partially of ectodermal origin, consisting of fibrous contributions from the inner
retinal wall as well as contributions from the atrophy of the hyaloid
artery.

The Cornea

The cornea is a continuation of the sclera over the outer surface of
the lens (Figs. 21–9; 21–12). Proliferation of the mesoderm over the
outer surface of the lens leaves a cavity between the cornea and the
lens. This is the *anterior chamber* of the eye. The anterior chamber

of the eye is separated from the outer lens epithelium by the pupillary membrane (Fig. 21–9).

Of course, both the cornea and the lens must be transparent in order to transmit the light rays through to the retina. It is generally stated that the cells of these structures can carry out their function only after they acquire transparency during development. Since embryonic tissues are generally already transparent, it should rather be stated that these particular tissues retain their embryonic condition of transparency.

The pupillary membrane, as mentioned previously, is a temporary structure that is normally resorbed during the sixth month. Following its resorption, the anterior chamber then becomes confluent with the space between the iris, the lens, and the suspensory ligament. This space is the *posterior chamber* of the eye (Fig. 21–9). Both the anterior and the posterior chambers are filled with a fluid *aqueous humor*.

The cornea and the sclera show the same radius of curvature in early stages. However, beginning at four months, the radius of curvature of the cornea decreases and, as a result, the corneoscleral boundary is easily distinguished. Failure of development of the correct curvature of the cornea results in improper focusing of the image on the retina. The entire focusing apparatus is, of course, dependent on the position, shape, and curvature of the cornea, the lens, and the retina, all of which play a part in the formation of the point retinal image.

The Eyelids

The eyelids develop as folds of ectoderm that grow toward each other over the surface of the cornea during the second month (Fig. 21–11). These folds meet and their epithelial layers fuse (Fig. 21–9; 21–12). Very soon after this fusion, invagination of the common epithelium indicates the beginning of the formation of the hair follicles of the eyelashes, those of the upper lid developing slightly in advance of the lower. The eyelashes differentiate exactly as hair on any other part of the ectodermal surface. Three types of glands develop in the eyelids (Fig. 21–13). Associated with and opening into the lumen of the hair follicles are sebaceous glands (*glands of Zeis*) and the modified sweat *glands of Moll*. In addition, about 30 large sebaceous glands develop from the epithelium just anterior to the posterior lid margin. These are the *tarsal* or *Meibomiam glands*. By the end of the fifth month, the adhesion between the upper and lower lids begins to break down and the lids are separated completely during the seventh month.

The stratified columnar epithelium covering the inner surface of the eyelids, which is continuous with the corneal epithelium, is the

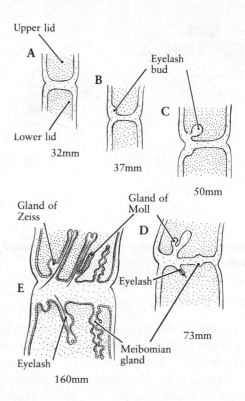

21–13 Development of the eyelashes and associated glands during the time the eyelids are fused. (From I. Mann, 1964. The Development of the Human Eye. British Medical Journal, London.)

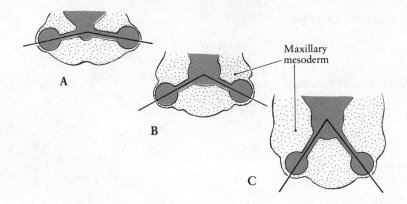

21–14 Decrease in the angle of the optic axis during development. A, 8 mm, 160°; B, 16 mm, 120°; C, 40 mm, 72°. (After I. Mann, 1969. The Development of the Human Eye. British Medical Journal, London.)

conjunctiva. The *conjunctival sac* is the space between the cornea and the conjunctiva (Fig. 21–12).

Positional Changes of the Eyes

At the time of the outgrowth of the optic cup, the right and left optic stalks lie in the same straight line forming an angle of 180°. By the middle of the second month, the angle has been reduced to 160° (Fig. 21–14). As a wedge of maxillary mesoderm pushes upward posterior to the eyes, the optical axes continue to converge, the highest rate of convergence occurring during the third month when the angle is reduced to about 105°. At birth it has been reduced to about 71°, only slightly less acute than in the adult (Fig. 21–14). This decrease in the angle of the optical axis allows for the overlapping of the visual fields and the development of binocular vision characteristic of mammalian species.

Abnormalities in the Development of the Eye

Coloboma is a term applied to the presence of a notch or gap in the retina, the choroid, or the iris, or in several of these structures. Most colobomata may be presumed to be the result of a failure of complete closure of the optic fissure. The notch may be extensive, involving all three of the above structures; or, it may involve the iris alone. Coloboma of the iris alone occurs as often as not in some plane other than that of the optic fissure and in these cases may have a different developmental origin from defects that involve both the iris and the choroid.

Opacity of the lens may occur at any time in fetal or postnatal life. The high incidence of congenital cataracts in children whose mothers had contracted German measles early in pregnancy has already been discussed.

Many bizarre abnormalities of the eye are known but they are, fortunately, rather rare. *Cyclopia* is a condition in which only a single median eye (or two eyes in various degrees of fusion) are present. *Anophthalmia* is the complete absence of the eye and may be the result either of the failure of the optic vesicle to evaginate from the forebrain or of its atrophy, after its evagination. *Microphthalmia* is a reduction in the size of the eye and is often accompanied by the formation of optic cysts—herniations of the retina into the scleral sac—which, in some cases, may be larger than the microphthalmic eye itself.

THE EAR

As does the eye, the ear also represents a composite organ to which contributions are made from a variety of sources. The ear consists of three separate parts, the *inner* ear, the *middle* ear, and the *outer* ear, each from a different origin. The major portion of the inner ear, which represents the actual organ of hearing, the *cochlea,* and the organ of equilibrium, the *semicircular canals,* the *sacculus* and the *utriculus,* is derived from an ectodermal *otic placode.* The inner ear thus serves two functions—equilibrium and hearing. In the lower vertebrates, the inner ear is solely an organ of equilibrium to which the higher vertebrates have appended the organ of hearing. The middle ear, the transmitting apparatus, consists of three ear bones, formed from mesoderm of the first and second visceral arches, enclosed in a cavity that is an extension of the first pharyngeal pouch. The external ear is a fleshy cartilaginous structure derived from visceral arch mesoderm surrounding the first visceral furrow, which persists as the external auditory meatus.

The Inner Ear

The optic placode is the first sensory placode to develop. It is externally apparent in the early somite embryo as a thickening of the ectoderm at the level of the middle of the hindbrain. Before the end of the third week, in the nine somite embryo, it is quite prominent (Fig. 21–15 A). The auditory placode invaginates to form the *auditory pit* during the fourth week (Fig. 21–15 B) and by the end of the first month has sunk completely below the surface to form the *auditory vesicle (otocyst)* (Fig. 21–15 C). The otocyst lies directly caudad of and in contact with the facioacoustic ganglion.

During the fifth week, the otocyst begins to elongate dorsoventrally, and from the part of the vesicle just dorsad of its point of detachment from the epidermis, an appendage forms. This rounded

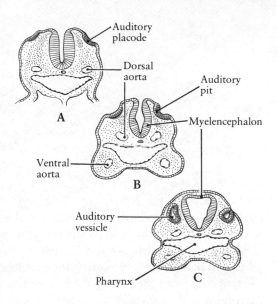

21–15 Formation of the auditory vesicle in the early human embryo. A, 9 somites, 20 days; B, 16 somites, 23 days; C, 30 somites, 30 days.

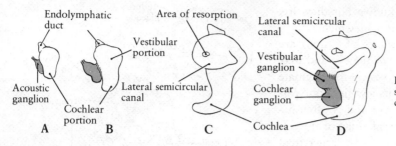

A B C D

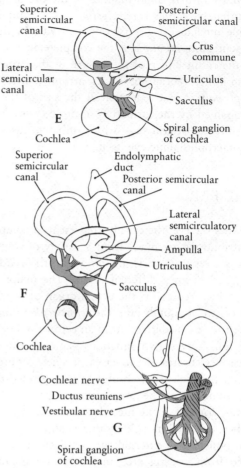

E

F

G

21–16 Development of the inner ear. A, 6 mm; B, 9 mm; C, 11 mm; D, 13 mm; E, 20 mm; F, 30 mm; G, 30 mm. A–F are lateral views. G is a medial view.

protuberance is the forerunner of the *endolymphatic duct* (Fig. 21–16 A,B). It develops rapidly, its dorsal tip expanding and its ventral portion contracting. By the end of month two (20–30 mm), the tip has widened to form a flat pouch, the *endolymphatic sac,* while the narrow ventral portion forms a tube, the endolymphatic duct, opening into the part of the otocyst that will develop into the *sacculus* and the *utriculus* (Fig. 21–16 E–G).

From the beginning of its dorsoventral expansion during the fifth week, the otocyst may be divided into two areas. One is a large triangular dorsal portion to which the endolymphatic duct is attached, the *vestibular pouch.* It will form the semicircular canals. The other, ventral to the vestibular pouch, is more slender and flattened. It is the *cochlear pouch,* and it will form the cochlea (Fig. 21–16 A,B). The meeting place of these two regions is called the *atrium* and will give rise to the sacculus and the utriculus.

During the sixth week, the vestibular portion develops three disc-like expansions oriented perpendicularly to each other, one in the superior, one in the posterior, and one in the lateral plane (Fig. 21–16 D). With the absorption of their central portions, these discs are converted into canals, the semicircular canals (Fig. 21–16 E). Each semicircular canal develops one bulbar end, the *ampulla.* The superior and posterior canals share an arm in common, the *crus commune,* and each develops its ampulla at the other end. The lateral canal develops its ampulla at its rostral end (Fig. 21–16 F). Sensory receptors, called *cristae,* develop within the ampullae. They respond to the movements of the fluid within the semicircular canals.

The utriculus and the sacculus begin their differentiation later than the semicircular canals, during the middle of the second month (Fig. 21–16 E). Each develops sensory receptors, *maculae,* which initiate impulses recording the position of the head. Both the cristae and the maculae are innervated by nerve fibers from the vestibular division of the acoustic ganglion (Fig. 21–16 D-F).

The cochlear portion of the inner ear also begins its development during the middle of the second month at a time when the semicir-

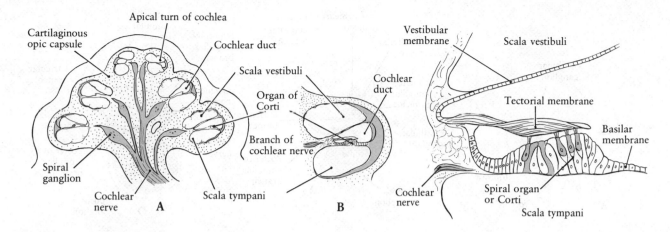

21–17 A, section through the cochlea of a four-month-old fetus; B, enlargement to show the relation of the cochlear duct to the scala vestibuli and the scala tympani.

21–18 Section through the spiral organ of Corti of a 250 mm fetus.

cular canals are almost completely formed. At six weeks, the cochlear duct appears as an elongated tube that bends rostrally at its ventral end (Fig. 21–16 C). During the second half of the month, the duct elongates at a rapid rate, and the original bending is continued to produce a spiral duct with two-and-a-quarter turns. The original broad connection to the vestibular portion of the otocyst is gradually reduced to a small canal, the *ductus reuniens,* uniting the dorsal portion of the cochlear duct to the sacculus (Fig. 21–16 G).

The cochlear duct represents only a part of the definitive organ of hearing. The mesenchyme surrounding the duct differentiates into a cartilaginous capsule enclosing the membranous cochlear duct. During the third month, the cartilaginous capsule undergoes resorption; the cochlear duct is now surrounded by an open space, the *perilymphatic* space, filled with a fluid, the *perilymph.* The cochlear duct is triangular with the base of the triangle attached to one wall of the perilymphatic space and the apex stretching across the space to attach to the opposite wall (Fig. 21–17 B). The perilymphatic space is thus divided into two passages by the cochlear duct. One of these passages, the *scala vestibuli,* ends at the *oval window* between the inner and middle ear, the region to which the malleus bone of the middle ear abuts. The other, the *scala tympani,* ends at the *round window* between the inner and the middle ear. The structure that supports the cochlear duct and separates the scala vestibuli and the scala tympani is the *basilar membrane.* The organ of hearing (the *organ of Corti*) rests on this membrane (Figs. 21–17; 21–18). The sensory receptors of this organ consist of a number of rows of

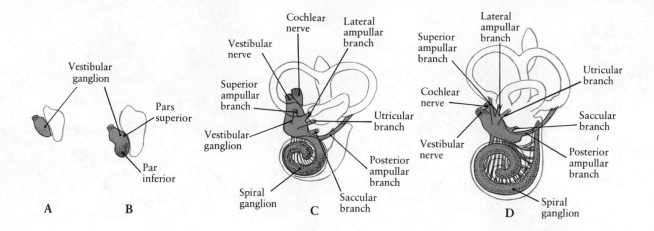

A   B

C

D

21-19 Differentiation of the left acoustic ganglion and nerve. The vestibular ganglion is finely stippled and the spiral ganglion is coarsely stippled. A, 4 mm; B, 7 mm; C, 20 mm; D, 30 mm.

neuroepithelial elements called *hair cells,* which are covered by a *tectorial membrane* adhering to the tips of the hair cells (Fig. 21–18). Wavelike motion of the perilymph imparted to it by the ear ossicle at the oval window result in vibrations of the basilar membrane and consequent stimulation of the hair cells. Nerve impulses are then initiated in the nerve fibers surrounding the bases of the hair cells.

The sensory receptors of the inner ear are supplied by nerve fibers from the acoustic division of the facioacoustic ganglion. The more caudal portion of this ganglion is the acoustic division that is seen in contact with the rostral portion of the developing inner ear during the fourth week (Fig. 21–16). The superior portion of the acoustic ganglion supplies fibers to the semicircular canals, the sacculus and the utriculus. It consists of two divisions, a superior one supplying the ampullae of the superior and lateral semicircular canals and the utriculus, and an inferior one supplying the sacculus and the ampulla of the posterior semicircular canal (Fig. 21–19). These fibers converge to form the vestibular part of the acoustic nerve.

The inferior portion of the acoustic ganglion differentiates into the *spiral ganglion,* whose fibers supply the hair cells of the spiral organ of Corti. As the cochlear duct develops its typical spiral pattern, the spiral ganglion conforms to this same pattern (Fig. 21–19 C,D). The centrally directed fibers from the spiral ganglion form the cochlear division of the acoustic nerve.

The Middle Ear and the External Ear

At the time that the inner ear is developing as the sound receiving element of the organ, the middle ear cavity (*tympanic cavity*) and

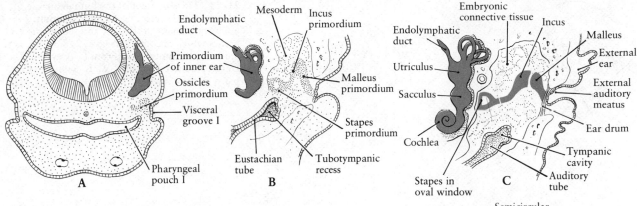

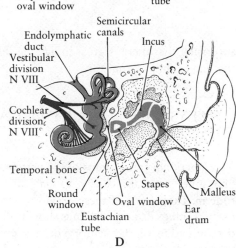

21–20 Schematic diagrams of four stages in the development of the middle ear. (From B. Patten, 1968. McGraw-Hill Book Company, New York.)

the middle ear ossicles are developing as the sound transmitting element of the system. The tympanic cavity is derived from the first pharyngeal pouch. This pouch, which appears at about three weeks, grows laterally and makes temporary contact with the inpocketing that is the first visceral furrow (Fig. 20–20). Shortly, this contact with the ectoderm is lost and the distal portion of the first pouch expands, forming the primodium of the tympanic cavity, the *tubotympanic recess*. The more proximal region of the pouch remains narrow, forming the *auditory (Eustachian) tube* (Fig. 21–20 B), the channel by which the middle ear is connected to the pharynx. At the same time, the mesenchyme just above the tympanic cavity lateral to the developing otic vesicle shows three areas of condensation resulting from the proliferation of the mesenchyme of the first and second visceral arches (Fig. 21–20 A,B). These represent the precursors of the three middle ear bones, the *malleus,* the *incus,* and the *stapes.* The first two are derivatives of the first arch, and the stapes is a derivative of the second arch. The ear ossicles remain embedded in mesoderm until the eighth month when the connective tissue surrounding them begins to undergo resorption and the tympanic cavity enlarges to envelop them (Fig. 21–20 C). At birth, there is still some unresorbed mesoderm around the ear ossicles (Fig. 21–20 D).

The *tympanic membrane* (*eardrum*) is a derivative of the closing plate between the first pharyngeal pouch and the first visceral furrow. The first visceral furrow thus becomes the *external auditory meatus* (Fig. 21–20).

The *auricle* (*pinna*) develops from swellings formed as mesenchymal proliferations of the first and second visceral arches surrounding the first visceral furrow (Fig. 21–21). Three *auditory hillocks* are first arch derivatives and three are second arch derivatives. Fusion of these individual hillocks and their further growth forms the auricle. In view of the number of growth centers involved, it is not

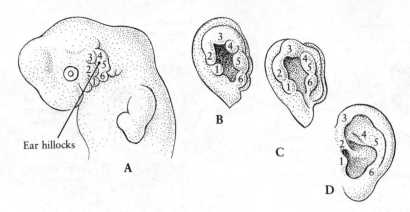

21–21 Development of the human auricle. A, 11 mm; B, 13.5 mm; C, 15 mm; D, adult. 1–6, auditory hillocks of the first and second visceral arches which become 1, tragus; 2, 3, helix; 4, 5, antihelix; 6, antitragus. (From L. Arey, 1974. Developmental Anatomy. W. B. Saunders Company, Philadelphia.)

surprising that there is great individual difference in the shape and the size of the external ear.

ANALYSIS OF SENSORY ORGAN DEVELOPMENT

The functional components of the vertebrate eyes, olfactory organs, and inner ears are chiefly specializations of the embryonic ectoderm. Rudiments of these organs are morphologically detectable as thickenings or outpocketings shortly after gastrulation. However, determination of the sensory organs probably occurs either just prior to or during the process of gastrulation itself. The development of all these organs is always dependent upon a complex of embryonic inductions, often involving several different tissues. Indeed, a part of an organ developing as the result of an induction may then itself subsequently act as an inducing stimulus.

The initial or primary inductor of the inner ear is the deuterencephalic portion of the roof of the archenteron (i.e., chordamesoderm). As previously pointed out, its presence is required for the development of the rhombencephalon or hindbrain. The hindbrain acts as a secondary inductor and stimulates the overlying ectoderm to thicken as the auditory placode. Adjacent, underlying mesenchymal tissue also appears to be necessary to effect this step in inner ear development. Once the inner ear vesicle forms from the placode, it acts as a tertiary inductor by stimulating mesenchyme cells, which originate from sclerotomes, to aggregate and differentiate as a cartilaginous capsule surrounding the inner ear. If the ear vesicle is extirpated shortly after its formation, this capsule fails to develop. Mesenchyme of neural crest or subcutaneous origin is not capable of reacting to induction by the inner ear vesicle. This incapability suggests that only a specific type of mesoderm is responsive to the inducing stimulus.

Similarly, there are several sources of induction for the nose rudiment. There is an early induction by the anterior end of the chordamesodermal mantle and a later induction by the prosencephalon or forebrain. Although direct causal relationships can be experimentally demonstrated in the development of the olfactory and inner ear rudiments, little is known about the mechanisms controlling the inductions and the bases for the differentiation of the sensory cells.

Next to the brain, the vertebrate eye is probably the most complex organ with respect to its development. Originating from several tissue sources that are dependent for their differentiation upon a complicated chain of inductions, a number of cell types are functionally unified into an organ of unusual efficiency. The early development of the eye, particularly the retina–lens complex, provides a useful model system in several animal species for investigating the relationships between the phenomena of embryonic induction, morphogenesis, and cell differentiation.

Recall that the early rudiments of the whole eye are the primary optic vesicle, which is an outpocketing of the prosencephalon, and the lens placode, which is a thickening of the embryonic ectoderm (Fig. 21–22). Vital staining experiments have shown that the cells destined to form the optic vesicle lie well forward in the neural plate (Fig. 21–22 A). Presumptive lens material is localized lateral to and slightly anterior to the optic vesicle rudiments (Fig. 21–22 B). In the case of the eye vesicle rudiment, its expression is dependent upon an inductive influence originating from the anterior end of the roof of the archenteron (i.e., archencephalic inductor). The determination of the optic vesicle appears to be irreversibly set by the end of the neural plate stage. If the eye rudiment is excised at this time and transplanted with some surrounding mesenchyme, it will differentiate in normal fashion into retina, iris, and so on.

As in the case of many organ primordia (Chapter 13), the early eye rudiment shows the property of self-regulation. That is, a part of the rudiment has the ability to develop as a whole. For example, the eye rudiment at the neural plate stage or the optic vesicle stage can be dissected into two halves in the frog. Each half will develop into a complete, though smaller than normal, eye. Even at the early optic cup stage, a piece of presumptive pigmented epithelium, following its removal and transplantation into the vicinity of an eye in another embryo, will form a whole eye (Fig. 21–23). These experiments also indicate that the individual parts of the eye are not determined at the same time that the eye as a whole is determined.

The lens originates as a disc-shaped thickening in the skin ec-

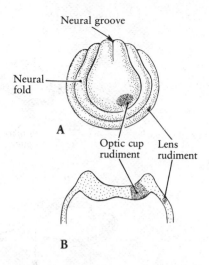

21–22 Location of the presumptive optic cup and presumptive lens in the neurula stage of an amphibian. A, dorsal view; B, transverse view. (After H. Spemann, 1938. Embryonic Development and Induction. Yale University Press, New Haven.)

21–23 Transplantation of a large piece of pigmented epithelium into the vicinity of a normal eye of another embryo develops into a complete eye with pigment coat and retina. (After N. Dragomirow, 1933. Wilhelm Roux' Arch. Entwicklungsmech. Org. 129, 522.)

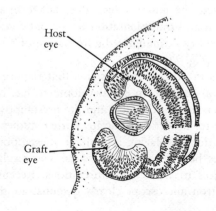

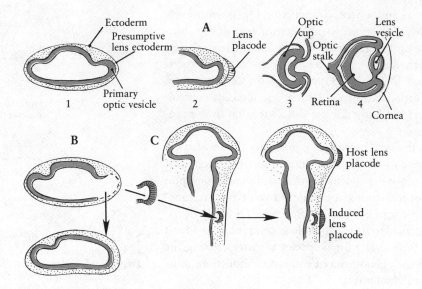

Ectoderm
Presumptive
lens ectoderm
A
Lens
placode
Optic
cup
Optic
stalk
Lens
vesicle

Primary
optic vesicle
1
2
3
Retina
4
Cornea

B
C
Host lens
placode

Induced
lens
placode

toderm overlying the primary optic vesicle. In most vertebrates, the differentiation of the lens from competent head ectoderm depends upon a prolonged inductive influence principally from the optic vesicle. Additional inductive stimuli from other head tissues are now recognized in amphibian, avian, and mammalian embryos. For example, the tip of the foregut and heart mesoderm are, in addition to the optic vesicle, required for normal lens expression in the salamander. The direct causal relationship between the presence of the primary optic vesicle and lens development has been experimentally demonstrated in several ways (Fig. 21–24). If the optic vesicle is removed, the skin ectoderm does not form a lens (Fig. 21–24 B). Excision and transplantation of the optic vesicle beneath the flank of an embryo stimulates the formation of a lens in an abnormal position (Fig. 21–24 C).

As in other organ systems that require embryonic inductions, a major question in eye development has been whether contact between the optic vesicle and the presumptive lens ectoderm is necessary for induction to occur. Earlier studies attempted to resolve this question by placing cellophane sheets, porous membranes, or agar slices between the two tissues. The results were inconclusive and subject to varying interpretations. Recent investigations with the electron microscope clearly demonstrate that an interspace, several

21–24   Diagram to show the importance of the optic vesicle in lens induction. A, 1–4, steps in the normal development of the optic cup, lens, and cornea. Transverse views through the prosencephalon; B, extirpation of the primary optic vesicle before it approximates the presumptive lens ectoderm results in the absence of lens development; C, transplantation of the primary optic vesicle beneath the flank ectoderm of a second embryo at a comparable stage of development induces an accessory lens. A, 1–4 and B, transverse views; C, dorsal view.

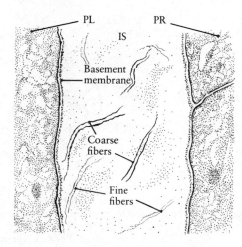

microns in width, does exist between the presumptive lens and the presumptive retina during the induction process (Fig. 21–25). This space in the chick embryo is acellular, lined by basal lamina on both sides, and contains a fibrous, hyaluronate material closely resembling the composition of the vitreous body. Hence, it appears that only a close approximation of presumptive neural retina and presumptive lens ectoderm is required for a successful lens induction to occur.

During the inductive period, the lens placode becomes invaginated to form the lens vesicle (Fig. 21–26). Shortly after closure of the vesicle, the epithelial cells that form its posterior wall begin to elongate to form the lens fibers. The same induction that is

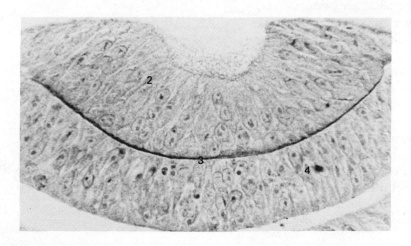

responsible for determination of the lens as a whole is also involved in the differentiation of the lens epithelial cells into lens fiber cells. Epithelial cells of the lens vesicle, when grafted in the vicinity of either presumptive retina or the epithelium of the inner ear vesicle, may develop lens fibers (Fig. 21–27). Details on the morphological, cytological, and biochemical transformation of lens epithelial cells into lens fibers cells have to a large extent been worked out by using the adult lens. The adult lens is solid, avascular, and composed of the following (Fig. 21–28): a single layer of epithelial cells; a zone of cellular elongation (or equatorial region) comprised of cells that are in the process of becoming fiber cells; and inner fiber cells. Fiber cells are laid down continuously in the zone of cellular elongation after the embryonic lens has formed. The fiber cells formed during embryonic growth compose the central or nucleus region, while the newly formed fiber cells are located in the cortex of the lens. With lens fiber formation, the cell loses its replicative ability and enters a stationary phase of the cell cycle.

Since fiber cell formation is a terminal step in the differentiation of a specific cell type, the lens has been an ideal system for the study of the interrelationships between morphogenesis, cellular differentiation, and protein synthesis. Lens epithelial cells are characterized by their cuboidal shape, their basophilic staining properties, and their ability to undergo mitosis. Their transformation into fiber cells is accompanied by physical changes in shape, an increase in the population of ribosomes, and the synthesis of structural proteins termed *lens crystallins*. Three major groups of these proteins have been identified in adult lens cells: *alpha crystallins, beta crystallins,* and *gamma crystallins*. Techniques of column chromatography, electrophoresis, and immunofluorescence have established that these crystallins are indeed restricted to the lens (i.e., they are tissue specific) and have rather limited distributions within the lens. In the mouse, for example, the alpha and beta crystallins are primarily found only in the lens epithelial cells. All three types of crystallins are synthesized in the lens fiber cells. Hence, the gamma crystallins (also found in frog, newt, and cow) are tissue-specific proteins whose synthesis is associated with fiber cell differentiation.

The site of the first appearance of crystallins during lens development strongly suggests that their synthesis is a direct response to induction. Studies by Zwaan and his colleagues on the chick embryo have shown that *delta crystallin,* the primary lens fiber protein of the adult bird lens, appears at about the time when the lens placode begins to invaginate from the ectoderm. Beta crystallin is detected at approximately 56 hours of development, but it is not present in substantial amounts until the lens vesicle stage (80 hours). Alpha crystallin can first be identified at the lens vesicle stage. The delta

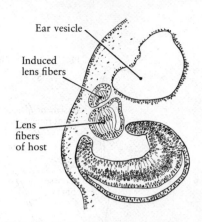

21–27 Epithelial cells of the lens vesicle when grafted in the vicinity of the inner ear vesicle may be induced to form an additional mass of lens fibers (arrow). (After N. Dragomirow, 1929. Wilhelm Roux' Arch. Entwicklungsmech. Org. 116, 633.)

21–28 Diagram of the structure of the lens of a typical adult vertebrate. (See text for additional details.) (From J. Papaconstantinou, 1967. Science 156, 338. Copyright 1967 by the American Association for the Advancement of Science.)

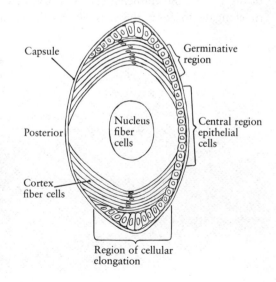

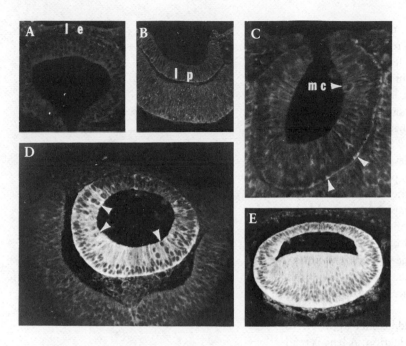

21–29 Immunofluorescence is a technique in which a specific tissue protein is visually localized by reacting it with a fluorescein-labeled antibody made against the antigen. A, optic vesicle and its area of contact with the presumptive lens ectoderm (le) in a 9.25-day-old mouse embryo. Note that no lens crystallins are detected; B, section through the lens placode (lp) and optic cup of a 10.5-day-old mouse embryo; C, invaginated lens of an 11.0-day-old embryo. Note that crystallins are present in the cytoplasm of a few of the innermost cells (arrows) but not in apically situated mitotic cells (mc); D, 11.5-day-old embryonic mouse eye showing strong fluorescence in cells along the interior wall of the lens vesicle and in mitotic cells (arrows); E, all lens cells fluoresce in a 12.5-day-old mouse eye. (From M. van de Kemp and J. Zwaan, 1973. J. Exp. Zool. 186, 23.)

crystallin would appear to be a fetal protein because its distribution in the adult lens is restricted to the lens nucleus. Immunofluorescence methods have shown that crystallins in the chick and mouse are initially detected in those cells of the invaginating lens placode and newly formed lens vesicle that lie directly opposite to the central area of the presumptive neural retina (Fig. 21–29). Comparisons of mitotic activity and DNA formation with the immunofluorescent data suggest that the chick lens primordial cells produce delta crystallins while they are part of a replicating population of cells, and that their synthesis is initiated during the S or early G_2 phase of the cell cycle.

The induction of the lens is particularly complex, encompassing a spectrum of events which includes changes in individual cell shapes, accumulation of ribosomal RNA, and the initiation of tissue-specific protein syntheses. It is not surprising, therefore, that the nature of the stimulus responsible for the induction and the mechanism by which it influences its target cells are poorly understood. An early hypothesis was that the lens inductor was a chemical agent, presumably RNA of the messenger type. This was based upon the observation that during lens induction the RNA content in the presumptive retina cells decreased while that in the proximal lens cells increased. There is no substantive proof, however, that RNA macromolecules pass from the eye cup cells to the lens rudiment cells. On the basis of more recent studies, particularly by Zwaan and his co-investigators, there is increasing evidence that the extracellular matrix in the interspace between the presumptive lens and the optic vesicle may play an important role in delimiting the lens territory, fixing the dimension of the lens, and controlling changes in cell and organ shapes, as well as in providing a specific stimulus for the synthesis of the tissue-specific lens proteins. At this time, however, it cannot be completely ruled out that possible substances diffusing from the neural retina or other tissue sources may be involved in lens induction.

The lens also exerts an influence over the development of the eye. Acting with the primary optic cup, the lens is primarily responsible for the induction and maintenance of the cornea. This can be demonstrated by transplanting the retina–lens complex beneath the skin in another part of the embryo and observing the development of an accessory cornea; or it can be demonstrated by replacing the normal cornea with skin from another part of the embryo and observing transformation of the graft into cornea. In contrast to the neural plate and lens ectoderm, the competence to form corneal tissue remains for a long period of time.

Lens regeneration experiments offer an additional approach to the study of problems associated with lens induction. A lens is readily regenerated in some vertebrates, particularly salamanders and the African clawed toad (Xenopus). Generally, the capacity to regenerate lens tissue is highest after the period of embryonic development (i.e., young larval or adult stages). Lentectomized larvae of Xenopus and the newt regenerate lenses from the outer cornea and iris epithelium, respectively. Based upon several lens regeneration experiments with Notophtalamus, Reyer and his colleagues maintain that a neural trophic factor may act as a lens-inducing agent. When they implanted dorsal iris tissue into the undifferentiated cellular mass (blastema) of a regenerating forelimb, frequent lens regeneration was observed. However, no lenses were noted when dorsal iris tissue was implanted into regenerating forelimbs from which the nerves had been removed.

REFERENCES

Coulombre, A. J. 1965. The eye. In: Organogenesis. Eds., R. L. DeHaan and H. Ursprung. New York: Holt, Rinehart and Winston.

Hendrix, R. W. and J. Zwaan. 1974. Changes in the glycoprotein concentration of the extracellular matrix between lens and optic vesicle associated with early lens differentiation. Cell Differ. 2:357–362.

Mann, I. 1964. The Development of the Human Eye. New York: Grune & Stratton.

Papaconstantinou, J. 1967. Molecular aspects of cell differentiation. Science 156:338–346.

Silver, P. H. S. and J. Wakely. 1974. Fine structure, origin, and fate of extracellular materials in the interspace between the presumptive lens and presumptive retina of the chick embryo. J. Anat. 118:19–31.

Topashov, G. V. and O. G. Stroeva. 1961. Morphogenesis of the vertebrate eye. Adv. Morphog. 1: 331–378.

Twitty, J. 1955. Eye. In: Analysis of Development. Eds., B. H. Willier, P. A. Weiss, and J. Hamburger, Philadelphia: W. B. Saunders.

van de Kemp, M. and J. Zwaan. 1973. Intracellular localization of lens antigens in the developing eye of the mouse embryo. J. Exp. Zool. 186:23–32.

Yntema, C. L. 1955. Ear and nose. In: Analysis of Development. Eds., B. H. Willier, P. A. Weiss, and J. Hamburger, Philadelphia: W. B. Saunders.

22

Development of the Somites

We have described the development of the somites into segmentally arranged masses of mesodermal cells connected laterally to the lateral mesoderm by way of the intermediate mesoderm (Chapter 8). In man, the first somite appears during week three of development and early in week five, when somite formation is complete, some 42 to 44 pairs of somites have formed. Although the number of somites that develop is subject to some variation, somite count in these early stages provides a reliable measure of developmental progress.

In the differentiation of each somite from the paraxial mesoderm, the cells at first appear very similar (Fig. 22–1 A) but soon exhibit a wide range of developmental potentialities. Shortly after it first forms, each somite's boundaries become more regular and its cells increase rapidly in number and assume a radial orientation around a small central lumen, the *myocele* (Fig. 22–1 B). Further development consists of a lengthening of the somite in a dorsoventral direction and a flattening in a lateral direction accompanied by the formation of a slit-shaped myocele (Fig. 22–1 C,D). At this time, three regions of the somite may be recognized and named on the basis of their prospective fate (Fig. 22–1 C,D). In the most medial and ventral region, the cells lose their epithelial appearance and migrate away from the main body of the somite toward the notochord and the neural tube as a mass of mesenchyme. This region, which will give rise to skeletal material, is the *sclerotome.* A dorsal intersegmental artery runs between adjacent sclerotomes. The most superficial cells lying in a ventrolateral position beneath the ectoderm make up the *dermatome,* which will develop into the connective tissue of the epidermis and the subcutaneous tissue beneath it. In all probability some of the cells of the region marked off as the dermatome may also contribute to the formation of skeletal muscle. The third region is the *myotome,* which forms a platelike group of spindle-shaped cells medial and dorsal to the dermatome. It will form skeletal muscle. The further development of these three regions will be considered separately.

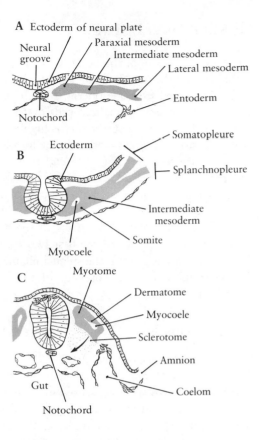

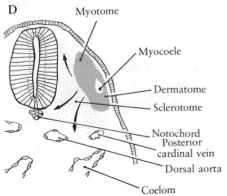

22–1 Diagrams of the early differentiation of a somite. A, beginning of somite formation from the paraxial mesoderm; B, formation of the myocoele; C, beginning of the migration of sclerotome cells toward the notochord; D, further migration of the sclerotome masses.

MUSCLE DEVELOPMENT

The muscular tissue of the body, with the exception of that found in the iris and the muscles associated with the sweat and mammary glands is derived from mesoderm. Muscle tissue is developed from primitive myoblasts, specialized cells that will differentiate fibers in which the function of contractility is highly developed. On the basis of their histology, origin, and ultimate location, three types of muscle tissue are recognized: (1) *skeletal* muscle, which is attached to and serves to move the bones of the body; (2) *smooth* muscle, which is found in the alimentary, respiratory, and urogenital tracts and in the walls of blood vessels and the ducts of glands; and (3) *cardiac* muscle, found in the walls of the heart. We will consider mainly the development of the first two types in this section. Cardiac muscle develops from the splanchnic mesoderm that surrounds the heart tube. The development of the heart was described in Chapter 17.

Skeletal Muscle

Skeletal muscle develops from three different regions of mesoderm. The axial (trunk) muscles, and probably the muscles of the limb girdles, develop from the myotomes of the somites. Most of the muscles of the head region develop from the visceral mesoderm of the visceral arches and the muscles of the limbs develop from local accumulations of cells of the lateral mesoderm.

The Development of a Myotome

Each myotome increases in size and, at five weeks, divides into a smaller group of cells located dorsally, the *epimere,* and a larger ventral group of cells, the *hypomere,* thus establishing an *epaxial* and *hypaxial* column of myotomes (Fig. 22–2). At the same time, each spinal nerve growing into its respective somite divides into a *posterior primary division* and an *anterior primary division* that establish permanent connections with the epimere and the hypomere, respectively (Fig. 22–2).

The epaxial musculature subdivides further into deep and superficial portions. The deep portion may fuse over a few consecutive somites but, in general, retains its original segmental arrangement giving rise to short intervertebral muscles. The superficial portion fuses over a large number of consecutive segments and then, by longitudinal splitting, develops the long extensor muscles of the head and trunk (Fig. 22–3).

The hypaxial musculature extends into the lateral and ventral body wall. The myoblasts of the more cranial hypomeres give rise

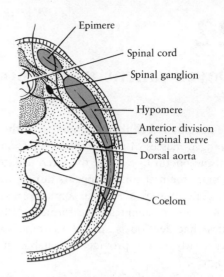

22–2 Division of the myotome into a dorsal epimere and a ventral hypomere in the five-week-old embryo. The posterior primary division and the anterior primary division of the spinal nerve supply the epimere and the hypomere, respectively.

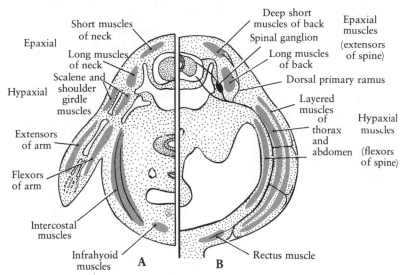

22–3 Diagrams of the arrangement of the primitive muscle masses derived from the epimeres and the hypomeres. A, section through the shoulder region; B, section through the trunk region.

to the scalenes, shoulder girdle muscles, and intercostal muscles (Fig. 22–3 A). The more caudal hypomeres form the broad, coat-like-layered muscles of the thoracic and abdominal walls and the longitudinally running rectus abdominis (Fig. 22–3 B). The hypomeres of the lumbar somites form the muscles of the pelvic girdle.

Muscles of the Limbs

The limb buds in man form during the second month as ectodermal outpocketings of the body wall filled with mesenchyme. Condensations of the limb bud mesenchyme form premuscle masses near the base of each limb bud. The superior limb buds form opposite the last six cervial and the first two thoracic myotomes and the inferior limb buds develop opposite the second to the fifth lumbar and the first three sacral myotomes. Branches of the spinal nerves supplying these myotomes extend into the premuscle masses and, as the limb elongates and the muscles differentiate, the nerves retain these early connections. The muscles develop into a ventral limb flexor group and a dorsal limb extensor group (Fig. 22–3 A). Anterior and posterior branches of the spinal nerves supply the flexor and extensor groups, respectively. Thus, in the superior extremity, the median and ulnar nerves, from the anterior division, innervate the flexor muscles while the radial nerve, derived from the posterior division, innervates the extensor muscles.

Although it has been shown that the fin musculature of fishes is derived from extensions of the myotomes into the developing fins, evidence for a myotomal origin of the limb musculature in the tetrapods is not convincing. Most embryologists consider that these muscles differentiate in situ from limb bud mesenchyme, probably of lateral plate origin. An analysis of the morphogenesis of the vertebrate limb has already been presented in Chapter 13.

Tongue Muscles

Cranial to the cervical somites, four *occipital somites* develop. The first occipital somite then disappears, and the myotomes of the remaining three differentiate into the intrinsic muscles of the tongue. The migration of the myoblasts from the occipital myotomes to the floor of the oral cavity to form the tongue muscles has not been observed directly. However, the hypoglossal nerve has been shown to grow into the occpital somites, and the innervation of the tongue muscles by this nerve indicates the origin of these muscles from the myoblasts of the occipital somites.

Eye Muscles

The intrinsic muscles of the eye appear to develop in situ from head mesenchyme. The three muscle masses from which they develop can be considered as three pairs of *head (preotic) somites,* even though typical somites do not develop in the head region of any mammalian embryo. In the shark embryo, in which head somites do differentiate, the myotome portions of the three somites in this region develop into the intrinsic eye muscles and are supplied by cranial nerves III, IV, and VI. Thus, in the mammal the three mesenchymal masses that give rise to the eye muscles and that are, in turn, supplied by the same three cranial nerves, represent the differentiation of what is, at least phylogenetically, head somite material.

Visceral Arch Muscles

The development of the muscles derived from the visceral arches has been described in Chapter 14.

Smooth Muscle

The smooth muscle of the alimentary tract arises independently of the somites as a differentiation of the splanchnic mesoderm covering the alimentary tract. From it are developed the circular and longitudinal muscle coats of the tract as well as the muscularis mucosa, the thin layer of muscle found in the mucosa of many parts of the gut. The smooth muscle of the trachea and the bronchi develop in the same manner.

Other smooth muscle is found as part of the coat of the vessels of the circulatory system. In those vessels that develop in the splanchnopleure, such as the allantoic and vitelline vessels, the muscle is also of splanchnopleuric origin. However, it is probable that, as the blood vessels extend into the somatopleure of the body wall and limb buds, the muscles developing in the walls of these vessels arise from the surrounding somatic mesoderm. The smooth muscle of some parts of the urogenital system is also derived from somatic mesoderm and it is not unreasonable to consider that mesenchyme anywhere in the body is capable of forming this type of muscle.

Myogenesis

Muscle cells and tissues have been a favored material in cell differentiation studies because they possess a highly specific morphology and identifiable markers of their differentiated state, such as myosin and actin. Also, the differentiation of skeletal muscle cells in cell culture from isolated embryonic myogenic cells closely parallels the developmental sequence observed in vivo. The cell culture system for analyzing muscle development offers several advantages over the study of muscle in the intact embryo. In contrast to the embryo in which muscle tissue is complicated by many distinct cell types, including nonmyogenic cells, cell suspensions of embryonic muscle can be prepared which are relatively homogeneous. These cells can be manipulated experimentally to give a greater degree of synchrony of development than in the embryo. In this section, we will consider primarily the events leading to the differentiation of skeletal muscle because this cell type, in contrast to smooth and cardiac muscle cells, has been rather extensively studied. The salient features of skeletal myogenesis can be arranged in the following chronological sequence: the formation by proliferation of presumptive myoblast and myoblast cells; the synthesis of myosin, actin, and other associated muscle-specific molecules; and the fusion of myoblasts into multinucleated cells termed *myotubes* that continue synthesis of contractile proteins and their assembly into myofibrils.

The differentiation of the skeletal muscle cell can be considered to consist of two primary events. There is a beginning period when presumptive myoblast cells, which originate chiefly from the mesoderm of the lateral plate or somites, increase by cell mitoses (Fig. 22–4 A). These cells are observed to increase at a constant exponential rate in culture. At a rather predictable time, the mononucleated myogenic cells cease to divide and fuse to form multinucleated cells containing many nuclei with a common cytoplasm (Fig. 22–4 B-D). The number and size of these cellular syncytia increase very rapidly for the first 48 hours after the fusion process begins. Although details of the signal—or signals—that initiate the fusion between myoblasts, or between myoblasts and myotubes, are still unclear, observations on the behavior of muscle cells in culture suggest that fusion is a two-step process. There is an initial cell rec-

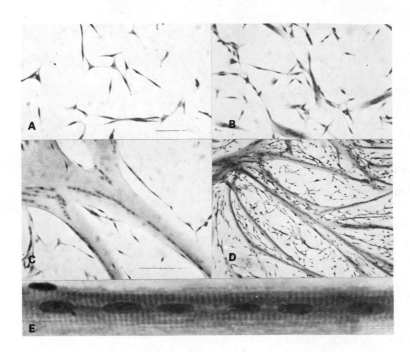

22–4 Photomicrographs of quail muscle cells in culture. A, mononucleated myoblasts recognizable by their characteristic bipolar shape; B, the beginnings of the formation of myotubes from fusing myoblasts; C, a higher magnification of the fusion process; D, extensive formation of myotubes; E, cross-striations in a multinucleated myotube. (From I. Konigsberg and P. Buckley Ahrens, 1974. Concepts of Development. J. Lash and J. Whittaker, eds. Sinauer Associates, Sunderland, Mass.).

ognition by primed homotypic (similar) cells. This has been shown by labeling fibroblasts, chondroblasts, and liver cells with tritiated thymidine and then mixing these nonmyogenic cells with unlabeled myoblast cells that are in the process of fusion. Labeled nonmyogenic cells are never incorporated into myotubes, indicating that there is a very precise system of recognition sites on the surfaces of myogenic cells about to fuse. The second step appears to involve rearrangements in the membrane surfaces of myogenic cells, for several collisions precede a period of stationary contact before myoblasts fuse either with each other or with myotubes.

Skeletal muscle is an unusual tissue in that it is formed by the physical fusion of its constituent cells. Initially, it was thought that the myotubes were formed by mitosis of a single muscle cell without subsequent division of its cytoplasm. A subject of considerable controversy has been the relationship between the event of fusion, the cell cycle, and cytodifferentiation. Fusion of the mononucleated myogenic cells appears to be tightly coupled to the mitotic cycle. Bischoff and Holtzer (1969) have determined from analysis of myogenic cell cultures that myoblasts fuse only when they are in the G_1 phase (before DNA synthesis) of the cell cycle. Once fusion has taken place the nuclei of myotubes do not synthesize DNA and hence do not divide, except under certain abnormal conditions. That fusion results in the cessation of DNA synthesis and cell division may be easily demonstrated by the fact that prefused myoblasts

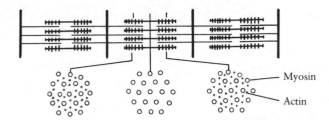

22–5 Diagrammatic representation of a part of a myofibril showing the arrangement of actin and myosin-containing filaments. Note the hexagonal array of actin filaments around the myosin filament. (From A. Huxley, 1969. Science 164, 1356. Copyright 1969 by the American Association for the Advancement of Science.)

contain DNA in two amounts corresponding to 2N and 4N, while the multinucleated cells or fused myoblasts show only a single amount corresponding to 2N. The latter is the amount of DNA present in the G_1 or postmitotic phase of the cell cycle. Also, myotubes never take up tritiated thymidine, indicating that they are no longer synthesizing DNA.

Sharp differences of opinion exist over whether myoblasts withdraw from the mitotic cycle before fusion or are withdrawn as a consequence of the fusion process. Holtzer and his collaborators (1972) believe that myoblasts are taken from the proliferation pool before fusion. They base their position on the observation that tritiated thymidine-labeled nuclei of myoblasts first appear in myotubes only after a postmitotic gap period about twice as long as the normal time of the G_2 of the dividing myoblast. Hence, a premitotic event occurs which programs the cell to withdraw from proliferative activity and fuse with other similarly programmed cells. Konigsberg and his associates (1974) believe that the hypothesis of Holtzer is difficult to test directly since it is impossible to determine if a particular myoblast would or would not have divided if it had not fused. There is agreement that myoblasts about to fuse spend an increased period of time in G_1 of the cell cycle. Presumably, during this time there are laid down surface molecular configurations that allow homotypic cells to recognize each other.

The second phase of the differentiation of the skeletal muscle cell takes place after the fusion of myoblasts into myotubes. Myosin, actin, and other proteins characteristic of this tissue type accumulate rapidly after fusion. Myosin and actin self-assemble into the thick and thin myofilaments, respectively, which characterize the myofibrils of muscle tissue (Figs. 22–4 E, 22–5). There is evidence that myosin is synthesized on polysomes containing 50 to 60 ribosomes. Approximately 200 molecules of myosin self-assemble to form a thick filament about 150 Å in diameter and 1.6 micrometers in length. Considerably less information is available on the formation of the thin or actin filament. Once assembled, however, thin filaments form a hexagonal array around each myosin filament (Fig. 22–5). The earliest myofibrils have very few myofilaments. Additional filaments are added at the circumference of a growing myofibril until the fully mature state is reached.

Since fusion inhibits DNA synthesis, one might logically ask whether this step in muscle differentiation initiates the synthesis of the muscle-specific contractile proteins. Two particularly useful tools in detecting minute quantities of myosin are the electron microscope and use of fluorescein-labeled antibodies prepared against myosin. Analysis of various types of muscle cells using these techniques suggests that the synthesis of myosin is initiated at variable times during the development of a muscle cell. For example, the mononucleate myoblasts of early chick somite tissue not only accumulate myosin before their fusion, but organize the protein into recognizable filaments. By contrast, leg muscle cells from older chick embryos clearly do not begin the production of myosin until after the fusion of myoblasts. The messenger RNAs coding for myosin are present in the prefused rat myoblast, but their translation is delayed until myotube formation. This suggests that specific biosynthesis of myosin is regulated at the translational level and linked to myogenic fusion.

The relationship between cell division and the differentiation of cell types has been and continues to be the subject of heated debate between investigators. During the differentiation of a cell type, there is an initial period in which cell numbers increase by the ordinary mitoses of stem cells. Subsequently, cytodifferentiation follows in which the proteins or *luxury molecules* that characterize the terminal cell type are synthesized. Cells then are differentiated into types on the basis of the types of luxury molecules they produce (i.e., myosin in muscle, hemoglobin in red blood cells, etc.). It is generally held that the differentiated state is accompanied by a loss in capacity for the synthesis of DNA and for further proliferative activity.

How is a population of dividing cells able to integrate the synthesis of their luxury molecules into its economy? On the basis of studies with erythrogenic, myogenic, and chondrogenic cells, Holtzer and his collaborators have proposed that the cell cycle plays an obligatory role in organizing and channeling the differentiation of these cell types. Holtzer distinguishes two types of cell cycles in cell populations. First, there is a proliferative cycle that results in daughter cells whose patterns of protein synthesis are identical to those of the parent cell. The sole function of proliferative cell cycles is to increase cell numbers. Second, there is a *quantal cell cycle* that produces daughter cells capable of synthesizing protein patterns very different from the parent cell. That is, there is a reprogramming of genes in the progeny cells. With regard to muscle tissue, the quantal scheme would postulate that the presumptive myoblast passes through an obligatory S phase (DNA synthesis) at which time the genome is reprogrammed. The daughter or myoblast cells are then "postmitotic" and capable of overt differentiation (i.e., fusion and synthesis of muscle-specific proteins). The transition to the terminal myoblast capable of cytodifferentiation is coupled to this single, critical round of DNA synthesis. According to the quantal concept, a cell cannot synthesize cell-specific proteins until the terminal quantal mitosis has occurred.

An opposing view is that DNA synthesis is not obligatory for muscle cell fusion to occur because myoblasts are capable of additional proliferative cycles if provided with the proper conditions. Konigsberg (1971), for example, has reported that a rapidly dividing population of presumptive myoblasts produces a diffusable, *conditioned medium factor*. These myogenic cells will rapidly fuse if cultured in the medium factor. In studies with the base analogue cytosine arabinoside, which blocks DNA synthesis, myogenic cells grown in this compound will fuse although taking a longer period of time than similar cells in control cultures. Myogenic cells treated with cytosine arabinoside fuse more rapidly than control cells when the conditioned medium factor is added to the culture. The implication from these studies is that changes in the external milieu rather than a critical mitosis or intrinsic program regulate the differentiation of muscle cells.

With the critical role of mitosis in mind, Holtzer (1970) has speculated that obligatory, quantal mitoses establish cell lineages early in development around the time of gastrulation. Further quantal mitoses, interspersed with a variable number of proliferative mitoses, produce intermediate, genetically unique populations of precursor cells. As a result of these series of stepwise changes in the genome, cells acquire the synthetic machinery to synthesize the proteins of the terminal cell type. Contrary to the view that differentiation involves a gradual narrowing down of synthetic abilities from "undifferentiated" cell patterns to cell-specific patterns, the quantal scheme proposes that there is the sequential acquisition of a specified series of synthetic pathways by depressions of portions of the genome.

A model for the establishment of the muscle cell lineage, shown in Figure 22–6, proposes the existence of several discrete, discontinuous populations of cells which act as precursors to the myoblast cell. One or two quantal divisions interspersed with proliferative cycles are envisaged as setting up the broad determinations of ectoderm, endoderm, and mesoderm. Further quantal mitoses within the mesodermal population create lineages leading to cartilage, muscle cells, and so on. Within the myogenic line of cells, alpha myogenic and beta myogenic cells would be early precursor cells to

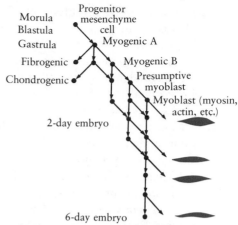

22–6 Holtzer's concept of the role of quantal mitoses in the origin of cell lineages and the differentiation of the myoblast cell. A vertical mitosis is proliferative and perpetuates the phenotype. A horizontal mitosis is quantal and alters the phenotype of the daughter cells. (From H. Holtzer, 1970. Cell Differentiation, Ole A. Scheide and Jean De Vellis, eds. © 1970 by Litton Educational Publishing, Inc. Reprinted by permission of Van Nostrand Reinhold Company.)

the stem or presumptive myoblast cells. These are transient populations and cease to perpetuate their own phenotypes since they give rise to higher levels of differentiation. The presumptive myoblasts can either proliferate into more presumptive myoblasts or undergo a terminal quantal mitosis to initiate the terminal differentiative step. All horizontal shifts between cell "compartments" presumably involve the selective derepression of batteries of genes.

Skeletal muscle and cardiac muscle cells share several common features during their myogenesis. The myoblasts of both cell types undergo a mitosis to produce daughter cells that cease to synthesize DNA and commence to rapidly translate for actin, myosin, and other muscle-specific proteins. While these programs are apparently initiated concurrently in the G_1 phase of daughter cells of skeletal tissue, the decision to shut down DNA synthesis is delayed for one or two division cycles in cardiac muscle cells.

CONNECTIVE AND SUPPORTIVE TISSUE

The connective and supportive tissues of the body are derived from embryonic mesoderm. Part of this mesoderm appears in the segmentally arranged somites that give rise to the axial skeleton and its muscles. However, everywhere between the epithelial layers of the endoderm and the ectoderm another kind of mesodermal tissue is present as a loose aggregation of cells. This is the mesenchyme. The mesenchymal cells in the embryo are stellate in shape and form a loose network, the interstices of which are occupied by a structureless intercellular matrix or ground substance. The branching processes of the mesenchymal cells are adherent rather than continuous, as has been shown by extensive observations of tissue cultures. This loosely arranged material of the early embryo soon differentiates in a number of different directions that will result in the formation of connective and supportive tissue. Its development in any direction is distinguished not so much by the differentiation of the cells as by what takes place in the intercellular matrix. The matrix is characterized by the presence of fibers of three different kinds, *reticular*, *collagenous*, and *elastic*. The cells that form these fibers are called *fibroblasts*. Fiber formation occurs as an organization of the ground substance in close proximity to the cell surface. Intercellular material, including the fibers, is nonliving and dependent for its continuous existence upon the presence of the cells of the connective tissue.

The type of connective tissue that remains most like the embryonic mesenchyme is the reticular connective tissue, which forms the

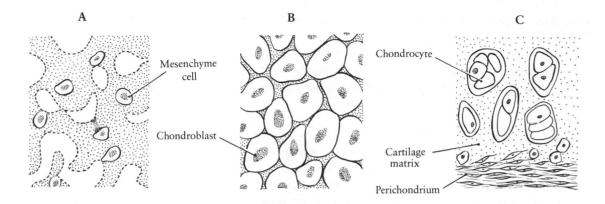

A   B   C

Mesenchyme
cell

Chondroblast

Chondrocyte

Cartilage
matrix

Perichondrium

22–7   Three steps in the histogenesis of cartilage from embryonic mesenchyme.

supporting framework in many lymphoid organs. *Tendons* and *ligaments* are connective tissue developments in which the collagenous fibers are closely packed in a parallel orientation. *Fascia* is connective tissue with a loosely arranged network of both collagenous and elastic fibers. *Supportive tissue,* cartilage and bone, is also an important derivative of the embryonic mesoderm. Although cartilage and bone contain the same kinds of fibers present in other types of connective tissue, the major change in the formation of these tissues is an increase in the hardening and strengthening of the intercellular matrix.

The Differentiation of Cartilage

Cartilage begins to develop during the second month when, in dense aggregations of mesenchyme cells, *centers of chondrification* appear. In these aggregations the cells, *chondroblasts,* are closely packed and their processes are withdrawn (Fig. 22–7 A,B). This precartilage mass increases in size and is molded into the shape that the cartilage will eventually take. Increasing amounts of matrix now appear and the cells are forced farther and farther apart, each cell surrounded by matrix and enclosed in its own separate compartment. Young chondroblasts may divide once or twice and, in mature cartilage, the division products then occur as isolated groups of two to four cells embedded in the matrix and separated by it from other similar groups (Fig. 22–7 C). Each cartilage is covered by a tough connective tissue sheet of *perichondrium.* Continued growth of cartilage may occur either by appositional or interstitial growth. In the former, new chondroblasts are differentiated from the connective tissue of the perichondrium and these cells add new matrix to the surface. A small amount of interstitial growth may also occur by the addition of new material on the inside of the structure, thus resulting in internal expansion. The definitive cartilage is avascular and the *chondrocytes* are supplied by the diffusion of substances through the matrix.

During fetal life the major portion of the skeleton is cartilaginous, but cartilage persists in the adult only in certain restricted areas such as the articular surfaces of the long bones and in the respiratory tract.

The Role of the Notochord in Cartilage Differentiation

The cartilage of the vertebral column is formed from somite mesoderm. Early experiments indicated that vertebral chondrogenesis is dependent upon an inductive influence from the embryonic notochord or spinal chord. When grown alone, somites from early chick embryos do not form cartilage but do so if cultured with either embryonic notochord or spinal cord. More recent experiments, however, have shown that under the proper culture conditions embryonic somites can form cartilage under their own power. The mass of the cultured material is important. Individual somites or small numbers of somites seldom form cartilage matrix. Even mature chondrocytes that are actively synthesizing cartilage will lose their typical shape when cultured in small groups of cells and become fibroblastlike, and although they continue to synthesize DNA and divide, they no longer form cartilage matrix. However, if entire rows of somites from a number of embryos are cultured together in a tightly packed mass, they will synthesize cartilage without any outside influence. The cells in the densely packed center of the culture aggregate, form connections with each other, and deposit large quantities of matrix. Cells on the periphery tend to flatten out and avoid forming close associations with each other. Hence they fail to synthesize matrix. Thus, the establishment of a dense aggregate of sufficient size is enough of a stimulus to trigger matrix formation. Indeed, the formation of a dense mass of precartilage cells is the first step in normal chondrogenesis.

However, under normal conditions, vertebral cartilage is formed by an interaction between the somite mesoderm and embryonic notochord and spinal cord. This interaction depends upon a diffusible substance, since it can take place through a Millipore filter and can be produced using tissue extracts. The nature of the substance has not been defined. Its action should be considered as a trigger mechanism rather than as an inductive one. Precartilage cells are already biased toward the synthesis of matrix and the notochord acts as a stimulus for the stabilization and enhancement of already existing pathways of differentiation. It is not an inducer of new activity. The stimulus could be in the form of the release of a block, which would then allow the accumulation of terminal products; or it might act as a repressor of other of some other of the cells potentialities such as myogenesis.

Biochemical Differentiation

One of the components of cartilage is chondroitin sulfate, repeating units of sulfated N-acetylgalactosamine and uronic acid, which, when occurring as side chains attached to a protein backbone, forms proteochondroitin sulfate. In the differentiation of cartilage, it would be interesting to determine at what time the metabolic pathways for the synthesis of chondroitin sulfate are established. The steps in its synthesis involve compounds which are reasonably specific and for which assays are available. All of the evidence indicates that low levels of chondroitin sulfate synthesis occur in the earliest somites formed as well as, surprisingly, in other embryonic tissues, including extraembryonic membranes. Levels of chondroitin sulfate increase during cartilage differentiation, and it is found in large quantities only in mature cartilage. Cartilage differentiation is thus often defined by the increasing amount of chondroitin sulfate measured by the uptake of radioactive sulphur.

Recently it has been determined that the synthesis of chondroitin sulfate and proteochondroitin sulfate may be more specific to cells that will differentiate into chondrocytes than had been reported previously. Analysis of proteochondroitin sulfate synthesized by chick chondrocytes in vitro has shown it to be chromatographically heterogeneous with two distinct peaks. The first represents about 90 percent of the total, the second about 10 percent. It was then suggested that the proteochondroitin sulfate seen in the first peak represented a cartilage-specific molecule, while that seen in the second was a more widespread nonspecific molecule. One would then expect that the chondroitin sulfate seen in the early somite would be the latter, nonspecific kind and that, as the cartilage differentiated, the specific variety would appear and increase. In fact, analysis of explants from stages 23 and 24 of chick limb buds cultured for different lengths of time shows a striking change in the elution profile of proteochondroitin sulfate over a period from 18 hours to nine days (Fig. 22–8). In the analysis, three peaks appear, peaks Ia and Ib representing monomer and aggregate forms of the cartilage-specific molecule and peak II representing the widespread molecule. In the material cultured for 18 hours, peaks Ia and Ib represent about 22 percent of the total and peak II the remainder. After two and nine days of culture, the peaks remain qualitatively alike, but there is a quantitative increase in peaks Ia and Ib and a decrease in peak II so that at nine days peak II contains only about 11 percent of the total. Thus, cartilage differentiation is marked by a dispro-

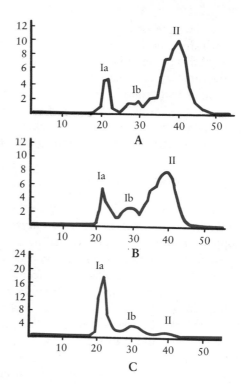

22–8 Elution profiles of proteochondroitin sulfate obtained from cell cultures of stage 23–24 chick limb buds. Abscissa: effluent volume; ordinate: percentage of total dpm. A, after 18 hours of culture. Only 22% of the activity is found in the cartilage-specific molecule (I_a and I_b); B, after two days of culture. Activity is shifting from the cartilage-nonspecific to the cartilage-specific molecule; C, after nine days of culture. About 90% of the activity is now found in the cartilage-specific molecule. (From P. F. Goetinck, J. P. Pennypacker, and P. D. Royal, 1974. Exp. Cell Res. 87, 241).

portionate increase of a particular molecule of proteochondroitin sulfate, which is specific for cartilage matrix. The presence of small amounts of this material in the precartilaginous mesoderm may represent the same situation seen in the presence of myosin in the limb bud at stages before any myoblasts can be identified morphologically. Both cases would involve an initial biochemical differentiation, the establishment of specific metabolic pathways, which underlies and presages the final morphological differentiation.

The Differentiation of Bone

The differentiation of bone proceeds by two methods, *intramembranous* and *endochondral* ossification. However, the microscopic organization of bone formed by both of these methods is the same. Intramembranous ossification occurs mainly in the development of the bones of the skull, particularly in those bones that form the vault of the cranium. Intramembranous bone differentiates from loose aggregates of embryonic connective tissue. In its formation the matrix between the cells first accumulates bundles of collagenous fibers and then the cells become oriented in epithelial-like layers along these fibers (Fig. 22–9). These cells are *osteoblasts* (bone-forming cells) whose function is to lay down the intercellular matrix that is first known as *osteoid*. Later, this matrix is hardened by the deposition of calcium salts, presumably through the activity of the osteoblasts. As the bone matrix is formed, the osteoblasts become bone cells, *osteocytes*, trapped within the matrix (Fig. 22–9). They are retained in small spaces called *lacunae*. The connective tissue covering the bone, *periosteum*, continues to supply new osteoblasts, which replace those that have been engulfed, as the bone increases in size. Since materials cannot diffuse through the calcified bone matrix, the osteoblasts depend for their existence on an intricate network of small channels, *canaliculi*, which interconnect their lacunae and provide a passage to the main central canals, the *Haversian canals* (Fig. 22–10). Bone is laid down in the form of sheets called lamellae. The major part of the bone is made up of lamellae arranged concentrically around a central Haversian canal containing the nerves and blood vessels that supply the bone. *Endosteal* and *periosteal* lamellae are those that are found parallel to the inner surface of the bone surrounding the marrow cavity and those that are found parallel to the outer surface of the bone, respectively (Fig. 22–10).

The largest part of the skeleton develops by the replacement by bone of a previously existing cartilaginous model, endochondral ossification (Fig. 22–11). In a typical long bone, *primary centers of ossification* arise in the center of the shaft. Here, the cartilage cells

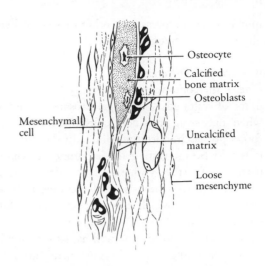

22–9 Differentiation of membrane bone.

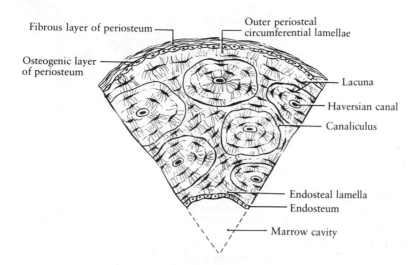

Fibrous layer of periosteum

Outer periosteal circumferential lamellae

Osteogenic layer of periosteum

Lacuna

Haversian canal

Canaliculus

Endosteal lamella

Endosteum

Marrow cavity

22–10 Cross section of the shaft of an adult long bone showing the arrangement of the Haversian, endosteal, and periosteal lamellae.

hypertrophy, much of the matrix is resorbed, and calcium salts are deposited in the remaining matrix. The result is the formation of branching trabeculae of calcified cartilage. Connective tissue of perichondrial origin and blood vessels grow into the center of ossification to begin the formation of the marrow cavity. These connective tissue cells become osteoblasts, which then deposit bone on the spicules of calcified cartilage. Continued resorption of the spicules and enlargement of the marrow cavity occurs. The shaft of the bone with its marrow cavity is now known as the *diaphysis*.

The ends of the long bones, the *epiphyses*, generally do not develop centers of ossification until after birth. When they do, the same processes that have previously taken place in the diaphysis of the bone now occur in the epiphyses. Between each epiphysis and the diaphysis, a plate of cartilage persists which allows for the fur-

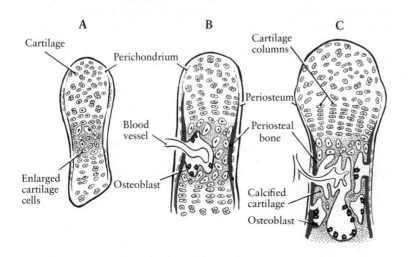

A   B   C

Cartilage

Perichondrium

Cartilage columns

Periosteum

Periosteal bone

Blood vessel

Enlarged cartilage cells

Osteoblast

Calcified cartilage

Osteoblast

22–11 Diagram of endochondral ossification in the diaphysis of a long bone.

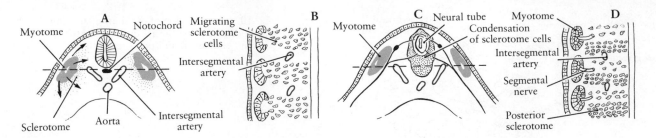

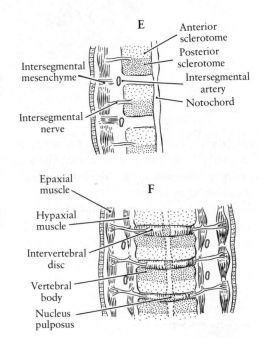

ther increase in the length of the bone during postnatal life. Closure (ossification) of this *epiphyseal–diaphyseal plate* of cartilage precludes any further elongation of the bone. However, a layer of cartilage persists over the ends of the bones, providing a surface for articulation.

Development of the Axial Skeleton

The axial skeleton of the embryo is simply the notochord. This primary skeleton persists as the only adult axial skeleton in *Amphioxus* and also makes up a large part of the adult skeleton of the cyclostomes. In all other vertebrates, the notochord is replaced by a stiffer, either cartilaginous or bony, skeleton. In mammals, the axial skeleton consists of the skull, the vertebral column, the ribs, and the sternum.

The skull: As we described previously, most of the bones of the skull develop by intramembranous ossification in local accumulations of embryonic connective tissue.

The vertebrae and the ribs: The vertebrae and the ribs develop from the sclerotomes of the somites. During the fourth week, the cells from each sclerotome migrate in three different directions (Fig. 22–12 A): (1) ventromedially to surround the notochord; (2) dorsally to cover the neural tube; and (3) ventrally into the ventral body wall.

At each segmental level, the sclerotomal mass surrounding the notochord consists of a loosely arranged cranial portion and a densely arranged caudal portion (Fig. 22–12 B,D). These two portions of the individual sclerotome then undergo a rearrangement in which the denser caudal part of one sclerotome joins the looser cranial half of the sclerotome just caudal to it. The fused cranial and caudal parts of the adjacent sclerotomes will form the body of one vertebra. This then explains why the intersegmental arteries (which originally ran between the adjacent segmentally arranged sclerotomes) now pass over the center of the bodies of the vertebrae and why the spinal nerves (which originally grew toward the center of

22–12 Diagrams of four stages in the formation of the bodies of vertebrae (B, D, E, F). A, diagram of a transverse section through a four-week-old embryo; C, diagram of a transverse section through a five-week-old embryo. Dotted lines in A and C represent the level of the frontal sections diagrammed in B, D, E, and F. Since the vertebrae form by the fusion of caudal and cranial parts of adjacent scleotomes, the spinal nerves, originally oriented toward the center of a somite, now pass between the bodies of the vertebrae.

each somite) now run between the bodies of adjacent vertebrae (Fig. 22–12 F).

A small cranial part of the dense caudal portion of the original sclerotome moves craniad and becomes located opposite the center of the adjacent myotome. This part of each sclerotome differentiates into an *intervertebral disk*. The only parts of the notochord that persist in the adult are the remnants of this structure, which are incorporated into the intervertebral disks where they form the gelatinous center of the disk, the *nucleus pulposus*.

The cells of the sclerotome that migrate dorsally to surround the developing neural tube differentiate into the *neural arch*, with its central canal through which the spinal cord passes, and into the spinous and transverse processes of the vertebrae.

The cells of the sclerotome that migrate ventrally form the costal processes of the vertebrae and, in the thoracic region, the ribs.

The mesenchymal masses that are differentiating into the vertebrae begin cartilage formation during the second month and the cartilaginous models begin endochondral ossification in the late embryonic period. Ossification is not complete until about the mid-twenties of postnatal life.

The sternum. The sternum, the midventral line of bones to which the ribs attach, develops in the second month from local condensations of mesenchyme as a longitudinally oriented pair of sternal primordia, which are at first widely separated from one another and have no connections with the ribs. The ribs soon attach to the developing paired sternal bars that then unite with each other progressively in a craniocaudal direction. The cartilaginous model begins ossification during the fifth month, but all of the centers of ossification are not present until after birth.

Development of the Appendicular Skeleton

The *appendicular skeleton* consists of the shoulder (pectoral) and hip (pelvic) girdles and the bones of the limbs. The bones of the appendicular skeleton develop in association with the limb buds. As do the muscles of the limbs, the bones also develop some distance from the somites; and although the bones of the respective girdles probably develop from somite sclerotome, the limb bones differentiate from the unsegmented lateral mesoderm.

The mesenchymal condensations that will form the cartilaginous models of the girdles and the limbs are present early in the second month, begin to calcify at about seven weeks, and show centers of ossification by eight weeks. Differentiation in each limb proceeds in a proximodistal direction, and the superior extremity develops somewhat in advance of the inferior. In general, the larger bones are the first to chondrify and the first to ossify. Most of the limb bones show primary centers of ossification before birth, but in most of them ossification in the epiphysis does not begin until after birth.

REFERENCES

Bischoff, R. and H. Holtzer. 1969. Mitosis and the processes of differentiation of myogenic cells *in vitro*. J. Cell Biol. 41:188–200.

Holtzer, H. 1970. Myogenesis. In: Cell Differentiation, pp. 476–503. Eds., O. A. Schjeide and J. de Vellis. New York: Van Nostrand Reinhold.

Holtzer, H., H. Weintraub, R. Mayer, and B. Mochran. 1972. The cell cycle, cell lineages, and cell differentiation. Curr. Topics Dev. Biol. 7:229–256.

Konigsberg, I. R. 1971. Diffusion-mediated control of myoblast fusion. Dev. Biol. 26:133–152.

Konigsberg, I. R. and P. A. Buckley. 1974. Regulation of the cell cycle and myogenesis by cell-medium interaction. In: Concepts of Development, pp. 179–193. Eds., J. Lash and J. Whittaker. Stamford, Conn.: Sinauer Associates.

Levitt, D. and A. Dorfman. 1974. Concepts and mechanisms of cartilage development. Curr. Topics Dev. Biol. 8:103–149.

Lipton, B. H. and A. G. Jacobson. 1974a. Analysis of normal somite development. Dev. Biol. 38:73–90.

Lipton, B. H. and A. G. Jacobson. 1974b. Experimental analysis of the mechanisms of somite morphogenesis. Dev. Biol. 38:91–103.

O'Neill, M. C. and F. E. Stockdale. 1972. A kinetic analysis of myogenesis *in vitro*. J. Cell Biol. 25:52–65.

Yaffe, E. and H. Dym. 1973. Gene expression during differentiation of contractile muscle fibers. Cold Spring Harbor Symp. Quant. Biol. 37:543–547.

23

The Integumentary System

The integumentary system of the adult vertebrate consists of two morphologically distinct layers and their associated appendages, such as hairs, feathers, scales, and glands. The superficial layer, or *epidermis,* is a stratified squamous epithelium that develops from the surface ectoderm. The deeper layer, or *dermis (corium)*, is a connective tissue originating from mesoderm. An acellular basement membrane lies between the epidermis and the dermis.

Study of the integument and its maturation is particularly intriguing. As a tissue with a permanent germinal population that produces differentiating cells, the epidermis can provide a model system for examining complicated processes of differentiation involving sudden and marked changes in cell morphology. One approach has been to use the human fetal skin in an effort to resolve key questions regarding the postnatal skin since conditions in the fetus are in slower motion, so to speak, and therefore capable of closer analysis. More permissive legislation relating to the termination of pregnancy has greatly increased the availability of human fetal material for this purpose. As with events seen during the development of other organs, there is increasing evidence that interactions between epidermis and dermis play important roles in the differentiation of the skin and its appendages. The possibility has been raised that interference with these interactions may be a causative factor in epidermal abnormality and disease.

THE EPIDERMIS

In early embryos of most vertebrates, the cells of the ectoderm proliferate and form a protective, transitory epithelium known as the *periderm* or covering layer (Fig. 23–1 A,B). Cells in the basal region of the ectoderm will become the *generative* or *germinative (Malpighian) layer,* a zone destined to give rise to the stratified epithelium of the adult epidermis (Fig. 23–1 B–H).

The developing epidermis of human embryos and fetuses has recently received a significant amount of attention using new techniques for analysis, including transmission and scanning electron microscopy. The ectoderm of very young human embryos (less than 36 days old) is a simple epithelium whose plasma membranes facing

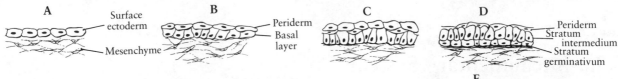

the amniotic fluid exhibit occasional microvilli (Fig. 23–1 A). Between 5 and 10 weeks, there develops a clear distinction between the periderm and the germinative layer of the epidermis (Fig. 23–1 B,C). There is an extensive elaboration of special intercellular contacts known as *desmosomes* during this time. The initial indication of desmosome differentiation is a localized increase in the density of apposed segments of the plasma membranes of adjacent cells.

Until recently, the periderm was generally viewed as a passive, protective covering for the rest of the epidermis while the latter was in varying stages of keratinization. Ultrastructural observations now tend to indicate that the periderm, over a limited period of time, probably functions actively in providing for and maintaining the well-being of the fetus. Cells of the young periderm are low cuboidal in sectional view and flat and polygonal in surface view. However, between 9 and 16 weeks of development, the cells of the periderm become very tall and elevated (Figs. 23–1 C–E; 23–2). The amniotic surface of each cell shows microvilli, globular projections, and various clefts and infoldings; these are all specializations designed to provide maximum surface area of the epidermis to the amniotic fluid. The microvilli in particular are currently thought to assist in the uptake and transport of glucose from the amniotic cavity into the fetus. Subsequently, the periderm undergoes regression with its cells becoming flattened, altered with respect to internal morphology (i.e., pycnotic nuclei), and sloughed off or desquamated into the amniotic cavity. The periderm is completely absent in embryos of approximately 23 weeks (Fig. 23–1 F,G).

A major question regarding the periderm has been whether it undergoes keratinization (i.e., cornification) prior to the final stages of regression. Most studies tend to indicate that the specific alterations in periderm cells are quite different from those involving the transformation of the underlying epidermal cells into keratinized squames. Additionally, cells of the periderm have never been observed to contain *keratohyalin granules*.

The epidermis becomes increasingly stratified as cells of the stratum germinativum actively divide and their daughter cells crowd toward the surface. By 12 weeks in the human embryo, for example, sections through the epidermis show that it consists of one layer of stratum germinativum, one to three layers of a *stratum intermedium,* and a simple periderm (Fig. 23–1 D). By about 25

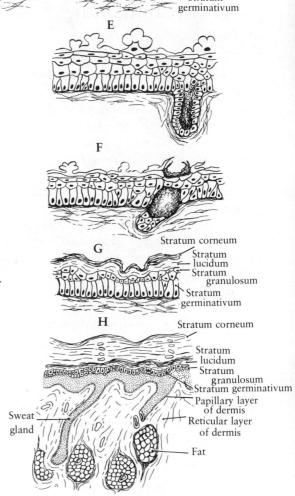

23–1 Schematic diagrams illustrating the development of the periderm, epidermis, and dermis in human embryos. A, indifferent ectoderm and mesenchyme (36 days); B, the early bilaminar epidermis with periderm flattened (36 to 55 days); C, periderm layer consists of elevated, domelike cells (55 to 75 days); D, appearance of intermediate layer in epidermis (65 to 96 days); E, periderm modified to form large clusters of simple and complex blebs (95 to 120 days); F, regression of the periderm (108 to 160 days); G, epidermis has characteristics of adult tissue type (160 days); H, the integument at birth. (A–G, after K. Holbrook and G. Odland, 1975. J. Invest. Dermatol. 65, 16.)

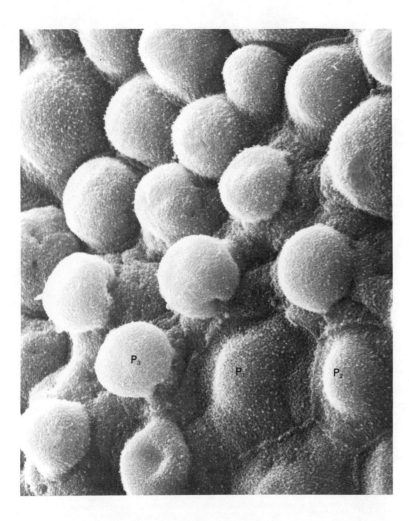

23–2 A scanning electron microscope view of the fetal skin at 88 days. Many of the peridermal cells are tall and elevated. Note the flat-surfaced cells (P_1), elevated cells (P_2), and cells with formed blebs (P_3). (From K. Holbrook and G. Odland, 1975. J. Invest. Dermatol. 65, 16.)

weeks, the fetal epidermis is completely keratinized and similar in organization to that of the adult, consisting of a basal, germinative layer, a *stratum granulosum* whose cells have distinct keratohyalin granules, a *stratum lucidum* (two to three layers thick) whose cells contain variable amounts of glycogen, and five or six layers of *stratum corneum* (Figs. 23–1 G,H; 23–3).

Stratification of the epidermal epithelium is accompanied by cytomorphic and differentiative changes that progressively transform cells of basal layer origin through a series of stages into the flattened, avital squames of the stratum corneum. The fully keratinized cell of the stratum corneum is one with a matrix of filaments embedded in an amorphous substance and arranged in bundles or fibrils. Whether epidermal keratinization is regarded as a process of differentiation or disintegration, it is a complex process involving synthesis of keratin proteins, keratohyalin granules, alterations in

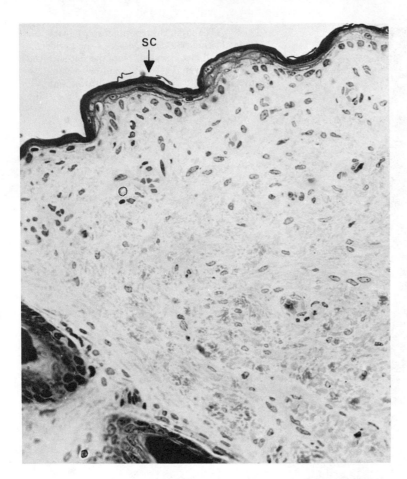

23–3　The human fetal skin at 185 days as shown by the light miscroscope. All layers of the epidermis are present. Note the absence of all periderm cells. SC, stratum corneum. (From K. Holbrook and G. Odland, 1975. J. Invest. Dermatol. 65, 16.)

the cell surface and the junctional complexes between cells, dehydration, and death of cells. The dynamic aspects of keratinization are poorly understood. Most investigators tend to believe that cytoplasmic filaments of the basal cells are prekeratin, fibrous proteins that become chemically and morphologically altered to yield the keratin bundles characteristic of the stratum corneum cells. There remain unresolved questions relating to the nature, origin, and fate of keratohyalin granules as well as their role in the cornification process. At the level of the light microscope, these granules are very distinct particles in the cytoplasm of cells comprising the stratum granulosum. Although initially believed to be precursors to the keratinous proteins, it is now suggested that keratohyalin granules may function in organizing and arranging the substance of the stratum corneum cell into its final keratin pattern.

Several other cells, which are generally termed *epidermal non-*

keratinocytes, can be identified in the developing human epidermis. Neural crest cells are known to migrate into the dermis and differentiate as *melanoblasts.* Subsequently, these invade the basal layer of the epidermis and, as *melanocytes,* specialize in pigment formation (Fig. 23–4). Brown and black melanin pigments (the *eumelanins*), which commonly make up the different body color patterns observed in vertebrates, are produced in special organelles (*melanosomes*) of the melanocyte cytoplasm by the oxidation of L-tyrosine in the presence of the enzyme *tyrosinase.* Active melanocytes have been observed as early as eight weeks in the human epidermis.

Merkel cells are intraepidermal elements generally considered to be integumentary mechanoreceptors (Fig. 23–5). Although once thought to be an epidermal keratinocyte, most workers now support the view that the Merkel cells, probably of neural crest origin, migrate through the dermis into the epidermis.

A particularly interesting cell type is the *Langerhans cell,* a squamouslike cell with distinctive granules (*Langerhans granules*) and present within the epidermis in a fully differentiated state by 14 weeks. The general function, the origin, and the fate of this cell remain a mystery. They have been implicated in immune reactions as well as in organizing the highly ordered, columnlike arrangement of epidermal keratinocytes.

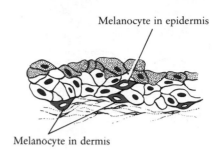

23–4   Early melanocytes entering the human epidermis from the dermis.

THE DERMIS

The dermis is derived from mesenchyme tissue beneath the surface ectoderm (Fig. 23–1). It is generally recognized that there are two sources for the mesenchyme. Most of the dermis differentiates from the somatic plate mesoderm. The remainder originates from the dermatome of the somite.

When fully developed, the dermis consists of a highly vascularized, fibroelastic connective tissue divided into *papillary* and *reticular layers* (Fig. 23–1 H). Differentiation of collagenous fibers and elastic fibers from mesenchyme is well established in human embryos of approximately 24 weeks. Dome-shaped thickenings of the dermis (*dermal papillae*) project into the basal layer of the epidermis; these alternate with downgrowths of the stratum germinativum termed *epidermal ridges* (Fig. 23–1 H). The unevenness of the dermoepidermal boundary is an effective structural adaptation that permits maximum resistance to forces of shear, thereby acting to maintain the structural integrity of the integument.

23–5   A Merkel cell (M) in the dermis of a 21-week-old human fetus. It is closely associated with peripheral axonal–Schwann cell complexes (S) in the skin. (From A. Breathnach, 1971. J. Invest. Dermatol. 57, 133.)

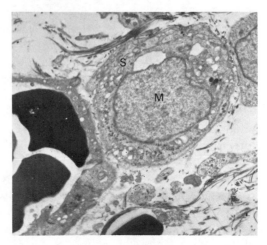

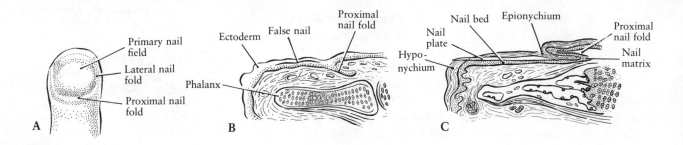

23–6 Development of the human nail. A, dorsal view of the tip of the fingernail at about 10 weeks; B, sagittal section through the fingernail at about 14 weeks; C, sagittal section through the fingernail at birth. (After L. Arey, 1974. Developmental Anatomy. W. B. Saunders Company, Philadelphia.)

THE CUTANEOUS APPENDAGES

The vertebrate skin displays an astounding degree of functional and morphological diversity. This is expressed by the presence of discrete, highly specialized structures or appendages, including a variety of glands (ranging from the mammary, sweat, and sebaceous glands of mammals to the preen or uropygial glands of birds), hairs, feathers, terminal phalangeal coverings (nails, hoofs, claws), and scales. The primordia of most of these appendages arise initially as localized thickenings of the epidermis. An exception is the scales of fishes, which are specializations of the dermal mesenchyme. Although the development of these integumentary derivatives has been rather carefully studied at the anatomical level, our knowledge regarding mechanisms underlying their differentiation is fragmentary.

The Nails

Each nail is initially foreshadowed by a thickened area of the epidermis (the *primary nail field*) on the dorsal side of the tip of each digit (Fig. 23–6 A). The nail field soon becomes more sharply defined with the appearance of elevated folds of the epidermis known as the *proximal* and *lateral nail folds* (Fig. 23–6 A,B). Although some keratinization of the nail field does take place, forming the so-called false nail (Fig. 23–6 B), the true nail or *nail plate* develops as the result of the proliferation, cornification, and consolidation of cells originating from the *nail matrix* or the germinative layer of the proximal epidermal nail fold (Fig. 23–6 C). The nail plate grows forward over the *nail bed* from the base of the terminal phalanx to reach the tip of the digit just before birth.

The periderm and the stratum corneum for a time constitute a covering layer, termed the *eponychium* (Fig. 23–6 C), for each nail plate. By the latter part of fetal life, this layer is lost except for fragmentary, keratinized portions near the margins of the nail (cuticle of the nail).

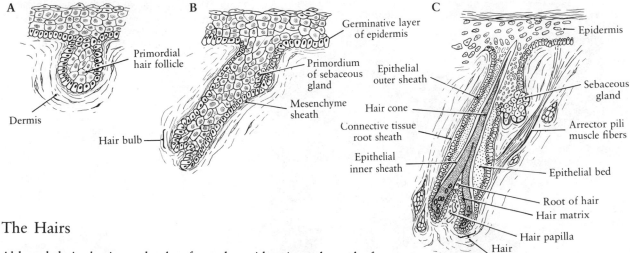

A, Primordial hair follicle, Germinative layer of epidermis, Primordium of sebaceous gland, Mesenchyme sheath, Hair bulb, Dermis

B, Germinative layer of epidermis, Primordium of sebaceous gland, Mesenchyme sheath, Hair bulb

C, Epithelial outer sheath, Hair cone, Connective tissue root sheath, Epithelial inner sheath, Epidermis, Sebaceous gland, Arrector pili muscle fibers, Epithelial bed, Root of hair, Hair matrix, Hair papilla, Hair bulb

23–7   Drawings to illustrate the successive stages in the development of hair. A, the early primordial hair follicle; B, beginning of the formation of the hair matrix of the hair bulb; C, hair cone formation. (From B. M. Patten, 1968. Human Embryology. Copyright © 1968 by McGraw-Hill, Inc. Used with permission of McGraw-Hill Book Company.)

The Hairs

Although hairs begin to develop from the epidermis at the end of eight weeks in the eyebrows, lips, and chin of human embryos, those of the general integument do not begin to appear until about the fourth fetal month. The primordium of each hair originates as a solid column of cells (*hair follicle*), produced by localized proliferation of the stratum germinativum, which pushes down into the underlying mesenchyme (Fig. 23–7 A). The deepest part of the hair follicle (*hair bulb*) quickly becomes enlarged into a club-shaped mass and then invaginated by a domelike mass of mesenchyme tissue (Fig. 23–7 B,C). A detailed view through the hair follicle at this time shows the moundlike mesenchyme, or *hair papilla,* capped by epithelial cells that, because they later give rise to the hair proper, constitute the *hair matrix* (Fig. 23–7 B,C). The tissue of the hair papilla is continuous with mesenchyme cells that invest the rest of the hair follicle; these mesenchyme cells will differentiate into the *dermal* or *connective tissue root sheath* (Fig. 23–7 C).

Proliferation of cells by the hair matrix produces a young, cone-shaped mass of cells (*hair cone*), which pushes toward the surface through the central cells of the hair follicle (Fig. 23–7 C). The more peripherally situated cells of this axial core will give rise to the *inner epithelial root sheath* while the remaining, centrally located cells will form the *hair shaft.* Above the region of the hair matrix, the cells of the hair shaft become keratinized and topographically organized into an *outer cuticle,* a *middle cortex,* and a *central medulla.* The peripheral cells of the original follicle wall will differentiate into the *outer epithelial root sheath* (Fig. 23–7 C).

Two thickenings of the outer root sheath appear on the lower side of the obliquely directed hair follicle (Fig. 23–7 C). The lower one is the *epithelial bud,* a region of rapid cell proliferation that contributes to the growth of the hair follicle. The upper swelling is the

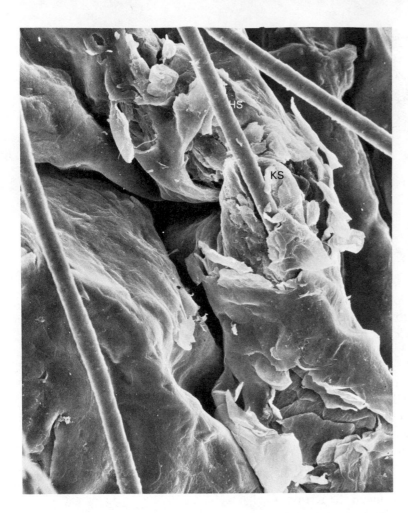

23–8 A surface view of the fetal skin at 23 weeks showing hair shafts (HS) and keratinized epidermal cells (KS). (From K. Holbrook and G. Odland, 1975. J. Invest. Dermatol. 65, 16.)

primordium of the *sebaceous gland*. Mesenchyme below the epithelial bed aggregates to form the *arrector pili muscle,* a bundle of smooth muscle fibers attached to the connective tissue root sheath of the follicle and the papillary layer of the dermis.

The first hairs to emerge in the fetal skin are rather slender and spatially close together (Fig. 23–8). They form a downy coat commonly termed *lanugo*. Hairs of this type are typically shed into the amniotic fluid by birth and replaced by fine *vellus hairs* characteristic of the prepuberal skin. Vellus hairs appear to be at least in part derived from new hair follicles.

The Sebaceous Glands

Most of the sebaceous glands arise as lateral evaginations from the outer epithelial root sheath of the hair follicle (Fig. 23–7 B,C). The

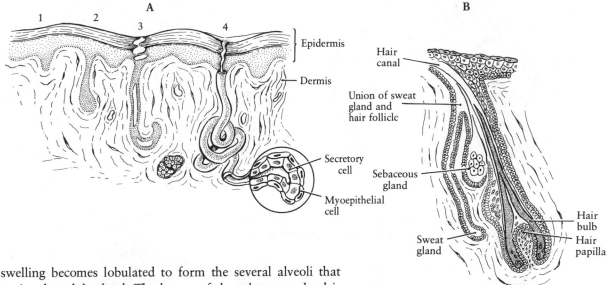

A

1   2   3   4

Epidermis

Dermis

Secretory cell

Myoepithelial cell

B

Hair canal

Union of sweat gland and hair follicle

Sebaceous gland

Sweat gland

Hair bulb

Hair papilla

23–9   A, successive stages in the development of the common eccrine sweat gland; B, an apocrine sweat gland developing in association with a hair follicle.

solid swelling becomes lobulated to form the several alveoli that characterize the adult gland. The lumen of the sebaceous gland is formed through breakdown of central sebaceous cells with the resultant oily secretion (*sebum*) passing into the amniotic fluid by way of the hair canal. The sebum mixes with desquamated peridermal cells to form *venix caseosa,* a whitish, cheeselike substance that acts as a protective coating for the fetal skin. Since the sebaceous gland is *holocrine* (i.e., the secretion consists of disintegrated gland cells), periodic replacement of secretory cells is required.

Sebaceous glands independent of hair follicles are found in the upper eyelids, external genitalia, and around the anus. They arise in a similar manner from epithelial buds of the epidermis.

The Sweat Glands

The ordinary eccrine sweat glands develop as solid, cylindrical downgrowths of the generative layer of the epidermis (Fig. 23–9 A). As each bud pushes into the underlying mesenchyme, the distal segment of the primoridum becomes coiled to form the secretory portion of the gland. Recent studies with the electron microscope show that lumen formation in sweat glands appears to be a complex process. Hashimoto and his colleagues (1966) have demonstrated that the lumen of the intraepithelial portion of the duct forms extracellularly by the separation of cells, while the lumen of the intradermal portion of the duct arises through the formation of cytoplasmic vesicles within the primordial cells. These vesicles break through the plasma membranes and coalesce. Epithelial cells in the secretory segment of the gland differentiate into *secretory* and *myoepithelial cells* (Fig. 23–9 A). Myoepithelial cells are of special

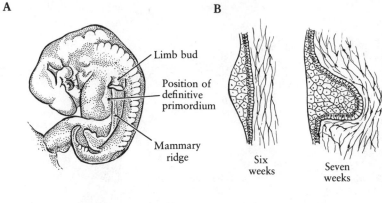

A

Limb bud

Position of definitive primordium

Mammary ridge

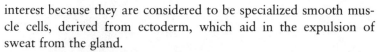

B

Six weeks

Seven weeks

Ten weeks

Sixteen weeks

interest because they are considered to be specialized smooth muscle cells, derived from ectoderm, which aid in the expulsion of sweat from the gland.

Apocrine sweat glands develop in association with hair follicles and have a distribution largely limited to the axilla, the pubic region, and the areola of the mammay glands. They develop from downgrowths of the stratum germinativum and as such open into the hair canal above the sebaceous glands (Fig. 23–9 B).

Actual secretion by sweat glands is probably neglible before birth.

The Mammary Glands

Although mammary glands do not normally function until adulthood, their primordia appear relatively early in mammalian development. The first visible evidence of mammary gland development appears in the form of a pair of epidermal thickenings along the ventrolateral body walls from the axillary to the inguinal regions (Fig. 23–10 A). These so-called *mammary ridges* or *milk lines* are particularly prominent in mammals with serially arranged mammary glands, such as the rat and cow. In humans, the milk ridges disappear rather quickly except in the pectoral region where the paired glands will develop.

The progressive development of the human mammary gland is shown in Figure 23–10 B–D. Localized proliferation within the mammary ridge produces, on either side, a lenticular-shaped epithelial mass of cells that extends down into the underlying dermis. Each mass continues to enlarge and gradually becomes globular in shape. During the fifth fetal month, 20 to 25 solid, epithelial cords bud off and push deeper into the mesenchyme. These cords of cells are the primordia of the *lactiferous ducts* (milk ducts). Each slowly acquires a lumen, branches at its distal end, and will serve as a focal

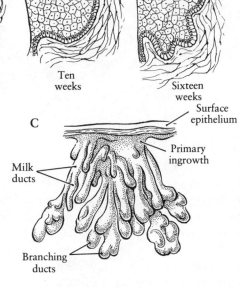

C

Surface epithelium

Primary ingrowth

Milk ducts

Branching ducts

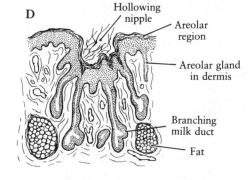

D

Hollowing nipple

Areolar region

Areolar gland in dermis

Branching milk duct

Fat

23–10 Development of the human mammary gland. A, the position of the mammary ridge at 6 weeks; B, a series of vertical sections through the epidermal gland primordium from 6 to 16 weeks; C, the appearance of the gland at 6 months; D, the mammary gland in vertical section at 8 months.

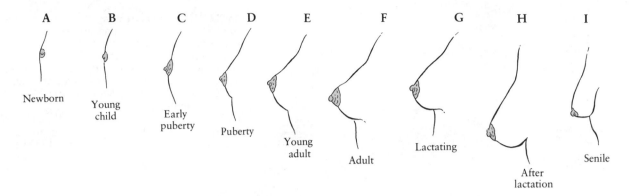

A Newborn
B Young child
C Early puberty
D Puberty
E Young adult
F Adult
G Lactating
H After lactation
I Senile

23–11 Sketches of the human breast in profile to show changes in contour with age and states of functional activity.

point around which a lobe of the mammary gland is organized (Fig. 23–10 C). Subsequently, the epidermis at the site of the origin of the gland becomes keratinized and hollowed out to form a shallow mammary pit into which the ducts open (Fig. 23–10 D). Shortly after birth, this same area will elevate into the *mammary nipple*. The areola of the gland will develop from the circular area of the epidermis around the nipple (Fig. 23–10 D).

Until pregnancy occurs, the mammary gland remains incompletely developed (Fig. 23–11). Most of the increase in the size of the gland in females with the onset of puberty is due to the accumulation of fat tissue between the duct system. Rapid proliferation of the terminal ends of the lactiferous ducts to form organizational units termed lobules and the secretory portions of the gland occurs during the last third of gestation. The mammary glands in males normally undergo little postnatal development.

DERMAL–EPIDERMAL INTERACTIONS AND THEIR ANALYSIS

At an early stage of development in all vertebrates, the general integument consists of a flat, two-layered epidermis, originating from embryonic ectoderm, and a dermis of uniform constitution derived from somatic mesenchyme. From this relatively undifferentiated state, an epidermis emerges whose cells are stratified, rigidly organized, and in varying stages of keratinization. Closer examination of the epidermis reveals that there are regional differences in its microanatomy, expressed primarily in terms of its thickness and degree of cellular stratification. Also, there are variations in the extent to which the epidermis is interrupted by the appearance of discrete, highly specialized cutaneous appendages, such as hairs, glands, and so on. Because the skin is the largest organ in the body and fulfills a spectrum of important physiological functions, there has been an

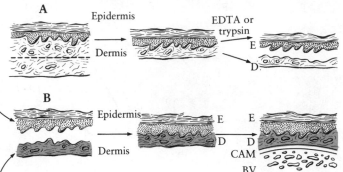

23–12 Diagram illustrating the steps in the recombination of skin components and the transplantation of resulting grafts to the chorioallantoic membrane. A, separation of skin components by EDTA or trypsin into isolates of epidermis (E) and dermis (D); B, recombinants of epidermal and dermal isolates are assembled under a microscope and placed on a portion of the chorioallantoic membrane (CAM) rich in blood vessels (BV). (After R. Biggaman and C. Wheeler, 1968. J. Invest. Dermatol. 51, 454.)

intense interest in the processes leading to the differentiation of the embryonic skin, particularly those responsible for the origin and maintenance of the various structural specializations associated with the epidermis.

As pointed out in previous chapters, one of the most fundamental processes in embryonic development is the interaction between populations of cells and tissues of diverse ontogenetic origins (i.e., presumptive neural ectoderm and chordamesoderm). The interaction typically leads to the expression of new, differentiated cell and tissue types. Based largely on the results of the studies with the chicken embryo, it is now generally agreed that: (1) reciprocal interactions between epidermis and dermis are required for normal skin development; and (2) regionally distinctive differentiations of the epidermis are determined under the influence of the dermal mesenchyme.

Techniques available for the study of dermoepidermal interactions in embryonic and adult tissues are similar to those employed to examine epitheliomesenchymal relationships in general (Chapter 13). Thin sections of different kinds of skin can be grafted into wounds that are prepared in the integument of genetically compatible hosts. For example, one can observe the in vivo response of epidermal epithelia excised from different sites (ear epidermis or cornea epidermis) as they grow over the surface of common mesenchyme that invades the wound bed. A particularly useful method for determining the interrelationships between epidermis and dermis is illustrated in the diagram of Figure 23–12. A section of skin is dissected out and cut into smaller fragments. The epidermal and dermal components of these fragments are then completely separated from each other by chemical (EDTA) or enzymatic (trypsin) treatment (Fig. 23–12 A). Heterotypic recombinant grafts, formed by bringing together the two tissues from different sources, are then transplanted to heterotopic sites in the same host or to the chorioallantoic membrane of an embryonated chicken egg (Fig. 23–12 B).

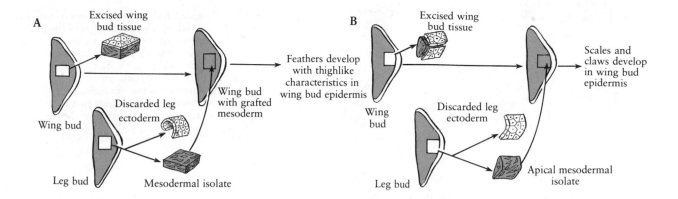

A

Excised wing
bud tissue

Wing bud

Wing bud
with grafted
mesoderm

Discarded leg
ectoderm

Mesodermal isolate

Leg bud

Feathers develop
with thighlike
characteristics in
wing bud epidermis

B

Excised wing
bud tissue

Wing
bud

Discarded leg
ectoderm

Leg bud

Apical mesodermal
isolate

Scales and
claws develop
in wing bud
epidermis

23–13 Diagram illustrating mesodermal control of the development of the epidermis in the chick, A, thigh mesoderm grafted into wing bud; B, apical mesoderm of leg bud grafted into wing bud. (From J. Cairns and J. Saunders, 1954. J. Exp. Zool. 127, 221.)

When the whole skin of embryonic chickens or fetal mammals is cultured, growth and differentiation of both epidermis and dermis generally resemble patterns observed in vivo. The criteria for epidermal growth and differentiation are the maintenance of a healthy stratum germinativum, indicated by mitotic figures in its cells, the formation of keratin, and the development of an organized stratum corneum. However, isolated grafts of epidermis (i.e., without dermis) in organ culture tend to curl up, remain largely undifferentiated, and eventually degenerate. Epidermis from isolates of very young chicken embryos has been shown to become completely keratinized; however, these same grafts show very few mitoses and little evidence of the tissue organization characteristic of normal epidermis. Isolated explants of dermis undergo necrosis rather rapidly without significant differentiation. When epidermis is recombined with its own dermis in culture, both layers survive and differentiate to produce a graft of normal whole skin.

A variety of studies have demonstrated that the mesoderm of the skin (dermis) controls and determines the regional differences in the epidermis. Particularly useful in establishing the importance of mesodermal control have been the feathers of the avian integument. Although all feathers are cutaneous specializations of the ectodermal layer, they show great diversity in their morphology and function over the body. Several types of experiments have shown that the type of feather formed in the skin is clearly governed by the dermal mesoderm. Saunders has demonstrated, for example, that grafts of ectoderm-free, prospective thigh mesoderm, following transplantation into a prepared site on the wing bud of a four-day-old chick embryo (Fig. 23–13 A), become covered with wing ectoderm. Feathers subsequently develop in the wing epidermis above the mesenchymal graft that display structural and organizational characteristics typical of feathers appearing on the thigh. Also, when transplanted to the wing bud, mesoderm from the distal end of the

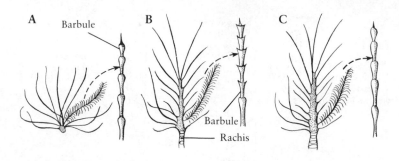

A   Barbule

B   C

Barbule

Rachis

23–14 A, a sketch of a young feather of the chick; B, a sketch of a young feather of the duck. Note the presence of the shaft or rachis; C, chick ectoderm in the presence of duck mesoderm forms a feather with a rachis. Note the morphology of an individual barbule of the feather in A and B. The barbules in the recombinant graft of C are of the chick type, indicating that there are genetic limitations in the response of the ectoderm. (After P. Sengel, 1971. Adv. Morphog. 9, 181.)

leg bud causes the wing epidermis to form scales and claws, epidermal specializations associated with the leg (Fig. 23–13 B). Similar studies have been conducted using recombinant grafts prepared from chicken and duck skin tissues. Again, the source of the mesoderm appears to control gross feather structure. A rigid, rodlike shaft forms the skeletal backbone of the early duck feather (Fig. 23–14 B). This structure is absent in the young chick feather (Fig. 23–14 A). When the mesoderm of a duck is combined with chick ectoderm, the feathers that develop in the epidermis are of the duck type with a central shaft (Fig. 23–14 C).

The importance of mesenchymal factors in influencing the expression of the epidermis has been clearly shown in a series of classic experiments by McLoughlin (1961). Isolated five-day-old chick limb epidermis was explanted in vitro with mesenchyme excised from several sources, including gizzard, proventriculus, and heart (Fig. 23–15). The response of the epidermis to stimulation by the mesenchyme was different and very specific in each of these heterotypic recombinants. With gizzard mesenchyme, the epidermis failed to keratinize, but its cells were induced to secrete mucus and sometime form cilia. This is a marked alteration in the prospective fate of the epidermis, which normally would produce only keratinous proteins. Explants of heart mesenchyme became subdivided into two zones: a central region of myoblast cells surrounded by a region of fibroblast cells. The epidermis was prevented from keratinizing on the region of myoblasts and spread into a simple squamous epithelium; however, the epidermis keratinized heavily on heart fibroblasts. On proventriculus mesenchyme, the epidermis was initially prevented from keratinizing and secreted mucus, but after approximately seven days its cells became keratinized. The latter suggests that the mesodermal influence must be continuous in order to maintain the modified differentiation of the epidermis. Studies by Briggaman and Wheeler (1968) using recombinant grafts of human skin have demonstrated that the dermis is continuously required to conserve and maintain the stable adult features of the

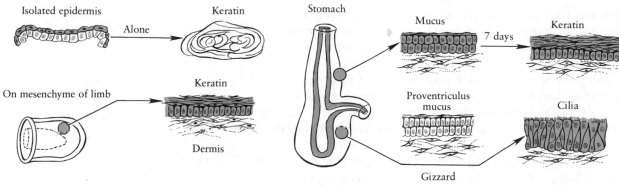

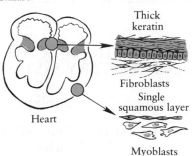

23–15 Drawings to show the differentiation of isolated embryonic chick limb epidermis (A) when combined with mesenchymes of different sources (B). (After C. McLoughlin, 1963. In Cell Differentiation, Symposia of the Society for Experimental Biology, No. 17.)

integument. Hence, dermoepidermal interactions are not restricted to the embryonic period.

Other studies on the chick embryo, particularly by Lawrence (1971), have shown that the epidermal comb is determined by the fourth day, that the determinative influence resides in the mesenchyme, and that phenotypic control is exerted by the mesenchyme. Additionally, tissue experiments using recombinant grafts of comb, feather, and scale region of epidermis and dermis indicate that the inducing capacity of the dermis and the competence of the epidermis vary with developmental age.

How does the dermal mesenchyme act to enable the epidermis to acquire its specific properties? If mesenchyme tissues are the inducers of epidermal specificities, how are their instructions transferred to the epidermis? Unfortunately, answers to these questions are incomplete and far from being satisfactory. This is undoubtedly related to the fact that responses by the epidermis to mesenchymal stimuli involve a complex of processes, including determination, mitosis, morphogenesis, and cytodifferentiation. Because the epidermal responses are so varied, it is unlikely that they are produced as the result of the same inductive mechanism.

Although the dermis is normally required for the proper orientation of epidermal cells and the proliferation of cells in the stratum germinativum, other substrates, such as freeze-thawed dermis, collagen gel, and Millipore filters, appear to support and sustain these activities in explants of embryonic epidermis. Hence, living dermal cells and direct contact between epidermis and dermis do not appear to be required during the interaction. Various other observations strongly suggest that the mesenchyme exerts its influence through the basement membrane and the extracellular matrix between epidermis and dermis. For example, at a specific time in development, the capacity to synthesize DNA and to divide becomes restricted to the stratum germinativum of the epidermis. The cells above this layer are no longer in contact with the basement membrane and undergo cytodifferentiation. It has been suggested that the basal layer retains its competence to divide in response to a growth factor that passes through the basal lamina.

Other factors or agents may also be involved in epidermal differentiation. Large amounts of vitamin A suppress keratinization of the epidermis and promote the development of a mucus-secreting epithelium. If the vitamin-treated explants are returned to a normal culture medium, there is production of a squamous, keratinized population of cells. The concentration of this agent may act directly upon the basal cells to influence their pathway of differentiation.

MALFORMATIONS OF THE INTEGUMENTARY SYSTEM

Disturbances in Keratinization

There are several integumentary disorders that represent departures from normal levels of keratinization in the epidermis and its appendages. A particularly interesting, though rare, hereditary disorder is *congenital ectodermal dysplasia*. It is characterized in severe cases by the absence or hypoplasia of the eccrine sweat glands, the sebaceous, and mucus glands; hair and teeth may be defective or completely absent. Early diagnosis of the malformation is essential since the absence of sweat glands severely disturbs thermoregulation.

Occasionally, the skin may become over keratinized (*hyperkeratosis*) during early infancy. Frequently under these conditions, the stratum corneum cracks into numerous scalelike thickenings. This disorder, termed *ichthyosis simplex,* is transmitted by a single autosomal gene.

Hypertrichosis is a condition in which there is an overabundance of hair in regions where hair is normally sparse. It can be traced to the development of supernumerary hair follicles and/or the abnormal persistence of fetal hair follicles. *Hypotrichosis* is the converse disorder.

Abnormalities of the Mammary Glands

Absence of the mammary glands (*amastia*) or mammary nipples (*athelia*) are rare. More common are supernumerary breasts (*polymastia*) and supernumerary nipples (*polythelia*). Extra breasts and nipples develop from accessory mammary epithelial buds that develop along the mammary ridges, particularly in the vicinity of the normal pair of glands. Aberrant mammary glands and nipples have

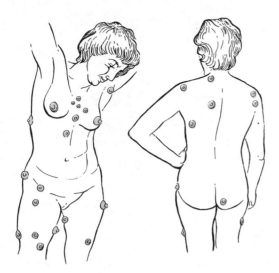

23–16 Abnormalities in the development of breasts and nipples. Schematic diagrams summarize, on a single individual, abnormal locations where supernumerary gland development has been reported in the literature.

been reported at sites far from the conventional positions of the paired mammary ridges (Fig. 23–16).

REFERENCES

Breathnach, A. S. 1971. Embryology of the human skin. A review of ultrastructural studies. J. Invest. Dermatol. 57:133–143.

Briggaman, R. A. and C. Wheeler. 1968. Epidermal-dermal interactions in adult human skin: Role of dermis in epidermal maintenance. J. Invest. Dermatol. 51:454–465.

Cairns, J. and J. Saunders. 1954. The influence of embryonic mesoderm on the regional specification of epidermal derivatives in the chick. J. Exp. Zool. 127:221–248.

Dodson, J. W. 1967. The differentiation of epidermis. I. The interrelationship of epidermis and dermis in embryonic chicken skin. J. Embryol. Exp. Morphol. 17:83–105.

Hashimoto, K., B. Gross, R. DiBella, and W. Lever. 1966. The ultrastructure of the skin of human embryos. J. Invest. Dermatol. 47:317–335.

Holbrook, K. and G. Odland. 1975. The fine structure of developing human epidermis: Light, scanning and transmission electron microscopy of the periderm. J. Invest. Dermatol. 65:16–38.

Lawrence, I. 1971. Timed reciprocal dermal-epidermal interactions between comb, mid-dorsal and tarsometatarsal skin components. J. Exp. Zool. 178:195–210.

McLoughlin, C. B. 1961. The importance of mesenchymal factors in the differentiation of chick epidermis. II. Modification of epidermal differentiation by contact with different types of mesenchyme. J. Embryol. Exp. Morphol. 9:385–409.

Rawles, M. 1963. Tissue interactions in scale and feather development as studies in dermal-epidermal recombinations. J. Embryol. Exp. Morphol. 11:765–789.

Index

Amphioxus (continued)
    endoderm formation, 137
    gastrocoele, 137
    gastrulation, 137–138
    meiosis, 57
    mesoderm formation, 138
    nervous system, early development, 137–138
    notochord, 138
Amphimixis (syngamy), 81
Ampulla, 552
Androgen, 16, 482
    sex reversal, 479, 480–481
Angioblast, 398
Angiocardiography, 442
Angiogenesis, 398–399
Animalization, 202, 206
Animalizing agents, 204, 206, 207
Animal plasm, 103
Animal polar plasm, 45, 196
Animal pole of egg, 44, 97, 196, 201, 203, 205
Annelids, 47, 57, 197, 207
    cleavage, 128–129
    nurse cells, 47
Annulate lamellae, 40
Anophthalmia, 551
Anoxia, 378, 380
Anterior cardinal vein(s) (*see* Cardinal veins)
Anterior intestinal portal, 160, 352, 406, 410, 411
Anterior neuropore, 138
Antibodies, 306
Anticodon, 107
Antifertilizin, 82, 94
Antigen(s), 237
Antral fluid, 59
Anus, 591
Aorta(ae), 402, 420–426, 432, 448
    arch, 428
    ascending, 421, 428
    branches, 429–433
    descending, 442
    dorsal, 367, 427–429, 431, 433
    stenosis, 448
    transposition, 447
Aortic arch(es), 403, 406
    anomalies, 449–450
    fifth, 427
    first, 403, 426–427
    fourth, 421, 427–429, 431
    second, 427
    sixth, 374, 421, 427–429, 449
    third, 421, 427, 429
Aorticopulmonary septum, 420, 424, 447, 448
Aortic sac, 374, 420, 426–429
Apical cap, 243–245
Apical ectoderm maintenance factor (*see* Mesodermal maintenance factor)
Apical ectodermal ridge, 315–319
Apical tuft, 197, 199, 200, 201, 203, 204

Arbacia, 42, 58, 101, 107, 198–199
Appendix, 355
Appendix testis, 472
Aqueduct of Sylvius, 513
Archenteron, 7
    amphibians, 221, 225, 232, 556
    echinoderms, 136, 201, 202, 206
Archicerebellum, 519
Area opaca, 124, 170
Area pellucida, 124, 224, 405
Areola, 592, 593
Arrector pili muscle, 590
Artery(ies)
    allantoic (*see* Artery, umbilical)
    axillary, 433, 440
    basilar, 431
    brachial, 433
    brachiocephalic, 428
    carotid
        common, 428
        external, 427
        internal, 427, 431
    caudal, 433
    coeliac, 432
    costocervical, 431
    epigastric
        inferior, 431
        superior, 431
    femoral, 433
    hyaloid, 542
    iliac
        common, 433
        external, 433
        internal, 433
    inferior gluteal, 433
    innominate, 428
    intercostal, 429
    internal ophthalmic, 547
    interosseous, 433
    intersegmental, 403, 430, 432, 433, 580
    of limbs, 433
    lumbar, 429
    maxillary, 427
    mesenteric
        inferior, 432
        superior, 432
    ovarian, 433
    peroneal, 433
    phrenic, inferior, 431
    popliteal, 433
    pulmonary, 420, 421, 423, 424, 426, 428, 429, 442, 448, 449
    radial, 433
    renal, 431
    sacral, middle, 433
    sciatic, 433
    spermatic, 431
    subclavian, 428, 431, 449

Epicardium, 424–425
Epidermal non-keratinocytes, 586, 587
Epidermal ridges, 587
Epidermis, 219–221, 223, 232, 237, 238, 246, 301, 316, 322, 324, 326, 583–587, 588, 589, 593, 596, 597
Epididymis, 16, 469
Epigenesis, 5, 6, 181–183
Epiglottis, 350, 369
Epimyocardium, 406–408, 410, 412, 421, 424
Epiphysis, 524
Epiploic foraman, 391
Epithalamus, 523, 524
Epithelial-mesenchymal interactions, 300, 308–313, 313–321, 357–358, 405, 406, 593–598
Epithelium, 299
    anterior lens, 546
    morphogenesis, changes in cell shape, 300–303, 308–313
Eponychium, 588
Epoophoron, 472
Erythrocyte(s) (see also Erythropoietic cells), 400
Erythropoiesis, 399–402
Erythropoietic cells, 399–402
Erythropoietin, 255, 400, 401
Escherichia coli, 257
Esophageal atresia, 379
Esophageal mesentery, 386, 387, 389
Esophagus, 351–352, 368, 379, 389, 390
    remodeling by cell death, 324, 325
Estrogen, 63, 64–66, 73, 74–75, 255, 259, 260, 261, 479
Estrous cycle, 63–67
    anestrus, 63
    diestrus, 63
    estrus, 63–64
    follicular phase, 64, 66
    luteal phase, 64, 66–67
    metestrus, 64
    proestrus, 63
Ethylenediaminetetraacetic acid (EDTA), 173, 316, 599
Eumelanins, 587
Evans blue, 206
Evocation, 227, 234
Evocator
    direct, 234
    indirect, 234
Excretory system, 451–458
Exocoelomic cavity, 269
Exocoelomic membrane (see Yolk sac, primary)
Exogastrula, 163, 165
Exogastrulation, 202, 204
Experimental (artificial) activation, 93, 102, 108
External genitalia, 16, 17, 19, 591
    development, 475–477
        hormonal control, 482–483
External respiration, 365, 367
Extracellular matrix, 300, 304, 307–313, 377, 397, 408
Extraembryonic blood vessels, 398

Extraembryonic coelom, 383
Extraembryonic membranes, 384, 388
Eye(s), 305, 541–551, 556–561
    anterior chamber, 550–551
    developmental abnormalities, 550–551
    positional changes, 550
    posterior chamber, 549
Eyelids, 541, 549–550, 591

Face, 333–336
Fate maps
    amphibian, 139–140
    bird, 153, 155–156
    fish, 146–149
Feather development, 583, 595–596
Fertilization, 81–115
    acrosomal reaction, 88–91
    activation of protein synthesis, 105–109
    cytoplasmic reorganization, 102–103
    egg-sperm interacting substances, 82–87
    egg membrane penetrating substances, 84–87
    metabolic changes, 103–109
    permeability changes, 103, 105–106
    response of egg, 91–113
    sperm activation, 81, 83
    sperm agglutination, 83–84
Fertilization membrane, 58, 94, 96, 98, 99, 187
Fertilization wave, 94
Fertilizin theory, 82–84
Fetal-maternal immunological reactions, 289
Fibroblasts, 305, 307, 308, 424, 570, 574, 596
Fields, 314, 315
Filopodia, 168–169, 170, 171, 172, 305, 306
Fishes
    accessory envelopes, 61
    blastoderm, 122, 146–149, 167–170
    blastodisc, 122
    cleavage, 121–122
    cortical reaction, 96, 97
    development of organ rudiments, 146–149
    fertilization, 97
    gastrulation, 146–149
    neurulation, 149
    oxygen consumption in oocytes, 104
    respiratory organs, 366, 367
    yolk, 48, 50
Fissure(s)
    anterior median, 494
    lateral (Sylvian), 530
    optic (retinal), 542
    posterolateral, 518
    prima, 518, 519
    secunda, 518, 519
Fistula, urachal, 458
Flask cells, 164–167, 171, 216, 217
Flexure(s)
    brain, 512

Tetralogy of Fallot, 448, 449
Thalamus, 523, 524–525, 529
    dorsal, 524–525
    intermediate mass, 525
    ventral (subthalamus), 524
Theca folliculi, 39, 60
Theories of cleavage, 129–130
Thoracic ducts, 445
Thorotrast, 378
Thymidine-³H incorporation, 109, 323, 571
Thymus, 259, 344
Thyroid gland, 299, 301, 302, 326, 344–348
    bird, 346–348
    human, 345–346
Thyroid hormone (*see* Thyroxin)
Thyroxine, 326, 327
Tight junctions, 168
Timing hypothesis, 176–177
Tissue sorting and assembly, 173–176, 327, 329, 330
Tongue, 348–350
    nerve supply, 349, 534, 537
Tonsil(s)
    lingual, 344, 350
    palatine, 344
    pharyngeal, 344
Tooth bud (tooth germ), 339
Topographic terminology, 13
Totipotency, 193, 201, 202, 208
Trabeculae carneae, 421
Trachea, 302, 307, 368, 370, 377, 379
Tracheal mesoderm, 375, 376
Tracheobronchiolar ridge (*see* Laryngotracheal ridge)
Tracheoesophageal fistula, 379
Tracheoesophageal septum, 368
Tract(s)
    corticobulbar, 523
    corticopontine, 523
    corticospinal, 523
    optic, 538–539
        establishment of central connections, 509–511
Transcription, 106–107, 242, 243, 245, 254, 257, 258, 260, 261, 326, 402
Transfer RNA, 107, 185, 237, 252
Translation, 241, 243, 326
Translational inhibitors, 105
Transplantation, 219, 222–224, 243, 244, 314–318, 320–323, 328, 404, 557, 558, 562
Transverse septum, 383–388, 394, 409, 412, 413, 435
Tricuspid valve, 419
Trigone, 457
Triiodothyronine, 326
Triturus, 53, 55, 101, 189, 214, 219, 220, 221, 234, 237, 301
Trochophore larva, 197
Trophoblast, 125–126, 265–266, 292–294
Truncus arteriosus, 409, 420, 426, 427, 429
Trypsin, 108, 173, 206, 234, 311, 329, 594

Trypsinlike enzyme (TLE) (*see* Acrosomal proteinase)
Tryptophan, 207
Tubercle
    genital, 476–477
    Müller's, 457, 470, 471
Tuberculum impar, 348, 349
Tubule(s)
    collecting, 455
    distal convoluted, 455
    mesonephric, 453–454, 455, 469, 472
    proximal convoluted, 455
    seminiferous, 16, 33, 467
Tubulin, 187, 188
Tubuli recti, 16, 467
Tunica albuginea, 466, 467
Tunica (processus) vaginalis, 474–475
Tympanic cavity, 344, 554
Tympanic membrane, 555
Tympanic recess, 555
Tyrosinase, 587

Ulna, 320, 323
Ultimobranchial body, 345
Umbilical arteries, 403, 426, 432, 442, 443
Umbilical cord, 393
Umbilical veins, 403, 413, 433, 434, 435, 442, 443, 444, 436
Urachus, 458
Ureter, 454
Urethra, 19, 458, 477, 478
Uridine-³H incorporation, 53, 245, 248
Urogenital folds, 438
Urogenital ridge, 454, 466, 470
Urogenital sinus, 457, 458, 470, 471
Urogenital system, 451–488
Uropygial gland, 588
Uterine tubes, 19, 60–61, 256, 259–261, 276, 299, 325, 470
Uterovaginal canal, 470, 471
Uterus, 19, 471
Utriculus, 551, 552
UV irradiation, 234, 244
Uvula, 338

Vagina, 19, 470, 471–472
Vagina masculina (*see* Prostatic utricle)
Vasa efferentia, 16, 469
Vascular system
    abnormalities, 446–450
    arteries, 425–433
    heart, 404–425
    primitive, 402, 403
    veins, 433–440
Vas deferens, 16–17, 456, 469
Vegetal body, 197

Yolk platelets, 48, 50
  proteins, 50
Yolk plug, 148
Yolk production
  autosynthesis, 49
  heterosynthesis, 49
Yolk sac, 171, 384, 397–399, 429, 432, 433, 436
  human
    primary, 269–270
    secondary, 270

Yolk stalk, 325, 327, 353, 356
Yolk vesicles, 49

Zeugopodium, 320
Zone of polarizing activity, 320
Zona pellucida, 39, 61, 97, 99, 101, 266
Zona radiata, 45
Zona reaction, 99
Zygote, 92, 101